DYNAMICS OF DISEASE TRANSMISSION AND CONTROL

Dr. Kedir Yahya Yasin

ALLIED HEALTH PRESS

Dynamics of Disease Transmission and Control

Author: **Dr. Kedir Yahya Yasin**

Allied Health Press
4164 Lakeshore Road
Burlington ON L7L 1A4
Canada
www.alliedhealthpress.com
Email: orders@arclereducation.com

ISBN: 978-1-77956-791-8

ABOUT THE AUTHOR

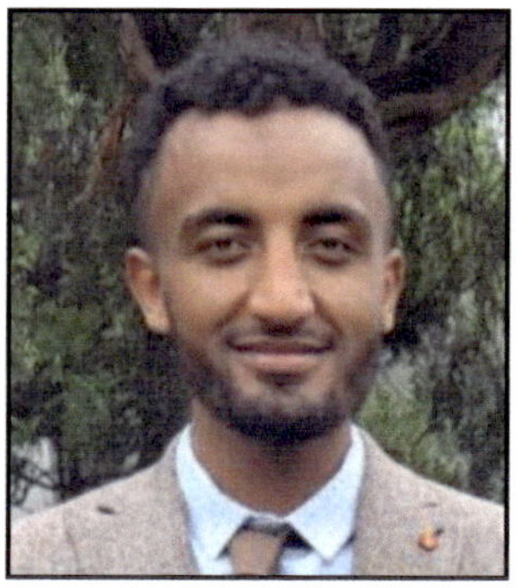

Dr. Kedir Yahya is a young medical doctor who is currently working in Asella teaching and referral hospital. He embarked on a journey to explore various fields within the medical landscape. With a versatile skill set and a commitment to lifelong learning, he has made significant contributions to healthcare across diverse specialities. Whether it's clinical practice, research, or teaching, he continues to strive for excellence in improving patient care and advancing medical knowledge.

Brief Table of Contents

Detailed Table of Contents

CHAPTER 3

The Epidemiological Triangle 65

CHAPTER 4

Mathematical Foundations for Disease Modeling 95

CHAPTER 9

Vaccination and Herd Immunity 241

CHAPTER 10

Intervention Strategies and Disease Control 271

CHAPTER 11

Modeling Epidemics and Predicting Outbreaks 299

CHAPTER 12

Antimicrobials and Resistance 329

CHAPTER 15

Public Health Policy and Future Directions 423

LIST OF FIGURES

LIST OF ABBREVIATIONS

ACD	Acute Chagas Disease
ACE	Adverse Childhood Experience
ACIP	Advisory Committee on Immunization Practices
ACT	Advancing Care Coordination & Telehealth Deployment
AHC	Accountable Health Communities
AI	Artificial Intelligence
AIC	Akaike Information Criterion
ALS	Amyotrophic Lateral Sclerosis
AML	Acute Myeloid Leukemia
AMR	Antimicrobial Resistance
AMS	Antimicrobial Stewardship
ANC	Antenatal Care
ANN	Artificial Neural Network
ASEAN	Association of Southeast Asian Nations
ASF	African Swine Fever
AST	Antimicrobial Susceptibility Testing
BDV	Border Disease Virus
BIC	Bayesian Information Criterion
BRAIN	Biomedical Risk Assessment Intelligent Network
CAB	Community Advisory Board
CBDA	Compressive Big Data Analytics
CBPR	Community-Based Cancer Prevention
CBPR	Community-Based Participatory Research
CCHF	Crimean-Congo Haemorrhagic Fever
CDC	Centers For Disease Control and Prevention
CER	Comparative Effectiveness Research
CGM	Continuous Glucose Monitoring
CHIKV	Chikungunya Virus
CLL	Chronic Lymphocytic Leukemia

CMMI	Center For Medicare and Medicaid Innovation
COI	Conflicts of Interest
COIR	Community-Based Outbreak Investigation and Response
CP	Clinical Pharmacist
CTO	Clinical Trials Organization
CUD	Cannabis Use Disorder
DAA	Direct-Acting Antiviral
DALY	Deaths and Substantial Disability-Adjusted Life-Year
DEDIPAC	Determinants of Diet and Physical Activity
DR	Diabetic Retinopathy
DSN	Disease Surveillance Networks
EWS	Early Warning Systems
FETP	Field Epidemiology Training Program
FLAPS	Farm Location and Agricultural Production Simulator
FMD	Foot-and-Mouth Disease
GAM	Generalized Additive Model
GBD	Global Burden of Disease
GIS	Geographic Information Systems
GLASS	Global Antimicrobial Resistance Surveillance System
GNP	Gelatin Nanoparticle
HBV	Hepatitis B Virus
HCP	Healthcare Professional
HD	Huntington's Disease
HGT	Horizontal Gene Transfer
HL	Health Literacy
HPAI	Highly Pathogenic Avian Influenza
HPSR	Health Policy and Systems Research
HPV	Human Papillomavirus
HRS	Health Recommender Systems
ICT	Information and Communication Technology
ICU	Intensive Care Unit
IHR	International Health Regulations
IMD	Invasive Meningococcal Diseases
INLA	Integrated Nested Laplace Approximation
IPTp	Intermittent Preventive Treatment

IS	Infective Spondylodiscitis
IVM	Integrated Vector Management
LMICs	Low- and Middle-Income Countries
MAE	Mean Absolute Error
MAPE	Mean Absolute Percentage Error
MCC	Matthews Correlation Coefficient
MDR	Multidrug Resistance
MDR-TB	Multidrug-Resistant Tuberculosis
MFS	Major Facilitator Superfamily
MLP	Multilayer Perceptron
MMR	Measles, Mumps, And Rubella
MRC	Medical Research Council
MRSA	Methicillin-Resistant Staphylococcus Aureus
MR-SIR	Model Like the Multi-Risk Sir
MSI	Musculoskeletal Injuries
NAP	National Action Plan
NCD	Non-Communicable Diseases
NDIS	National Disability Insurance Scheme
NGO	Non-Governmental Organization
NGS	Next-Generation Sequencing
OD	Oropharyngeal Dysphagia
ODE	Ordinary Differential Equation
PCOR	Patient-Centered Outcomes Research
PCR	Polymerase Chain Reaction
PGIS	Participatory Geographic Information Systems
PG-PHASE	Pathogen Genomics in Public Health Surveillance Evaluation
PORT	Postoperative Radiotherapy
PPDM	Post-Pancreatitis Diabetes Mellitus
PPP	Public-Private Partnership
PRRS	Porcine Reproductive and Respiratory Syndrome
RBPM	Blood Pressure Monitoring
RCT	Randomized Controlled Trial
RPAS	Remotely Piloted Airdesign Systems
RVF	Rift Valley Fever
SADC	Southern African Development Community
SARS-CoV-2	Severe Acute Respiratory Syndrome Coronavirus 2

SCD	Sickle Cell Disease
SCRIBE	Single-Case Reporting Guideline in Behavioral Interventions
SEIA	Susceptible–Exposed–Infected–Asymptomatic
SIR	Susceptible, Infectious, Recovered
SSI	Surgical Site Infections
SVM	Support Vector Machine
TB	Tuberculosis
UHC	Universal Health Coverage
UN	United Nations
UNASUR	Union of South American Nations
UNDAF	United Nations Development Assistance Framework
VBD	Vector-Borne Disease
VCI	Vulnerable–Contaminated–Immuned
VCT	Voluntary Counselling and Testing Point
VL	Visceral Leishmaniasis
VPDs	Vaccine-Preventable Diseases
WASH	Water, Sanitation, and Hygiene
WBE	Wastewater-Based Epidemiology
WDD	Wheat Dwarf Disease
WGS	Whole-Genome Sequencing
WHO	World Health Organization
XAI	Explainable Artificial Intelligence
ZCL	Zoonotic Cutaneous Leishmaniasis
ZVL	Zoonotic Visceral Leishmaniasis

PREFACE

The spread of disease-causing agents among individuals has shaped the trajectory of human history, influencing societies, economies, and even the texture of day-to-day life. From pandemics of yore that reshaped empires to pandemics in recent times challenging global public health systems, understanding how disease transmits within populations is a scientific inquiry and an immediate practical issue. Transmission dynamics are based on countless variables—pathogen biological characteristics, human behavior trends, environmental variables, and community structural attributes. Knowledge of these determinants allows public health workers to predict new dangers, design effective interventions, and distribute resources in a manner that will optimize impact.

In addition to immediate outbreaks, studies on disease transmission inform long-term control and prevention measures. Mathematical models translate complex biological and social processes into quantitative terms, enabling the extrapolation of epidemic trends and the evaluation of intervention scenarios. In turn, surveillance networks and outbreak investigations yield real-time data that ground theoretical frameworks in observed reality. Together, surveillance and modeling create a feedback loop where prediction drives action and field information refines understanding. In this era of worldwide travel, environmental disruption, and emerging microbial threats, this synergy is vital to protecting human health at the local, national, and global levels.

Dynamics of Disease Transmission and Control was conceived to bring unity to these disparate approaches. It offers an integrated treatment that begins with fundamental principles of infectious disease and moves steadily toward applied strategies of prevention and mitigation. Along the way, emphasis is placed on linking theory to practice: readers will find brief explanations of fundamental concepts, step-by-step walkthroughs of modeling techniques, and concrete examples taken from real outbreaks. The organization of the text facilitates progressive learning, encouraging readers to develop foundational knowledge and then engage with more complex subjects in subsequent chapters.

It starts by defining a disease that is infectious and why its prevention needs specialized approaches (Chapter 1). A few basic epidemiological measures in particular—incidence, prevalence, and numbers of reproductions in the population—are defined in Chapter 2, laying out the primary variables used to identify the frequency and progression of disease. Chapter 3 introduces the epidemiological triangle, illustrating where host, agent, and environment converge to influence transmission potential. Mathematical tools come next: Chapter 4 covers calculus and probability background important for modeling, and Chapter 5 uses these tools to cover classical compartmental models (SIR, SEIR, and their generalizations). Chapter 6 discusses population heterogeneity, exploring the role of age structure, social contacts, and geographic distribution in epidemic dynamics. Chapter 7 gives special attention to vector-borne and zoonotic diseases and how the transmission cycles work when non-human hosts are included.

Chapters 8 and 9 become operationally concerned with disease control matters. Techniques for disease surveillance and outbreak investigation are outlined in Chapter 8, and Chapter 9 is concerned with vaccine policy, herd immunity levels, and planning for immunization programs. Intervention policies, ranging from quarantine and contact tracing to campaigns that change behavior, are appraised in Chapter 10 on quantitative grounds for the effectiveness. Chapter 11 demonstrates real-time application of modeling in predicting the emergence of outbreaks and informing policy. Chapter 12 discusses antimicrobial consumption and resistance: mechanisms of resistance emergence, strategies of stewardship, and worldwide aspects of drug resistance are described in great detail.

The third and final part of the book addresses broader concerns and emerging risks. Chapter 13 summarizes international models of health and the mechanisms of new pathogen dynamics, including coronaviruses and hemorrhagic fever viruses. Chapter 14 summarizes socioeconomic and behavioral determinants of disease spread and how poverty, misinformation, and cultural practices drive epidemic risk. Chapter 15 deals with public health policy and the future direction: the roles of international agencies, the coming together of digital technologies, and the vision for healthier, more resilient health systems round off the discussion.

This book is aimed at graduate students in epidemiology, public health professionals, infectious disease modelers, and policymakers requiring a practical, up-to-date guide to the control and understanding of infectious diseases. It will serve as a reference for researchers developing new models or evaluating intervention programs.

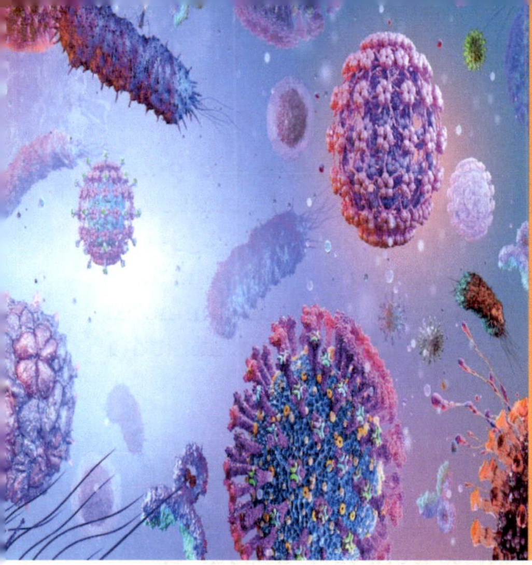

Chapter 1

INTRODUCTION TO INFECTIOUS DISEASES

Contents

Introduction

Knowing how an infection is transmitted is crucial to determining what diseases are involved. It typically begins when minute organisms—viruses, bacteria, fungi or even parasites—find their way into our bodies and cause symptoms. Sometimes it is as simple as a handshake or a cough, while at other times it floats through the air or catches a ride on insects. There are even cases where diseases jump from animals to humans, such as the recent COVID-19 pandemic, which reminds us that such spillovers are very much possible quite unexpectedly. Public health, for the most part, must be on guard—take SARS-CoV-2 as an example—to quickly grasp how fast these diseases can explode and trigger widespread problems (Murray et al., 2022). Infectious diseases do not just affect a person; they derail whole communities. They result in serious illness and numerous deaths, inundating hospitals, and hurting economies along the way. One of the biggest worries is antimicrobial resistance (AMR), which, in straightforward terms, makes treating infection much harder and makes hospital stays and expenses longer and higher, respectively. Some research even credited AMR with nearly 4.95 million deaths in 2019—a grim reminder that we must have intervention strategies that work and we must have them now (Gorbalenya et al., 2020). As you think about it, grasping the big picture of these diseases helps in developing smart policies that keep the public's health in equilibrium. At the same time, our definition of what an infectious disease constantly evolves as science learns more and new insects arise. We no longer just name the microbe alone—we now bring in environmental factors, genetics, and even human behavior to understand transmission. With the world so connected, these diseases easily leap borders, sometimes making containment difficult. It is interesting to think about how our own adaptability and that of pathogens co-evolve in this confused dance. As science evolves, so does our approach to preventing, diagnosing, and curing these infections; this evolving knowledge is of the utmost significance for global health and for reducing risks in most cases (Gorbalenya et al., 2020; Murray et al., 2022) (Figure 1.1).

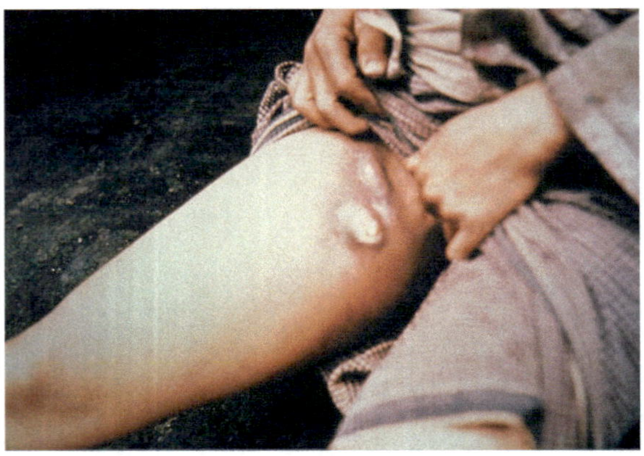

Figure 1.1. Understanding how infections spread is key to figuring about diseases.

Source: By Photo Credit:Content Providers(s): CDC - This media comes from the Centers for Disease Control and Prevention's Public Health Image Library (PHIL), with identification number #2047.Note: Not all PHIL images are public domain; be sure to check copyright status and credit authors and content providers.العربيّة | Deutsch | English | македонски | slovenščina | +/−Transferred from en.wikipedia to Commons., Public Domain, https://commons.wikimedia.org/w/index.php?curid=6286382

Explanation of Infectious Diseases

Infectious illnesses are chaotic and difficult to pin down—they originate from various sources and spread in ways that are not always predictable. Viruses, bacteria, fungi, and parasites each have their own idiosyncrasies, which typically means they affect how infection becomes established and produces disease in unexpected ways. For instance, SARS-CoV-2 continues to evolve at a fast pace, which typically makes it difficult to contain from further spreading, while bacteria such as Streptococcus pneumoniae, in most instances, develop drug resistance and prove to be even more challenging to contain. Diseases spread by air, by insects, or simply through close proximity, so each community and environment appear to have their own set of challenges in keeping them under control. Taking the larger perspective, socio-economic influences also have a tremendous impact on the way these diseases spread and affect communities. In regions with poor healthcare—consider regions of sub-Saharan Africa, for example—the combination of bad sanitation, thin healthcare infrastructure, and lower educational resources tends to allow infections to rage out of control, so early detection and rapid response is a genuine challenge. The COVID-19 crisis, say, has sort of brought these imbalances to the fore; some models even show that notwithstanding monumental challenges, many sub-Saharan countries registered lower infection rates than anticipated, a suggestion of local trends and policy decisions possibly at play (Evans et al., 2020). There is also the Global Burden of Diseases (GBD), Injuries, and Risk Factors Study, which, in most instances, indicates that whereas in the past infectious diseases were the leading cause of high mortality, these days non-communicable disease is now front and center in most areas (Roth et al., 2018). Nevertheless, the relentless tenacity of these infections, particularly in low-income countries, forces us to remain vigilant even as progress with vaccines and public health brings some easing. In the end, addressing both communicable and non-communicable diseases requires a wide-ranging, adaptable health system—one that can change and keep up with the way diseases progress (Figure 1.2).

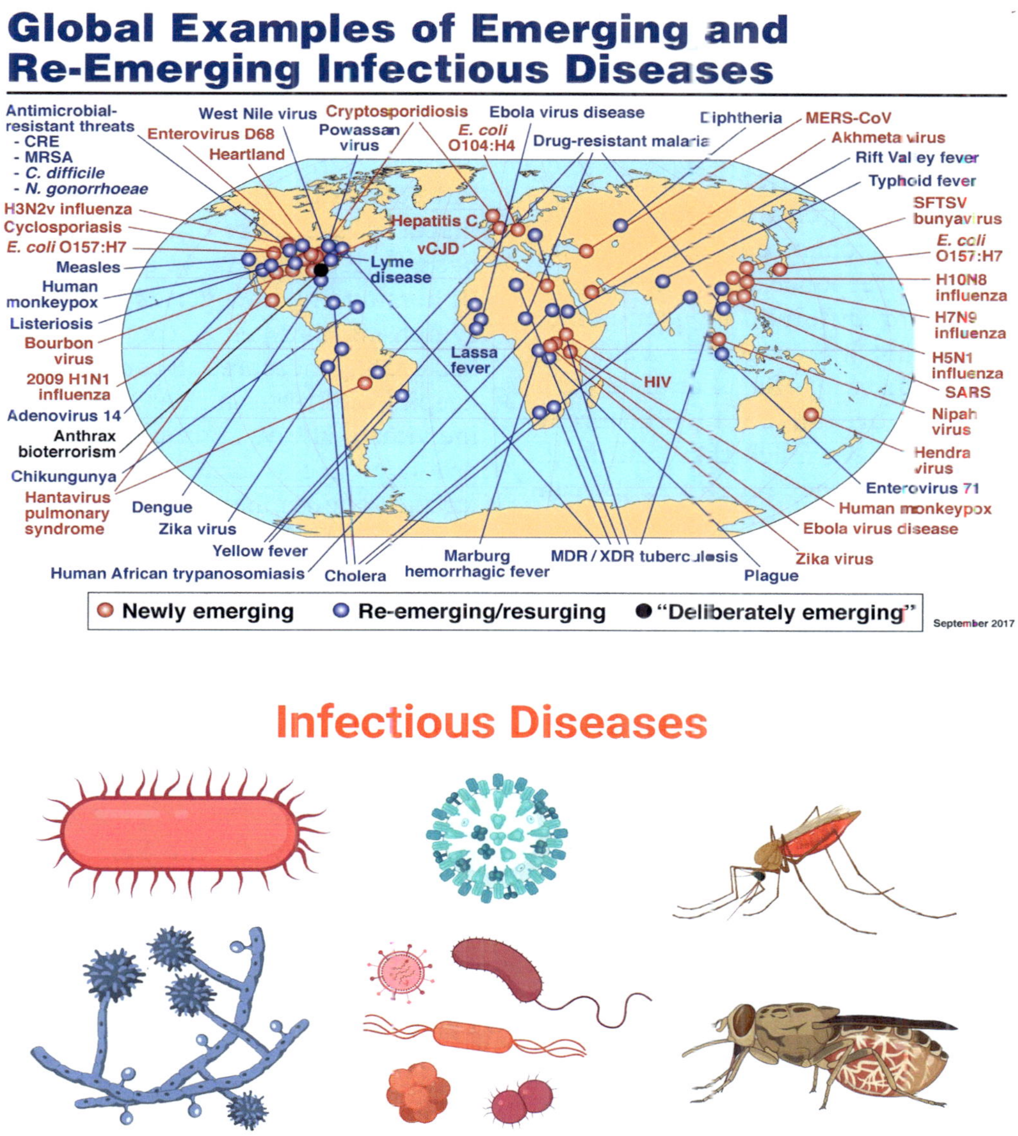

Figure 1.2. Infectious diseases.

Source:By Anthony Fauci (Q573246) - https://www.niaid.nih.gov/sites/default/files/main%20map.jpg, Public Domain, https://commons.wikimedia.org/w/index.php?curid=89608427

Types of Pathogens Involved

Pathogens are all shapes and sizes, each performing in its own unique manner and spreading in its own unique way. Bacteria, for instance, are small one-celled organisms that can exist on their own but at times create huge health problems. Escherichia coli and Streptococcus pneumoniae, for instance, employ some nifty sticking techniques to attach themselves to our tissues, which then triggers an infection. In recent studies, researchers have noted—even if only generally speaking—that certain proteins on a bacterium's surface help it grip host cells, setting off the whole cascade of illness. This messy dance between bacterial clinginess and host response shows how these microbes adapt to different environments, making it clear that knowing their behavior is key to fighting diseases (Bagel et al., 2023). Viruses, however, are an entirely different animal. They don't have much they can do in the first place because they require a host cell to multiply, and that necessity comes with a peculiar set of problems. These agents trigger everything from the common cold to pandemics such as COVID-19. Incidentally, viruses do mutate very fast; new varieties emerge—Delta, Omicron, etc.—and that fast change does make vaccine work and antiviral strategies so difficult. Classic control measures (such as live-attenuated vaccines) sometimes pose safety concerns, and so scientists now look at concepts that incorporate nanotechnology to enhance diagnosis and therapy. Overall, it appears that controlling these viral threats requires a combination of new and old approaches (Sharifi et al., 2023). Fungi also have a significant role to play, particularly if one's immunity is anything but optimal. These eukaryotic cells can either eat dead stuff or, with an opportunity provided, turn into opportunistic pathogens, consider Candida albicans. They frequently evade our immune system by growing into biofilms, which just complicates the process of treating them. In most cases, the battery of enzymes they create breaks down host tissue and increases infections. As antifungal resistance increases, it has become quite apparent that excavating further into how these fungal cells function is necessary to design successful therapies. This demands constant, if somewhat fractured, investigation of the contribution that fungi make toward disease and public health implications from this.

Importance of Understanding Infectious Diseases

Public health and awareness of infectious diseases are two things that go hand in hand—a relationship we often take for granted. Understanding how germs spread, recognizing symptoms, and just having a general sense of basic safety measures all count when it comes to keeping outbreaks in check. And now, with more individuals always in transit, diseases previously grounded in one corner can break out suddenly far and wide, reminding us (again, in the majority of instances) that it's all about catching things early. For instance, when novel germs emerge and are not yet comprehended, "outbreaks occur easily. Breaking these facts down clearly prepares individuals and constructs a faster, community-focused response. In brief, education and awareness first is key to minimizing the real-world effect on public health. Exploring how infections work provides healthcare professionals with the insight they require to design specific solutions. Our everyday interactions with nasty insects are dirty and require a combination of knowledge from disciplines such as microbiology, epidemiology, and even intelligent public policy. Consider the worldwide battle against viruses—you can't just examine a virus's biology; you have to look at the social and cultural imperatives that influence how we behave for our health. By relying on evidence-based practices, physicians and other providers can better customize prevention strategies. This strategy is especially crucial in areas with their own unique challenges (such as merging issues such as infections with cardiovascular issues), where understanding the blend of pathogens and risk factors results in smarter management as a whole. In the end, these discoveries enhance our combined capacity to address both ongoing and emerging infectious dangers. Recently, more people are struggling with allergies, chronic diseases, and infections simultaneously, which truly underscores the importance of a wide, overarching health strategy. Many studies indicate that understanding how both our surroundings and our DNA influence these matters is essential in keeping individuals healthy. For example, certain allergy research reveals unexpected connections to infection epidemics—suggesting that carefully managed exposure to specific germs could even modulate immune function in the most vulnerable individuals. Such concepts open the door to prevention strategies that are customized to the specific needs of various populations. Overall, combining a balanced perspective on health with a good grasp of infectious threats not only addresses the short-term issues but also lays the groundwork for better, long-term results. In most instances, the control of infectious diseases becomes part of a greater puzzle in addressing the broad array of health issues we now confront (Figure 1.3).

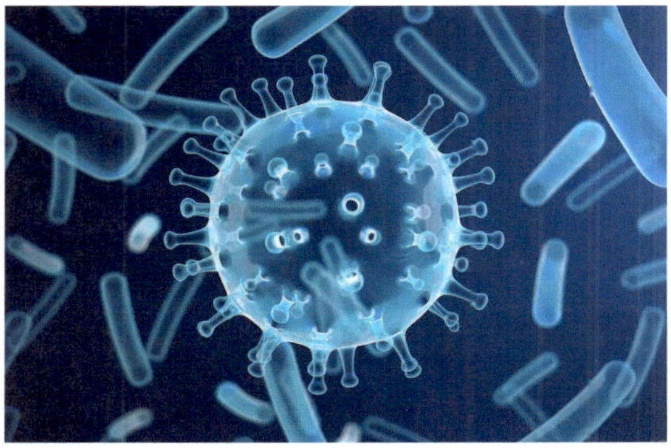

Figure 1.3. Public health and knowing about infectious diseases.

Source: Sysmex Europe. (n.d.). Infectious Disease.

1.1. Historical Context

History plays a crucial role when dealing with infectious disease. Previous outbreaks, societal changes, and medical advancements have all contributed to shaping the way that disease is transmitted. Centuries-old outbreaks, altered public health strategies and methods of disease control, remind us that the past is always relevant, particularly when we look at issues such as antimicrobial resistance (AMR). Consider, for instance, the two bacteria Neisseria meningitidis and Neisseria gonorrhoeae; they have approximately 80–90% of their genetic material in common, which practically makes them appear like distant cousins. Whereas AMR was previously almost unheard of in Neisseria meningitidis, Neisseria gonorrhoeae is beginning to develop growing resistance—quite in general, we currently require new, creative treatment concepts to keep up with these progressing threats (Marshall et al., 2024). Politics and social forces also have a huge influence on how we manage infectious diseases. Public health programs around the world have yielded variable results—most often a function of regional leadership and politics. Take China's health poverty reduction programs: they illustrate how a methodical, nearly grassroots, strategy can enhance access to health care, but at the same time reflect persistent problems with new infections as well as diseases making a comeback. Chronic illnesses are even surfacing among young people nowadays, making it a further level of sophistication to deal with infections. The transformation of healthcare policies from the latter part of the 20th century to the present day, in most instances, is one of ongoing transformation and adjustment that is informative for learning lessons that can be applied to future policy (Xu et al., 2024). Travel, commerce, and technology have shaken things even more fundamentally in our understanding of disease dynamics. People, goods, and information (and sometimes ideas) move so fast these days that pathogens can spread rapidly across borders. The 1918 influenza, for instance, shows us that when nations share resources and coordinate responses, they can better manage widespread crises. As disease agents evolve and adapted, the need for robust vaccination campaigns and rebeginning research into antibiotics becomes increasingly evident, particularly against resistant variants such as Neisseria gonorrhoeae. In total, reconstructing these chronicled events is quite important for informing current public health strategies and for enhancing the resilience of our healthcare infrastructures to whatever's on the horizon (Marshall et al., 2024).

1.1.1. Major Pandemics and Their Impact

Pandemics have left their imprint on history in ways that extend far beyond mere tragic loss. The 14th-century Black Death, for instance, killed so many in Europe that a critical labor shortage arose, surprisingly disrupting the ancient feudal system. This collapse, in a way, prepared the ground for the emergence of the working class and an emerging middle class. Then there is the HIV/AIDS epidemic of the late 1900s; it not only compelled health policy changes, but also reoriented society's perceptions of sickness and exclusion. Overall, these occurrences illustrate that pandemics are potent forces for change, reshaping social, economic, and political structures while changing public health strategies and cultural perceptions of disease. More often than not, infectious diseases appear to erupt from a sloppy combination of social currents and ecological adjustments. Epidemics such as HIV/AIDS and pandemic flu usually start where humans interact with animals—this fuzzy edge is where zoonotic transmission usually gets activated. Recently, such phenomena as widespread deforestation and rapid urbanization have only made that border more dangerous, facilitating pathogens to jump species more easily. And with international trade and travel in high gear, germs have easy rides across countries, making the outbreaks even harder to contain. Understanding such dynamics is certainly pivotal for establishing public health systems to respond early, and that explains why there has been increased demand for comprehensive monitoring and preventive actions against zoonotic diseases (Carroll et al., 2012).

Today, most experts contend that we require new, creative strategies to avoid and contain pandemics in our globalized world. In the past, reactions have been largely reactive, but there is a strong appeal to move toward identifying threats early. This involves turning up the surveillance and digging deeper into how diseases are transmitted from animals to humans—hopefully catching them before they get out of hand. Since our global surveillance systems are still not perfect, supporting community activity and disseminating public health knowledge may be game-changers (Djoko et al., 2010). And by embracing emerging technology, such as improved mathematics models and better diagnostics—we have a better chance of seeing how these dangers travel. All things being equal, shifting from a reactive approach to one of prevention could very well be the solution to creating enduring resilience.

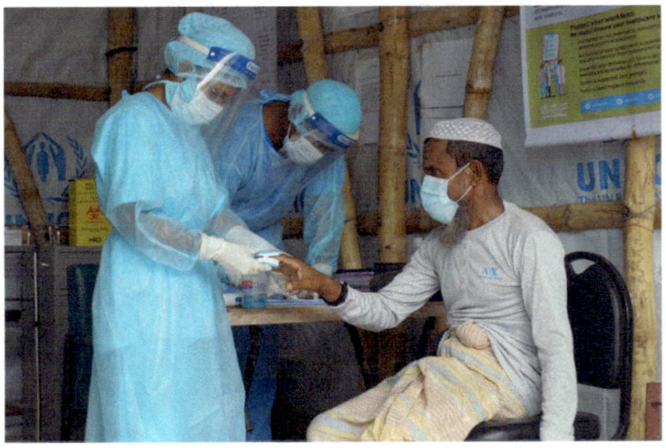

Source: World Health Organization. (n.d.). The COVID-19 Patient's Condition is Assessed by the Triage Team Comprising a Nurse and a Medical Assistant.

1.1.2. Evolution of Medical Understanding

Over time we've observed how our perception regarding diseases–particularly those that are contagious–has turned on its head with scientific and technological developments. Ancient times had people attributing illness to a supernatural power or a disturbance of bodily humor, so treatments and public health initiatives were quite limited. Then in the late 1800s, when folks discovered that germs cause illness, everything shifted; sanitation, vaccines, and basic health measures became the new norm, setting a rough foundation for modern microbiology. Researchers started moving from merely watching how people fell sick to digging deep with experiments and data, marking a real turning point in medicine. Most times the transition was slow and a little unclear, but it changed our style forever. In recent years, however, new infectious dangers have compelled a rethinking of disease dynamics. The COVID-19 pandemic, for example, more or less overturned outdated models and challenged scientists to apply advanced computing techniques to map virus transmission and even predict the way outbreaks were likely to unfold. Models like SEIR have been made to work approximating such as reproduction numbers and mortality rates–assisting policymakers, though sometimes prematurely, in gearing up responses. In general terms, as knowledge increases, so do our procedures, keeping our method keep step with emerging issues (Zanella et al., 2021). AI and machine learning have now joined the fray, introducing a new spin on estimating infectious threats. These technologies enable researchers to experiment with and iterate upon existing models, frequently boosting precision and dependability in directions even experienced specialists can't predict. For instance, certain techniques of deep learning used on epidemiological data are now able to predict future trends of infection and mortality rates to an extent never previously possible. This marriage of technology and classical medical understanding sort of illustrates the reason why it is imperative to combine disciplines when confronted with public health emergencies. As researchers continue to unravel the idiosyncratic behaviors of pathogens and how our bodies react to them, this constant refinement in medical knowledge continues to be an essential component in addressing existing as well as forthcoming outbreaks (Stochitoiu et al., 2020).

1.1.3. Role of Public Health in Disease Management

In managing disease and outbreaks, public health is still an important player that combines various strategies to reduce risks and protect our communities. Diagnostic tests, for instance, have truly stepped-up in times of crisis such as the COVID-19 pandemic—they identify the virus early so physicians know exactly how to respond promptly. Lab results, by revealing precisely what is happening, provide healthcare teams with a means to counteract issues arising. At other times, even something so out-of-the-blue as monitoring wastewater provides hints on trends in disease and what resources may be required in the future. All of this combined, though, not only allows us to cope with what is going on at present but also creates some sort of pre-existing support system for any future epidemics (Lippi et al., 2025). Recently, shifts in population composition, particularly with increased immigration—have put an entirely new spin on public health issues. Studies indicate that diseases such as chickenpox and measles have been more prevalent in establishments catering to these expanding populations. Paying close attention to the ways that diseases manifest ensures that health officials can customize responses to suit special local conditions. For example, accelerating the effort of vaccinations and making seeing a doctor simpler can prevent impending outbreaks before they reach epidemic size, ensuring the most vulnerable aren't left out. Such practical practice not only increases individualized health outcomes but enhances the broader ability of whole populations to withstand infections as well (Khan et al., 2025). Some public health efforts extend beyond tests and numbers—they also emphasize a lot of education and engaging people. Plain, common-language explanations of items such as vaccines and proper hygiene habits can empower people to protect themselves. Awareness campaigns that are designed to spread the word about the goodness of immunizations have proven to be effective, in reducing the transmission of disease. In addition, when there is a collaboration between public health organizations, physicians and community organizations (sometimes in surprise combinations), they tend to fill the gaps in care, particularly in underserved communities. This brings these collaborations to reality and disseminates health know-how not just to manage existing health problems but also to lay the groundwork to address any future emergencies, demonstrating once more how crucial public health is in ensuring everyone's safety—although sometimes the message gets a little confused (Figure 1.4).

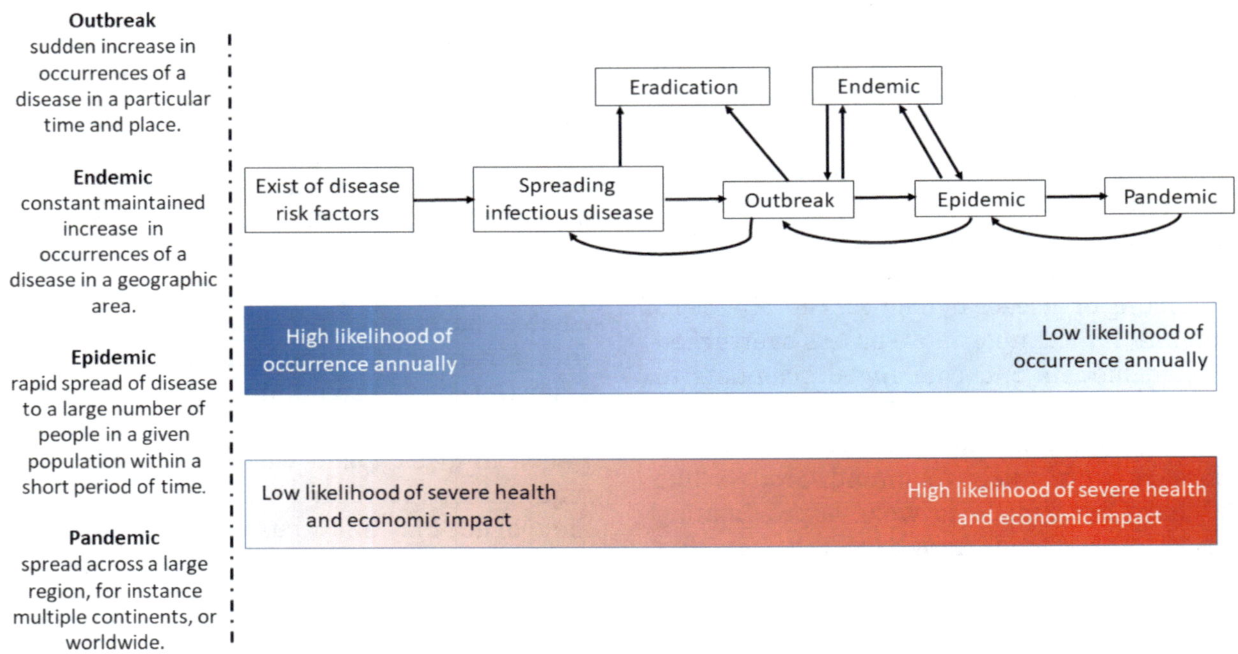

Figure 1.4. Role of public health in disease management.

Source: By Alaa Najjar - Own work, CC BY-SA 3.0, https://commons.wikimedia.org/w/index.php?curid=88074490

1.2. Transmission of Infectious Diseases

Public transport does more than just get people from here to there—it powers the workaday beat of bustling cities by cradling millions in transit, but in the process can also create issues with spreading germs. Consider a packed subway where individuals sit shoulder to shoulder; these types of areas can very rapidly become infection hot spots. Research, on average, highlight the fact that although individuals exhibit no indication of illness, silent travel accounts greatly for how pathogens pass through such networks. There exists a kind of modeling theory called the susceptible–exposed–infected–asymptomatic (SEIA) framework—a mechanism for simulating true-world exposures rather than, well, another technological buzz phrase, which sets such concepts quite well in line. Running simulations that replicate daily travel can surprisingly shed light on important aspects that accelerate disease transmission and, in the end, inform public health actions in our cities (Zhou et al., 2024). In nature, dynamics of disease transmission ultimately become intricately embedded with how species interact. Current studies tend to indicate that changes in our climate can both initiate the emergence and the resurgence of infectious diseases among animal populations. Consider Hawaii: there, the introduction of malaria—its vector insect-borne—has caused spectacular declines in indigenous bird populations. As it happens, even modest environmental changes can make wildlife vulnerable to these aggravating pathogens. As researchers observe the ways that genes respond under these stresses, they begin to see the body's underlying and reinforced defenses. This type of profound, molecular glimpse reminds us just how knotted disease transmission can become, while also encouraging us to smarter, more adaptive approaches to maintaining biodiversity (Paxton et al., 2023). Unraveling the numerous layers through which disease propagates requires integrating meticulous epidemiological modeling with old-fashioned ecological observation. Cities and nature spaces alike present a rich variety of avenues through which germs travel, some quite unanticipated. In most instances, pinpointing those who carry diseases without being symptomatic provides us with a crucial clue regarding the larger picture—information that could well redefine future public health initiatives. While doing that, conservation programs must also consider how our evolving environment places wildlife in danger as well. When you combine insights derived from urban health research with new insights borrowed from nature, you have a surprisingly comprehensive map that addresses both human and animal domains. Ultimately, going this comprehensive route is rather nearly essential to developing strategies that counteract the transmission of diseases in all types of settings (Paxton et al., 2023; Zhou et al., 2024).

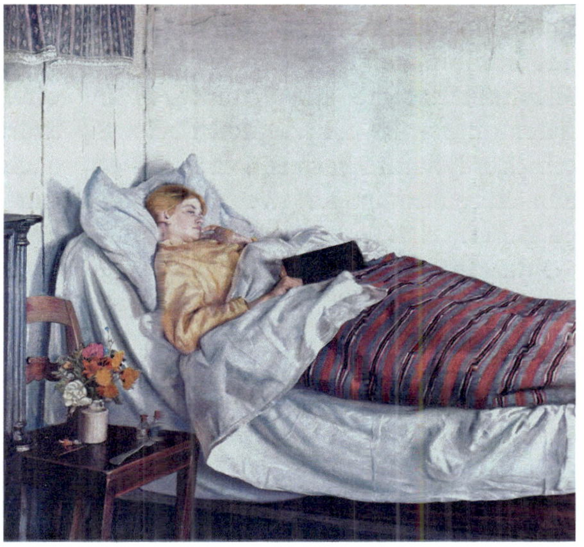

Source: By Michael Peter Ancher - The Yorck Project (2002) 10.000 Meisterwerke der Malerei (DVD-ROM), distributed by DIRECTMEDIA Publishing GmbH. ISBN: 3936122202., Public Domain, https://commons.wikimedia.org/w/index.php?curid=147457

1.2.1. Modes of Transmission (Direct and Indirect)

Infectious diseases spread in strange, sometimes unpredictable manners—and this impacts public health. Direct spread occurs when germs hop directly from person to person via physical contact, whether it is a handshake, a kiss, or even sex. Consider sicknesses such as the flu and COVID-19: small droplets in a cough contain germs that can ignite an outbreak in seconds, for the most part. Simple steps such as maintaining one's own personal hygiene, staying vaccinated, and conducting community health campaigns slow the transfer of this type. An understanding of how these direct routes function provides a sort of platform for controlling outbreaks and reminds everybody, in the majority of circumstances, that it is social responsibility that counts. At times, however, things are not that simple. Germs can transfer indirectly as well, riding shotguns without any sort of face-to-face contact. In such situations, factors such as tainted surfaces, water, or airborne particles come into play. Surfaces, commonly referred to as fomites, can unwittingly transport viruses and bacteria to a new individual, increasing the risk of infection. Even minute vectors like insects may facilitate the transfer of such threats (vector control does indeed become very important here). The complicated, rather complex nature of indirect spread explains why having strong sanitation and regular health screenings is just as vital in preventing disease. A general understanding of both direct and indirect pathways is crucial for healthcare professionals and policymakers alike. For example, in the context of the COVID-19 crisis, experiences gleaned from earlier outbreaks contributed decisively to framing how patients were quarantined and isolated, with the dynamic between the two approaches being crystal clear (Peeri et al., 2020). Even the nuanced relationship between our microbiome and infection shows that such factors as lifestyle, age, and genetic risk factors can genuinely complicate these dynamics (Cryan et al., 2019). Recognizing that disease transmission is not one-dimensional nudges our healthcare systems toward a more combined, out-of-the-box approach to protecting public health (Figure 1.5).

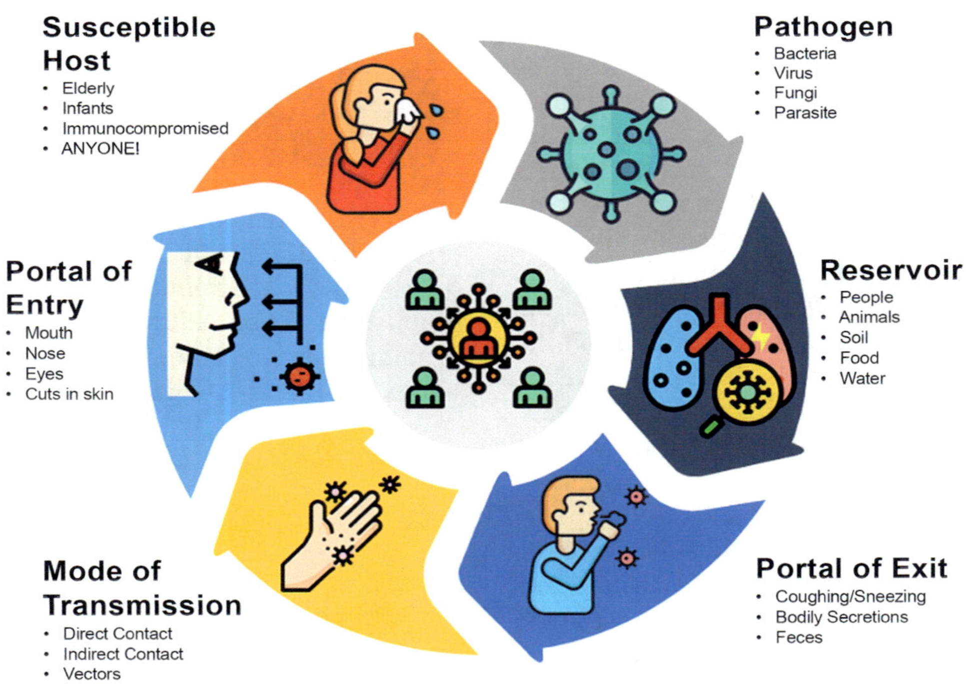

Figure 1.5. Modes of transmission (direct and indirect).

Source: Texas Health and Human Services. (n.d.). Chain of Infection.

1.2.2. Factors Influencing Transmission Rates

When looking at how infections spread, it seems everything boils down to a mix of who you are and the kind of life you live. In places where health services are struggling—think Afghanistan—the lack of solid medical infrastructure can push illnesses like Hepatitis C into higher gear. One study, for example, suggests that factors like age, gender, and even how much schooling someone's had are not just numbers; they shape who ends up getting sick. Generally speaking, younger folks—especially men with limited education—tend to show higher infection rates. Their everyday habits and how easily they pick up reliable information seem tied straight to their increased risk, pointing to a clear need for public health moves that focus on prevention and treatment options for HCV (Danish et al., 2025).

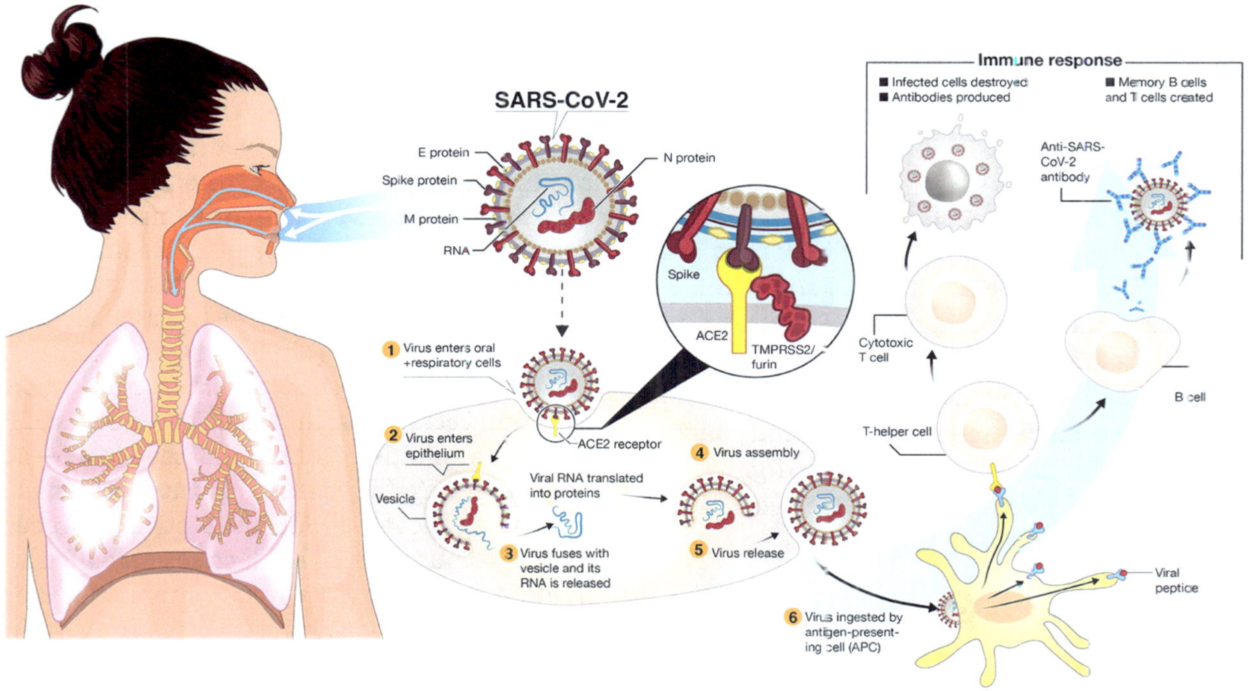

Figure 1.6. Factors influencing transmission rates.

Source: By Colin D. Funk, Craig Laferrière, and Ali Ardakani. Graphic by Ian Dennis - http://www.iandennisgraphics.com - Funk CD, Laferrière C y Ardakani A (2020) Una instantánea de la carrera mundial de vacunas dirigidas contra el SARS-CoV-2 y la pandemia COVID-19. Parte delantera. Pharmacol. 11:937.Funk CD, Laferrière C and Ardakani A (2020) A Snapshot of the Global Race for Vaccines Targeting SARS-CoV-2 and the COVID-19 Pandemic. Front. Pharmacol. 11:937.https://doi.org/10.3389/fphar.2020.00937, CC BY 4.0, https://commons.wikimedia.org/w/index.php?curid=99473789

Then there is the impact of where you work and what you do. Environmental settings and job roles play a big part in transmission dynamics, too. Take illnesses spread by vectors—like Crimean-Congo Hemorrhagic Fever, where close interaction with animals and nature is essential. People working in agriculture, animal care, or meat processing often find themselves right in harm's way, constantly exposed to infected animals or ticks. Global patterns generally show that where you have lots of livestock, CCHF tends to appear more often—whether through tick bites or coming into contact with contaminated blood. This kind of work-based risk clearly underlines the need for customized health interventions that educate high-risk groups on safer practices (Srivastava et al., 2024). Looking at viruses from another angle, the ever-changing genetic makeup of pathogens makes the fight against them even trickier. This gene variability does not just tweak how aggressive an infection can get; it also messes with our vaccines and antiviral treatments. For instance, the Crimean-Congo Hemorrhagic Fever virus itself shows a wide range of genetic differences that affect not only how it spreads but also how hard it is to manage from a public health standpoint. In most cases, understanding these genetic twists is key to crafting better treatment plans, smarter vaccines, and diagnostic tools. Clearly, a deep dive into how environmental, social, and genetic factors combining is essential for lightening the burden of infectious diseases worldwide (Srivastava et al., 2024) (Figure 1.6).

1.2.3. Role of Vectors in Disease Spread

Infectious illnesses usually conceal a dirty combination of elements, and one of the most important characters in this soap opera is the vector. Mosquitoes, ticks, and even fleas—all small arthropods—tend to be nature's messengers transporting germs from host to host. Consider Aedes aegypti, for instance; this insect, primarily responsible for transmitting dengue and Zika viruses, is an obvious indication that our environment truly determine how such carriers transmit illness. Hot weather and pools of standing water increase breeding among mosquitoes, which in turn increases the number of such diseases. Urban expansion, surprisingly enough, at times has the consequence of bringing about exactly the right sort of habitat for these creatures, facilitating their population growth and increasing the likelihood of outbreaks. Overall, understanding the ins and outs of vector behavior is fairly important because clever interventions in managing them can reduce transmission and keep individuals healthier. There is also an increasing perception that the issue of AMR complicates things even further with regard to such diseases. In most areas where vectors transmit the pathogens, individuals not only have to deal with viruses but also contend with bacterial infections that disregard our standard antibiotics. The double whammy increases the health threats, particularly in poorer communities where medical attention is already thin. Such statistics even identify insects such as Escherichia coli and Klebsiella pneumoniae as significant drivers of increased mortality rates in these contexts because of their recalcitrant resistance patterns (Murray et al., 2022). As these carriers reproduce, the interaction among AMR and vector-transmitted diseases demands a strategy as multi-faceted as the issue itself—not only targeting the control of the vectors, but also being clever about antibiotics. In recent times, serious public health crises globally shed light on how necessary it is to monitor vectors that may be harboring reservoirs for emerging diseases. When pathogens jump from animals to humans—a phenomenon that is becoming more frequent—it becomes apparent that observing these carriers in the wild is more crucial than ever. Consider COVID-19: its quick transmission among humans reminds us that zoonotic jumpovers can happen at any time, with bats frequently being cited as a probable source (Shereen et al., 2020). These events necessitate looking beyond the biological functioning of vectors and into how they interact with wildlife and ourselves. All of these combined indicate why it is so crucial to continue studying vector behavior and ecology if we are to be prepared for whatever new dangers come our way.

1.3. Symptoms and Diagnosis

Infectious disease is not straightforward; its presentation comes in a myriad of hazy forms that make it difficult to the diagnose from the outset. The signs can oftentimes be evasive—imagine a patient like infective spondylodiscitis (IS) where pain in the back and fever could very well be explained away as simply part of usual aches, not necessarily some severe condition. It is usually necessary for clinicians to dig a little deeper and not overlook such fine cues, employing cautious examinations that serve to raise the red flag in the event. Rapid detection, particularly with new imaging techniques such as MRI or CT scans involved, can guide the treatment in the desired direction (Milinkovi et al., 2024).

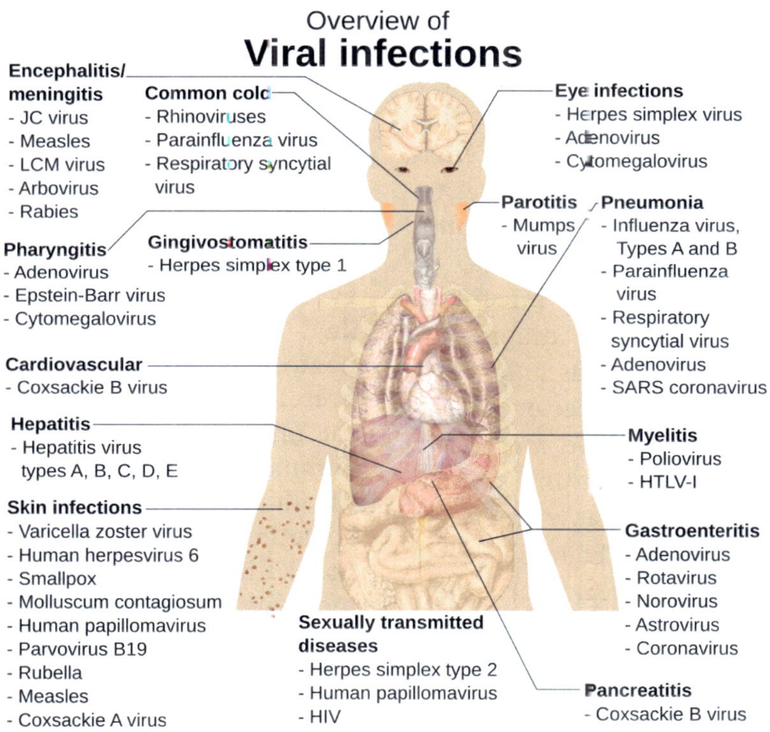

Figure 1.7. Infectious diseases are not straightforward.

Source: By Mikael Häggström - All used images are in public domain.ReferencesMainly Chapter 33 (Disease summaries), pages 367-392 in Fisher, Bruce; Harvey, Richard P.; Champe, Pamela C. Lippincott's Illustrated Reviews: Microbiology (Lippincott's Illustrated Reviews Series), Hagerstwon, MD: Lippincott Williams & Wilkins, pp. 367–392 ISBN: 0-7817-8215-5.For common cold: National Institute of Allergy and Infectious Diseases (NIAID) > Common Cold. Last Updated December 10, 2007. Retrieved on 4 April, 2009For exclusion of CMV among the main viral STDs: Lucile Packard Children's Hospital > Sexually Transmitted Diseases (STDs) Retrieved on 5 April, 2009</ref>, Public Domain, https://commons.wikimedia.org/w/index.php?curid=6416102

Furthermore, as infectious illnesses may strike suddenly, gradually develop, or persist in the long term, monitoring the length of symptoms and their quality is crucial when developing diagnostic approaches. In locations where infections strike drastically, newer methods of detecting illnesses are causing ripples. Automated Polymerase Chain Reaction (PCR) methods like TrueNat have transformed the diagnosis of tuberculosis (TB). Conventional sputum microscopy merely fails to deliver on sensitivity and specificity, especially in endemic areas. When such newer techniques are placed alongside traditional ones, physicians end up receiving results that are faster and more accurate, which opens the door to more prompt interventions (Padmaja et al., 2024). Interestingly, TrueNat does not merely verify the presence of Mycobacterium TB—it also detects drug susceptibility patterns, a determining factor in choosing effective treatments. Knowledge of how symptoms and testing procedures fit together is, in most instances, the key to better infectious disease management. Ongoing diagnostic advances coupled with an increasingly keen eye for clinical signs can result in better patient outcomes and, in the end, reduced morbidity. Prompt and correct diagnosis not only refines treatment but also serves to slow infection spread in communities. As has been observed with IS, combining microbiological information with what patient's report can indeed guide the way toward more targeted therapies and individualized care plans (Milinkovi et al., 2024). Consequently, pushing research to refine these testing techniques is essential—especially in resource-limited regions where the challenge of infectious disease is most pressing (Figure 1.7).

1.3.1. Common Symptoms of Infectious Diseases

Infectious diseases appear in a combination of symptoms that make them difficult to identify and treat. You may experience a fever, a little exhaustion, or even soreness in one location—all indicating that an infectious process may be at work. Fever, for instance, is one of the simple responses by the body; it is a natural defense mechanism to hinder the villains from rushing around by increasing the temperature. And, you know, the specific signs just vary so greatly depending on whether you are working with bacteria, viruses, or fungi. There's a study, which reported non-specific symptoms, such as backache with fever—are fairly prevalent in diseases like IS, which commonly confounds early diagnosis and prolongs treatment. In general, because each infection appears to have its own individual character, understanding these chaotic symptoms is the way to manage them effectively. Getting a diagnosis in a hurry can make a big difference, particularly when symptoms come on abruptly. Frequently, an acute onset appears to bring about increased neutrophil levels, demonstrating how the immune system is resisting. One cohort study even indicated that patients ill for over 15 days wound up with considerably increased neutrophil counts than those with a rapid, acute presentation — in general terms, that indicates the immune system's prolonged struggle with chronic infections. The longer and more severe the illness, the harder the outcome of treatment sometimes is, for instance, in extremely long hospitalization periods and sometimes increased mortality. This emphasizes how both the patients and medical professionals need to be vigilant for these repeated symptoms. Reminding them of the common fever and tiredness, most infections also present with gastrointestinal discomfort like nausea, vomiting, and diarrhea, which can thoroughly disrupt daily life. Specifically in instances such as hepatitis B virus-associated acute-on-chronic liver failure, these symptoms can disrupt nutrition and general well-being – a risk not to be neglected. The connections between these symptoms and additional complications require complete, diligent clinical examination to determine the optimal treatment measures. As our models for treatment evolve, becoming aware that these symptoms have multiple layers assists in creating better strategies and, in the end, improved results for patients. Overall, knowledge of these complicated presentations is at the forefront of both day-to-day medical practice and research (Figure 1.8).

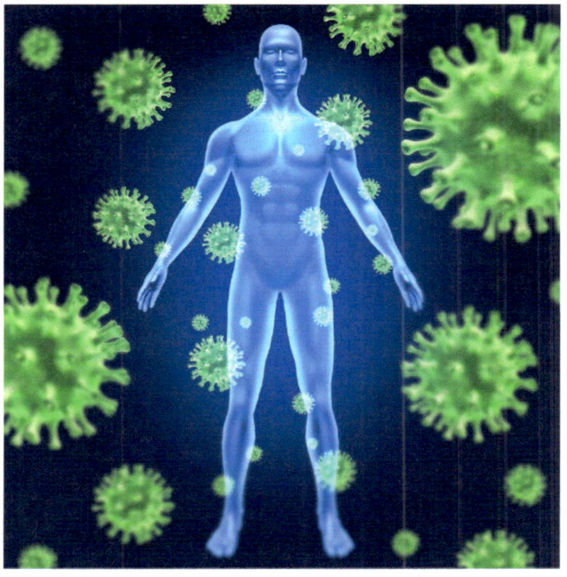

Figure 1.8. Common symptoms of infectious diseases.

Source: Fairview Rehabilitation. (2020). Infectious Disease Types. Fairview Rehabilitation.

1.3.2. Diagnostic Methods Used in Healthcare

New technologies to screen for infections have revolutionized how we respond to new pathogens. PCR is one of them—it rapidly detects the genetic signatures of viruses and bacteria, which came in particularly handy during the SARS-CoV-2 pandemic, when rapid test results enabled the implementation of rapid response strategies. In most instances, laboratories are now experimenting with isothermal amplification methods that are said to yield even faster results without requiring a lot of specialized equipment. Not only do these new methods facilitate the easier spotting of pathogens, but they also assist in monitoring AMR, a significant issue for public health in low-resource settings (Murray et al., 2022). Testing our own immune system is another important part of the equation. Consider serological tests such as ELISA and LFIA, for example; these detect antibodies that have formed following an infection. These tests are genuine workhorses for research that measures how much of the population has been exposed to a disease agent and even informs vaccination planning. While these are not typically the first resort for diagnosing an individual during an illness, they serve to fill in the blanks by providing fragments of information about an individual's history of infections and general immunity. Nevertheless, it is best that such techniques are accurate—false negatives and positives can thoroughly confuse the information and disrupt public health responses (Murray et al., 2022).

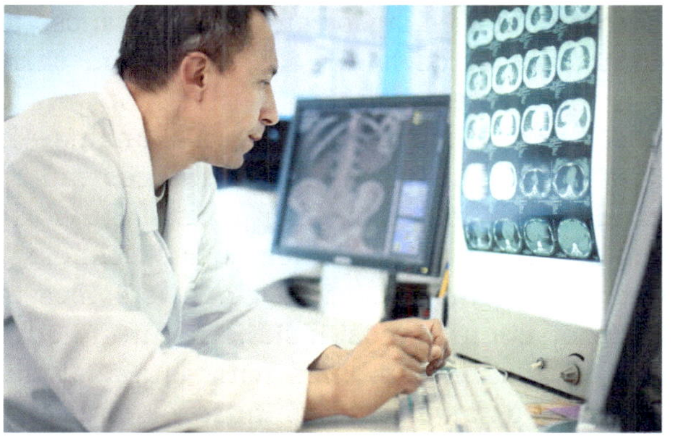

Source: Health Images. (2019). Radiologist.

Occasionally, taking a sneak peek inside the body with pictures provides the best image. X-rays, CT scans, and MRIs are all tools of a set that reveal how far an infection has reached—this is particularly useful when dealing with pneumonia or abscesses. Imaging not only assists in diagnosing, but it also enables doctors to track the progress of the disease and determine whether or not treatments are having an effect. When used in conjunction with lab results, these visual hints contribute to a complete, though occasionally unattractive, clinical picture—especially when symptoms don't tell the whole tale. And, in general, the addition of artificial intelligence (AI) to radiology is promising; it has the potential to enhance diagnostic accuracy and automate workflows, promoting quicker, better-informed decisions in patient care (Murray et al., 2022).

1.3.3. Importance of Early Detection

Infectious disease outbreaks have been occurring too often lately, and that certainly highlights early detection systems. These arrangements, otherwise performing a sort of first line of defense function, allow healthcare teams to catch infections in their tracks before they get out of hand—serving to slow the spread and soften the total burden on public health. Consider dengue fever, for example; in the tropics, the ubiquitous presence of Aedes mosquitoes combined with environmental changes can cause instances to burst unexpectedly. In general, a good early warning system, such as the customized surveillance plans envisioned in Panama—is essential, and these types of measures can be readily implemented in other parts of the world with the same type of problems. New technology is also changing the game when it comes to early detection. In most instances, cutting-edge tools such as AI combined with data analytics now give a far clearer glimpse of emerging trends. While usual public health tactics tend to be bogged down with passive surveillance and fragmented sources of data, breakthroughs in machine learning and predictive modeling truly assist in crunching massive datasets to predict potential dangers. By drawing upon such advances, health systems can detect infections faster, which, in turn, allows for more rapid and more precise responses. Such a proactive approach not only ramps up disease control but also strengthens resilience within health systems, preparing them for outbreaks before they have a complete impact (Eze et al., 2024). Ultimately, early detection is not merely a matter of the immediate battle against infections—it is a pillar of successful public health policy. Detecting and isolating diseases in a timely manner not only saves lives but also reduces the significant economic impact of widespread outbreaks. The exorbitant expenses associated with holding up responses, both in terms of healthcare expenditure and social disruption, truly highlight the necessity of investing in these alert systems. When healthcare players come together and fund enhanced infrastructure, it sort of paves the way for an integrated strategy toward managing health threats spontaneously as they evolve, leading the way toward a healthier, resilient society (Eze et al., 2024).

1.4. Treatment Options

Infectious diseases require not only textbook knowledge but also a feel for the treatment options that rely heavily on the pathogens in question and host response. There is more than one solution to these problems—consider prevention, direct therapy, and providing additional supportive care. Consider the case of poultry; diseases such as Newcastle disease and highly pathogenic avian influenza have the potential to destroy flocks, resulting in massive financial losses and even pose threats to food availability (Grace et al., 2024). Biosecurity and vaccination are central to preventing these diseases, but smallholder farmers have a problem with limited resources and inadequate veterinary access. For the most part, prevention combined with practical treatment truly remains at the core of alleviating the burden of these diseases. Considering forms of treatment involves truly focusing on what kind of insect you have in mind. Viral infections, for example, can be particularly difficult because antivirals tend to fail and may not strike the target as desired. Conversely, bacterial infections typically leave the way open for antibiotics—although these must be treated with care to prevent the development of AMR (Grace et al., 2024). The development of resistant strains throws a spanner into the works, rendering continuous surveillance and judicious, intelligent use of antibiotics essential. Technologies such as gelatin nanoparticles (GNPs) also enter the picture here; they provide the nifty potential for controlled, sustained drug release over time. Though these technological advances are in their infancy, they highlight the continued necessity for new studies and innovative treatment strategies. There is also something appealing about mixing the old with the new when combating infectious diseases. For instance, ethnoveterinary methods—which tap into local wisdom and are sometimes more within reach for rural folks (Grace et al., 2024)—could help where high-tech options are not available. Still, it is important to check these alternative methods thoroughly to see if they work as well or are as safe as our more established norms. Merging conventional approaches with innovations such as GNPs could even chart new territory in the management of disease. Eventually, getting policy-makers, scientists, and providers speaking the same language is critical to developing solutions to treatment that translate across diverse settings, although there may be a few speed bumps along the way (Figure 1.9).

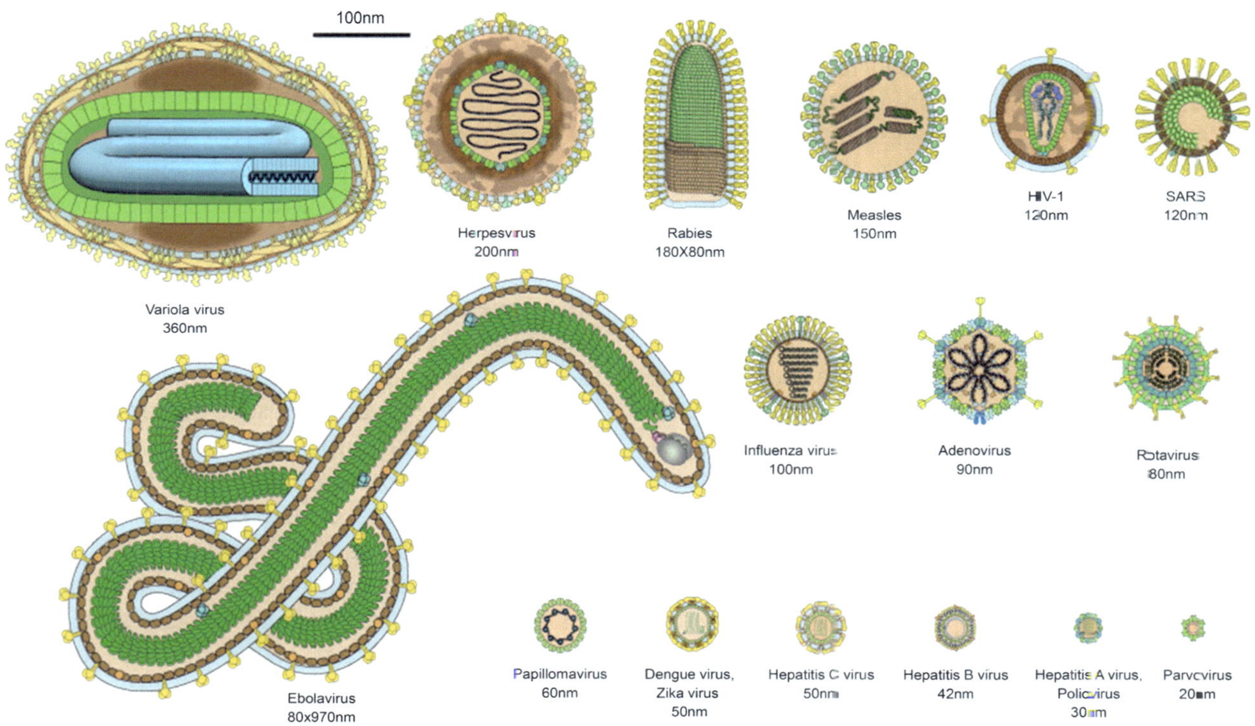

Figure 1.9. Infectious diseases demand not just a textbook understanding but also a hands-on feel for the treatment alternatives that depend a lot on the pathogens involved and how hosts react.

Source: By ViralZone, SIB Swiss Institute of Bioinformatics: Human virus relative size - https://viralzone.expasy.org/resources/Virus%5Fsize.png, CC BY 4.0, https://commons.wikimedia.org/w/index.php?curid=99667474

1.4.1. Antimicrobial Therapies (Antibiotics, Antivirals)

Infectious diseases have evolved throughout history, and consequently, new methods of coping with them have been developed–primarily through antimicrobial therapies. Physicians now resort to antibiotics and antivirals to combat a broad spectrum of bacterial and viral infections that represent serious public health concerns. However, the advantages of these drugs are being undermined by an increasing pattern of AMR; in many instances, microbes have begun to resist, weakening treatments, prolonging diseases, and increasing costs as well as morbidity and mortality rates. This alarming trend, driven by the misuse and at times reckless use of these drugs in humans and animals alike, necessitates immediate worldwide action and improved education to guarantee these life-saving drugs are used appropriately (Aminu et al., 2024). In the case of child care, the judicious use of antimicrobials is strictly essential due to their increased susceptibility to infections. One study at the Helsinki University Hospital, for example, found that approximately 17% of children who received treatment for blood culture-positive infections went on to be inappropriately prescribed antimicrobials (Laine et al., 2017). This indicates that not only do incorrect matches between infections and treatments fail to function as needed, but it makes the door wide open for resistance–an issue that can snowball if physicians fail to exercise additional caution when prescribing. Hospitals implementing sound antimicrobial stewardship (AMS) programs can contribute to developing a culture of more prudent prescribing, which in turn facilitates improved infection control and eliminates harmful side effects. The scenario of today's war against infectious diseases is far from straightforward. It demands a combination of keen monitoring, comprehensive studies, and continuous learning regarding antimicrobial therapy. In general, having a better understanding of how AMR functions will be the most important factor in guiding future drug development and public health policies on the right track. Scientists are now committed to seeking out alternative treatments and prevention strategies–an endeavor that is still pretty much necessary, particularly in the face of resistant pathogens that could erode previous global health advances. In a world where the character of infections is continuously changing, a strong dedication to reasonable and knowledgeable use of antimicrobials will be essential to attaining improved health outcomes and maintaining the present treatments effective (Laine et al., 2017).

1.4.2. Supportive Care and Symptom Management

Successful infection management is not necessarily about a magic bullet treatment—it oftentimes requires good supportive care to alleviate symptoms and enhance recovery. Simple maneuvers such as reducing fever with antipyretics and keeping patients hydrated play an enormous part, particularly when confronted with viral outbreaks where specific antiviral medications are not available. Consider, for instance, a case of Chandipura virus: keeping a child hydrated and lessening fever are now essential moves because high fever and neurological conditions can put a child's health in harm's way. For the most part, such daily habits tend to prevent cascades of complications, which explains why healthcare personnel tend to resort to supportive care measures to regulate both acute as well as chronic infectious challenges (Deshwali & Sharma, 2025). Other times, symptom control becomes an actual balancing act. With the likes of Lassa fever, even asymptomatic patients who may be detected only by routine contact tracing may require close observation to prevent the disease from spreading quietly in the background. Ribavirin, the antiviral drug that is typically first line, is usually complemented by supportive care measures to provide patients with the best possible chance at recovery when symptoms arise. But treatment decisions can become complicated, particularly when economic and social aspects strike hard against vulnerable populations. Usually, this implies that providers, government programs, and community organizations must sort things out together in an imperfect dance, pointing to the more-than-one-aspect nature of supportive care. Finally, it is not only the body that requires care—the patient's mind and social health count as well. Working through infections, especially where symptoms are bad or hospital stays are prolonged, can be emotionally draining as much as physical. Hospitals commonly discover that intermixing mental health services and social support has the effect of keeping patients on their treatment regimens, ultimately creating improved outcomes. This entire concept—that good care extends beyond the meds and penetrates into all aspects of a patient's life—is being recognized more each day, reaffirming the necessity of integrated strategies in addressing infectious diseases (Deshwali & Sharma, 2025).

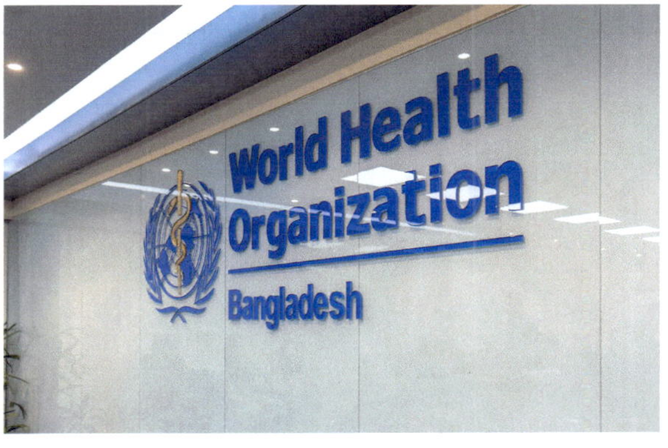

Source: By Jubair Bin Iqbal - Own work, CC BY-SA 4.0, https://commons.wikimedia.org/w/index.php?curid=129796877.

1.4.3. Challenges in Treatment (Resistance, Side Effects)

Tackling infections these days isn't quite as clear-cut as it used to be—drug resistance is the monkey wrench that's thrown into the works. Former tactics that would decimate pathogens in no time now falter when confronted with resistant bacteria and viruses that just won't budge. Take, for instance, TB, and the difficulty is easily seen; with emerging multidrug-resistant strains, the traditional treatments are suddenly rendered ineffective, and physicians are forced toward brutal, sometimes downright poisonous, options. Worse yet, most locations, particularly in developing parts of the world—lack even the lab infrastructure for standard drug-susceptibility testing, so delayed diagnoses allow drug-resistant TB strains to spread uncontrolled, which throws global health initiatives into a pretty big stir (Abubakar et al., 2012). On top of that, the majority of drugs come with a baggage of side effects that just make treatment more difficult. Most drugs have side effects that are easily enough to deter patients from continuing treatment. Serious side effects such as organ impairment or disabling symptoms then arise, rendering continued long-term therapy, such as the endurance programs needed for TB—extremely difficult to adhere to. This reduction in adherence to treatment not only reduces the overall efficacy of treatments but also provides a breeding ground for even more resistant pathogens, sabotaging our worldwide battle against infections (Abubakar et al., 2012).

There is some hope, however, with the latest drug delivery mechanisms. Nanotechnology, for example, shows promise in enhancing drug absorption with terrible side effects held at bay. Employing nanoparticles as carriers of medications can equate to delivering the treatment exactly where it is required, releasing it gradually, and even lowering the amount of medicine patients need to take. This new strategy addresses the two problems simultaneously—improving how well medicine works and lowering the likelihood of resistance. It could very well revolutionize the game of infectious diseases, particularly when it comes to TB, and with the global urgency on that front, rest assured more studies are certainly required to tap all that nanotechnology and other innovations have to offer (Kumar et al., 2011).

1.5. Prevention Strategies

Tackling infectious disease requires a robust, ahead-of-time prevention game plan. Vaccines get top billing in this case—producing vaccine shots that will reduce the dissemination of those frontline pathogens identified by the WHO as top concerns is an actual game changer. It has been well established in a plethora of research that understanding what ignites the infection, transmission mechanisms, and subsequent events when the infection does get underway informs a great deal of how vaccines get designed and delivered. Current R&D activities have identified many potential candidates that, with some aggressive preclinical work, may enhance our capacity to deal with novel threats. Utilization of animal models also has a large role to play; such models allow us to replicate human infections in manners that serve to plug the loopholes in our present countermeasures. On the whole, advancing vaccine strategies quite literally comprise the pillars of our struggle against infectious diseases (Wang et al., 2024). In addition to vaccines, other methods also have a critical role in infection prevention. Scientists are expanding into novel biomaterials – chitosan, for example, is highly popular with a great many because it is both friendly to the body and degradable. Such specific ncharacteristics make chitosan not just a good vector for drugs and vaccines but even a direct antimicrobial agent. The increasing interest lies in modifying chitosan-based configurations to make them more potent against pathogens. In general, with its demonstrated ability to provide a push for the immune system, chitosan may play an important role in preventing as well as curing infections. Further research on these materials may trigger creative answers that nicely supplement conventional practices, enhancing our multi-layered protection against infectious disease (Sinani et al., 2024). Tech developments and public health initiatives also blend in to further support prevention tactics. Contemporary surveillance systems enable us to identify outbreaks earlier—which, in most situations, is paramount for dampening disease spread. AI currently assists in sifting through epidemiological data, identifying patterns and even anticipating potential outbreaks so we can intervene before matters take hold. Community outreach and education are still important as well; when individuals become educated on vaccines and proper hygiene, the general public's health receives a pleasant boost. When health professionals, policymakers, and the general public collaborate—albeit at times in a slightly disconnected manner—it creates a stronger, more adaptable strategy. Ultimately, an intermingling of scientific advances and community engagement is our best hope for staying in front of infectious disease (Wang et al., 2024) (Figure 1.10).

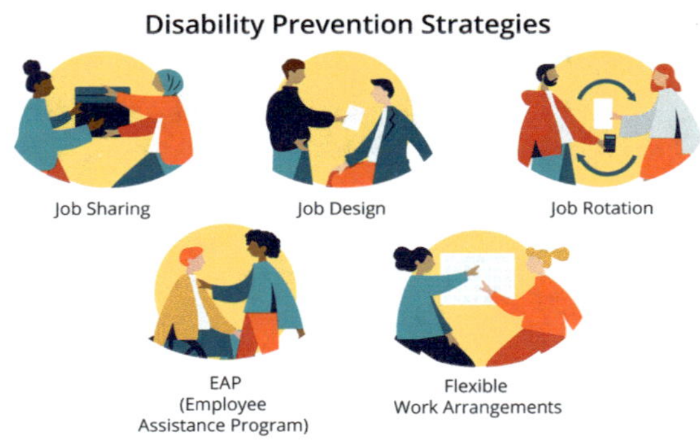

Figure 1.10. Prevention strategies.

Source: Giles, A. (2022). Disability Prevention Strategies. Canadian Health and Safety Workplace Fundamentals. eCampusOntario.

1.5.1. Vaccination and Its Significance

Vaccines revolutionized everything in public health. History teaches us these small shots eradicated illnesses that used to spread wildly. Smallpox disappeared and polio was almost forgotten because populations united and vaccinated. New technologies, such as the mRNA strategies employed in more recent COVID shots, demonstrate we are constantly coming up with new ways to approach new dangers. Germs continually evolve, and therefore we must continually research vaccines, which in most instances fortifies our defenses for the future (Khuroo et al., 2020). Herd immunity is effective when sufficient individuals receive their vaccinations so that even those who are unable—to include little children or people who have compromised immune systems—are safeguarded. Granted, contracting an illness may at times result in natural immunity, but that path has dangers that are not truly justified. Shots inoculate entire neighborhoods and reduce the possibility of large outbreaks. The COVID scenario, for example, clearly illustrated how high vaccination levels slow down the virus, reduce hospital pressures, and ultimately save lives. This new emphasis on immunization has prompted several governments to promote large-scale vaccination campaigns (Roth et al., 2018). Despite all these advantages, many are still reluctant to have vaccines. Confused messages, safety concerns, and misinformation tend to rattle people's confidence and create space for contagions to set in. To meet this, communities require frank discussion and clear science-based information—although the information may not always be flawless. Health agencies and authorities need to come together to execute campaigns not only defining how vaccines work but also reminding us that taking care of yourself takes care of everyone else. Against the present-day more challenging health issues, the establishment of vaccine trust continues to be a central aspect of keeping communities healthy and having a quality life across the world (Khuroo et al., 2020).

1.5.2. Public Health Initiatives and Education

Infectious diseases are a true mystery. They require a combination of efforts—public health campaigns and daily education—that truly strike at the very foundation of how germs are transmitted. When groups come to understand the fine points of transmission, it tips them into small yet significant habit adjustments. Campaigns emphasizing staying clean and being vaccinated, for instance, have improved community health in ways that are difficult to overlook. These types of programs also demonstrate flexibility, adapting spontaneously to fit the cultural nuances of various groups, as we experienced during the COVID-19 pandemic. For the most part, by keeping communication simple and straightforward, public health leaders assist individuals in adopting habits that reduce infection risks (Gausman et al., 2020). Mixing education into public health initiatives better illustrates the disparate means by which individuals confront health issues. Balanced programs show that variables such as restricted access to healthcare and varying education levels can determine who becomes hardest-hit by infections. This sort of everyday observation tends to be the foundation for measures intended to safeguard vulnerable communities. It should be noted that when resources are distributed more equitably, even those on the margins get the education and care they deserve. In this manner, connecting education and health has a tendency to mobilize community action, gradually moving toward improved outcomes and alleviating the overall disease burden (Ahorsu et al., 2020). Partnership of public health organizations with schools and other educational centers tends to ignite an authentic passion to prevent diseases and encourage well-being. Schools then become vibrant hotspots where teachings on how infection occurs equip the students with weapons to make sound health decisions. These programs don't merely dump facts on individuals—they give people confidence and encourage young people to take charge of themselves and others. Occasionally these programs over-spill into the wider community, inviting families and local institutions to join them and create a source of support. To some degree, when all members participate—even if it does seem somewhat scattered here and there—public health campaigns blend into society, igniting long-term cultural changes toward maintaining good health (Gausman et al., 2020).

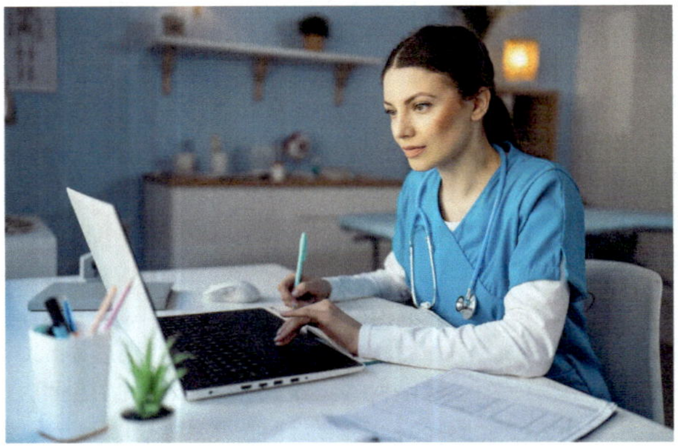

Source: Fortune. (2023). Online Master's in Public Health Methodology. Fortune.

1.5.3. Personal Hygiene and Lifestyle Choices

Personal cleanliness, way of life choices, and infection transmission have turned into a very popular topic among public health experts nowadays. Individuals who understand how to repel disease do things that work during difficult times of health. One of them, combining Protection Motivation Theory concepts with a more expansive interpretation of the Theory of Planned Behavior, discovered that knowledge about COVID-19 had directly captured how exposed people felt and how dangerous they perceived the illness to be, encouraging them to adhere to simple safety habits and in the majority of instances enhancing belief within those practices (Prasetyo et al., 2020). It demonstrates that easy habits such as frequent hand washing, mask wearing, and distancing can reduce outbreaks, so steady health education is darn important. Self-care isn't all about being squeaky clean. The way we eat, travel or even acquire habits such as smoking and drinking all factor into our body's capacity to ward off illness. The pandemic has shaken things up so thoroughly that sectors such as restaurants and hotels have been forced to reframe their entire strategy—customers now demand the best sanitation practices. Hotel management studies, for instance, have found that the perception of cleanliness among guests has changed, forcing establishments to raise their game (Jiang et al., 2020). This new order, in the majority of instances, binds individual behavior with what is practiced in public spaces, as everyone begins to expect that public places look and feel as clean as home. Among all this chaos, the blend of daily hygiene and lifestyle choices we make creates a surprisingly complex connection with disease transmission. As communities struggle and adjust to constant health panics, grasping what drives our daily choices is becoming ever more important. A balanced formula that blends simple speeches about staying clean, some community support, and thoughtful adjustments to our environments may be the secret to healthier public health. By creating awareness and pushing our habits toward better behaviors, it becomes feasible to not just fight today's outbreaks but also prepare for what might be coming next. Overall, these well-informed decisions—flawed and human as they can be—go a significant way in protecting not just individuals, but the population as well, from infections.

1.6. Global Impact of Infectious Diseases

Infectious diseases not only impact personal health—they drive economies and direct the path of world advancement. According to a 2017 Global Burden of Diseases (GBD), Injuries, and Risk Factors study, nonfatal conditions are increasingly becoming an issue, especially with our growing elderly population and increased lifespan. As life becomes longer, circumstances previously being skipped along enter in, and so non-communicable disease begins to emerge along with the familiar infections—meaning a sort of double whammy for areas that then fall behind catching up with public health demands. Evidence (James et al., 2018) suggests just how knotted things become when health systems have to manage a broad range of problems, all whilst attempting to maintain care for all. Economic consequences are another wake-up call in this blend. Infectious diseases ripple economic markets worldwide, and in the majority of instances, increasing antibiotic resistance, as highlighted in Aslam et al. (2018), makes it all the more threatening. While bacteria develop resistance to multiple medications, fewer treatment options remain, costs increase, and recuperation is slower. Nations already struggling with shaky healthcare infrastructure get shoved further still when epidemics strike hard and up-to-date care costs an arm and a leg. This conflict not only interferes with individual well-being but also hampers economic progress, as the productivity of labor decreases in conjunction with mounting disease burdens. Confronting these fiscal burdens clearly necessitates a collaborative effort that transcends healthcare, industry, and policymaking. Then there is the broader picture when looking at global safety and public health policies. A highly interconnected world means outbreaks can jump borders faster than expected—recent pandemic responses have underscored this truth. As nations become more aware of emerging risks, they are starting to work together on monitoring, research, and control activities, basically accepting that diseases do not stick to neat national lines. Widespread evidence from research such as the GBDs only serves to underscore the importance of having an adaptable, team-oriented approach to these dangers. Measured gains in vaccine and treatment technology, combined with continuing efforts to battle AMR (Aslam et al., 2018), are squarely crucial to reinforcing our defenses. As nations come together, they not only strengthen their own health security but they also create a more resilient and flexible global health network (Figure 1.11).

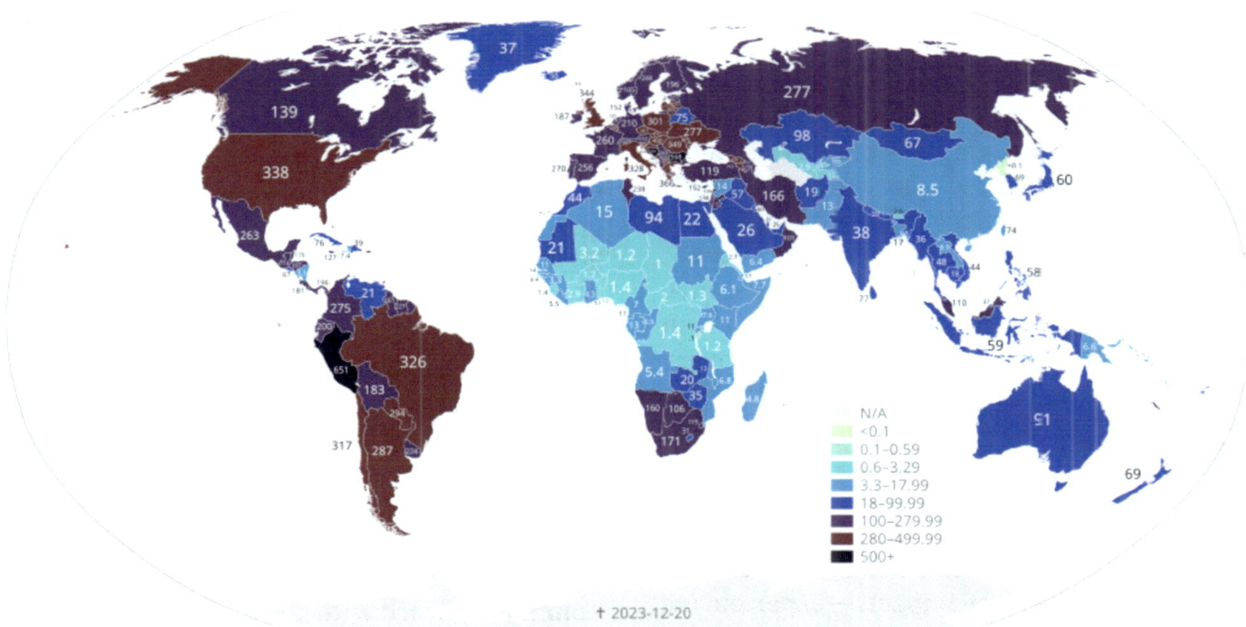

Figure 1.11. Global impact of infectious diseases.

Source: https://en.wikipedia.org/wiki/File:COVID-19_Outbreak_World_Map_Total_Deaths_per_Capita.svg

1.6.1. Economic Consequences of Outbreaks

Infectious disease outbreaks don't only cause health scares; they also disrupt our economies in a myriad of unexpected ways. When a pathogen gains traction, disruptions appear everywhere—commerce, labor, and even the food supply chain get thrown out of whack. Companies lose some of their luster as consumers hold back on spending, and industries such as tourism and hospitality take an even harder hit. Governments typically intervene with quarantines or travel restrictions, which ironically enough can add additional economic burden. For most developing countries with already overextended health systems, these problems tend to create a cycle of underdevelopment and poverty. These costs do not just disappear in the long run. Nations will oscillate between spending a lot on emergency measures and attempting to strengthen preventive measures, with less room for investment in education or vital infrastructure. This perpetual fiscal balancing act tends to exacerbate vulnerabilities, laying the groundwork for subsequent outbreaks. While scaling up health surveillance and early warning systems may assist in reducing the overall cost of managing serious crises, most governments forego the short-term payoff of such investment, particularly where infectious disease is viewed as a chronic, endemic threat (Ayala et al., 2017). Mostly, this perspective implies redirecting health expenditure as an ongoing venture rather than a temporary solution in a state of crisis. How outbreaks ripple through society truly highlights how intricately linked global health is with economic prosperity. When pandemics strike, they tend to magnify inequalities and lay bare vulnerabilities in our systems. Marginalized communities bear the brunt of the worst impacts—experiencing skyrocketing unemployment, less secure access to basic services, and an increasing concern about what the future will bring. Addressing these imbalances requires an integrated strategy that links together health efforts with overall economic policy. By doing so, policymakers can establish a more adaptive, responsive structure that not only protects public health but also maintains the economy above water (Ayala et al., 2017).

1.6.2. Social Implications and Stigma

Infectious diseases have a way of exposing more than mere biological issues—they usually expose underlying social fissures such as stigma. Individuals with conditions like TB or sexually transmitted infections typically end up on the receiving end of social judgment, which only serves to exacerbate their plight. In some cases, fear of being judged causes them to procrastinate seeking assistance, and in most cases, that procrastination tends to snowball into poorer health outcomes. This delay not only harms personal well-being but also perpetuates a cycle of misinformation and cultural confusion regarding the diseases. In most communities where health concepts are closely married to cultural assumptions, the bite of stigma is felt particularly acutely, and therefore focused public health intervention becomes needed to break these barriers (Ibrahim, 2025). It is important to understand how stigma becomes entangled with unequal health opportunities if we are to create plans that do work. Stemming from root social problems such as racism and economic disparity, stigma tends to prevent individuals from receiving the care they require. Although treatments are available in contemporary times, the potential of some of these is lost due to the negative sentiments associated with the disease. In the majority of instances, this implies that any attempt to combat an infectious disease must also tackle the associated stigma. Certain breakthrough initiatives, such as combining community work with clear public education—can erode damaging stereotypes and help foster a more equitable health environment (Zelner et al., 2023). To implement effective solutions, we have to acknowledge that stigma is an intricate, multifaceted problem. Cultural pressures and widespread misinformation have huge roles to play in determining the way that individuals perceive infectious disease. Sensitive health education schemes can empower communities to challenge their ingrained prejudices and initiate debates regarding what constitutes an infection. And then, policymakers must drive wider changes that not only address the medical aspects but also seek to combat the social beliefs that perpetuate stigma. Through the implementation of these concepts, public health professionals can gradually establish a more nurturing environment in which those who are afflicted can feel cared for, and through this, healthier outcomes and improved overall sense of community well-being may be achieved (Ibrahim, 2025) (Figure 1.12).

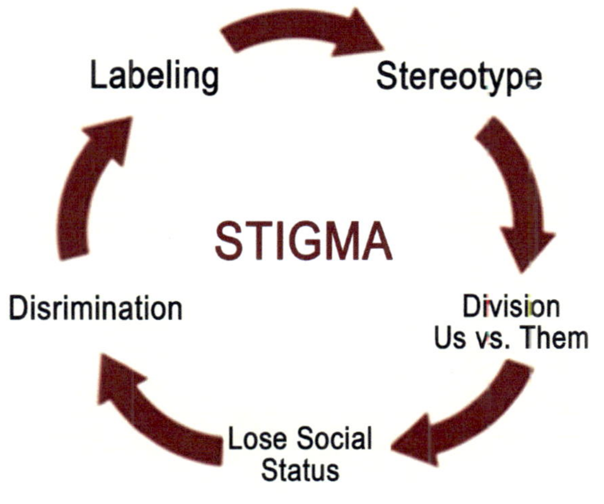

Figure 1.12. Social implications and stigma.

Source: Clayton, H. (2020). Ending stigma: let us talk about effects of stigma surrounding suicide. Cognitive Approaches to Combatting Suicidality (CARMS), University of Manchester.

1.6.3. Global Health Organizations and Their Roles

Global health communities have always been correct during combating infectious danger—it is not simply a function of policy but of actual, on-the-ground work. Organizations such as the World Health Organization (WHO) and the Centers for Disease Control and Prevention (CDC) establish guidelines, monitor outbreaks, and even connect countries at times in ways that extend beyond typical boundaries. Zoonotic diseases, those diseases that spread from animals to humans—comprise approximately two-thirds of the challenge we are experiencing. This truth, as a general rule, has engendered attempts at expert sharing among nations. Take, for instance, some programs operated by Michigan State University (Ghimire et al., 2022) designed to equip experts with know-how necessary for epidemic conquest. To sum it up, when countries come together under one coordinated global effort, they're more equipped to deal with unforeseen outbreaks. Occasionally, magic occurs when private and public halves shake things up a little. Collaborations among government agencies and private firms have increasingly become critical, not only for developing medicines but for fending off illness in areas where resources are limited. If one examines more closely, these partnerships speak volumes of an unusual blend of motivation—clinical trial groups and public health organizations alike joining forces, particularly in parts of the Global South (Brown & Frame, 2009). Such collaboration, in the process, not only drives innovation but somehow smoothes out sustainability problems that arise in drug discovery. It is a framework that, although a bit unpredictable, builds a stronger response capacity by nurturing mutual understanding among different communities. Beyond the here-and-now battles, there is also a long-term strategy building up. Global health organizations are investing in research and training to boost future preparedness. They introduce extensive courses and other capacity-building initiatives aimed at new infectious diseases, which ultimately enhance both the national and regional health systems. Data from such collaborative efforts highlight the imperative of continued education and information sharing—pre-eminent principles for remaining prepared in the long term. For example, numerous online courses in zoonotic diseases (Ghimire et al., 2022) have attracted learners from across the globe, showing how crucial knowledge dissemination can be. And increasingly, it is apparent that health, trade, and environmental challenges all become intertwined, making way for interdisciplinary solutions that, though occasionally a bit messy, provide a more holistic and resilient reaction to global health threats.

CLOSER LOOK

Antimicrobial Resistance (AMR)

Antimicrobials–such as antibiotics, antivirals, antifungals, and antiparasitics–are medicines for preventing and treating infectious diseases in people, animals, and plants. AMR happens when bacteria, viruses, fungi, and parasites are no longer able to respond to antimicrobial medicines. Due to drug resistance, antibiotics and other antimicrobial medicines lose their effects and infections become hard or impossible to treat, putting more people at risk of disease transmission, serious illness, disability, and death.

AMR is an inevitable process that occurs over a period of time due to gene changes in microorganisms. The emergence and growth of AMR are facilitated by human activities, primarily the incorrect and excessive use of antimicrobials in the treatment, prevention or regulation of infections among humans, animals, and crops.

A Global Concern

Antimicrobial drugs are the foundation of contemporary medicine. The development and dissemination of drug resistance pose a threat to our capability to treat minor infections and to carry out life-saving operations such as cancer chemotherapy and cesarean section, hip replacement, organ transplantation and other operations. Drug-resistant infection also affects the health of animals and plants, lowers productivity in farms, and compromises food safety.

AMR comes with high costs to both health systems and national economies at large. For instance, it generates demand for more costly and intensive care, impacts patients' or caregivers' productivity through increased hospitalization time, and damages agricultural output.

AMR is an issue for every nation at every level of income. It spreads across country borders. Factors that contribute to this include insufficient access to clean water, sanitation, and hygiene (WASH) for animals and humans; weak infection and disease prevention and control in households, health facilities and farms; weak access to affordable and quality vaccines, diagnostics, and medicines; limited awareness and knowledge; and insufficient enforcement of pertinent legislations. Individuals in low-resource environments and vulnerable populations are particularly affected by both drivers and impacts of AMR.

SUMMARY

Human health and the transmission of infectious diseases is a challenging business that we cannot simply sweep under the rug. Humans continue to travel across borders—usually in fairly harsh conditions—and with that migration, the likelihood of infections occurring is always present. For instance, migrants from regions such as North Africa frequently end up in horrible living quarters and high stress levels, which makes them more susceptible to contracting diseases. In general, how our social and political environments determine these risks is not clear-cut; it is a combination of environmental danger and human conflict, all leading to the requirement for adaptable and broad public health measures (Türkmen et al., 2022). Separately, new concepts in medicine are turning out to be more than a game-changer, particularly when dealing with difficult skin infections. Studies now, in many instances, reveal that nanoscale drug delivery systems—not necessarily something you witness daily—truly assist in bringing drugs further into deeper skin layers more efficaciously. These techniques, it appears, turn the odds against resilient germs such as MRSA, somewhat revolutionizing our previous treatments. It is a thrilling mix of everyday medicine and cutting-edge techniques that pushes us into new avenues in dealing with infection (Türkmen et al., 2022). Ultimately, both the achievement of progress on the frontiers of medical technology and the complexities confronting mobile populations demand cooperation. Policymakers, health professionals, and researchers must get together and pool what they know to prevent illnesses among the most at-risk while adopting these innovative treatments. Collaborating resources and thoughts—even though this may be at the expense of having some duplicated efforts along the way—could potentially lay the foundation for improved strategies that satisfy both human and technical aspects of combatting infections, particularly where brutal migration conditions present additional layers of risk (Angeletti et al., 2020).

Infectious diseases strike a blow to world health, and we must examine their real cost and how they evade our medicine. Recent studies indicate that AMR continues to increase as an important threat, contributing significantly to illness and premature death. To illustrate, an estimated 4.95 million individuals died of bacterial AMR in 2019–a figure that reached low-resource settings in particular. Lower respiratory infections, for example, accounted for more than 1.5 million fatalities, ranking as one of the most virulent offenders. This harrowing statistic, as disturbing as it is, illustrates unequivocally that there is a crying need for new, efficient means of avoiding and curing infections, particularly considering that insects such as Escherichia coli and Staphylococcus aureus continue to exacerbate the crisis (Murray et al., 2022). There is also emerging awareness of the way our microbiota is involved in infections and highlighting the gut-brain axis. In a general sense, the trillions of microbes that cover and inhabit our bodies don't just keep stomachs functioning but can also influence neuropsychiatric disorders. How these small creatures build communities rely on a multitude of variables, from how one is born, to environmental pressures, to antibiotic exposure, to make a messy complex that appears in such age-related and neurodegenerative diseases. The above multi-faceted link between infection and mental state means we need to think about both simultaneously when designing healthcare policies, rather than categorizing treatment under one umbrella (Cryan et al., 2019). Addressing the complexity of infectious diseases and AMR requires a response as diverse as the issues. Relying solely on classic epidemiological tests will not be sufficient; we must also investigate new, novel treatments. The devastating impact of AMR, particularly on the most vulnerable—underscores the necessity of policies that are shaped to local contexts, aimed at preventing and controlling infections. Concurrently, novel understandings of the microbiota-gut-brain axis open up exciting therapeutic opportunities that could, for instance, redefine the way we treat conditions ranging from autism to Alzheimer's. Through the identification of how microbial disease and infection are connected, future studies could create approaches that treat not only the clinical aspect of disease but also enhance general health and community resilience (Cryan et al., 2019; Murray et al., 2022).

KEY TERMS FROM THIS CHAPTER

Pathogen	Infection	Host
Virulence	Transmission	Reservoir
Vector	Contagious	Epidemiology
Incubation period	Carrier	Zoonosis
Immunity	Antibiotic	Antiviral
Antifungal	Antimicrobial resistance (AMR)	Endemic
Epidemic	Pandemic	Vaccination
Innate immunity	Adaptive immunity	Opportunistic infection
Nosocomial infection (HAI)	Quarantine	Isolation
Biosecurity	Outbreak	Diagnosis

REFERENCES

1. Abubakar, I., Atun, R., Chakaya, J., Cox, H., et al. (2012). Drug-Resistant Tuberculosis—Current Dilemmas, Unanswered Questions, Challenges and Priority Needs. https://core.ac.uk/download/9839026.pdf (accessed on 6 May 2025).

2. Ahorsu, D. K., Lin, C. Y., Imani, V., Saffari, M., Griffiths, M. D., & Pakpour, A. H. (2020). The Fear of COVID-19 Scale: Development and initial validation. International Journal of Mental Health and Addiction, 20, 1537–1545. https://doi.org/10.1007/s11469-020-00270-8.

3. Aminu, R., Apollos, S. D., Enesi, K. O., Kwaga, J., et al. (2024). Antimicrobial Resistance as a Global Public Health Threat: The Way Forward. https://core.ac.uk/download/618203595.pdf (accessed on 6 May 2025).

4. Aslam, B., Wang, W., Arshad, M., Khurshid, M., Muzammil, S., Rasool, M. H., Nisar, M. A., et al. (2018). Antibiotic resistance: A rundown of a global crisis. Infection and Drug Resistance, 11, 1645–1658. https://doi.org/10.2147/idr.s173867.

5. Ayala, A., & Gostin, L. O. (2017). Global health security in an era of explosive pandemic potential. Journal of National Security Law & Policy, 9(1), 53–72. https://core.ac.uk/download/74539397.pdf (accessed on 6 May 2025).

6. Brown, C. J., & Frame, P. (2009). Communities of Practice in The Public-Private-Partnership Sector for Neglected Diseases Drug Development: The Importance of Mindset Mapping. https://core.ac.uk/download/1639972.pdf (accessed on 6 May 2025).

7. Carroll, D., Daszak, P., Karesh, W. B., Lipkin, W. I., et al. (2012). Prediction and prevention of the next pandemic zoonosis. The Lancet, 380(9857), 1956–1965. https://doi.org/10.1016/S0140-6736(12)61684-5.

8. Deshwali, Zahid Hussain, and Vikas Sharma. 2025. "A Review on Chandipura Virus: Outbreaks and Emerging Infectious Disease for Children in India". Asian Journal of Research in Infectious Diseases 16 (1):1-12. https://doi.org/10.9734/ajrid/2025/v16i1413. (accessed on 6 May 2025).

9. Djoko, C. F., Fair, J. N., Lebreton, M., Pike, B. L., et al. (2010). The origin and prevention of pandemics. Clinical Infectious Diseases, 50(12), 1636–1640. https://doi.org/10.1086/652860.

10. Gausman, J., & Langer, A. (2020). Sex and gender disparities in the COVID-19 pandemic. Journal of Women's Health, 29, 465–466. https://doi.org/10.1089/jwh.2020.8472.

11. Ghimire, R. P., Maredia, K. M., & Wilkins, M. J. (2022). Virtual training for managing emerging zoonotic diseases including COVID-19. Journal of International Agricultural and Extension Education, 29(1), 57–75. https://doi.org/10.4148/2831-5960.1019.

12. Grace, D., Knight-Jones, T. J. D., Melaku, A., Alders, R., & Jemberu, W. (2024). The public health importance and management of infectious poultry diseases in smallholder systems in Africa. Foods, 13. https://www.semanticscholar.org/paper/c3deddc7ba59ad563d6ff215ea783ddf143b921e (accessed on 6 May 2025).

13. Grimaldo Ureña, Y., Díaz, Y., Pascale, J. M., López-Vergès, S., & Sánchez-Galán, J. E. (2025). A framework for the early detection and prediction of dengue outbreaks in the Republic of Panama. Frontiers in Tropical Diseases. https://www.semanticscholar.org/paper/c3f4c8ef0129622b9bcd2b4a676a1ef93e738eae (accessed on 6 May 2025).

14. Ibrahim, Ibrahim Awad Eljack. Unveiling the Hidden Barriers: A Review of Stigma Associated with Infectious Diseases and Its Impact on Prevention and Control. Journal of Pharmacy and Bioallied Sciences 17(Suppl 1):p S166-S168, May 2025. | DOI: 10.4103/jpbs.jpbs_52_25 (accessed on 6 May 2025).

15. Jiang, Y., & Wen, J. (2020). Effects of COVID-19 on hotel marketing and management: A perspective article. International Journal of Contemporary Hospitality Management, 32(8), 2563–2573. https://doi.org/10.1108/ijchm-03-2020-0237.

16. Khan, M., Vergara-Mojica, S., Zodo, A., Ali, M., & Mena Lora, A. M. (2025). P-1311. Infectious diseases trends in migrant populations at a safety-net community hospital in Chicago. Open Forum Infectious Diseases, 12. https://www.semanticscholar.org/paper/7c876cc73a48b593 8c4b22bc9021d45378692873 (accessed on 6 May 2025).

17. Khuroo, M. S., Khuroo, M. S., Khuroo, M. S., Sofi, A., & Khuroo, M. S. (2020). COVID-19 vaccines: A race against time in the middle of death and devastation! Journal of Clinical and Experimental Hepatology, 10, 610–621. https://doi.org/10.1016/j.jceh.2020.06.003.

18. Kumar, M., Kumar, N., Kumar, P., Kumar, A., et al. (2011). Nanotechnology: A focus on treatment of tuberculosis. International Journal of Drug Delivery, 3, 25–42. https://core.ac.uk/download/233973368.pdf (accessed on 6 May 2025).

19. Laine, N. (2017). Use of Antimicrobials in a Tertiary Children's Hospital. https://core.ac.uk/download/132491357.pdf (accessed on 6 May 2025).

20. Lippi, G., Henry, B., & Mattiuzzi, C. (2025). The crucial role of laboratory medicine in addressing future public health infectious threats: Insights gained from the COVID-19 pandemic. Diagnostics, 15. https://www.semanticscholar.org/paper/d00e97f9e8624cc05b84972fa7477095cff4f3d4 (accessed on 6 May 2025).

21. Prasetyo, Y. T., Castillo, A. M., Salonga, L. J., Sia, J. A., & Seneta, J. A. (2020). Factors affecting perceived effectiveness of COVID-19 prevention measures among Filipinos during Enhanced Community Quarantine in Luzon, Philippines: Integrating Protection Motivation Theory and extended Theory of Planned Behavior. International Journal of Infectious Diseases, 99, 312–323. https://doi.org/10.1016/j.ijid.2020.07.074.

22. Shereen, M. A., Khan, S., Kazmi, A., Bashir, N., & Siddique, R. (2020). COVID-19 infection: Emergence, transmission, and characteristics of human coronaviruses. Journal of Advanced Research, 24, 91–98. https://doi.org/10.1016/j.jare.2020.03.005.

23. The Writing Committee of the Report on Cardiovascular in China, & Hu, S. (2023). Report on cardiovascular health and diseases in China 2021: An updated summary. Journal of Geriatric Cardiology: JGC, 20(6), 399–430. https://www.semanticscholar.org/paper/b3da8bacf180f6e35d727cc389a5a67cf39fb90d (accessed on 6 May 2025).

24. Xu, L., You, X., Cui, Y., & You, J. (2024). Health poverty alleviation in China from the perspective of historical institutionalism: Policy changes and driving factors. Frontiers in Public Health, 11. https://www.semanticscholar.org/paper/212670f9f11e443875ea48617f0e7c6f76200ea2 (accessed on 6 May 2025).

25. Zelner, J., Naraharisetti, R., & Zelner, S. (2023). Invited Commentary: To Make Long-Term Gains Against Infection Inequity, Infectious Disease Epidemiology Needs to Develop a More Sociological Imagination. American journal of epidemiology, 192(7), 1047–1051. https://doi.org/10.1093/aje/kwad044 (accessed on 6 May 2025)

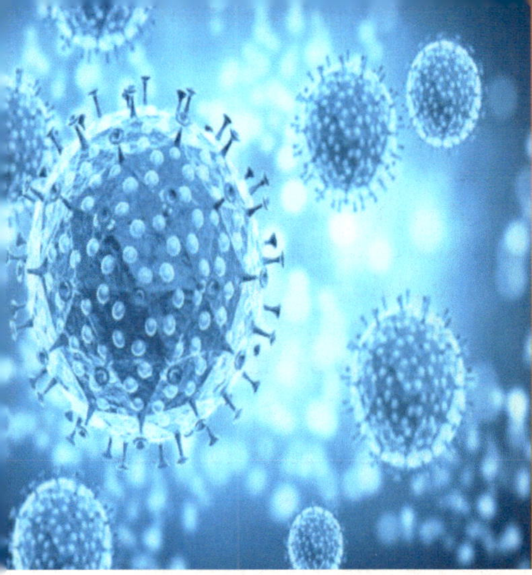

Chapter 2

BASIC EPIDEMIOLOGICAL CONCEPTS

Contents

Introduction

Epidemiology is an important field of research that examines the cause, effect, and distribution of disease and health conditions within populations. Fundamentally, epidemiology is an inquiry into disease distribution and causative factors for the development of disease. By studying populations, and not individuals, epidemiologists aim to identify the determinants of the occurrence of health events. It plays a crucial role in the determination of risk factors, public health planning, and healthcare policymaking. Knowledge of disease transmission patterns as well as sociocultural determinants of these patterns constitutes an integral part of effective disease control and prevention. The complete definition of epidemiology also includes, in addition to outbreak investigation, chronic disease etiology, psychiatric disease, and environmental determinants of health. Epidemiologists use multiple techniques, such as observational studies, clinical trials, and statistical analysis, to collect data on disease effects on different populations of individuals. This multi-faceted methodology allows researchers to establish associations between environmental exposures and disease, and assess the success of interventions in lowering disease rates. The fusion of these varied data sources and approaches gives epidemiology the ability to inform evidence-based practice, whereby public health interventions are grounded in good scientific information. Additionally, epidemiology is a cross-disciplinary field, learning from medicine, sociology, and environmental science to gain fused public health strategies.

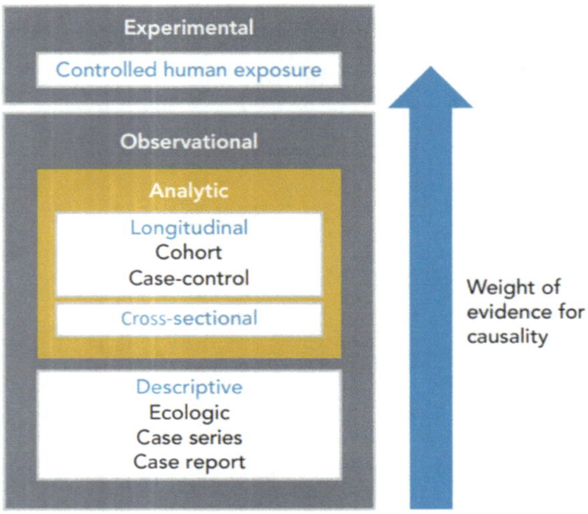

Figure 2.1. Epidemiology serves as a critical field of study that investigates the patterns.

Source: By National Institute for Occupational Safety and Health - https://www.cdc.gov/niosh/docs/2020-106/pdfs/2020-106revised032020.pdf, Public Domain, https://commons.wikimedia.org/w/index.php?curid=150471869

The definition of epidemiology is widened to include descriptive and analytical branches. Descriptive epidemiology concerns itself with the who, what, when, and where of health occurrences, whereas analytical epidemiology tries to demonstrate causal association and correlation using stringent testing and evaluation. By precise definition and elaborated explanation of disease trends, epidemiologists play a very important role in enhancing population health, eradicating health inequalities, and strengthening healthcare facilities. Therefore, the science of epidemiology is required to help prepare the healthier and more robust populations required in today's complex health environment (Figure 2.1).

Epidemiology provides a basis for health behavior education, the disease causes, and the many determinants of public health. Epidemiologists are trained to professionals who often working in interdisciplinary teams, examining the distribution and determinants of health-related states or events among a defined population. By dissecting data using many different methods, epidemiologists seek to determine patterns in health data, demonstrating the influence of socio-economic, environmental, and behavioral determinants that cause impacts on health outcomes. The critical analysis and interpretation of the determinants are significant in the context that they form the building blocks of policy formulation for disease prevention and health promotion. The use of epidemiology, therefore, not only reveals the intricate health dynamics that influence health but also reveals a scientific foundation that guides the practice of public health and health intervention for preventing health inequalities and promoting community wellness. One of the greatest strengths of epidemiology is its reliance upon data taken from a wide variety of sources including clinical research, questionnaires, and public health data. Epidemiologists apply an extensive range of statistical techniques to analyze this information, making conclusions that are employed in informing local and global health policy. Built environment research, for example, focuses on how the urban planning decisions influence health behavior, notably avoiding obesity. Interdisciplinary collaboration among disciplines such as urban planning, public health, and the behavioral sciences enriches a holistic understanding of the contribution of environmental determinants toward exacerbating health issues. A critique argues that interdisciplinary collaboration facilitates the assessment of the built environment and generates practically relevant outcomes set to enhance public health issues, particularly those of non-communicable diseases (NCDs) (Davis et al., 2016). In summary, the value of epidemiology is more than data analysis; it is a higher dedication to supporting public health based on evidence. With the health profile steadily shifting with new threats such as pandemics, chronic disease, and health inequity, the efforts of epidemiologists are more critical. This field not only enables determinants to appreciate their complex interaction with health but also enables a shared forum from many disciplines where new health solutions could potentially lie. Additionally, conferences like the Advances in Teaching and Learning Day also serve to highlight the continued need for teaching and the transmission of knowledge in this arena, once more reinforcing the importance of interdisciplinarity in the resolution of contemporary public health problems (Phelps et al., 2004). The continued evolution of epidemiology thus bears witness to its vital role in the building of healthier futures.

Importance of Epidemiology in Public Health

Epidemiology is the cornerstone of public health because it gives primary information on determinants and distribution of states of health among populations. It is extremely important to know disease patterns and trends for the disease prevention and control authorities. For instance, the chikungunya virus (CHIKV) has highlighted the importance of extensive epidemiological studies since outbreaks are disseminated across targeted populations, like what happened in Brazil, where a massive outbreak from 2014 to 2018 was attributed to a novel ECSA genotype. This incident demonstrates how epidemiological research follows the introduction and transmission of infectious diseases to allow their impact to be contemporaneously minimized by public health interventions In the context of a dynamic health situation, especially in regions where emerging diseases are known, strong epidemiologic frameworks are needed to make interventions that are effective and offer evidence for the allocation of resources in public health policy (Naveca et al., 2019). Apart from that, the utility of epidemiology cannot be exaggerated in chronic diseases, where data about prevalence and risk factors are vital to worldwide health systems. The increased prevalence of conditions like diabetic retinopathy (DR) highlights the necessity of stringent epidemiological research. Effective planning, execution, and evaluation of DR public health policies depend on the existence of up-to-date information on the burden of DR at the global level. Systematic review and meta-analysis methodology, as has been debated in recent literature, can provide up-to-date and context-specific estimates that guide healthcare providers and policymakers. This kind of information is critical in designing sufficient prevention and care intervention addressing the diverse needs of diverse populations. Epidemiological studies, as such, stand in an activated position to address NCDs and render interventions evidence-based and community-level (Cheloni et al., 2019). Further, the application of novel techniques for epidemiology reflects how this science is progressing and becoming more applicable in contemporary public health. Application of digital epidemiology and genome sequencing, as evident from the study of the CHIKV outbreak, portrays how the incorporation of conventional protocols with techno-tools improves disease surveillance. These new methods not only enable the detection of disease outbreaks but also reveal their possible progression, facilitating timely intervention. With infectious and chronic diseases further evolving in correlation with globalization and climatic shifts, the integration of such technologies within the discipline of epidemiology will be inevitable. This transformation can substantially enhance the ability of public health systems to effectively counter current threats, thereby protecting population health and developing health infrastructure in response to future health and outbreak threats (Naveca et al., 2019) (Figure 2.2).

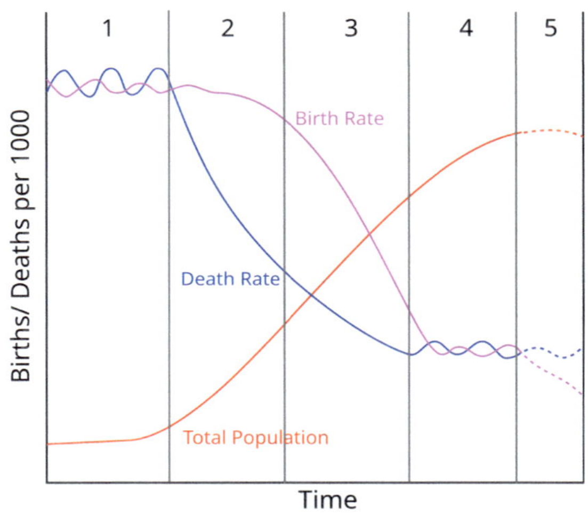

Figure 2.2. The epidemiology in public health.

Source: By Stage5.jpg: en:User:Charmed88derivative work: NikNaks93 (talk) - Stage5.jpg, Public Domain, https://commons.wikimedia.org/w/index.php?curid=5841448

Key Terms and Concepts in Epidemiology

Epidemiology, or the investigation of the determinants and distribution of states related to health, has several terms and concepts that are most important to know to understand population health. Among the basic concepts in epidemiology is the incidence and prevalence concept. Incidence is the number of new disease cases within a given time period and gives evidence of disease incidence risk. Yet, prevalence is employed to quantify instances that co-exist at one point in time and will be employed to estimate the intensity of disease prevalence among the population. These definitions are important as they will inform public health intervention and resource allocation. For example, a high incidence rate may indicate immediate preventive measures are required, whereas a high prevalence may necessitate long-term treatment programs. These estimates are of unparalleled importance to health officials in policy formulations informed of their own scope of work, delivering better population health outcomes (Carmalt et al., 2018). The epidemiologic triad is another basic epidemiologic concept outlining the host, agent, and environment interaction in disease causation. This kind of model is core to comprehending how different variables affect the outcome of health. The host is that population or individual that is under risk of disease and the agent is the etiological agent of the disease, i.e., bacteria, viruses, or lifestyle. The environment encompasses extrinsic influences on the transmission of disease, e.g., access to healthcare and socio-economic level. Based on the research of this triad, epidemiologists can identify possible interventions that will most probably break the chains of disease transmission and, thus, support public health programs that hold morbidity and mortality at a bare minimum. This integrative approach enables health administrators to develop detailed policies that rely on a high frequency of epidemiological determinants (Anderson et al., 2005). Besides these principles, the significance of spatiality in epidemiology has also increased over time, particularly with regard to geographic disease spread. Spatial analysis considers how the distribution of disease changes in space, and how it translates into the pattern of outbreaks and environmental hazards. Through studying spatial flows, epidemiologists can make sense of the disconnection involved in infectious disease, tracing out the linkages between epidemic occurrences and local conditions. Population density, for instance, may lead to quicker disease spread. Learning about this spatial aspect also means learning about the interrelation between social and cultural determinants, affecting health behavior and vulnerability to disease. Spatiality in epidemiologic studies, therefore, advances the understanding of health risk and facilitates more effective public health interventions and policy (Anderson et al., 2005).

2.1. History of Epidemiology

The history of epidemiology is inherently entangled with the history of public health practice. Its beginnings trace back to ancient Greece, where health and disease patterns among populations were first identified. The word epidemic literally originally came from the Greek *epi*, on or above, and demos, people, and referred to the early conceptualization of disease spread. Great minds like Hippocrates established early theories proposing that environmental influences and lifestyle habits have a considerable impact on determining health outcomes. As time passed, the discipline of epidemiology developed along with science and medicine, especially between and following the Renaissance era, when scientific observation was extremely appreciated for its ability to discern disease patterns and guide public health measures. The history of epidemiology therefore provides some indication of its importance in creating policies for disease control and prevention. The revolutionary period in the field in the 19th century saw the contributions of the pioneering epidemiologists. John Snow's examination of a cholera epidemic in London has been referred to as a landmark in the methodology of epidemiology. With careful mapping and investigation, Snow determined that contaminated water supply was the cause of the outbreak and thus proved the role of environmental factors in disease transmission. The event highlighted the need for evidence-based practice and spurred on the formation of sanitation reform and modern public health practice. In addition, Louis Pasteur and Robert Koch s establishment of germ theory further advanced the discipline, establishing a scientific underpinning for research in infectious disease and causative microbes. These advances cemented epidemiology's central position in informing health policy designed to enhance population health outcomes. By the 20th century, epidemiology broadened its focus to include a wider array of health-related issues beyond infectious disease, such as chronic disease and social determinants of health. Advances in sophisticated statistical techniques and epidemiological research, such as cohort and case-control studies, allowed more comprehension of how different variables affect health outcomes within different populations.

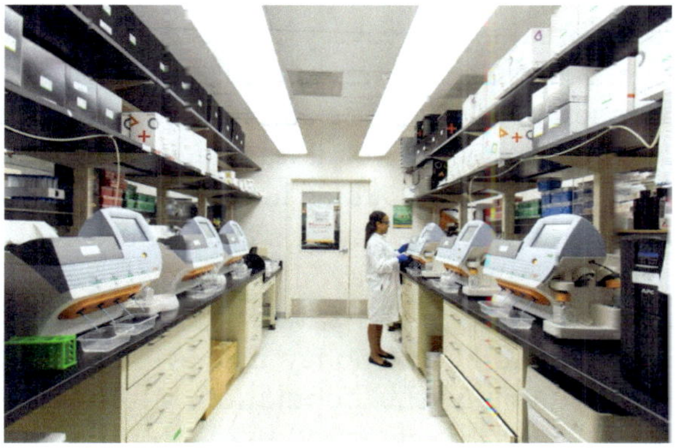

Source: National Cancer Institute. (2020). DNA Genotyping and sequencing. *Unsplash.*

When scientists began using whole-genome sequencing (WGS) and phylogeographic techniques to study viral diseases, they came to see that they learned more about complex transmission dynamics. For instance, newly emergent pathogens like the rabies virus uncovered the significance of genetic heterogeneity in the understanding of diseases' spread and control. As emphasized in recent studies, the complex interaction between environmental, social, and biological determinants remains to test public health interventions, calling for a multidimensional epidemiology response placed in the context of history and employing novel methodologies (Biek et al., 2015; Cortey et al., 2016).

2.1.1. Early Contributions to the Field

The initial work in epidemiology established the model for the investigation of the determinants and distribution of events and states related to health. The initial epidemiology pioneers, including John Snow, were interested in linking the outcomes of diseases with environmental factors, such as his study of cholera in London in the mid-19th century. Snow's conscientious investigations set contaminated water sources as the leading route of cholera infection, a groundbreaking discovery that conflicted with current miasma theories of disease etiology. His approach not only made empirical observation and the acquisition of data more significant but also required public health measures to be based on epidemiologic evidence. These initial endeavors played a crucial role in medical paradigm shifts, which contributed to better public health policy and overall health improvement of the population. After World War II, British scientists made tremendous contributions that studied health issues in the tropics. The Witness Seminar on June 3, 1999, concentrated a lot of information on how African medical research evolved with focus on the contribution of the Medical Research Council (MRC). The organization made a significant contribution toward the research of the vector-borne diseases (VBDs), malaria and sleeping sickness that largely plagued postcolonial societies. The collaboration of British researchers highlights that African health workers enabled effective disease control interventions and impacted treatment approaches, which spilled over into Africa and ultimately to health practice in the UK. The connection reinforced the global nature of epidemiology and reaffirmed the wisdom in gaining knowledge on variable environmental and sociocultural contexts in avoiding infectious diseases (Reynolds et al., 2001). Moreover, the transition from colonial medical practice to independent practice created an unprofessional environment for instruction and research in Africa. Through the focus on nutrition, non-infectious diseases, and vector-borne diseases, researchers sought to develop context-specific interventions for the unique issues that were faced by newly independent nations. The results of these early epidemiological studies not only improved health outcomes in local populations but also stimulated global controversy regarding health equity and social determinants of health. The work of early epidemiologists thus helped to emphasize the worth of participatory research that synthesizes local realities and knowledge, enriching ultimately epidemiology as a science. These early contributions still resonate in the application of contemporary epidemiology as they necessitate a comprehensive response to understanding and fighting health disparities (Reynolds et al., 2001).

2.1.2. Major Historical Outbreaks and Their Impact

19th century, have informed public health policy and epidemic response. The cholera outbreaks yielded high death rates and showed that urban water supply and sanitation systems are susceptible to vulnerabilities. Measures of response were modified as time passed by improving knowledge of how cholera is transmitted, allowing for more effective interventions across different cohorts. Based on a historical review, it has been noted that even with the implementation of primary and secondary control measures in outbreaks, statistical overviews have largely revealed low but steady achievements in occurrence and death rate decline (Carneal-Frazer et al., 2019).

This is a demonstration that there is a need for ongoing study into the efficacies of past interventions in the expectation that they will effectively guide public health policy at present. VBDs like yellow fever, plague, and malaria have equally well-documented historical importance, extending beyond simple health issues to impact social and political environments. The infections have been drivers of populations, which in turn usually lead to decreasing populations due to uncontrolled morbidity or disabling chronic illness. Additionally, VBDs have differentially affected communities based on existing immunity and social determinants, exacerbating disparities and informing resilience in populations. For example, plague epidemics have in the past facilitated the concentration of power among ruling classes and the exclusion of sufferers, epitomizing universal themes of classism and racism in times of public health crisis (Athni et al., 2021). The dynamics reflect how VBDs become interwoven in the fabric of social development, triggering reform in governance and reshaping traditional communal exchanges. Examination of the effects of these past outbreaks demonstrates that they have spurred essential public health and medical awareness growth. Outbreaks have encouraged creative solutions like better sanitation, disease monitoring, and vaccine production. The intersection between epidemiology and societal reaction has hastened the creation of health policies to prevent and reduce the occurrence of outbreaks. Such previous pandemics' lessons are thus crucial knowledge for public health environments today. By studying how previous outbreaks influenced societal responses and guided the next interventions, we learn better to respond to current and future health threats. This process of learning from experience during each cycle emphasizes the importance of broad epidemiological knowledge for the safeguarding of global public health (Figure 2.3).

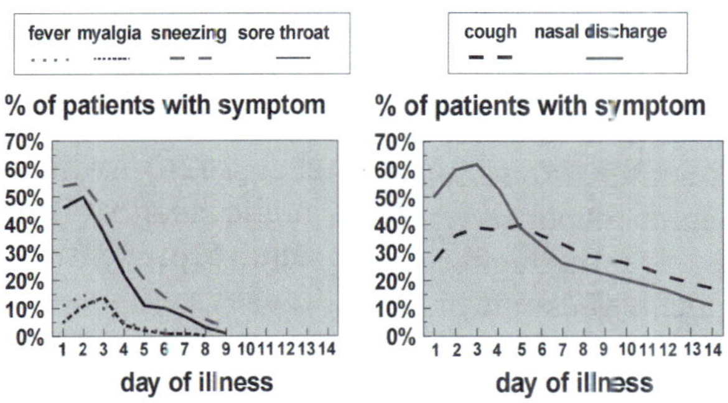

Figure 2.3. The major outbreaks of infectious diseases.

Source: By US Government - The Centers for Disease Control and Preventionhttps://www.cdc.gov/getsmart/community/materials-references/print-materials/hcp/child-rhin-vs-sinus.pdf, Public Domain, https://commons.wikimedia.org/w/index.php?curid=54272465

2.1.3. Evolution of Epidemiological Methods

Technological advances have augmented the advancement of epidemiological techniques hard, and disease patterns are being analyzed by researchers with unrestrained accuracy. Infection transmission dynamics have been understood with more sophistication thanks to statistical models, and outbreaks can be examined in a more advanced manner. Aggregate data were typical in conventional epidemiological techniques, and this can mask the complexity of the spread of disease. By contrast, modern approaches utilize precise genetic, temporal, and spatial data to reconstitute transmission events. Working within new frameworks, scientists can detect undetected cases and map transmission lines more effectively, refraining from the older models' assumption of a unique source of infection (Hampson et al., 2014). This move toward greater methodology is another step in the ongoing development of epidemiological practice to serve public health. Along with epidemiological studies is the integration of next-generation sequencing (NGS) into public health practice, revolutionizing the scope of microbial genomics. The application of WGS enables comprehensive analysis of bacterial pathogens, with lucid results on patterns of transmission as well as resistance patterns. As shown by several studies, WGS's capability to identify outbreak sources as well as track the development of virulent strains has been invaluable (Boon et al., 2019). Its potential to one side, utilization of WGS in routine practice is hindered by issues like data integration and contextual quality. However, the transition from early research to routine practice is a milestone for epidemiology, making it possible to usher in a new era where genomic data informs outbreak investigations and public health response with greater evidence. This passage through the history of epidemiological techniques not only tells us about developments in technology but also about the necessity for interdisciplinary cooperation. As disease patterns become more and more complex with the pressures of globalization and environmental change, the techniques employed must follow suit. Epidemiologists are increasingly having to work alongside geneticists, bioinformaticians, and public health officials to be able to extract the maximum use out of new technologies. These collaborations are essential in bridging the challenges of incorporating genomic data into conventional epidemiologic models. By seeking synergy among disciplines, researchers can take disease surveillance and control to its extremes, ultimately maximizing population health benefits (Boon et al., 2019). This shift accentuates the need to evolve means of addressing the health issues of the contemporary age effectively in an attempt to make epidemiology a critical area of study in the eradication of infectious diseases.

2.2. Types of Epidemiological Studies

Epidemiological research is important to account for public health patterns, and it can be generally classified into descriptive and analytical studies. Descriptive epidemiology seeks to describe the distribution of the disease and health outcome in populations, frequently measuring indicators such as age, sex, geography, and time. This study will yield crucial trends and patterns, and it is then possible to develop hypotheses about potential risk factors. For example, a descriptive study can monitor higher Brazilian beach tennis players' rates of injury and call for further research on certain protective and causative factors like duration of exposure and previous injuries, as revealed by the analysis of Rodrigues et al (2024). By the application of these methods, public health officials can identify areas that require preventive actions and interventions. Conversely, analytical epidemiology extends beyond the cause and determinants of health events to examine these through complex observational and experimental design. The most common analytical designs are cohort, case-control, and cross-sectional studies. Cohort studies, for example, may follow a cohort of subjects over time to determine the effect of risk factors on the development of specific conditions. New evidence on post-pancreatitis diabetes mellitus (PPDM), with a focus on population studies within the framework of the COSMOS program, represents the pinnacle of premier analytic efforts in this field. This initiative acknowledges the epidemiologic contribution of finding multiple risk factors, burden patterns, and PPDM morbidity outcomes, upholding the directives of stringent methodologies in investigating diffuse health phenomena, as asserted in Cho et al. (2024). Finally, randomized controlled trials (RCTs) are the most advanced type of epidemiological research, especially in proving causation between exposures and health effects. RCTs entail random assignment of the subjects to intervention and control groups to test interventions in a rigorous manner. The studies form a critical part of proving effective measures against disease prevention and health promotion. For instance, in exploring injury prevention among sports participants, an RCT can contrast the effect of different training timetables or rehabilitation regimens on rates of injury for sporting activities such as beach tennis. By planning these trials with meticulous care and strict adherence to ethical principles, investigators can produce evidence useful for public health policy and clinical practice. While the epidemiological science continues to develop, various forms of study are still required to improve knowledge and encourage better population health (Figure 2.4).

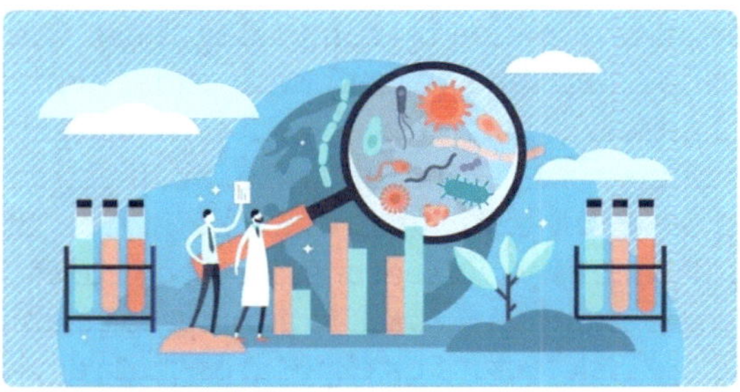

Figure 2.4. Types of epidemiological studies.

Source: VectorMine. (n.d.). Epidemiology vector illustration: flat tiny bacteria pandemic outbreak research. *Shutterstock*.

2.2.1. Descriptive Studies and Their Purpose

Descriptive studies serve a core function in epidemiology in terms of describing general states related to health and their pattern of distribution in populations. Descriptive studies differ from analytical studies, where the goal is to determine causality, since they have been conducted to describe systematically health effects in the context of person, place, and time. Descriptive studies make it possible for researchers to determine patterns and trends that can guide subsequent research into the etiology of public health. Descriptive studies are particularly useful in environments such as military recruit training, where knowledge of the incidence and nature of musculoskeletal injuries (MSIs) among troops will contribute to the identification of areas of intervention and training improvement design (Lovalekar et al., 2024). Therefore, such studies guide the creation of evidence-based guidelines for improving overall public health efficacy. Descriptive studies also work well in evaluating conditions such as Haglund's syndrome, whose descriptive demographic, clinical, and procedural information provides clear evidence regarding the conditions weather. Compilation and comparison of heterogenous patient cohorts' data enable researchers to note variability in surgical outcomes concerning the characteristics of patients and treatment protocols. Through descriptive statistics, meaningful observations like complication rates by different surgical methods may be inferred (Kutzer et al., 2024). Implications may guide clinical decision-making and refinement of patient care protocols, thereby validating the place of descriptive studies in clinical practice as well as epidemiology. Finally, the scope of descriptive studies includes health disparities detection and utilization of targeted interventions. Through a snapshot of health status, such studies can shed light on the prevalence of disease in different groups of people and thus improve insight into possible social determinants of health. An example is identifying the higher cumulative incidence of MSIs among female Marine Corps recruits compared with men to inform the realignment of training programs to close such disparities (Lovalekar et al., 2024).

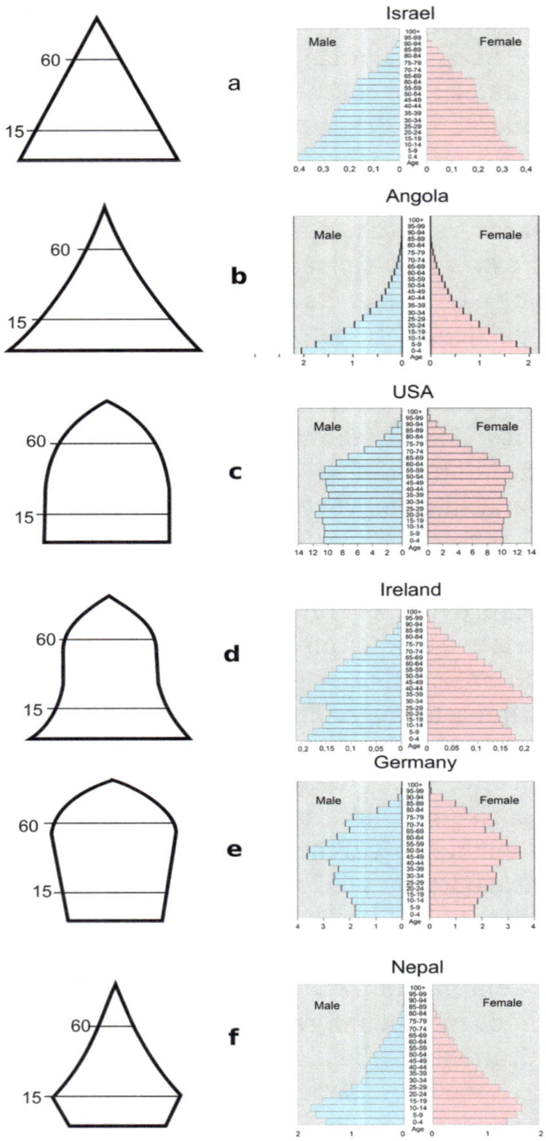

Figure 2.5. Descriptive studies serve a fundamental role in epidemiology by providing a comprehensive overview of health-related states and their distribution within populations.

Source: By Kopiersperre - de:Datei:Grundformen Altersstruktur.svg from Rosso Robot after Friedrich Burgdörfer: Volk ohne JugendFile:Israelpop.svg, File:Angolapop.svg, File:Uspop.svg, File:Irelandpop.svg, File:Germanypop.svg and File:Nepalpop.svg from Delphi234, CC BY-SA 3.0, https://commons.wikimedia.org/w/index.php?curid=34973828

Secondly, the above information can inform future research studies with the purpose of preventing risks and improving health by highlighting the role of descriptive studies in the ongoing development of epidemiological science and public health policy (Figure 2.5).

2.2.2. Analytical Studies: Cohort, Case-Control, and Cross-Sectional

It is necessary to know various study designs of analysis for examining health-related outcomes in populations. Among these, cohort studies are particularly helpful as they follow up on a group of individuals over time to analyze associations between risk factors and health outcomes. This kind of design separates subjects into exposed and non-exposed subjects and tracks the incidence of disease events in them. The longitudinal cohort study design allows temporal relationships to be established and gives insight into causation. Although they can produce strong data, cohort studies are extremely resource- and time-consuming, with a tendency toward participant loss and potential biases in follow-up assessments. Case-control studies offer an alternative by comparing those with a specified outcome (cases) with those without it (controls). This retrospective investigation is valuable when the outcome in question is rare or when exposures must be investigated simultaneously. Researchers select cases by outcome and then go back to attempt to establish possible risk factors or exposures that resulted in the condition. While case-control studies are generally cheaper and faster compared to cohort studies, they have the risk of recall bias and selection bias, thus compromising the validity of their findings. This makes precise definitions of cases and controls critical in ascertaining the reliability of results. Cross-sectional analyses present another perspective by measuring at a single point in time, giving a snapshot of the relationship between outcomes and exposures among a population. The design works best in determining the burden of disease and risk factors, allowing researchers to observe patterns and associations. Cross-sectional analyses do not address causality directly, however, as they cannot define the direction of the observed associations. They are often limited by their failure to account for temporal changes in exposure or outcome. Therefore, while cross-sectional studies may provide valuable initial data that can inform more detailed research, their findings must be interpreted cautiously, with recognition of the inherent constraints of the approach. In veterinary science, the use of instruments such as the STROBE statement ensures that research designs are conducted with thoroughness and in a rigorous manner, resulting in the enhancement of the quality of epidemiological reporting in the field (Cevallos et al., 2016; Ersbøll et al., 2016).

2.2.3. Experimental Studies and Clinical Trials

Clinical trials and experimental trials are fundamental components of epidemiological research, providing rigorous methods for cause-and-effect investigation of health conditions and exposures. Clinical trials are usually carried out in the form of random assignments of study subjects into intervention and control groups to minimize bias and enhance the reliability of results. In controlled settings, researchers can establish the efficacy of treatments, preventive measures, or interventions through systematic means. For instance, the development of scientific evidence concerning the contribution of vitamin D supplementations to the risk of breast cancer illustrates how RCTs operate in epidemiology. That knowledge derived from such studies helps make better-informed public health advice and policy for bettering population disease outcomes (Avenell et al., 2013). In addition to disease impacts for a single person, clinical trials and experimental studies play a critical role in medical guideline design and public health program design. By their rigorous insistence that benefits outweigh potential expenses before a novel treatment being approved for use by regulatory bodies, clinical trials protect against ineffective yet apparently beneficial regimens. Furthermore, the trials typically involve a variety of design features, including stratification and blinding, to reduce confounding variables that can skew results. For example, the Single-Case Reporting guideline In Behavioral interventions (SCRIBE) 2016 requires transparency and specificity in reporting single-case experimental designs. Adopting standard reporting guidelines like SCRIBE will enhance the replicability of studies and result in more informed decision-making for researchers and healthcare providers (Albin et al., 2016). Finally, the amalgamation of clinical trials and experimental research as a foundation for public health practices provides solid bases for evaluating interventions in disease prevention and treatment. These methods not only guide clinical practice, but also contribute to the development of epidemiological theory and models. Furthermore, the incessant innovation of trial design, such as adaptive trials and the incorporation of biostatistics, is constantly refining our understanding of health dynamics among populations. By embracing experimental studies and clinical trials, epidemiologists are better placed to address health disparities and implement evidence-based interventions that enhance the well-being of different populations (Avenell et al., 2013; Albin et al., 2015).

2.3. Epidemiological Measures

Epidemiological markers play a significant role in demarcating determinants and distribution of health-related illnesses among specific populations. They comprise sets of indices, such as case fatality rates, mortality rates, prevalence, and incidence, which constitute vital instruments for researchers and practitioners in the field of public health. Incidence refers to the rate of new cases of disease within a population over a specified time, while prevalence measures the total number of cases, both old and new, at a specific moment. Combined, the two statistics reveal the dynamic of the diseases so that epidemiologists can identify patterns, assess risk factors, and measure the effectiveness of interventions. As has been demonstrated through social epidemiology, understanding of the role of social and economic determinants—like income inequality and absolute poverty—has increasingly become essential in the interpretation of such epidemiological information (Link et al., 2008). Furthermore, modern epidemiology has employed advanced methods of refinement to traditional measures.

For instance, the integration of NGS in public health practice has revolutionized epidemiologists' surveillance and control work against many pathogens. The new approach enhances the understanding of outbreaks primarily by WGS, allowing accurate source tracing and timely detection of new health threats. By effective utilization of WGS, researchers are in a better position to unravel complex transmission dynamics, follow drug resistance, and assess the efficacy of public health interventions. The shift to the application of such sophisticated technologies points toward the imperative of the maintenance of high-quality contextual information, which with effective epidemiological measures, can significantly improve plans for disease control (Boon et al., 2019). Overall, the development and implementation of epidemiological measures are the foundations of continuing to advance public health programs and improve population health outcomes. Through the provision of critical data to clinicians and policymakers, these initiatives guide the allocation of resources, the planning of health programs, and the implementation of preventive strategies. The continued emphasis on a convergence of social determinants of health and innovative use of emerging technology, as the field evolves, will further illuminate researchers' and practitioners' understanding of disease trends and health inequity. Finally, the focus on holistic and multi-dimensional epidemiological interventions will not only improve the health of an individual but also ensure a healthier population in general, showing the interdependence of determinants of health in populations (Link et al., 2008; Boon et al., 2019) (Figure 2.6).

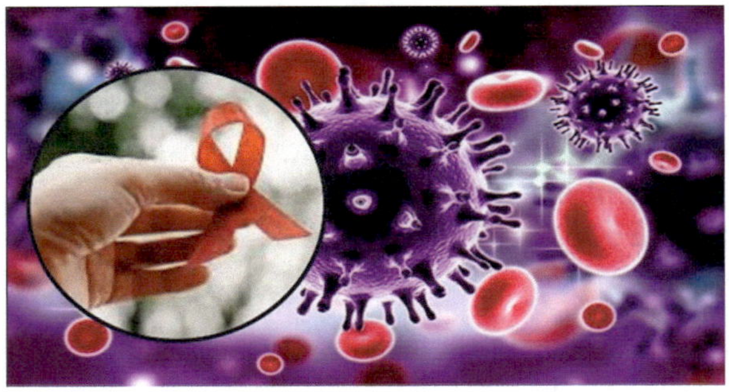

Figure 2.6. Epidemiological measures.

Source: National Institute of Health and Family Welfare (NIHFW). (n.d.). *Course Image: Epidemiology and Control of HIV*.

2.3.1. Incidence and Prevalence Rates

The field of epidemiology must understand rates of prevalence and incidence because the rates provide critical information about the frequency and distribution of disease among populations. Incidence is the count of new instances of disease in a period of time, typically expressed as per 100,000 persons per year. Conversely, prevalence is the total number of all cases that exist in the population at present, both old and new, at a specific point in time. Not only do these numbers determine public health requirements, but they also assist in allocating healthcare resources. For example, diseases like Amyotrophic Lateral Sclerosis (ALS) illustrate a striking incidence rate of approximately 2 per

100,000 per year in Europe, with a matching prevalence of approximately 6 per 100,000, and they illustrate both the burden and the requirement for specialist healthcare provision to be localized to affected areas (Bianchi et al., 2025). The incorporation of incidence and prevalence rates also underscores the necessity for understanding population demographics as well as disease course. Incidence analysis provides data regarding the risk of acquiring a disease, which varies widely with age, geography, and genetic factors. For instance, ALS has documented increased incidence in the 60–79 years age group, indicating the necessity for age-segregated epidemiological studies. Prevalence rates, however, can be used to account for survival rates after diagnosis. In ALS, survival rates at varying time intervals after disease onset are useful in indicating the impact of the disease on quality of life and health needs (Bianchi et al., 2025).

Thus, studies about the rates assist in setting public health policy on disease prevention and control measures. Also, the incidence-prevalence relationship is of staggering proportions in terms of planning for healthcare and resource allocation. High incidence with low prevalence might mean a short duration of disease or high mortality, whereas a high prevalence rate might mean stable status or dropping incidence as a result of efficient treatment and management measures. For example, the prevalence of diagnosed Huntington's disease (HD) in various countries has been estimated at 3.5 per 100,000 in Brazil to 8.2–9.0 per 100,000 in the USA and some parts of Europe, which not only reflects the burden of disease but also the healthcare system that can manage chronic diseases. Based on these principles, epidemiologists and policymakers can effectively respond to the public health subtleties, creating interventions that address existing as well as future needs of the affected populations.

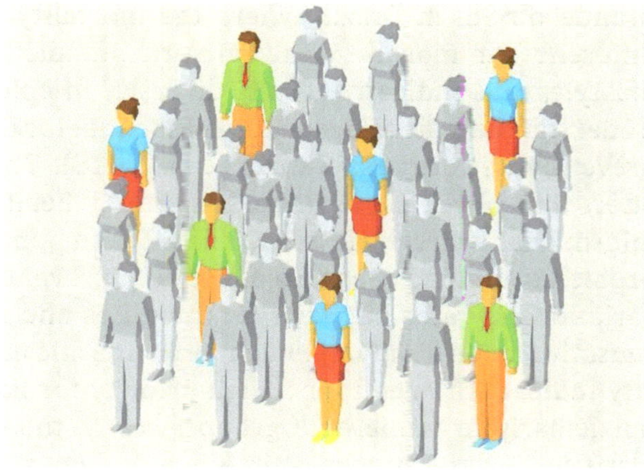

Source: Technology Networks. (2021). *Incidence vs Prevalence*

2.3.2. Mortality and Morbidity Rates

Mortality and morbidity rates are the basis of the concept of epidemiology because they provide evidence of the health status of populations. Mortality rates, commonly expressed as deaths per 100,000 population for a specified time, are a critical measure in assessing the impact of disease and health intervention. For instance, examination of mortality data might show trends with specific risk factors, groups, or regions. A study in Ardabil city highlighted the significance of tracking burn injury mortality rates, identifying a higher rate among women (1.86 deaths per 100,000 person-years) than men (0.88) for the period 1997–2006. The disparity highlights gender and age roles in shaping outcomes for health and the need for targeted public health interventions to counteract hazards from specific injuries in those at risk. Morbidity rates, which determine the prevalence of disease among a specific group, complement mortality statistics by giving a better idea of public health concerns. They enable researchers to measure the influence of diseases that significantly reduce the quality of life, even if they do not lead to death. For example, esophageal malignant neoplasia presents with high morbidity and mortality, particularly in certain regions such as Rio

Grande do Sul in Brazil, where the mortality rate is far greater than the national average. Such differences in mortality rates are attributable to socioeconomic status, access to medical care, and lifestyle, thus indicative of the diversity in epidemiological complexities of different communities. Understanding these dynamics is essential for developing effective public health policies and cancer prevention strategies (Gurski et al., 2018). The interplay between mortality and morbidity rates offers a comprehensive understanding of health issues facing populations. Collectively, these rates inform healthcare professionals (HCP) and policymakers about the magnitude and severity of health problems, guiding resource allocation, prevention measures, and treatment options. Furthermore, variations in rates between communities and regions call for ongoing research to understand the causative factors and implement area-specific interventions. For instance, studies on burns in Ardabil city indicate the need for a high priority for having educational programs to reduce such injuries, particularly in vulnerable groups. Lastly, the continuous monitoring of mortality and morbidity statistics is very important in epidemiology, informing the future direction of health interventions and fostering improved community health outcomes (Figure 2.7).

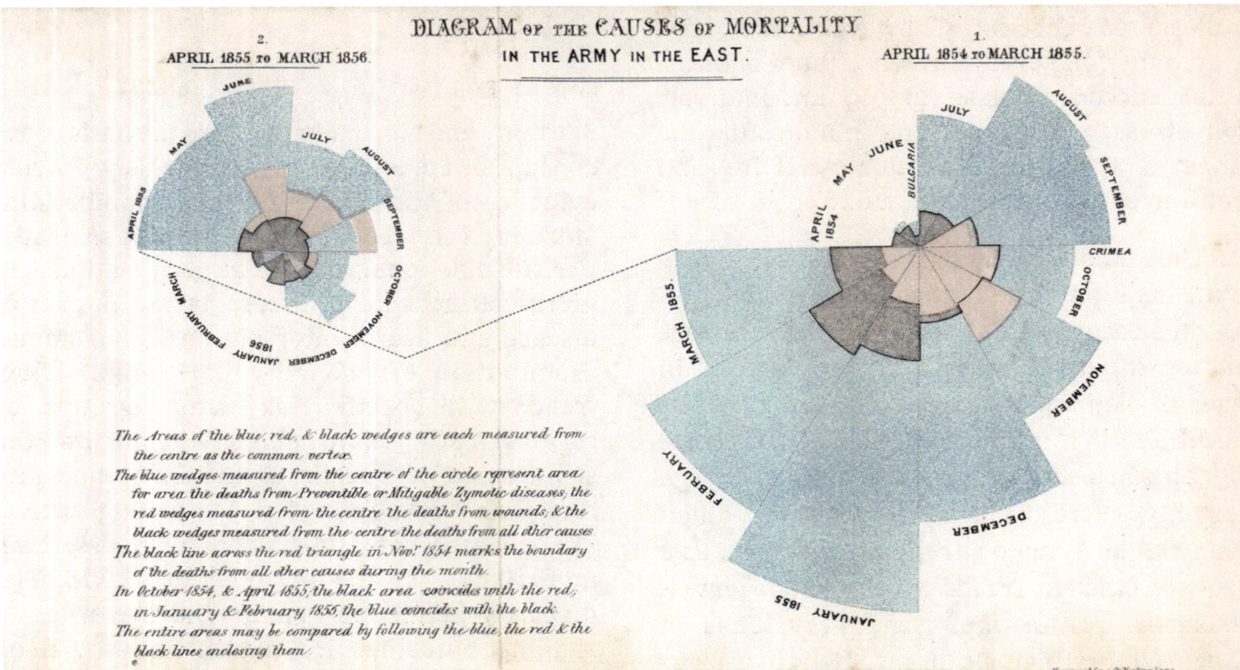

Figure 2.7. The mortality and morbidity rates.

Source: https://en.m.wikipedia.org/wiki/File:Nightingale-mortality.jpg

2.3.3. Risk Factors and Their Assessment

Risk factor measurement is an important aspect of determinants and distribution of health status understanding. Through such identification of risk factors, researchers can initiate intervention programs to control or stop disease. Risk factors are either non-modifiable or modifiable; genetic vulnerabilities can't be altered, yet dietary intake, physical exercise, and toxin exposure are modifiable factors. The interaction of these disparate risk factors forms an interlaced web that determines individual and population health outcomes. Epidemiologic studies employ various methodologies to analyze their interactions, surveying data with cohort, case-control, and cross-sectional study designs to eventually reveal seminal pathways toward disease formation. One of the most important applications of risk factor evaluation is the promise of public health action. The resources could be prioritized and programs implemented in high-priority groups through the identification of risk factors for that matter. For example, knowledge of psychosocial risk factors for chronic inflammation can guide workplace interventions to reduce not only individual risk but also population health problems in general. Prioritizing systematic reviews and meta-analyses allows scientists to synthesize evidence across multiple studies, enhancing risk factor estimates. An ecological perspective enables the creation of lucid connections between occupational stressors and health outcomes and eventually leads to the creation of effective preventive measures and better health practices in any environment (Emiko et al., 2018). Epidemiologic techniques are applied in animal welfare evaluation as well, where the determination of risk factors could make it possible to introduce measures to improve the required standards of care. Through the use of human epidemiological models, scientists can explore determinants of unusual behavior or maladjustment in a large range of species. Integration of epidemiological study designs, for instance, enables systematic assessment of animal welfare within compound environments like farms or zoos. The adoption of this view advances the argument of animal welfare through evidence-based reasoning that benefits the health of individual animals as well as improves industry best practices. Mathematical modeling also enhances risk estimates through approximations of outcomes in different management contexts, thereby allowing animal welfare scientists to better address animal welfare problems (Mata et al., 2022).

2.4. Data Collection Methods

In epidemiology, the approach to data collection forms an essential component of precise measurement of health events. Quantitative and qualitative methods form big categories of research approaches to data collection in which every one of them contributes differently to research studies. Quantitative methods, for example, surveys and observational studies, are characterized by the systematic collection of numerical data where researchers can assess statistical patterns and associations. For example, the Epidemiology of Critical Care after Surgery study is an example of a sound quantitative design through its prospective data collection regarding patient outcomes, surgical types, and morbidity indicators among others (Farmer et al., 2017). Employing methods like multilevel regression and propensity score matching, researchers can adjust for confounding variables and account for interactions between interventions and outcomes and thus make the findings more valid and reliable. Qualitative methods, however, provide rich detail that might be lost with traditional quantitative methods. Qualitative approaches involve nonnumeric data collection, for example, interviews and focus groups, which seek to expose individuals' own experiences and understanding of health concerns. There is more of an inclination to apply more qualitative data in environmental health studies because it provides more insight into the impact of social determinants on health outcomes. Through questioning respondents' and participants' perceptions and reasons, qualitative analysis confirms the complexity of health behavior and pathways of exposure. This focus in general helps to accentuate the excellence in combining quantitative with qualitative evidence toward crafting a more holistic picture of public health issues. Further, the combination of qualitative and quantitative data collection procedures can yield more insight into epidemiological events. The use of mixed methods will help in allowing for triangulation whereby findings will be validated through several different data sources and viewpoints. These are especially critical within settings where health inequities exist because they ensure a thorough examination of the determinants driving such inequities. By combining quantitative trend health information with qualitative perspectives on lived experiences, epidemiology is capable of becoming fairer in its resolution. As is evident from most studies, including that of environmental health, this thorough review can very considerably improve the effectiveness of public health interventions as well as policymaking, with an outcome toward improved health in vulnerable individuals (Figure 2.8).

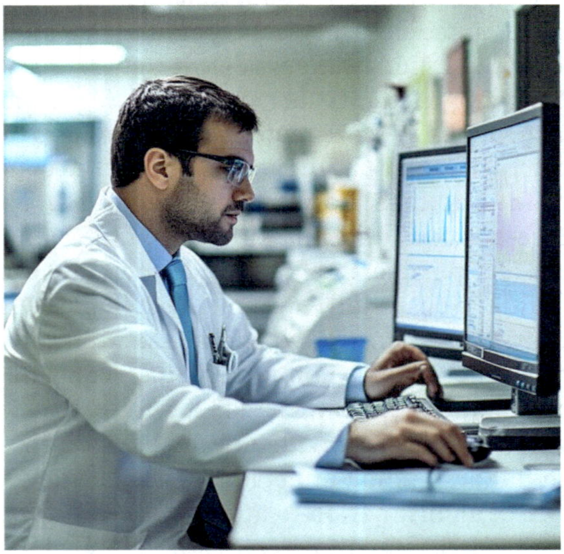

Figure 2.8. In the realm of epidemiology, data collection methods play a crucial role in the accurate assessment of health-related events.

Source: Freepik. (n.d.). *Healthcare Professional Analyzing Epidemiological Data on a Computer.*

2.4.1. Surveys and Questionnaires

Surveys and questionnaires are easy epidemiological tools for measuring and gathering data on health-related attitudes, behavior, and outcomes within groups of population. Their utility is the capability of getting quantitative and qualitative data in populations of large numbers and hence enable detection of public health trends and risk factors. Using standardized templates with preformatted questions applied, the tools standardize the responses and thereby make them comparable across various groups of the population. In addition, surveys can be designed to pose certain epidemiological inquiries, e.g., the prevalence of chronic diseases or the effect of environmental determinants on health. These are the characteristics that highlight the extent of the contribution of questionnaires and surveys to public health intervention and the way of good intervention that responds to the needs of heterogeneous populations. Albeit having many advantages, the application of questionnaires and surveys has its disadvantages. The validity of the information obtained from these devices is dependent on many conditions such as question wording, respondent comprehension, and survey conduct. Question wording that is not precise can result in skewed responses or misinterpretation, thus tainting the validity of conclusions. Representativeness of the sample is also crucial; if there is an underrepresentation of certain groups, conclusions derived might not apply to the population. These constraints usually require data to be triangulated, wherein survey results are complemented by qualitative techniques, e.g., interviews or focus groups, to give a more complete report of health problems at stake. So although surveys and questionnaires are highly useful, care should be taken in their use. In the quest for new approaches, participatory techniques have been useful additions to conventional survey techniques. Participatory mapping, for instance, enables community members to participate directly in the mapping of determinants of health in their surroundings, enriching data collection while ensuring participant ownership. Participatory geographic information systems (PGIS)-based research has established how results based on feedback from the community can reveal newly identified public health issues, i.e., usability of parks in areas plagued with crime. This approach not only improves the intensity of information gathered but also opens up opportunities for people to engage in policy reform advocacy and health equity, proving the potential to combine qualitative findings with epidemiological insights. Through the complementarity of traditional surveys with participatory methods, public health scientists can develop more robust, context-driven data that guide effective action toward health advancement in vulnerable populations (Douglas et al., 2020).

2.4.2. Surveillance Systems and Registries

The function of surveillance systems and registries is of paramount relevance to the recording, analysis, and reporting of health data in a bid to facilitate public health decision-makers make the correct decisions. It is meant to provide routine information on health status, determinants of risk, and outcomes, thus offering clear insights into trends and patterns of disease. For example, cancer surveillance in the United States, from the Surveillance, Epidemiology, and End Results Program data and other registries, assists in monitoring the incidence and mortality rates of different cancers over a period of time. This ongoing monitoring further enables health workers not only to identify high-risk groups but also to assess the success of prevention and control programs. Substandard data collection undermines public health programs and therefore the necessity of having strong surveillance systems to counter new health threats. Surveillance systems are also important in reacting to public health emergencies like antimicrobial resistance (AMR). Emerging studies have unveiled the massive burden AMR puts on global health, and therefore the necessity of having large-scale data collection systems in place. The statistical model predictions that were created to estimate deaths and disability-adjusted life-years due to AMR from various pathogens show that approximately 4.95 million of the deaths linked to AMR took place in the year 2019 alone, and that is a portrayal of the burden caused by AMR, especially among the low-resource countries. Surveillance systems are therefore crucial in tracking the disease burden and uncovering new threats, which is crucial in the planning of specific interventions. As we continue to grapple with infectious disease challenges, the inclusion of new surveillance methods becomes even more critical to public health readiness and response. Lastly, advances in technology in surveillance, including electronic health records and mobile health technology, have transformed data collection quality and validity. Tracking of disease outbreaks in real-time is facilitated by the advances, and it legitimates a more responsive public health response. Ongoing inspection of cancer incidence data, as described in reports by the American Cancer Society, uncovers patterns and allows for preventive solutions to reduce risk. For instance, enhanced treatment interventions have resulted in spectacular reductions in lung cancer death rates, illustrating the effect of surveillance data on policy and clinical practice. Through the support of surveillance networks and registries, public health organizations can optimize health effects through timely evidence-based decision-making, in turn maximizing community health and resistance to new health threats (Figure 2.9).

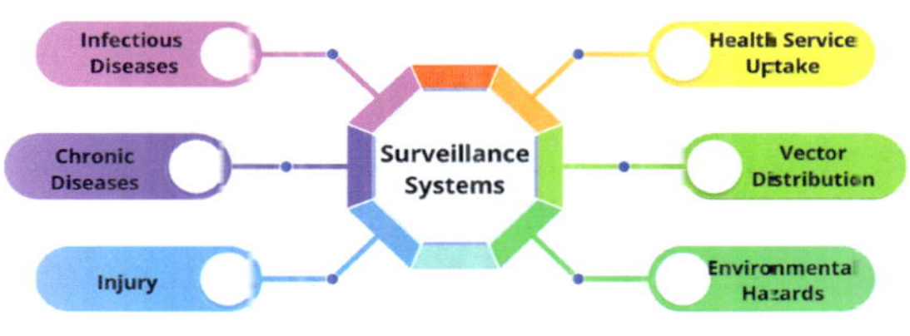

Figure 2.9. The role of surveillance systems and registries in epidemiology.

Source: Public Health Prepared. (2022). *Evaluating Public Health Surveillance Systems*. Public Health Prepared.

2.4.3. Use of Secondary Data Sources

Secondary data sources play a crucial role in research design in epidemiology. Secondary data are those data that already exist for non-research purposes, including surveillance data, hospital discharge data, and public health databases. Secondary data sources are a necessary tool for epidemiologists, providing the capability to examine trends in population health without having to devote time gathering primary data. The capacity to combine secondary data improves the range and effectiveness of epidemiological analyses, allowing the investigator to study large cohorts and mixed sets of data, thus shedding light on the determinants and trends of disease in various populations and geographic locations. Progress in the integration of divergent secondary data sources over the past few years has highlighted their role in enhancing disease surveillance. For example, in the Veneto, Italy study, it was found that integration of various data systems, i.e., mandatory notifications and laboratory surveillance, immensely improved the identification of invasive meningococcal diseases (IMDs) between the years 2007–2014. The combined system had a greater sensitivity of 94.7%, which proved how precise data integration will provide more precise epidemiological estimates. By collating data from different sources, epidemiologists can have a wider perspective on the occurrence and trend of disease, which ultimately helps in early and well-informed preventive actions for public health (Baldo et al., 2017). Secondary sources of data also help in theoretical model building in epidemiological studies. For instance, generation interval analysis of disease transmission, as argued in SIR epidemic models, is very much dependent on the availability of data to estimate parameters like the mean generation interval and the reproductive number. The two indicators are vitally important in the prediction of the course of infection spread as well as in the design of appropriate public health interventions. By applying past epidemic data, researchers can model transmission scenarios and improve the prognostic value of their models and inform public health policy effectively (Kenah et al., 2008). The capacity to draw pertinent conclusions from available data highlights the pivotal role played by secondary data sources in influencing epidemiological knowledge and practice.

2.5. Role of Epidemiology in Disease Prevention

The function of epidemiology in the prevention of disease lies at the hub of understanding how health issues can be effectively solved at the individual and population levels. Epidemiology offers the tools by which factors related to risk for disease can be delineated, thus facilitating effective interventions. Through the employment of epidemiological evidence, health workers are capable of undertaking preventive interventions in specific groups or communities, thus averting health disparities and enhancing health outcomes. This preventive intervention not only contributes to the absence of no disease outbreaks but also to the health literacy (HL) of populations, ultimately providing a well-designed strategy in epidemiology with the capability for healthcare workers to convert raw data into fruitful health policies and programs, underscoring the importance of prevention in public health programs. In addition, health administration education that incorporates population health concepts focuses on the changing health delivery system. The transition from fee-for-service to value-based care requires an integrated comprehension of epidemiological principles by the next generation of health leaders. As indicated by recent studies, the integration of population health models in curricula brings forth a more responsive and productive workforce capable of solving intricate public health issues. Discussing population health curriculum development prepares future administrators to adopt epidemiological practice as part of their professional practice. With the healthcare systems prioritizing disease prevention over treatment, integration of epidemiology and health administration is crucial when developing evidence-based approaches to preventing health threats as well as enhancing community health (Carmalt et al., 2018). As the science of epidemiology comes of age, it has broadened its scope from chronic diseases to encompass the intricacies of infectious diseases in response to the latest public health issues arising. Emergence of new pathogens and re-emergence of previously existing disease have triggered a renaissance of infectious disease epidemiology. Study of disease patterns, risk factors, and patterns of transmission has evolved by using innovative methods and technology. Through digital and molecular analysis, health workers can further enhance their knowledge of pathogen dynamics, which in turn continues to guide public health intervention and policy decision-making. This reciprocal feedback process between epidemiology and contemporary technology underscores the necessity for integrative epidemiological education in equipping future public health professionals to address these multi-faceted challenges to disease prevention (Lewnard & Reingold, 2019) (Figure 2.10).

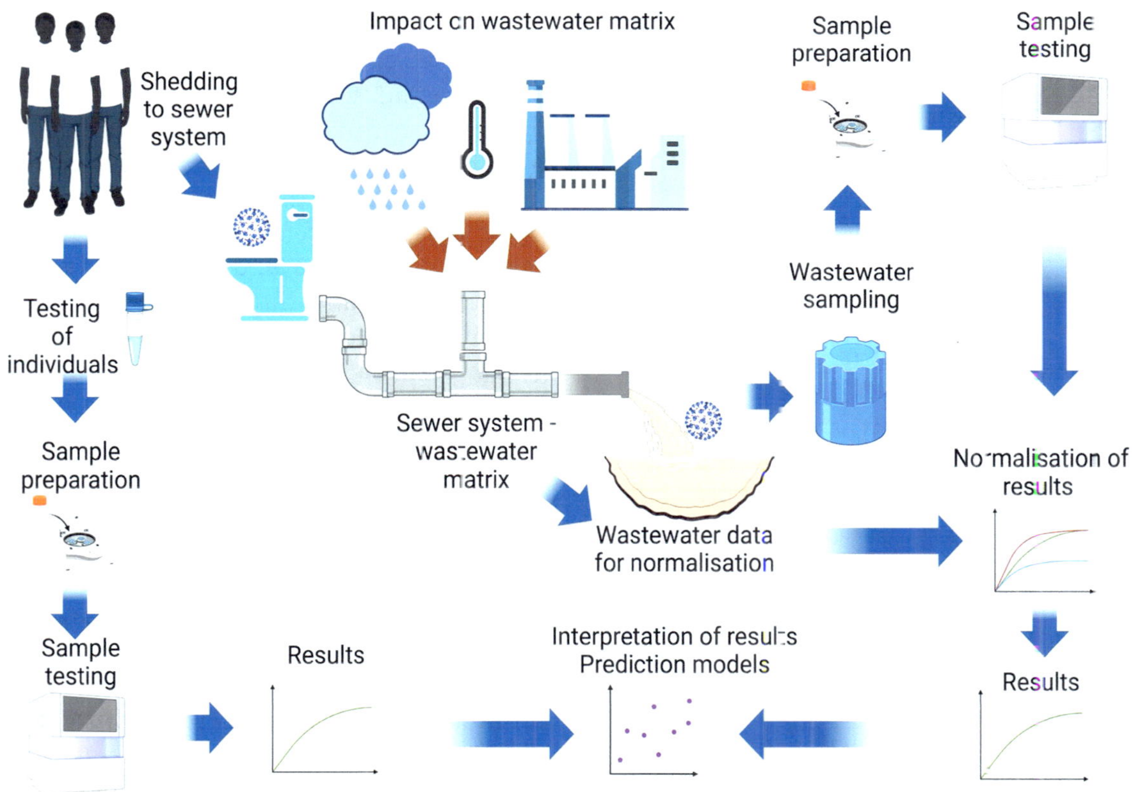

Figure 2.10. The role of epidemiology in disease prevention.

Source: Laicans J, Dejus B, Dejus S, Juhna T. Precision and Accuracy Limits of Wastewater-Based Epidemiology—Lessons Learned from SARS-CoV-2: A Scoping Review. Water. 2024; 16(9):1220. https://doi.org/10.3390/w16091220

2.5.1. Identifying Risk Factors for Diseases

Risk factor determination is one of the most important aspects of epidemiological investigations, as it enables public health practitioners and researchers to understand how conditions come to be and persist. Risk factors are categorized into various groups, ranging from behavioral to environmental, genetic, and socioeconomic. For example, lifestyle habits like inappropriate diet, physical inactivity, and smoking are central determinants of the disease burden of conditions like obesity and cardiovascular disease. Environmental risk exposures like exposure to toxins or residing in highly populated environments similarly increase health risks. Identifying these determinants allows epidemiologists to formulate aimed interventions that can reverse their influence, and in so doing, enhance population health status and decrease preventable disease healthcare spending. Risk factors identification also plays an important role in understanding complex conditions, such as obesity, which has declared as a pandemic globally. Obesity is not only the product of excess calories, as indicated by research, but is the outcome of a complex interplay between genetic, metabolic, environmental, and behavioral determinants (Gmitrzuk et al., 2024). The multifactorial nature of obesity highlights the critical need for broad-based epidemiological studies that investigate how risk factors interact. It is in these inter-relationships that the information required to develop effective public health interventions targeted at the causes of obesity as opposed to symptoms can be acquired. Through aggregation and examination of data on the risk factors, policy interventions can be channeled to ensure healthier living among vulnerable populations. In addition, methodologic advances in epidemiology, including cohort studies and case-control studies, have enhanced the precision in determining risk factors of disease. The study designs enable critical evaluation of temporal relationships between exposures and outcomes and illuminate causative associations. Lifestyle choice longitudinal studies and obesity, for instance, have yielded useful insights into early intervention in the prevention of future diseases (Jachymek et al., 2024). Epidemiology thus not only enhances our knowledge regarding disease causation but also forms the basis of public health disease prevention programs. Identification of risk factors is thus not only an academic exercise; it has significant health promotion and disease prevention planning consequences worldwide.

2.5.2. Developing Public Health Interventions

In epidemiology, the building of interventions is core to health prevention and the maintenance of well-being within populations. It is initiated by an in-depth understanding of determinants of health at the individual and population levels. Through the use of epidemiologic principles, researchers can grasp trends of disease occurrence and incidence, which are core in informing intervention interventions. Such interventions need to be multi-disciplinary, evidence-based from a range of disciplines such as behavioral science and socio-economic research, thereby tackling the complex and inter-connected determinants of health outcomes. Integrating different research strands allows for the improved development of interventions that not only are effective but also prove effective in the cultural setting as well as in regard to the particular needs of the populations in question. Thus, a sound epidemiological foundation for public health intervention is developed based on a sound structure bridging the practice and research gap (Hill et al., 2009). One of the most essential parts of the development of public health interventions is the assembly of evidence by diligent study. It then becomes clear that there is a need for a translational framework because it acts as a translator from research evidence to practice within real-world settings. By defying typical models that aim to institutionalize effective interventions, an enhanced model comes out that aims to maximize population health. This entails appreciating the place of individual and population determinants of health and adapting interventions so that they are adaptable in different settings. The emergence of intersectoral and non-linear alliances strengthens the effects of such strategies as actors across sectors bring expertise and resources. Focus on synthesis of evidence not only directs intervention development but also plays a critical role in policy influence for policy reformulation based on the latest findings (Hill et al., 2009). Furthermore, the need to mobilize resources toward funding applied public health research cannot be overemphasized. Provisions for funds must provide for a general research agenda that goes beyond phases of implementation and dissemination.

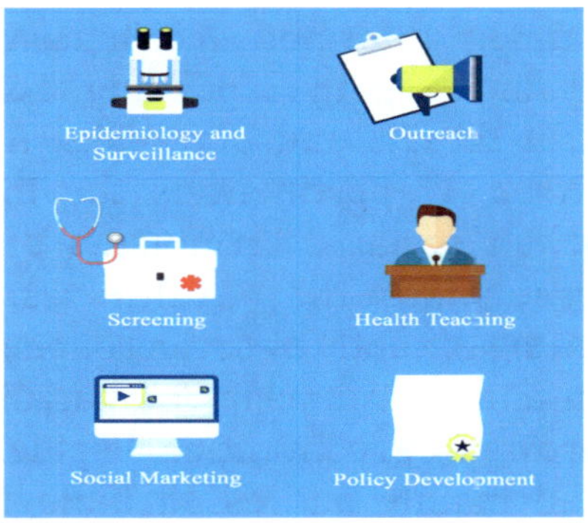

Figure 2.11. In the realm of epidemiology, the development of public health interventions is pivotal to mitigating health issues and enhancing community well-being.

Source: Everspring & Kent State University. (n.d.). *A Look at Public Health Interventions.*

Quoted in reviews of public health initiatives, there is a demand that is very evident to provide a plan for resource allocation in all phases of the research continuum such as discovery, application, and evaluation. This provides an environment in which there may be innovation in developing public health interventions. Through investing in evidence-based practice, policymakers are not only better placed to respond to new health issues as they arise but also to anticipate public health needs in the future. Therefore, strengthening the discipline of public health through organized research and mobilization of resources continues to be crucial for making sustainable gains in health for populations (Figure 2.11).

2.5.3. Evaluating the Effectiveness of Health Programs

The effectiveness of health programs takes center stage in the science of epidemiology because it has a direct impact on public health policy and resource allocation. Through the assessment of health programs, scientists can understand whether investments translate to effective changes in health outcomes. Cost-effectiveness analysis is a useful tool in deciding both the economic cost and the health benefit of a given intervention. For example, a national screening program based on the fecal occult blood test identified screening between 55 and 69 years as having the potential to save approximately 250 deaths per year at a gross cost of $A55 million with a gross incremental cost-effectiveness ratio of $A17,000/DALY. These results emphasize the significance of empirical data in informing health interventions and shaping policy decisions that yield maximum benefits to populations operating under budget restrictions (Stone et al., 2004). Another vital aspect in assessing health programs is the incorporation of comparative effectiveness research (CER). This approach enables the relative merits of other interventions or strategies to be made similar and thus presents evidence that guides the clinical actions and health policy. The creation of the Patient-Centered Outcomes Research (PCOR) Institute brought into focus the necessity of realizing the effects of health programs from the perspective of the patient. This effort intends to produce evidence regarding the performance of various health interventions in varied populations and circumstances. By prioritizing research to align with the pragmatic needs of patients in real life, CER increases the applicability and responsiveness of evidence to healthcare scenarios and inspires informed decision-making. Herein, PCOR plays a crucial function in directing resources to effective programs that enhance health outcomes (Brixner et al., 2018). Apart from this, the process of evaluating health programs should also include the general social determinants of health that have the potential to impact program performance. Health disparities are likely to have their foundation in systemic differences that impact quality and access to medical care services. As such, these types of evaluations may ignore the real effectiveness of health programs. Through the use of an equity lens within the evaluation process, programs are assured not to inadvertently perpetuate current health inequities. As such, evaluations are required to utilize methods that address demographic diversity, socioeconomic factors, and cultural needs. Through these considerations, epidemiologists can introduce health programs into the evaluation to understand better how interventions that are targeted help improve equity in health as well as bring about greater and lasting improvements in health in populations (Figure 2.12).

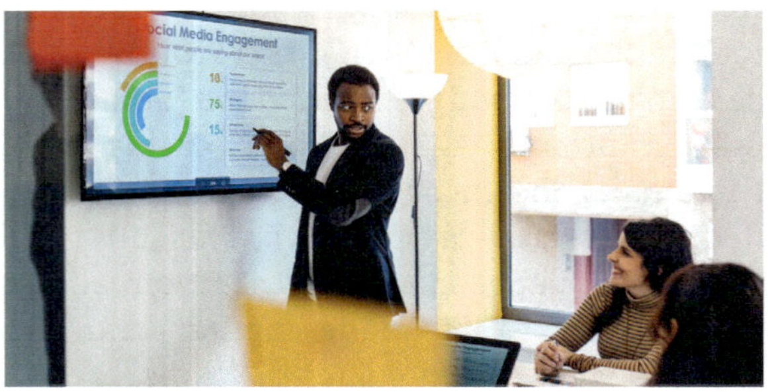

Figure 2.12. Evaluating the effectiveness of health programs.

Source: BrightPlan. (n.d.). *Evaluate Effectiveness.*

2.6. Current Trends in Epidemiology

The epidemiological context is constantly changing, as it is mirrored by the dynamic nature of public health issues. Among the trends is the growing application of sophisticated technology and data analytics in epidemiology studies. This is necessitated by the need to adequately analyze huge volumes of data so that epidemiologists can detect trends in disease transmission as well as intervention efficiency. For example, the creation of mobile health applications makes a critical contribution toward real-time data gathering, strengthening surveillance. Moreover, the application of Geographic Information Systems (GIS) enables spatial analysis, which results in improved health disparities knowledge among various populations. This technologization of research not only facilitates the work of research but also enables public health practitioners to provide timely informed decisions, which is extremely important in responding to emerging new health threats and outbreaks. A second trend extremely pertinent is the increased emphasis on social determinants of health, which recognizes that health results are influenced significantly by socioeconomic status, education, and environment. This paradigm shift is a departure from conventional epidemiology, which had mainly addressed biological and clinical issues of diseases. By questioning why social conditions affect health, epidemiologists can tackle the causative determinants of health inequalities. For example, current research has established that tobacco promotion, especially those targeting poor groups such as women and children, has been having critical impacts on health and needs vigorous public health intervention. As increasingly loud calls are made for tighter tobacco legislation, the role of the epidemiologist in aiding policy development with his/her evidence on social determinants of population health is strengthened (Allen et al., 2019). One of these trends not only enhances epidemiologic knowledge but also stimulates efforts toward health equity. Last, the capacity of the epidemiologist to react to emerging global health concerns most clearly demonstrates the field's flexibility. The COVID-19 pandemic has highlighted the need for strong epidemiologic models to generate timely information on patterns of transmission and infection prevention practices. In addition, incorporating international cooperation into epidemiological work has become imperative because diseases easily cross national borders. For instance, projects such as the UK's Exemplar Program proved the importance of having efficient integrated systems of communication in health facilities for managing out-of-hours care (Lattimer & Burgess, 2005). The experience made it evident how efficiently an integrated health service can minimize pressure on accident and emergency services and maximize the effectiveness of resource allocation. With advancing fields, such synergistic efforts will form the foundation for onward epidemiological studies, focusing on synergy between global health security and local practice.

2.6.1. Impact of Technology on Data Collection and Analysis

The evolution of technology has had profound impacts on data collection and study in epidemiology, making it possible to create more richer and detailed datasets. The use of digital technologies, for example, wearables and mobile applications, has made it possible to collect data in real-time from a diverse and large population and in finer patterns of behavior in health. Apart from that, it is easy to use technology to aggregate disparate data sources from electronic health data to social media usage to allow epidemiologists to perform strong analysis. Apart from providing a larger range of information, possessing a pluralist approach provides it with ease in detecting changing patterns of wellness among health, population patterns, or instances of an epidemic.

The application of sophisticated analytics, including machine learning and artificial intelligence (AI), also propels the capacity to derive useful insights from big datasets, demonstrating the pivotal role of technology in reshaping epidemiological practice. Beyond data collection, technology application extends to intricate analytical models capable of addressing complicated public health issues. For example, life course epidemiology emphasizes the need to examine long-term health consequences, which could be caused by many social, behavioral, and environmental factors, just as causal models are constructed in building science. These approaches correspond with technological developments that enable variables that were difficult to measure in the past to be taken into account. Through the application of multilevel models and simulation approaches, researchers are in a position to examine interactions among diverse determinants of health, thus yielding results that can inform effective intervention strategies. Based on the A People's Social Epi principles, the integration of social epidemiology with information and communication technology (ICT) and community-based participatory research (CBPR) provides a more inclusive data-analysis approach that also fosters collaboration among stakeholders and creates improved public health impacts (Allen et al., 2019). Furthermore, the expanded availability of information generated by technological processes poses challenges and opportunities for public health policy interpretation and application that are not easily compared to others. Data security and privacy issues become major concerns as massive amounts of personal health data are accumulated using a wide variety of digital modalities. Regulatory systems must be developed and modified to ensure that technology-driven data collection does not invade the privacy of people but enables valuable epidemiological data. Additionally, giving high priority to inter-disciplinary alliances can enhance the effectiveness of health interventions via the convergence of skills from various disciplines such as sociology, environmental science, and technology. As indicated while handling carbon emissions decrease, an understanding of the complex relationship between technology and social behavior is important for meaningful data interpretation (Bruhns et al., 2005). Accepting these developments in technology, along with prudent practices, is essential to raise the practice of epidemiology in effectively dealing with emerging health issues (Figure 2.13).

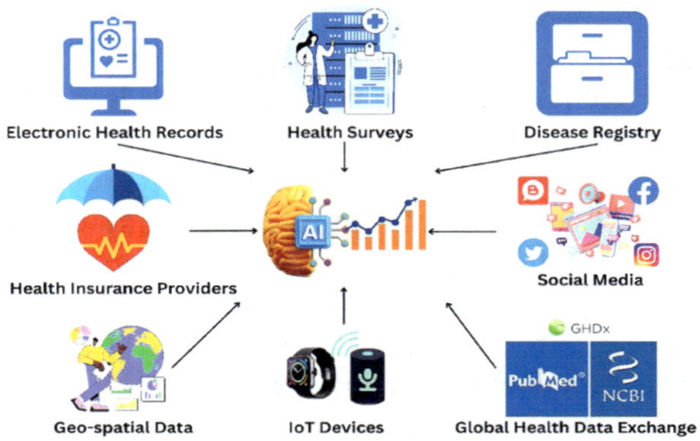

Figure 2.13. Impact of technology on data collection and analysis.

Source: Anjaria P, Asediya V, Bhavsar P, Pathak A, Desai D, Patil V. Artificial Intelligence in Public Health: Revolutionizing Epidemiological Surveillance for Pandemic Preparedness and Equitable Vaccine Access. Vaccines. 2023; 11(7):1154. https://doi.org/10.3390/vaccines11071154\ https://www.mdpi.com/vaccines/vaccines-11-01154/article_deploy/html/images/vaccines-11-01154-g001.png

2.6.2. Global Health Challenges and Epidemiological Responses

Epidemiologic interventions against global health issues commonly include the identification and control of infectious diseases that disproportionately burden target populations. Growing evidence has brought more attention to increasing infectious disease burdens of diseases such as tuberculosis (TB), which continues to be an international public health issue in the majority of the world and in particular in the Caribbean and South America. Early HIV testing and comprehensive care are emphasized in literature demonstrating marked advantage to early treatment and diagnosis. In addition, nosocomial infections, fueled by antibiotic-resistant microorganisms, represent an emerging threat to health systems. Resolution to these concerns will come in a multimodal approach that is dependent on strict infection control mechanisms, upgraded surveillance requirements, and international health agency coordination. There is an urgent need for focused epidemiological programs that target the most at-risk groups to better tackle the risk of infectious disease in the context of international health. A new international trend does not only refer to infectious disease but also to the use of psychoactive drugs and with a specific reference to cannabis. As cannabis legalization is on the increase globally for both medical and non-medical usage, the development of Cannabis Use Disorders (CUDs) assumes a critical public health significance. Epidemiological research has demonstrated that the prevalence of CUDs has mounted substantially throughout the last three decades, with High-Income North America reporting the peak occurrence. These results support the need to explore the interplay of substance use in the context of mental health. The 15–24-year age group is most impacted by CUDs and needs specific intervention and prevention. An understanding of such epidemiological trends and patterns is vital in the process of policymaking to avoid the social, economic, and healthcare effects of the use of cannabis at an international level (Shah et al., 2024). The interface between global health issues and epidemiological response goes beyond infectious disease and alcohol or other drug abuse disorders; it includes the general implications for healthcare systems globally. The escalating challenge of health disorders like chronic disease, mental illness, and emerging pathogens requires a paradigm shift in public health interventions. Successful epidemiological response must include prevention, surveillance, and education to reduce the long-term impact on populations. Technological innovation and data collation are of greatest significance since they sustain improved mechanisms for tracking disease patterns and inequities between and across population groups. Collaboration among nations and information exchange across health agencies can facilitate stronger responses and strengthen the resilience of public health systems. Finally, effective addressing of these varied global health issues is dependent on an integrated strategy that combines epidemiology, policy-making, and social mobilization (Justiz-Vaillant et al., 2025) (Figure 2.14).

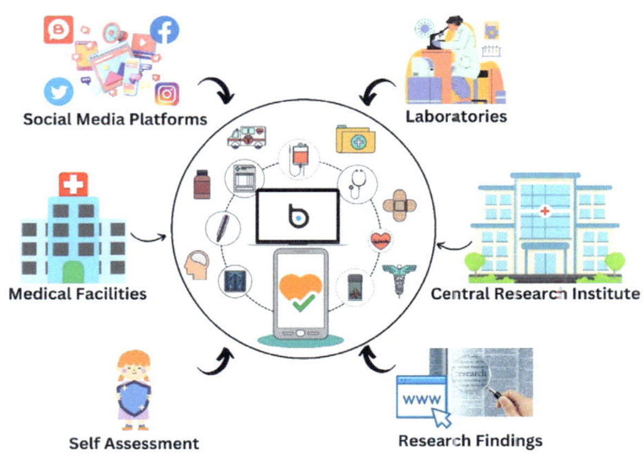

Figure 2.14. Global health challenges and epidemiological responses.

Source: Anjaria P, Asediya V, Bhavsar P, Pathak A, Desai D, Patil V. Artificial Intelligence in Public Health: Revolutionizing Epidemiological Surveillance for Pandemic Preparedness and Equitable Vaccine Access. Vaccines. 2023; 11(7):1154. https://doi.org/10.3390/vaccines11071154

2.6.3. The Role of Epidemiology in Addressing Pandemics

Epidemiology is a key tool in pandemic management because it is the theoretical basis of infectious disease transmission patterns. Through organized observation of disease trends, epidemiologists can trace the channels of transmission, risk factors, and susceptibility among populations. This information is of utmost importance to public health officials to employ successful interventions. For example, during the pandemic caused by COVID-19, epidemiological modeling predicted infection rates and effects of different public health interventions, including lockdown and vaccination programs. It became possible to analyze infection rate data and demographics to plan responses based on the greatest needs, thus reducing the virus transmission to a minimum. Since pandemics are defined by multifaceted interactions between biological, environmental, and social determinants, the interdisciplinary approach of epidemiology progressively assumes significance in developing effective countermeasures against their influence. The domain of epidemiology is also not just limited to immediate response activities but to shaping long-term public health policy as well. Epidemiologists measure the disease burden and describe intervention effectiveness, with direct implications for funding and resource allocation. For instance, the staggering numbers involved in AMR leading to millions of deaths in 2019 reflect the need for evidence-based policies on healthcare practice and antibiotic stewardship (Murray et al., 2022). Identifying trends and risk factors of pandemics allows epidemiologists to promote the shifts in the healthcare system toward immunity construction against future pandemics. These include investing in surveillance systems, high-quality data analysis, and increased access to healthcare among vulnerable groups, hence addressing the underlying causes of health inequities that could enhance the impacts of pandemics. Lastly, epidemiology promotes international cooperation and global health security since pandemics are a worldwide problem whose implications need concerted efforts. Epidemiologists can spread vital information and create universal guidelines for disease surveillance and outbreak through institutions like the WHO. Regular reporting of disease occurrence and risk factors is critical to the creation of strong evidence-based interventions that may be tailored to different regional environments (Feigin et al., 2021). With this unified framework, nations may learn from other countries' experiences, exchange innovations in intervention strategies, and join forces in fighting pandemics in large groups. This initiative focuses on building a strong epidemiological infrastructure able to offer backup in response to immediate outbreak situations as well as readying countries for possible future public health crises.

CLOSER LOOK

Morbidity

Morbidity is the occurrence of disease, illness, or any condition that affects health in a negative way. It does not include death—it's called mortality. Morbidity concerns whether diseases occur in many people and how serious they are, influencing the quality of life and function of individuals. There are two primary methods of measuring morbidity: incidence, which measures new cases over a while, and prevalence, which measures all present cases at a specific time. These metrics aid public health workers in disease trend tracking and healthcare need evaluation.

Morbidity may be caused by acute illness like infections or injury, or by chronic disease such as heart disease, diabetes, and mental illness. In most societies, NCDs are currently the main cause of morbidity as a result of aging populations and lifestyles.

Comorbidity—when an individual has more than one disease simultaneously—is prevalent and makes treatment more difficult. Knowledge of morbidity is necessary for planning health care, organizing resources, and structuring prevention. Morbidity is, in effect, a quantification of disease burden. Through the investigation, health systems can assist in enhancing the quality of life and decreasing the overall impact of illness within a given population.

SUMMARY

It is important to recognize the paramount importance this discipline holds in developing public health. Epidemiology is the backbone of health problem research, informing policy and directing disease prevention and health promotion interventions. By systematic examination of the determinants and distribution of health-related conditions, epidemiologists eliminate threats to public health and enhance community health outcomes. This empirical foundation undergirding evidence-based practice is of primary importance not only for health clinicians but also for policymakers responsible for dealing with the complexities of health environments. Ultimately, inferences derived from epidemiologic studies are imperative for grasping health disparities and preventing health inequities. Lastly, the evolution of epidemiologic techniques addresses its continued applicability to examining health issues in the present era. With an increase in technology as well as the study of data, the field has increased its tool kit to incorporate new methods like genomic epidemiology and electronic health surveillance. These technological advancements grant scientists greater power to detect trends and predict outbreaks and hence immediate responses to new health threats. These pre-emptive actions also can reverse the effects of vaccines, diet intervention, and taking up lifestyles, presenting an integrated approach to achieving health. As one can observe in the recent releases by expert groups such as the EWGSOP2, the need to accommodate new algorithms and definitions enforces the imperative of continuous refining of knowledge in health conditions. Flexibility lies at the heart of resistance to chronic disease and to significantly enhancing population health. Lastly, the overlap of epidemiology with interdisciplinarity makes it pivotal under the wider umbrella of public health. Interdisciplinary collaboration with sociology, environmental science, and health policy has enhanced epidemiological studies to provide an expanded perspective on determinants of health. By combining various views, scientists can more effectively address intricate health problems, for example, the interaction between lifestyle and environmental determinants of disease occurrence. However, despite these advancements, obstacles are yet to make epidemiological data available to practitioners and the public at large. Creating awareness and encouraging education on important findings is pertinent in bridging research and action. Therefore, as emphasized in individual guidelines and studies under conditions and health hazards, clear communication remains of importance in messaging to the general public and involvement in health promotion interventions, ultimately leading to better health outcomes for populations at large.

In the context of the place of Voluntary Counselling and Testing Points (VCTs) within the Polish landscape, perhaps one of the most significant aspects of public health programs is access and efficiency of HIV tests. In the last twenty years, VCTs have emerged as significant centers of operation, providing rapid, accurate, anonymous, and free HIV testing for adults of any nationality. Over the period between 2019 and 2023, about 157,833 people signed up to be tested at these sites, with more among foreigners, showing increased coverage among varied populations. More frequent testing among foreigners, who made up 6.45% of the testers, shows increased awareness and use of HIV prevention services. These figures show that VCTs are not only test sites but also sites for more general public health education and intervention initiatives to prevent HIV and other sexually transmitted diseases (Ański et al., 2024). Additionally, outcomes from the VCT tests reveal that a significant percentage of positive HIV infections were identified in these centers, representing approximately 26% of positive diagnoses between the years 2019 and 2023. The indicators show that the percentage of positive HIV diagnoses among foreigners who were tested was significantly higher at 5.08% than that of Polish nationals at 1.24%. This imbalance highlights the imperative for specialized public health interventions that respond to the specific needs of foreign communities. The results also bring to light the critical role of VCTs in early diagnosis and treatment, which are pivotal determinants in the care continuum for those living with HIV. These findings affirm the efficacy of VCTs to complement systematic healthcare policies in Poland and may be used as a model for such action globally (Ański et al., 2024). Concurrently, the incorporation of new technologies in the study and management of epidemics offers an alternative approach to improving public health. Remotely Piloted Airdesign System (RPAS) use in photogrammetry and lidar capture has grown with growing interest as a new method for collecting data for spatial epidemiology. With the evaluation of the geometric quality of RPAS surveyed data without depending heavily on ground control points, researchers have determined that the above procedures can achieve the high accuracies required for decision-making within health policy and resource planning. Quality assessment of RPAS data has important relevance in broader comprehension of geographic determinants of health outcomes, underscoring the unavoidable influence of technology in improving epidemiologic research. This use of sophisticated methodologies marks a change toward data-driven decision-making in public health with an interest in the necessity for ongoing adjustment and refinement in epidemiology practice.

KEY TERMS FROM THIS CHAPTER

- Epidemiology
- Prevalence
- Mortality
- Proportion
- Epidemic
- Surveillance
- Bias
- Incidence
- Morbidity
- Exposure
- Endemic
- Pandemic
- Confounding
- Causality

REFERENCES

1. Albin, R., Backman, C., Barlow, D. H., Douglas, et al. (2016). The Single-Case Reporting Guideline in Behavioral Interventions (SCRIBE) 2016 statement. *Canadian Journal of Occupational Therapy, 83*(3), 184–195. https://core.ac.uk/download/289166471.pdf (accessed on 6 May 2025).
2. Allen, A., Morello-Frosch, R., Mujahid, M., Petteway, et al. (2019). Toward a people's social epidemiology: Envisioning a more inclusive and equitable future for social epidemiology research and practice in the 21st century. *International Journal of Environmental Research and Public Health, 16*(20), 3983. https://core.ac.uk/download/323081131.pdf (accessed on 6 May 2025).
3. Anderson, M., Beck, U., Beck, U., Bouter, Brewster, D. D., Cann, A. J., Cannon, G., et al. (2005). Epidemic space. https://core.ac.uk/download/30636149.pdf (accessed on 6 May 2025).
4. Arcury, T. A., Evans, D., Haines, M. M., Halvorson, S. J., Higgins, J. P. T., Larsson, L. S., Lobdell, D. T., et al. (2010). Qualitative environmental health research: An analysis of the literature, 1991–2008. *Environmental Health Perspectives, 118*(8), 1146–1154. https://doi.org/10.1289/ehp.0901762.
5. Athni, T. S., Bharti, N., Caldwell, I. R., Caldwell, et al. (2021). The influence of vector-borne disease on human history: Socio-ecological mechanisms. *Ecology Letters, 24*(4), 829–846. https://core.ac.uk/download/573397409.pdf (accessed on 6 May 2025).
6. Stone, C. A., Carter, R. C., Vos, T., & John, J. S. (2004). Colorectal cancer screening in Australia: an economic evaluation of a potential biennial screening program using faecal occult blood tests. *Australian and New Zealand journal of public health, 28*(3), 273–282. https://doi.org/10.1111/j.1467-842x.2004.tb00707.x (accessed on 6 May 2025).
7. Avenell, A., Harstrick, A., Inanir, A., Kerst, A., Zittermann, A., Millen, A. E., Eliassen, A. H., et al. (2013). Vitamin D supplementation and breast cancer prevention: A systematic review and meta-analysis of randomized clinical trials. *PLoS One, 8*(7), e69269. https://core.ac.uk/download/16664256.pdf (accessed on 6 May 2025).
8. Baldo, V., Baldovin, T., Bertoncello, C., Cocchio, et al. (2017). Invasive meningococcal disease in the Veneto region of Italy: A capture-recapture analysis for assessing the effectiveness of an integrated surveillance system. *BMJ Open, 7*, e012478. https://core.ac.uk/download/80154796.pdf (accessed on 6 May 2025).
9. Bianchi, F., Minichilli, F., Pierini, A., Pieroni, et al. (2025). Amyotrophic lateral sclerosis: Results from Tuscany Registry of Rare Diseases. https://core.ac.uk/download/pdf/37831063.pdf (accessed on 6 May 2025).
10. Biek, R., Brunker, K., Cleaveland, S., Fooks, et al. (2015). Elucidating the phylodynamic of endemic rabies virus in eastern Africa using whole-genome sequencing. *Virus Evolution, 1*(1), vev011. https://core.ac.uk/download/42367711.pdf (accessed on 6 May 2025).
11. Bradford Hill, A., Lyon, A., Raffle, A., Wakefield, A., Lo, B., Committee of Inquiry into the Future Development of the Public Health Function, Cooksey, D., et al. (2009). A translational framework for public health research. *BMC Public Health, 9*, 116. https://core.ac.uk/download/80418.pdf (accessed on 6 May 2025).

12. Bruhns, H. R., Caeiro, J., Oreszczyn, T., Steadman, et al. (2005). Life course building epidemiology: An alternative approach to the collection and analysis of carbon emission data. https://core.ac.uk/download/1670910.pdf (accessed on 6 May 2025).

13. towardLattimer, V. and Burgess, A. (2005) Integrated out-of-hours care arrangements in England: Observational study of progress toward single call access via NHS Direct and impact on the wider health system. *Society for Social Medicine 49th Annual Scientific Meeting, University of Glasgow, UK. 14 - 16 Sep 2005*

14. Carneal-Frazer, N. D. (2019). *Analysis of Control Measures Used During Cholera Outbreaks Among Internally Displaced Persons* (Doctoral dissertation, Walden University). Walden Dissertations and Doctoral Studies, 6183. https://core.ac.uk/download/217235150.pdf (accessed on 6 May 2025).

15. Cevallos, M., Dohoo, I., Egger, M., Erb, et al. (2016). Explanation and elaboration document for the STROBE-Vet statement: Strengthening the reporting of observational studies in epidemiology—Veterinary extension. *Journal of Veterinary Internal Medicine, 30*(6), 1896–1928. https://doi.org/10.1111/jvim.14592.

16. Cheloni, R., Gandolfi, S., Signorelli, C., & Odone, A. (2019). Global prevalence of diabetic retinopathy: Protocol for a systematic review and meta-analysis. *BMJ Open, 9*, e022188. https://doi.org/10.1136/bmjopen-2018-022188.

17. Cortey, M., Drigo, M., Franzo, G., Hughes, J., et al. (2016). Phylodynamic analysis of porcine circovirus type 2: Methodological approach and datasets. *Data in Brief, 8*, 549–552. https://doi.org/10.1016/j.dib.2016.06.005.

18. Cruz-Jentoft, A. J., Bahat, G., Bauer, J. M., Boirie, Y., Bruyère, O., Cederholm, T., Cooper, C., et al. (2018). Sarcopenia: Revised European consensus on definition and diagnosis. *Age and Ageing, 48*, 16–31. https://doi.org/10.1093/ageing/afy169.

19. Davis, E. L., Glanz, K., Handy, S. L., Henderson, J., et al. (2016). Built environment assessment: Multidisciplinary perspectives. *SSM–Population Health, 2*, 24–31. https://doi.org/10.1016/j.ssmph.2016.02.002.

20. Douglas, J. A., Subica, A. M., Franks, L., Johnson, G., Leon, C., Villanueva, S., et al. (2020). Using participatory mapping to diagnose upstream determinants of health and prescribe downstream policy-based interventions. *Preventing Chronic Disease, 17*, 200123. https://core.ac.uk/download/362660306.pdf (accessed on 6 May 2025).

21. Farmer, L., Harris, S. K., Moonesinghe, S. R., Myles, P., et al. (2017). SNAP-2 EPICCS: The second Sprint National Anaesthesia Project—Epidemiology of Critical Care after Surgery: Protocol for an international observational cohort study. *BMJ Open, 7*(9), e017690. https://core.ac.uk/download/96627973.pdf (accessed on 6 May 2025).

22. Feigin, V. L., Stark, B., Johnson, C. O., Roth, G. A., Bisignano, C., Gebreheat, G., Abbasifard, M., et al. (2021). Global, regional, and national burden of stroke and its risk factors, 1990–2019: A systematic analysis for the Global Burden of Disease Study 2019. *The Lancet Neurology, 20*, 795–820. https://doi.org/10.1016/s1474-4422(21)00252-0.

23. Gmitrzuk, J., Jachymek, A., Jakubiec, J., Karasiński, D., et al. (2024). Obesity in adults: Causes, health consequences, and treatment methods. *Quality in Sport, 17*, 53051. https://core.ac.uk/download/620863033.pdf (accessed on 6 May 2025).

24. Gurski, R. R., Hoppe, L., Kuiava, V. A., Madalosso, C., et al. (2018). Epidemiological profile of esophageal cancer mortality in Rio Grande do Sul and its health regions. *Clinical and Biomedical Research, 38*(3), 213–217. https://core.ac.uk/download/303956442.pdf (accessed on 6 May 2025).

25. Hampson, K., Haydon, D. T., le Roux, K., Mollentze, N., et al. (2014). A Bayesian approach for inferring the dynamics of partially observed endemic infectious diseases from space-time-genetic data. *Proceedings of the Royal Society of London Series B: Biological Sciences, 281*(1782), 20133251. https://core.ac.uk/download/20480131.pdf (accessed on 6 May 2025).

26. Kenah, E., Lipsitch, M., & Robins, J. M. (2008). Generation interval contraction and epidemic data analysis. *Mathematical Biosciences, 213*(1), 71–79. http://arxiv.org/abs/0706.2024 (accessed on 6 May 2025).

27. Lewnard, J. A., & Reingold, A. L. (2019). Emerging challenges and opportunities in infectious disease epidemiology. *American Journal of Epidemiology, 188*(5), 873–882. https://doi.org/10.1093/aje/kwy264.

28. Mata, F. (2022). A framework for using epidemiology in animal welfare science. *Journal of Applied Animal Welfare Science, 26*(3), 361–373. https://core.ac.uk/download/596346861.pdf (accessed on 6 May 2025).

29. Murray, C. J. L., Ikuta, K. S., Sharara, F., Swetschinski, L. R., Robles Aguilar, G., Gray, A. P., Han, C., et al. (2022). Global burden of bacterial antimicrobial resistance in 2019: A systematic analysis. *The Lancet, 399*, 629–655. https://doi.org/10.1016/s0140-6736(21)02724-0.

30. Phelps, C. L. (2004). Advances in Teaching & Learning Day Abstracts 2005. https://core.ac.uk/download/46714715.pdf (accessed on 6 May 2025).

31. Ponikowski, P., Voors, A. A., Anker, S. D., Bueno, H., Cleland, J. G. F., Coats, A. J. S., Falk, V., et al. (2016). 2016 ESC guidelines for the diagnosis and treatment of acute and chronic heart failure. *European Heart Journal, 37*, 2129–2200. https://doi.org/10.1093/eurheartj/ehw128.

32. Reynolds, L. A., & Tansey, E. M. (2001). British contributions to medical research and education in Africa after the Second World War. https://core.ac.uk/download/30696175.pdf (accessed on 6 May 2025).

33. Siegel, R. L., Miller, K. D., Fuchs, H. E., & Jemal, A. (2021). Cancer statistics, 2021. *CA: A Cancer Journal for Clinicians, 71*, 7–33. https://doi.org/10.3322/caac.21654.

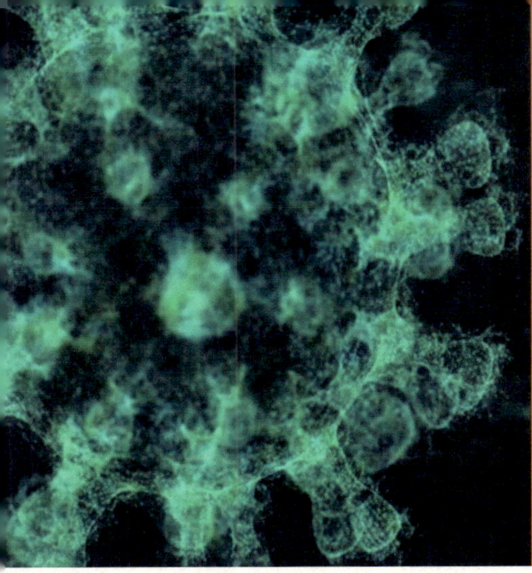

Chapter 3

THE EPIDEMIOLOGICAL TRIANGLE

Contents

Introduction

Knowing how disease transmission occurs is a large part of public health. Stepping into it, most specialists now rely on what is ordinarily referred to as the Epidemiological Triangle—a kind of map that tracks the dance among an infectious agent, its host, and the environment around them. All these components have their own significance in how diseases take hold and, in most instances, how they can be contained; , all of them do count. This triangle is not a neat outline hanging in textbooks—it is a working manual that epidemiologists apply, occasionally in extremely down-to-earth ways, to repel health threats. With concerns such as antibiotic resistance and disease emergence across species lines on the horizon, the model, in general, strikes even closer to the heart. By disentangling the dynamics between these three components, researchers can devise strategies that more precisely target what fuels the rate of disease in various populations. Sharing data, it turns out, is absolutely critical in utilizing something as the Epidemiological Triangle. More often than not, legal regulations established to safeguard personal data tend to cap the flow of the type of information that is capable of propelling good research; (Sethi et al., 2014) even go as far as to state that legislation intended to guard people can occasionally, albeit inadvertently, suffocate the broader sharing of information. For the most part, good epidemiological work relies on information flowing smoothly among all parties, combining privacy and the public good. As new technologies and tighter data analysis techniques build momentum, the drive to create systems that leave information open while remaining safe becomes even more urgent. Understanding, therefore, these challenges and confronting them directly can truly flip the script when it comes to both the study of diseases and the overall health of the public.

Recently, cutting-edge technology is finally beginning to revolutionize how we do epidemiology. By integrating smart systems into day-to-day research habits, specialists are now able to advance risk assessments to a whole new level of accuracy. Consider, the example cited in Culbert et al. (1993)—the so-called Biomedical Risk Assessment Intelligent Network (BRAIN) illustrates how much technology can transform our capacity to assess biomedical risks. As information from diverse sources converges, such systems provide information revealing how agents act on hosts in varied environments, directing more interventions in targeted ways. Such tech integration not only raises the bar in prediction but also triggers cross-disciplinary collaboration and, eventually, beefs up the entire framework applied to public health practice and research.

Definition of the Epidemiological Triangle

Grasping the Epidemiological Triangle is the first step in comprehending how illnesses function. Rather than perceiving it as a specific checklist, think of it as a mess of three important components—the agent, or the pathogen; the host, or rather the human, animal, or other organism that finds itself ill; and the environment, or all the external elements that can serve either to facilitate or to obstruct disease transmission. When you consider the way these pieces combine—sometimes in surprising combinations—scientists can identify weak links and figure out ways to prevent the spread. In most instances, this triangle provides public health experts with the type of solid framework they require to battle infections successfully.

This concept is more than mere classification. It is about grasping the interactions between such factors as vector changes and host behavior that can be pushed around by environmental change. Network theory, say, has become fairly significant; it allows researchers to explore the complex ways in which linked systems facilitate the spread of a disease throughout a population (Danon et al., 2010). To summarize, since the pathogens sometimes adjust their actions according to perceived threats, the entire situation becomes more complex, demonstrating that the one-size-fits-all will simply not work. Adding to this, how agents change to the environment is not simply individual cases—it indeed influences wider patterns of infection. Studies have even proposed that such agents can modify their contact networks subtly, inadvertently turning up a system's overall susceptibility (Muscillo et al., 2018). Such behavior of change encourages us to continue questioning our intervention strategies as static models may fail to capture the dynamic nature of disease transmission. Overall, understanding the profound, interwoven connections involved in the Epidemiological Triangle is critical to establishing public health policies and designing interventions that can match both local and international threats (Figure 3.1).

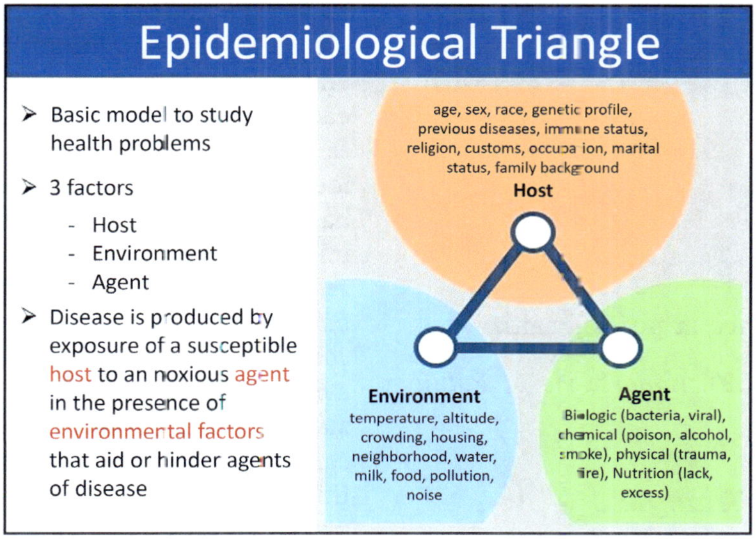

Figure 3.1. The epidemiological triangle.

Source: Unknown author. (n.d.). The epidemiological triangle. *Pinterest.*

Importance in Public Health

Many complex factors affect our health, and gaining mastery over these aspects influences public health actions. Consider the classic triangle concept—the agent, the host, and the environment—on which, most of the time, we're provided with suggestions on how to manage issues like malaria in hot regions. Malaria, which we know, poses enormous difficulties, and solving it usually involves monitoring vectors. Individuals employ measures such as insecticide-treated nets and even indoor residual spraying on occasion to ward off adult Anopheline insects, and these interventions can pay dividends in conjunction with policy initiatives meant to mitigate the impact of the disease. Sustainability is yet another perspective that cannot be overlooked. In pragmatic terms, public health measures must be regularly checked and adjusted. For example, insecticide resistance has notched up unnoticed as a cause for concern. Reports such as those from Tanzania's National Institute for Medical Research indicate that most of the malaria vectors remain susceptible, but there are isolated cases of resistance here and there. Following these trends is important since it informs decision-makers which chemicals are likely to be more effective on the ground. In general terms, as infectious diseases evolve over time, monitoring these variables becomes a paradigm for addressing other health issues where agents, hosts, and the environment combine in unpredictable patterns. Decision analysis also creeps into creating wiser public health decisions for diseases like malaria. Pricing the costs and benefits of such approaches as ITNs and ACTs is not mere bean-counting; it provides administrators with a better vision when it comes to doling out resources in an optimal manner. Applying this type of analysis—where concepts mix up study with actual need—smooths out some of that inherent randomness, and in most instances, it bridges the gap between study findings and grass-roots policy. By combining concepts from the epidemiologic triangle with a pinch of decision analysis, public health planners can alleviate the burden of infectious disease on societies globally, as highlighted in some of the more recent literature (Anderson et al., 2009; Batengana et al., 2011) (Figure 3.2).

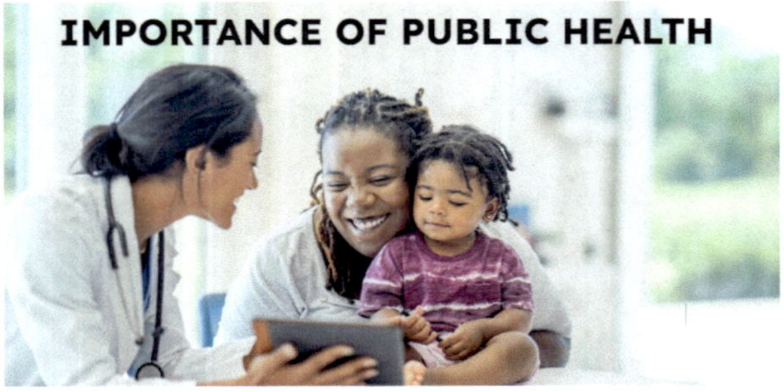

Figure 3.2. Importance in public health.

Source: Impofy. (2023). *Importance of Public Health.*

Overview of the Triangle's Components

Understanding how diseases spread hinges on three interlocking players—an insect (or pathogen), the person it infects, and the setting in which they meet. Often the culprit, be it a virus, bacterium, or parasite, can spark illness; its nasty characteristics, like how hard it hits or how it moves around, largely shape outbreak patterns. The individual isn't a passive "receiver" either—genes, daily routines, and immune system all combine together, which tends to make things a whole lot more complex. All this is saying is that understanding epidemics isn't about examining one piece of the puzzle, but getting a sense of how these factors bump up against each other in the real world. The environment around it, in some way or another, stage where an insect is encountered by the host. Weather, hygiene, and even ease of accessing a physician can help the disease settle in or control it. Consider a dense, polluted city—what goes on there can truly intensify infection spreading; but, in the sticks, problems may emanate from bothersome, vector-borne insects in an entirely different guise. Local considerations tend to prod public health practitioners to adjust accordingly, devising interventions and policies that are suitable to the place, and in some cases, even reducing disease rates in completely unanticipated manners. Stepping back and taking a look at how all of these pieces intersect, a better map for prevention and control begins to emerge. By modifying each corner of the triangle—the pathogen, the host, and the environment—officials can identify weak links where an outbreak could be halted in its tracks. For example, if one specific microbe appears to be the primary culprit, then efforts could then be directed to adjusting the environment by improving sanitation or vector control practices. And don't leave out community awareness; pushing people toward behaviors such as vaccination and healthier diets can seriously fortify their defense systems. Overall, this interlinked image compels us toward a more proactive stance, setting us apart from mere scrambling for solutions once the issue has already occurred.

3.1. The Components of the Epidemiological Triangle

To truly get a grip on how disease is transmitted between individuals, it is well worth investigating how the important components blend. Consider the epidemiological triangle as a mixture of three components. To start with, there is the agent—the nuisance microbe responsible for the disease. It might be a virus, a bacterium, or another small creature. Then there is the host, which refers to the individual or group that would become infected with the disease due to their genes, immune system, or general health. Finally, the environment plays the role of the setting in which the agent and host interact—it contributes to the likelihood that disease is transmitted. Seeing things in this manner, scientists can deduce the knotty dynamics of epidemics and calculate interventions that slice risks and advance public health. Focusing in on the agent, it is the match that ignites the entire trouble. Various germs—whether bacteria, viruses, or parasites—offer specific amounts of punch and means to spread. Most often, classifying things such as the way these threats evolve over time or become immune can uncover weak links in our healthcare systems. For instance, certain bacteria develop resistance to antibiotics, which completely alters the course of treatment that is available. Studies (Mavaddat et al., 2018) overall indicate that if we accurately predict and order risk factors, prevention measures, particularly in cases such as those of breast cancer, where the interaction between and host weaknesses exacerbates health inequities—receive an enormous impetus. So by digging into what these agents are doing, health professionals can concoct prevention regimens that suit the requirements of various populations quite nicely. Don't forget the host is just as important. It is not just a matter of our genetic blueprints; our habits in daily life, social status, and even what we are exposed to come into consideration. Sometimes having another condition—obesity or diabetes, for instance—can provide an added layer when infections present (Roth et al., 2018).

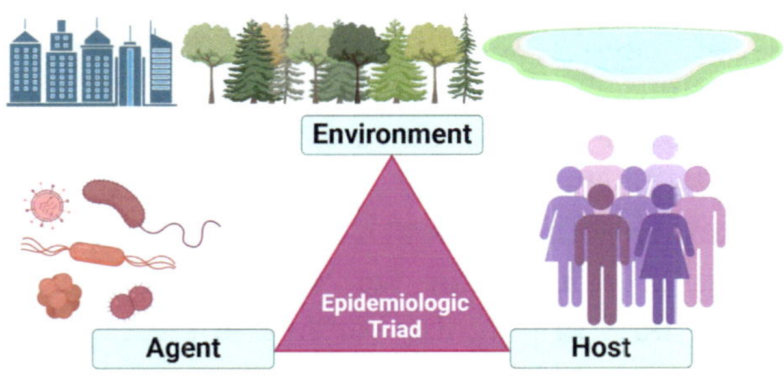

Figure 3.3. The components of the epidemiological triangle.

Source: Aryal, S. (2023). Epidemiologic triad: agent, host, environment. *Microbe Notes*.

By being sensitive to these differences among individuals, public health people can design specific interventions, such as vaccination campaigns or health talk in communities, that serve to harden up all individuals and reduce risk. Overall, fitting strategies to the individual combination of factors in every case is the secret to managing the tricky choreography of the epidemiological triangle (Figure 3.3).

3.1.1. Agent

Hosts, agents, and environments blend together in a manner that constitutes the center of what others refer to as the epidemiological triangle. Agents–that is, such things as bacteria, viruses, and parasites–are the living components that transmit disease, each with its own idiosyncrasies in how it infects and travels. Understanding what these agents do (and sometimes repeatedly doing so) is fairly crucial in attempting to institute public health solutions. One rather fascinating way to do it involves using agent based models that reproduce the complicated interplay among agents and their environment At other times, learning from such simulations can influence policies, such as those reports revealing how a small amount of false information can trigger vaccination decisions and disease trends generally. All these interconnected interactions provide researchers a better opportunity to predict outbreaks and fine-tune infectious disease responses, which can ultimately lead to better health outcomes (Chumachenko, 2025). Agent-based modeling is not merely monitoring disease transmission. Frequently, it delves deeper into agents interacting within their residence environments. Consider, for instance, research on tuberculosis (TB)—scientists sometimes employ multi-agent systems to follow the insidious paths infections travel in cities. Such research tends to rely on particular health information regarding individual agents, which captures variations in behavior, susceptibility, and local contact. Such a level of information sort of emphasizes the point that our social and environmental contexts play significant roles in how a disease unfolds. The findings of such simulations can also indicate how prevention and treatment strategies could be adjusted to address the special needs of various groups to reduce the spread of diseases such as TB (Semianiv et al., 2024). Including behavioral dynamics makes matters all the more serious for successful public health interventions. Research typically indicates that vaccine resistance is more than a mere glitch—it can direct epidemic trajectories. Agents, in other words, are not exclusively biological factors; they also reflect the frequently messy human perspectives and behaviors. For example, some agent-based models examine the influence of social networks and even a rumor storm on vaccination choices, demonstrating that it takes only a small shift in public sentiment to cascade into enormous changes in disease trends. By integrating behavioral elements into these models, we gain a more complete understanding of disease spread, one that can inform the development of communication and intervention plans. Since public health interventions more and more have to be adaptable, knowing even the slightest pieces of how agents behave is quite important for effective reactions to new health threats (Chumachenko, 2025).

3.1.2. Host

Recognizing how a host becomes part of the puzzle of infection is central to gaining control over disease behavior. Living organisms that are capable of harboring pathogens also come with their own idiosyncrasies - age, gender, genetic predisposition, and underlying health status all have roles to play in determining how bad an infection may end up being. For example, in COVID-19, older people and those with pre-existing medical conditions were well identified to be at higher risk. How a host responds to its environment as well as the disease cause quite accurately hits the nail on the head of the importance of public health actions focused on particular groups (Sabour et al., 2021). This sort of arrangement illustrates why paying attention to a host's profile is so important when determining methods to avoid disease. Zoning in just a bit more, the host is front and center of how infections occur. Pathogens tend to use various strategies to get in and replicate, and the immune system may either hold them at bay or, sometimes, assist them. Overall, a host's adaptive and innate immunity is likely to respond unpredictably to various invaders, and this influences the total effect of an epidemic.

Another threat is the emergent concern for antimicrobial resistance (AMR); habits such as overuse of antibiotics are likely to start an infection and reinfection loop. Different researches indicate that combining knowledge from disparate disciplines is required to bridge the chasm between host health preservation and resistance management (Aslam et al., 2018). Briefly, comprehending exactly how a host adapts and reacts is crucial to design treatments and prevention strategies. Delving into host–pathogen interactions occasionally reveal information that defies the standard treatment script. New options, such as employing probiotics or creating vaccines that stimulate a host's own immune systems—begin to gain traction as good methods to treat infections. Testing in various health settings has proven that these strategies can relieve the disease burden of infections previously treated primarily with antibiotics. As pathogens evolve continually, it is time we re-evaluate the role of the host in planning for health strategy. By emphasizing host resilience development and overall health, health authorities can deploy broader interventions that not only work against infections but also foster a more resilient immune environment in populations (Aslam et al., 2018). This transition indicates towardan integrated perspective of health that, in the majority of instances, is pivotal in addressing contemporary public health issues (Figure 3.4).

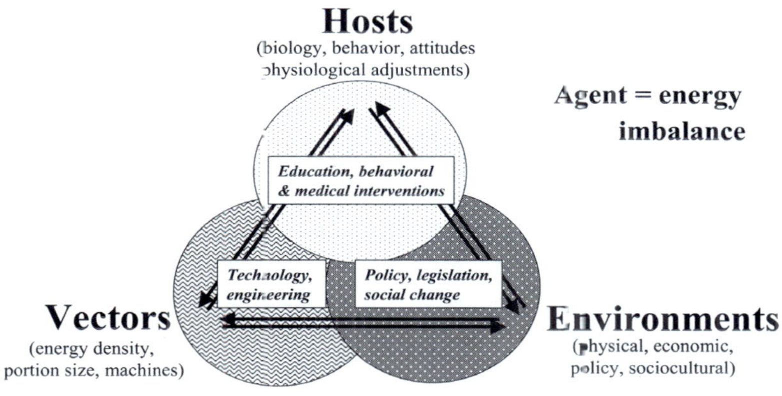

Figure 3.4. Understanding how a host fits into the puzzle of infections.

Source: https://www.ahajournals.org/cms/10.1161/01.CIR.0000140072.49273.6B/asset/e46a36df-154e-4e88-baa1-d2a3f06dd5f6/assets/graphic/38ff1.jpeg

3.1.3. Environment

Environmental changes and disease transmission appear to go hand in hand. Locations near us tend to lay the groundwork for germs to grow, with local conditions directly linking to how illness spreads within populations. For instance, when SARS-CoV-2 was detected in wastewater, it provided a preview of what viruses may be spreading even before major outbreaks occur. That quantifiable trace of viral RNA, often reflecting the documented COVID-19 instances (Wurtzer et al., 2020), prods public health teams to apply environmental indicators as leading indicators, particularly when lockdowns are occurring, and conventional data lags behind. Consider next how certain environments can predispose the emergence of drug-resistant pathogens. Abusing antibiotics in hospitals, farms, or even in more general community settings can provide the ideal environment in which these resilient organisms thrive. In most cases, if we ignore the role our environment has in developing resistance, our attempts to fight back may fail. Combating AMR, thus, is not merely a hospital problem—it needs to be married with what occurs in agriculture and nature in general (Aslam et al., 2018). This ugly but necessary link assists scientists in designing solutions that can potentially stem resistance while maintaining the effectiveness of our existing medicines. And then there is the less tangible side of the process: how our lifestyles and societal changes contribute to disease patterns. Urban sprawl, climate change, and habitat destruction can push disease carriers into new regions, making health responses more difficult. Environmental changes could instantly change where disease-carrying insects tend to congregate, presenting unexpected dangers. Since our societies expand into nature reserves, the likelihood of zoonotic disease increases, highlighting the inextricable links between our ecosystem and our general well-being. An environmentally conscious, forward-thinking method can turn these dangers back, ultimately affording us a greater chance to comprehend and contain the dissemination of disease in our globalized world.

3.2. The Role of the Agent

Epidemiology isn't merely labeling; it is unearthing the way that disease appears by examining the interaction between the agent, the host, and the environment. The agent—the insect or chemical itself—is at the core of the matter. Just think about how SARS-CoV-2 emerged: initially, it leaped from bats (or so we believe) into humans, flaunting its unexpected talent for adaptation. This realignment, most often, dictates that viruses aren't fixed things—they evolve, and so we must watch them all the while as we work to figure out how they traverse and wreak havoc in an increasingly global environment. Determining what precisely the agent is becomes essential if we are to design interventions aimed at their spread and effect, further emphasizing why understanding its mechanics is so critical in epidemiological practice. With time, our perception of these agents has changed significantly, and now their characteristics tend to determine the entire outcome of an outbreak—its intensity, its tempo, and much else. As an example, take the swift transmission of SARS-CoV-2 among humans: the virus's speedy human-to-human transmission demanded immediate reactions such as social distancing and accelerating vaccines. The agent is not merely some inert fragment of the jigsaw; it has an active role to play in the host-environment dance. Features such as pre-existing conditions within hosts can merge to shift disease outcomes. In the vast majority of cases, knowing this blend provides a more nuanced and diverse image for disease control and prevention, leaving new avenues for predicting future epidemics and smarter vaccine strategies. Control measures, also, have a great dependence on what the agent is like. At times, the precise manner in which we approach a disease—be it through tight lockdowns or widespread testing—is dependent on how virulent and contagious it is. COVID-19 has demonstrated how the responses can differ widely from region to region, all fueled by the virus's particular characteristics. In some ways, gaining control over what the agent does assists in determining not just treatment for the infected but also impacts overall public health practices and emergency measures. Research, then, must plunge into new concepts, from vaccine advances to therapeutic interventions, as well as fill the gaps in what we understand about these new threats. Overall, the agent's role in this entire triangle continues to be central; it not only directs responses to public health emergencies but also directs global efforts to contain infectious diseases effectively (Cantini et al., 2020; Ralph et al., 2020) (Figure 3.5).

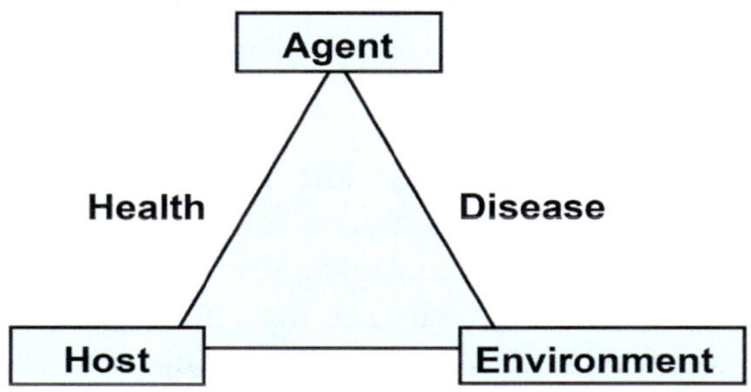

Figure 3.5. The role of the agent.

Source: Narayan, K. G., Sinha, D. K., & Singh, D. K. (2023). *Figure 3.1: Epidemiological Triad.* In *Veterinary Public Health & Epidemiology* (Chapter 3). Springer.

3.2.1. Types of Agents (Biological, Chemical, Physical)

Investigating the group of agents that cause the spread of disease is a fundamental activity in epidemiology. You have the pathogens like bacteria, viruses, and fungi that live and can infect, and the way these function is intertwined with the host's own vulnerabilities—factors that typically speed up or slow down an outbreak in ways that are not expected. For the most part, the behaviors of these microbes—how they replicate themselves, for example, or how they get around our body's defenses—play a big role in shaping the path of an outbreak. Some models even suggest that slight variations in how susceptible people are can change the severity of infections, with varying outcomes across different groups. Thus, essentially, being able to control such living things is the key when trying to solve public health issues in the best possible way (Goldsmith et al., 2020). Following are the chemical substances that also disrupt our health, especially in our environment. Think about toxins, pollutants, and other harmful chemicals that cause non-infectious diseases among communities. More recently, efforts have been made to study cumulative risk—attempting to see how one chemical exposure adds to the next, as well as social and even emotional stressors. By adding in non-chemical stressors, like a person's economic status, researchers sometimes have a better idea of why some groups are faced with greater challenges. To illustrate, when social stress is layered with chemical exposure, the resulting health effects can be even more complicated, enhancing the need for a multifactorial, tiered risk assessment approach (Adler et al., 2011). Physiological factors complete this scenario of health risks, including considerations like radiation, intense heat and cold, and even mechanical energy. These variables can dispense both acute and chronic health issues in manners that are not necessarily predictable. To truly determine their effect, you must examine both their direct impact and all the side effects that manifest within various environments. Add extreme ultraviolet radiation, which can increase skin cancer risk, or extreme weather that causes physical damage and also can add to psychological distress. All in all, if you look at the entire epidemiological triangle, it's clear that biological, chemical, and physical agents work within a general, sloppy environment that sets general community health. Understanding these interwoven forces is essential to uniting effective prevention and intervention strategies in public health.

3.2.2. Mechanisms of Transmission

Discovering how diseases are transmitted is the basis of containing outbreaks, particularly when you consider the old triangle of agent, host, and environment. Pathogens get around by various means: a quick handshake, airborne droplets wafting by, or even insects as carriers. It's complicated when these avenues blend with personal variables and the condition of the environment. Influenza, for example, tends to be a clear illustration; seasonal vaccination programs targeted toward specific age groups have spotty outcomes in reducing infection and mortality. At times, including children in vaccination drives has increased overall outcomes, as young individuals can fuel transmission, ending up reducing rates of illness and loss (Baguelin et al., 2013). Social contacts introduce another complication to modeling disease transmission. Network concepts have been influencing epidemiology nowadays by illustrating that the connections among individuals could either welcome the door to a disease or protect it. Experiments that map out how humans are connected tell us that certain individuals find themselves in pivotal places that influence whether outbreaks spread or not. Your position within a social network may tip the likelihood of getting infected or spreading one. Models that incorporate these network dynamics typically make more realistic predictions and inform intervention efforts in a more realistic manner—broadly speaking, this perspective enriches the image of transmission considerably (Danon et al., 2010). Combining various types of data further refines our understanding of disease flow. When laboratory findings align with clinical information and even with snippets of behavior, researchers are left with models that attempt to replicate the ways infections surge with time. With these diverse datasets pieced together, researchers can pick up on repeat patterns and tailor their approaches based on this. A review of influenza vaccination history in the UK revealed distinct disparities in infection prevention based on whether or not given groups were vaccinated. Overall, taking an approach that addresses several transmission routes—touching on the germ, the host, and its environment—is the only way we are going to be able to keep up with future outbreaks (Baguelin et al., 2013) (Figure 3.6).

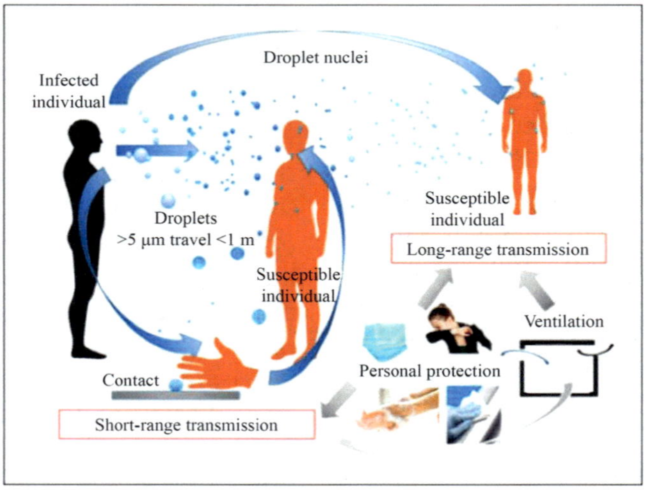

Figure 3.6. Mechanisms of transmission.

Source: Delikhoon M, Guzman MI, Nabizadeh R, Norouzian Baghani A. Modes of Transmission of Severe Acute Respiratory Syndrome-Coronavirus-2 (SARS-CoV-2) and Factors Influencing on the Airborne Transmission: A Review. *International Journal of Environmental Research and Public Health*. 2021; 18(2):395. https://doi.org/10.3390/ijerph18020395

3.2.3. Examples of Diseases Caused by Different Agents

The epidemiological triangle provides a sort of template for the way diseases travel, combining germs, individuals, and their environments in a manner that is not necessarily foreseen. Consider respiratory illness—it primarily originates with viruses such as influenza or bacteria such as *Streptococcus pneumoniae*. For the most part, how an individual's immune system responds—either over-responding or under-responding—can significantly alter how bad the disease becomes. People with compromised defenses tend to suffer more, and when you couple that with congested living, it's the perfect recipe for these insects to be mobile, as various studies in different parts of the world have reported (James et al., 2018). And then there is the entire universe of vector-borne diseases. Pestilences such as malaria and dengue fever both use the mosquito as a carrier; malaria is from Plasmodium spp., whereas one virus causes dengue. The triangle here indicates that transmission isn't solely dependent on one variable—it's based on how mosquito populations act, the weather at the time like temperature and humidity, and how susceptible people are to infection. For instance, excessive rains will increase mosquito breeding places, which in turn increases the number of these small transmitters and, before long, disease levels. In a majority of instances, applying a combination of methods to control these insects appears to be the cornerstone for stemming outbreaks (Aslam et al., 2018). Foodborne diseases introduce another angle to the scene. You have got a range of culprits here—from bacteria like Salmonella and *E. coli* to viruses such as norovirus—each taking its own route to affect the host. The triangle reminds us that food safety is not just about choosing one proper step; how food is handled, stored, and cooked can tip the scales. Occasionally, some undercooking or a slip-up resulting in cross-contamination provides these pathogens with a free ride, placing children and immunocompromised individuals at greater risk. In the majority of instances, comprehension of these overlapping factors is vital to public health initiatives for enhancing safety in our kitchens and decreasing outbreaks (James et al., 2018).

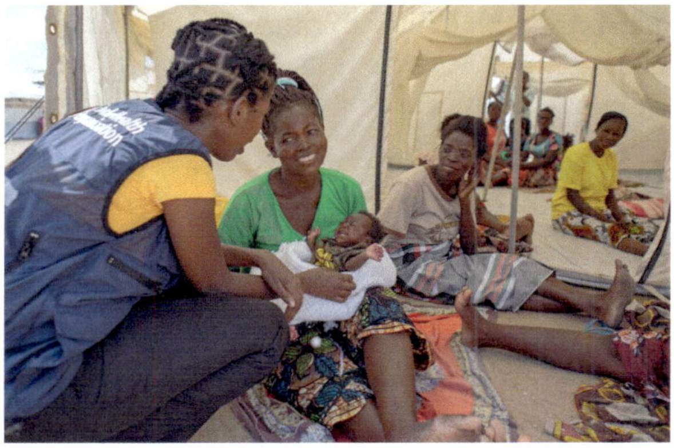

Source: World Health Organization (WHO). (2019). *Breastfeeding is Critical for Child Survival Following Cyclones in Mozambique*. WHO.

3.3. Understanding the Host

Emerging diseases reveal how pathogens and human hosts interact in fairly surprising combinations. Uncovering what drives a host to act has become key to public health. The immune system–that vital defense line–more or less determines how bad diseases like COVID-19 get. Nobody's immunity operates the same, so various individuals wind up with quite different fates. A study shows that SARS-CoV-2 infiltrates our cells through the Angiotensin Converting Enzyme-2 receptor; most of the time, this leads to the role of our genetic configuration in susceptibility and disease severity (Cantini et al., 2020). As scientists delve deeper into these host responses, they tend to discover new treatment concepts and improved ways of constructing vaccines, which cumulatively create a more effective framework for controlling diseases. Aside from genetics, underlying medical conditions contribute significantly to a host's susceptibility. Conditions such as diabetes, hypertension, and obesity, for instance, have been associated with poorer outcomes in diseases like COVID-19–supporting the notion that existing issues can increase risk. The combination of these conditions with the sheer virulence of the pathogen tends to blur the larger picture, and therefore health strategies must consider the entire tale of an individual's health and environment. Even a meticulous examination of patient information indicates that certain groups are particularly at risk, necessitating interventions attuned to the particular challenges faced by such groups (Ralph et al., 2020). This consciousness not only enhances our understanding of how disease acts but also informs the development of public health strategies that truly strike the right chord. Social and behavioral elements also influence the way hosts interact with infectious pathogens. Economic status, healthcare access, and even community participation influences how a host's system responds to an infection. Consider those marginalized communities–they tend to have higher rates of exposure through living and less access to preventive resources, which simply increases the chances of outbreaks. A comprehension of these social levels combined with biological characteristics provides helpful indications for reducing infection rates. During the COVID-19 pandemic, for example, healthcare providers have been struck reasonably hard, calling for judiciously targeted interventions to protect front-line workers (Cantini et al., 2020). In most instances, combining the biological with the social allows public health actions to address and eventually minimize the effects of infectious diseases while increasing general community welfare.

3.3.1. Factors Influencing Host Susceptibility

Epidemiology is a world where determining why some hosts are more susceptible to disease is the most important thing. Genetics can alter how our immunity operates—so a small difference is all the difference when combating germs at times. Meanwhile, the world has its own curveballs, such as certain pathogens truly flourishing when the weather changes, and these same seasonal fluctuations may also confuse a host's immune response. In general, understanding these gory details is important to consider when health strategies are being created because an assortment of pragmatic strategies can make hosts less appealing to incursive agents. Overall, such observations serve to streamline disease control and prevention by informing the public health interventions for each community's specific risk profiles. Socio-economic determinants also bear a surprisingly onerous burden of influence on how people who are exposed become so. People who are living in more precarious socio-economic conditions tend to be exposed more intensely to infectious agents due to less than ideal housing and reduced access to healthcare services. Even factors such as education and livelihood turn out to affect not only exposure levels but also the extent of individuals' knowledge of elementary hygiene. So far, the interaction of these social determinants tends to bring about a sort of susceptibility to whole populations, which in turn requires risk management approaches to span much ground. Others hold that closing socio-economic gaps can eventually reduce rates of susceptibility and enhance resilience to outbreaks. It would appear obvious that public health interventions must contain these socio-economic spices if they are to be effective at reducing infectious disease. Another spin on the story is behavior, inextricably entangled with genetics as well as environmental factors. The daily decisions—what we consume, the level of physical activity we maintain, or smoking—can change our immune status, increasing the risk to some and granting others a small measure of natural protection. Local action, such as smoking cessation programs or campaigns to increase nutritional education, can nibble away at these risks, albeit maybe slowly. Most models, in most instances, highlight how our own behavior and choices contribute significantly to how epidemics play out–human behavior does get a say after all. By considering these behavioral factors alongside biological and environmental ones, health experts can design strategies that ease individual vulnerabilities and concurrently boost community strength, forming a vital part of the overall picture in disease spread (Figure 3.7).

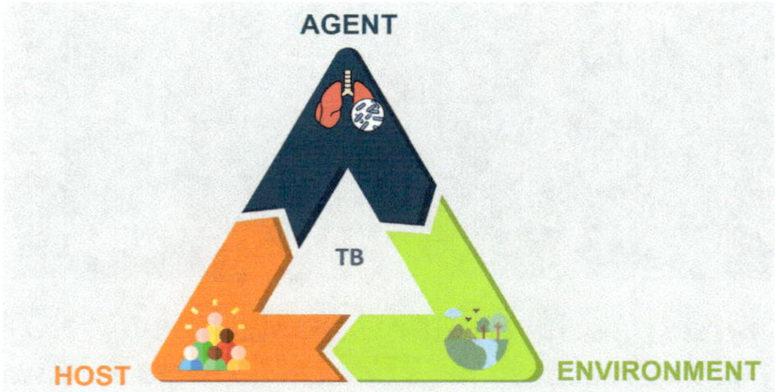

Figure 3.7. Host susceptibility.

Source: NTEP. (n.d.). *National Testing and Evaluation Project (NTEP).*

3.3.2. The Role of Immunity

At the center of chaotic interactions among our bodies, encroaching germs, and all that surrounds them, our defense systems bear a gigantic responsibility in determining the course of a disease. If our system is functioning as it should, it can cushion the impact of infections significantly, demonstrating that both our innate and acquired defenses play an important role. Take the SARS-CoV-2 Omicron variant – it unveiled some vulnerabilities in antibody neutralization, but studies find overall that T cells continue to put up a pretty good fight against different COVID-19 strains. That is to say, even if the virus adjusts itself slightly to evade antibody attacks, those innate cellular fighters still provide a reserve line of defense, rendering immunity an important component of the epidemiological equation (Keeton et al., 2022). Considered from the perspective of pathogen development, what is seen is that adaptive immune reactions within our populations are a large factor in directing that effort. History teaches us that most strains evolve by creating modifications, such as deletions or mutations—that enable them to evade detection by our immune system. Take the SARS epidemic, for example, which highlighted the ORF8 gene; mutations in that area appeared to increase the virus's ability to evade. This subtle balancing act of evading immune detection and remaining fit is important, now more than ever with new variants possessing changed immunogenic properties threatening our existing vaccines and requesting ongoing surveillance and new approaches (Su et al., 2020).

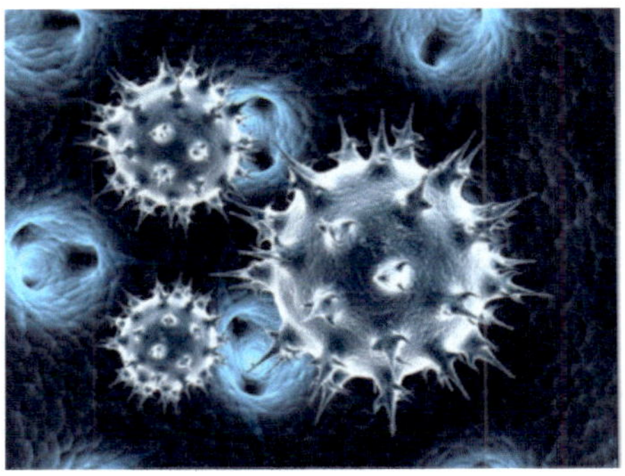

Source: https://vetmed.tamu.edu/research/wp-content/uploads/sites/64/2019/03/Research_Page3-e1551734898863.jpg

Our immune system's effect is not just about keeping an individual healthy—it spreads through communities and even influences public health policy. Vaccine campaigns to create group immunity rely on being able to understand how immune reactions can adjust this delicate balance. Having a vaccine not only safeguards the person but also assists in establishing a larger social barrier that reduces infection transmission. Even so, the emergence of variants that can evade immunity brings home the point that vaccine strategy must change on an ongoing basis. Finally, intelligent public health interventions are based on an intimate, perhaps imperfect, understanding of our defenses, and a critical element to enhance individual as well as population resilience against infection (Keeton et al., 2022).

3.3.3. Host Behaviors and Their Impact on Disease Spread

Host behaviors determine the spread of epidemics in ways that aren't always immediately clear. Individuals' personal responses—and even the way they respond together—can distort the course of disease transmission. For instance, when an individual becomes overwhelmed with too much health information, they tend to tune out, thereby reducing precautions; such message fatigue ultimately affects not just individual decisions but also the resilience of the larger community to infections (Fan et al., 2025). The balance between crisp messaging and inherent host response becomes a red-hot topic in studies, typically emphasizing a call for communications that capture interest without being excessive. And now agriculture adds its spin to these interactions. Consider wheat dwarf disease (WDD): wheat plants, with their special modes of responding to viral attacks, introduce another twist to the disease's saga. Some cultivars—*Complice* and *Filon*, for example—are predisposed to react to the virus and its insect vectors, such as the leafhopper *Psammotettix alienus*, in unusual fashions. These variations usually influence all from the survival of the insects to their rate of reproduction, providing useful hints and even a bit of odd insight into plant management and selecting the appropriate planting varieties (Armand et al., 2024). And then there is the big picture, where whole communities are involved in how diseases spread through populations. Vaccines, a little social distancing, and even the tone of public health messages can make a big difference. Usually, when people feel connected to and trust the advice they are given, disease transmission can slow down significantly. Other than that, consideration of cultural custom, socioeconomic level, and what information filters into the masses ultimately plays a factor–and how it's simply understood that aligning strategies for each community's atmosphere is where it's at (Fan et al., 2025). The constant tension between what is done by the host and disease behavior demonstrates occasionally, even incremental, mundane effort can make an enormous difference.

3.4. The Environment's Influence

Environmental conditions strike our health in all sorts of ways–it is not one thing but a combination of natural environments and the way people live their lives. For instance, in Syria there has been some discussion about increasing cancer rates; consider Al-Souida, where the topography and the exact location appear to increase disease incidence. In general, research indicates that factors such as what kind of rocks are in the area and even radiation, combined with what we eat or what hazards we encounter on the job, all contribute to why some communities wind up in worse shape health-wise. With a geographical information system, scientists have been able to plot clusters where various risks coincide with local cancer incidence, truly highlighting the significance of understanding these spatial connections (Deeb et al., 2012). Examining further infectious diseases, the landscape is equally complicated. Investigating endemic disease shows that how diseases spread can change wildly depending on a mixture of environmental and social variables. For example, when scientists reconstruct transmission events–for example, in rabies–they occasionally discover that nature itself segregates things into almost distinct cycles with hardly any crossover. By incorporating genetic hints, timing information, and where events occur, it has turned out (in the majority of instances) that urban sprawl and habitat reduction can accelerate or decelerate the spread of disease. This combination of elements serves to shed light on the serpentine routes down which diseases travel across various eco-settings, reminding us of the profound connection between surroundings and health outcomes (Hampson et al., 2014).

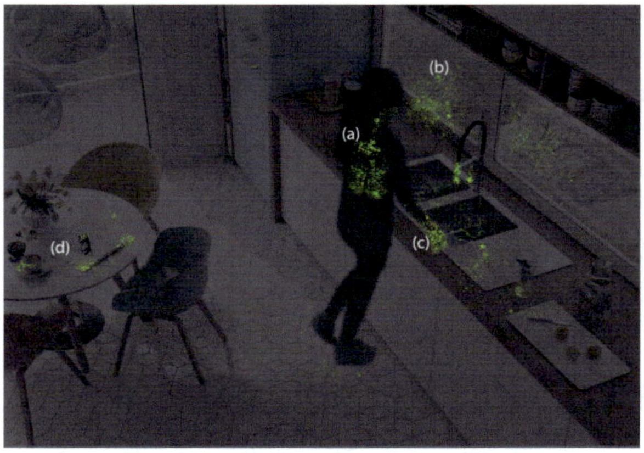

Figure 3.8. The environment's influence.

Source: Delikhoon M, Guzman MI, Nabizadeh R, Norouzian Baghani A. Modes of Transmission of Severe Acute Respiratory Syndrome-Coronavirus-2 (SARS-CoV-2) and Factors Influencing on the Airborne Transmission: A Review. *International Journal of Environmental Research and Public Health*. 2021; 18(2):395. https://doi.org/10.3390/ijerph18020395

Differences in health also tend to appear strongly by place, highlighting just how disproportionate environmental effects can be. Communities that lack ready access to clean water, adequate nutrition, or good healthcare find themselves grappling with increased environmental threats. Syria's cancer maps, for example, indicate that areas with greater pollution and unstable infrastructure are affected more—nearly as though economic and environmental difficulties are married. Cartographic resources in epi strive to expose these messy patterns, providing clues on how to customize interventions. In the end, policymakers who understand these dynamics (with all their ups and downs) have a better chance of trimming back the health consequences linked to our environment, opening doors to stronger, healthier communities (Deeb et al., 2012) (Figure 3.8).

3.4.1. Physical Environment (Geography, Climate)

Geography and climate influence the distribution of diseases. In areas with extremely fluctuating altitudes, weather patterns change abruptly—a situation that can accelerate the spread of diseases such as malaria. Consider Bududa district in Uganda, for instance; in that region, climate fluctuations have recently been associated with increased cases of malaria, even at about 1800 meters above sea level—a place where, Overall, such cases were not previously frequent. These regional anomalies, with a few exceptions, illustrate that certain weather patterns can facilitate the multiplying of disease vectors, and thus require public health interventions as anomalous as the regional weather (Aboda et al., 2012). Temperature fluctuations and unpredictable rain conspire to increase both the frequency and intensity of outbreaks. Studies overall suggest that intense rain, in creating almost perfect breeding grounds for mosquitoes, effectively allows malaria to seep into regions that hadn't had it before. Local people in some high-altitude areas may not have developed full immunity, and this can contribute to a combination of issues, such as increased illness and even increased mortality linked to malaria. It would appear to be obvious that incorporating climate data into our disease models is crucial for appreciating the way environmental components fit with human health. This combination, when you give it some proper thought, is the key to developing a good strategy that considers both the local landscape and the specific weather patterns. And then there is the entire issue of populations relocating due to these climate changes, something that further complicates the picture of disease spread. Populations sometimes move—whether temporarily or even permanently—due to changing conditions, but relocating to areas with greater densities of disease agents can elevate their risk of infections. Bududa district raises its head once more here; individuals migrating from higher elevations to lower ones tend to be less adapted to malaria, having neither experience nor the innate defenses that accompany prolonged exposure. Generally, this adaptive behavior highlights the complex loops between our environment, both climate and geography, and public health, and calls for epidemiological models that encompass all these aspects (Aboda et al., 2012).

3.4.2. Social Environment (Cultural Practices, Socioeconomic Status)

Social surroundings and daily conventions determine our health more than we realize. What individuals want to eat or how they raise their children commonly comes directly out of their financial status and the culture they came from. Study indicates that elements in the environment – particularly forces such as maternal education and income at home – ultimately direct nutrient outcomes, and children sometimes bear the brunt of it. When access to decent food and education is bad, health disparities only become bigger. Examining these intersecting social and cultural determinants is quite important when attempting to find public health solutions to address malnutrition (Lestari et al., 2021). History has a way of persisting in our health systems. Colonial domination, for instance, bequeathed practices that continue to play havoc with care today, and the HIV-1 epidemic reminds us of that earlier influence. Urbanization, driven by past colonial practices, displaced people and disintegrated customary health systems, resulting in patchy disease surveillance and sluggish responses to emerging threats. In most instances, placing our issues today side-by-side with a retrospect of social history reveals that historical influences still shape our current issues. It happens that knowing these historical colonial connections can go a long way in informing how we battle issues such as HIV/AIDS and even COVID-19 (Wu et al., 2023). When dealing with health issues, it is not merely a matter of medicine—it is a matter of incorporating cultural idiosyncrasies and economic realities into each step. Initiatives that directly address a community's peculiarities and incorporate targeted education for mothers on childcare and nutrition can have a significant impact. By integrating these realities into public health policy, decision-makers can more effectively target minimizing the harms associated with poverty and low education. In simple words, there needs to be an integrated and culturally sensitive effort because our social world contributes significantly to our health outcome—a large component of the muddled picture that defines today's Epidemiological Triangle (Lestari et al., 2021) (Figure 3.9).

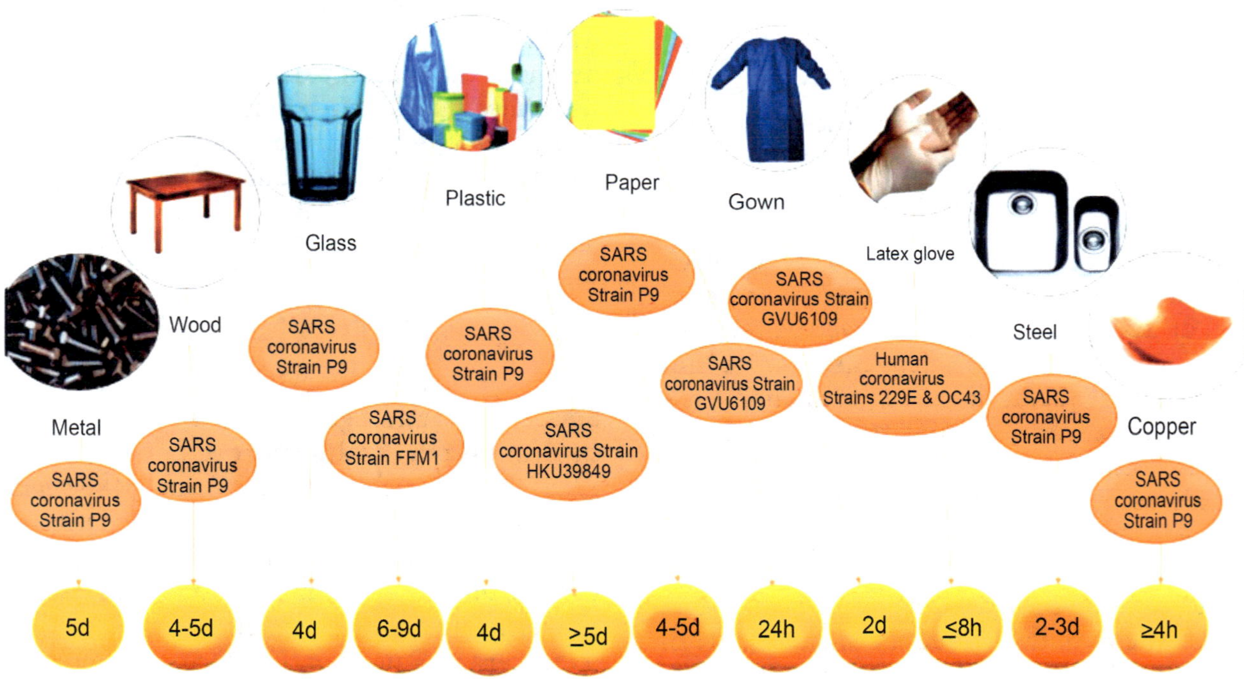
Metal
SARS coronavirus Strain P9
5d
Wood
SARS coronavirus Strain P9
4-5d
Glass
SARS coronavirus Strain P9
4d
SARS coronavirus Strain FFM1
6-9d
Plastic
SARS coronavirus Strain P9
4d
SARS coronavirus Strain HKU39849
≥5d
Paper
SARS coronavirus Strain P9
4-5d
SARS coronavirus Strain GVU6109
24h
Gown
SARS coronavirus Strain GVU6109
2d
Latex glove
Human coronavirus Strains 229E & OC43
≤8h
Steel
SARS coronavirus Strain P9
2-3d
Copper
SARS coronavirus Strain P9
≥4h

Figure 3.9. Social environment (cultural practices, socioeconomic status).

Source: Delikhoon M, Guzman MI, Nabizadeh R, Norouzian Baghani A. Modes of Transmission of Severe Acute Respiratory Syndrome-Coronavirus-2 (SARS-CoV-2) and Factors Influencing on the Airborne Transmission: A Review. *International Journal of Environmental Research and Public Health*. 2021; 18(2):395. https://doi.org/10.3390/ijerph18020395

3.4.3. Environmental Changes and Emerging Diseases

How our climate changes have disrupted ecosystems, and we're witnessing an increase in emerging diseases. Warmer temperatures and bizarre rainfall patterns are destabilizing landscapes, disrupting the fine balance between germs, their hosts, and the surrounding ecosystems. Occasionally such turns of events establish just the right context for germs that previously had not been a nuisance. For instance, a few more degrees can drive mosquitoes into new locations, allowing diseases like malaria and dengue to creep into areas not previously affected. Taming these shifts is critical, particularly when you consider models like the Epidemiological Triangle that illustrate how disease and environmental factors interact. The connection between our evolving environment and heart disease does illustrate just how older health threats can yield to new challenges. International research tends to indicate that a combination of environmental exposure, daily lifestyle activity, and changing climates all ultimately contribute significantly to the frequency with which heart issues arise and even add to increased mortality. Add in conditions such as high blood pressure, obesity, and physical inactivity—each of which can all deteriorate when the environment suffers—and things only get more complicated. As climate change disrupts the air, heat, and water quality, the likelihood of heart-related events compounds. Tackling these knotted pathways is key to public health initiatives seeking to reduce the burden of CVD and other emerging diseases (Tzoulaki et al., 2016). New plant illnesses also illustrate how intricate the connections are between environmental changes and general health. The relationship between an unstable climate and plant health is becoming increasingly apparent—for example, Sudden Oak Death could become more prevalent as temperatures increase. When both temperature and rainfall go off-pattern, it can disrupt how plants and their pathogens interact, and if plants become more vulnerable, huge agricultural problems can follow. Plus, climate change makes it harder to predict and manage these outbreaks, leaving us a bit uncertain about the best course of action. This unpredictability indicates that more research and various management approaches are needed, demonstrating why practitioners from various disciplines ought to collaborate to maintain plant health during these climatic variations. The impacts extend far, touching on food security and human well-being, and emphasizing just how important a stable ecosystem is to maintaining diseases at bay (Dobson et al., 2012).

3.5. Interactions Within the Triangle

Understanding how a host, an agent, and their environment combine to scramble disease transmission unlocks why we require a variety of public health strategies. These three actors—the human body, the pathogen, and the daily environment—intersect in ways that determine how infections emerge and spread. Consider COVID-19, for instance: the virus, individuals, and community environments all enter the scene in surprising ways that fuel transmission. Good contact tracing—much referred to in newer research—operates by rapidly identifying and quarantining cases; this truly demonstrates how the setting, with elements such as population density and shared social behaviors, can support or undermine such efforts (Keeling et al., 2020). Dealing with outbreaks means recognizing that nothing exists in a vacuum. More often than not, when bacteria are drug-resistant under duress, it makes treatment for humans and other hosts more difficult. The emergence of multidrug-resistant insects serves as a reminder that combating infections is not solely a matter of altering the behavior of hosts (such as receiving vaccinations or increasing hygiene) but also observing what's going on with antibiotics in agriculture and elsewhere (Aslam et al., 2018). Overall, this complex web requires a united response along healthcare, agricultural, and environmental fronts. How our globe changes—via urban sprawl, worldwide travel, and shifting climates—continuously rewrites the playbook for where germs congregate and breed. With more people on the move, diseases frequently flash from one region to the next faster than we anticipate. Health authorities currently rush to construct agile surveillance networks that integrate information about human habits and local environments. In the case of COVID-19, it has been important to pin down close contacts promptly, something that relies heavily on community cooperation and the environment where individuals reside (Keeling et al., 2020). Overall, allowing these interactions to inform our approach appears to be important to addressing public health crises in a more holistic, adaptable manner.

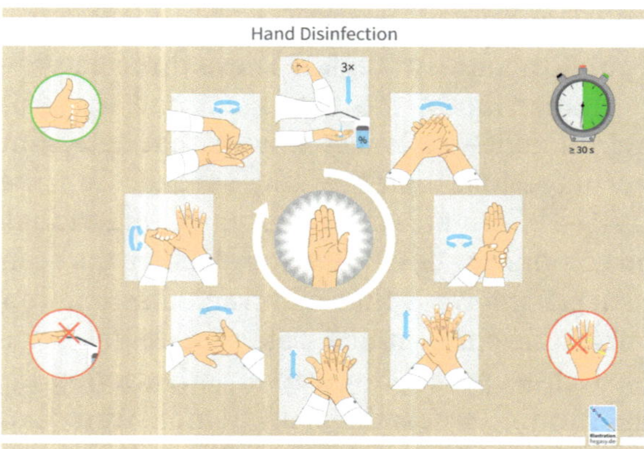

Source: https://commons.wikimedia.org/wiki/File:04_Hegasy_Hand_Disinfection_Wiki_EN_CCBYSA.png

3.5.1. How Agents Interact with Hosts

Hosts and agents coming together reside at the very core of infection transmission. Their combination isn't hypothetical–it carries real-world implications in what we refer to as the epidemiological triangle. Consider this: both living components and even nonliving factors such as weather or climate conditions adjust a host's chances of contracting an infection. I find myself often remembering studies of forest fungi, where how fast a disease travels through trees appears to rely entirely on weather and how crowded the forest is. At times these connections alter things radically—from a condition that is largely controlled to one that erupts instantly into an outbreak. Quantitative models can indicate such changes and provide hints on predicting or even preventing disease transmission, which is the reason why combining ecological indicators is crucial in such studies (Baggaley et al., 2018). Routes of transmission among agents and hosts remain fluid; they adapt to our social behaviors, environment, and even historical contexts. Consider HIV, for instance—its early history in Kinshasa shows how urbanization and colonial influence conditioned the pattern of the spread of the virus. There is something fascinating about the way in which human activity, such as traveling around or socializing, can either fuel or retard the progress of an infection. And how healthcare systems were established (which tended to be under colonial regulations) greatly influenced how communities coped with the crisis. These multi-layered interactions make us feel better about overall public health policies, particularly when new issues emerge, as we have experienced with COVID-19 (Wu et al., 2023). Ultimately, the messy interaction of agents and hosts means we've got to borrow ideas from various disciplines to understand disease transmission. Combining ecological models with the social sciences isn't a clever sleight of hand—it creates a richer picture of how infections spread through populations. Such a strategy even assists with identifying early warning signs of transitions between periods of calm and outbreaks, both on farmland and in woodlands. Checking on which hosts are most vulnerable is not only key for fighting disease; it also guides us in shaping ecosystems that can better handle stress. All these insights eventually help design public health measures that recognize the intricate dance between pathogens and their hosts, paving the way for smarter strategies against future outbreaks (Baggaley et al., 2018).

3.5.2. The Impact of Environmental Changes on Host-Agent Relationships

Environmental changes truly make a difference in the connections between living hosts and the small agents that impact us. At times, it is merely a matter of warmer days and monsoon alterations that make the scales tip—these changes can increase the level of disease carriers, such as when more mosquitoes appear in warmer, humid conditions that enable them to survive. You see, when nature gets a bit out-of-sync, the usual give-and-take between organisms and their hitchhiking microbes falls apart, and suddenly diseases find new ways to spread. Hosts, as it happens, require a suitable environment to the same degree as their unwelcome microbial visitors, and if that environment refuses to play along, then conflict is soon rife; generally, this is a reminder of just how essential our environment is to what others refer to as the Epidemiological Triangle.

Human beings, particularly many Indigenous communities, demonstrate in their own terms just how disrupted our health becomes by these changes in the environment. They rely on traditions—ancient, tried-and-true methods that combine local knowledge with hands-on approaches to gain sustenance and prosperity. Use the COVID-19 pandemic as a case in point; many Native communities leveraged ancient knowledge to adapt to sudden changes and climatic pressures. They even reverted to old habits—sustainable food gathering of medicinals, attempting to restore farming practices lost to history—to remain one step ahead of environmental mayhem. In most instances, these adaptive strategies reflect that examining the way local traditions blend with nature can influence public health policy, suggesting new paths for bettering our well-being when natural systems are in flux. And then there is the fascinating world of our gut microbiota that has a much more complex role to play than many would have thought.

Our microbiome, shaped by everything from what we're eating to the air we're breathing, maintains a delicate equilibrium that, when disturbed—a condition some refer to as dysbiosis, incidentally—can cause such conditions as heart or metabolic issues. Increasing evidence reveals, in the broadest terms, that if our sources of food become short or are disrupted because of changing conditions in the environment, such imbalance in the microbial communities within can make us more susceptible to chronic disease. All this amounts to indicating that in addition to the conventional host-agent equation, the micro-world within us necessitates as much consideration if at all we're to properly see the onset of disease and dissemination in our compound ecosystem.

3.5.3. Case Studies Illustrating These Interactions

The key to understanding how infections happen is examining how the environment, the disease agents, and the hosts combine. Consider the Zika outbreak in Brazil—social and environmental factors all contributed, so the crisis hit harder than anticipated. Scientists investigated how climate change, fast urbanization, and economic inequality left certain communities particularly vulnerable. For instance, the transmission of Aedes mosquitoes—those annoying Zika carriers—was contingent upon variables such as temperature, precipitation, and other random weather idiosyncrasies. Often enough, a minor environmental variation provides these agents with an edge during host infection, which contributes to a larger outbreak. So, actions such as reducing the mosquito population and increasing public health information naturally topped the list, demonstrating that you truly must approach diseases in terms of the entire picture. Another is from the Global Burden of Diseases Study, which revealed some interesting shifting health trends over time and between populations.

They mined enormous mounds of data—from official documents to oral autopsies—and broadly concluded that non-communicable diseases (NCDs) now claim a large proportion of global mortality. As societies change, so do health problems, and lifestyle and environmental determinants appear to be more influential than ever. Public health professionals, by examining these trends through a kind of epidemiological frame of reference, began identifying how ordinary behaviors combine with larger conditions to trigger these diseases. These findings, replicated in study after study, are a reminder that managing our health threats involves examining a messy mixture of variables, informing more focused strategies and policies.

And then there is the ominous issue of antibiotic resistance, where case studies demonstrate just how enmeshed things are. The misuse and overuse of antibiotics—usually the product of patchy healthcare systems and a lack of public enlightenment—allow bacteria to develop resistance overnight. Recent studies indicate that regions with intense agricultural and pharmaceutical use of antibiotics are even more at risk. The interaction between mundane human decisions, the small bacterial mutations, and environmental factors results in the proliferation of these persistent strains, forming severe public health problems. Overall, this situation illustrates that the traditional triangle of host, agent, and environment is more than a theoretical model—it nudges us toward holistic solutions such as improved medical practices, policy reform, and enhanced public education to address today's intricate disease issues.

3.6. Applications of the Epidemiological Triangle

How host, agent, and environment blend into the Epidemiological Triangle can truly highlight how to overcome cancer. In 2014 research in the United States, it was found that approximately 42% of all cancer cases—and around 45% of all cancer deaths—were associated with lifestyle habits that are alterable, such as smoking, obesity, and excessive alcohol consumption (Islami et al., 2017). As it happens, by unraveling these relationships, health workers can identify areas where easy interventions can take place. By focusing on lifestyle adjustments made on a daily basis and tiny modifications in our environments, public policies can reduce cancer statistics significantly. In most situations, this triangle works nearly as a guidepost, reminding us that addressing all three elements is of primary importance to the overall public good. And now, if you turn to infectious diseases, such as scrub typhus in the Asia-Pacific region, the tale emerges in much the same, though distinctively complex way. Its insect, *Orientia tsutsugamushi*, is only found in highly specific environments, which serves to highlight just how the agent and its habitat interact (Xu et al., 2017). Untreated, the mortality rate can reach as high as 70%; in the general sense, that makes familiarity with these bonds all the more important for public health interventions. Tactics here may range from controlling vectors to mobilizing communities around avoiding exposure. When you deduce the knotted relationships between the pathogen, its victims, and the environments it inhabits, researchers and administrators can develop more organic, grassroots methods of reducing infections. Even beyond that, the triangular model sets new avenues for improved tracking and research techniques. By taking a glimpse at the interaction between agent, host, and environment, it becomes simpler to determine which populations are most susceptible and what hazards are most in action. For example, the increasing prevalence of NCDs such as different cancers once again shows that our environment and individual behaviors are intricately interwoven (Islami et al., 2017). With health data—ranging from geographic idiosyncrasies to demographic facts—continuing to improve, so does our understanding of these connections. Overall, this framework not only supports the old-fashioned measures of public health but also generates new, sometimes unorthodox research concepts for eliminating diseases we could do without (Figure 3.10).

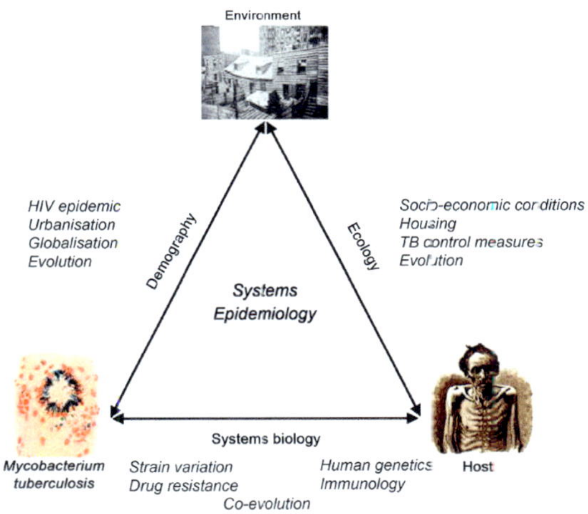

Figure 3.10. Applications of the Epidemiological Triangle.

Source: Gagneux, S. (2009). *A Systems Epidemiology Approach to Tuberculosis, Which Integrates Demography, Ecology, and Systems Biology*. In *The Changing Epidemiology of Tuberculosis*.

3.6.1. Disease Prevention Strategies

Host characteristics, local environments, and even the nature of infections all blend together in ways that make one easy prevention plan effective for nobody. Research indicates, more often than not, that when prevention efforts are tailored to the site, they are more effective. Alzheimer's disease, for instance—researchers have identified more than 200 factors that play a role, ranging from simple social backgrounds to more idiosyncratic psychological oddities. This complex web of factors means that a one-for-all approach simply won't cut it; rather, strategies must be attuned to the rhythm of each community. We even observe this trend with trends within certain developed areas, where reduced rates of dementia appear to be correlated with savvy public health initiatives designed to mitigate these threats (Contador et al., 2024). Knowing infectious disease now challenges us to think past curing one patient at a time. Take *H. pylori*, for instance: although the typical strategy historically emphasized individual therapy alone, in one recent Chinese study of 10,735 families, it was found that infection spread much more freely in and out of families due in large part to environmental factors they share. Typically, simply treating the individual is inadequate; it appears that a move toward family—even community—based care may be required to manage transmission (Zhou et al., 2023).

Community characteristics can reduce disease risks Programs designed to set out daily risks and promote better choices can enable individuals to gradually develop overall community resilience. When we consider the ways socioeconomic disparities shape behavior, it's easier to bring prevention plans together that not only reduce risks but also empower communities to rebound stronger. Also, when experts in various domains—health care, social services, and policy, just to name a few—share ideas, the quest for improved public health is pushed to a new level. With the emphasis on local action and solutions suitable for individual needs, there is the possibility of reducing both infectious and chronic diseases just that much more feasible, bringing it all back beautifully to the very central concepts of the Epidemiological Triangle.

3.6.2. Public Health Policy Development

Disease spread is not just about one factor – many different things end up playing a role, and this mix of influences calls for a pretty thoughtful public health plan. We need models that can roughly guess outbreak patterns so that interventions are not just shots in the dark. Consider Covasim, for example; the public health writing available demonstrates that by replicating the way COVID-19 spreads within communities – mixing in such things as simple demographic information and typical social interactions – it creates a snapshot that allows policy people to view how various measures could play out in given contexts. In short, these models highlight the importance of using real data to make decisions, particularly when you strip things down to the basics: germs, people, and the global environment. Science and informing the public are very important in creating sound health policies – genuinely, it is difficult to emphasize that enough. Go back to efforts such as the simultaneous effort against acid rain in the late 20th century; efforts such as that illustrate how science can push policy into action gradually.

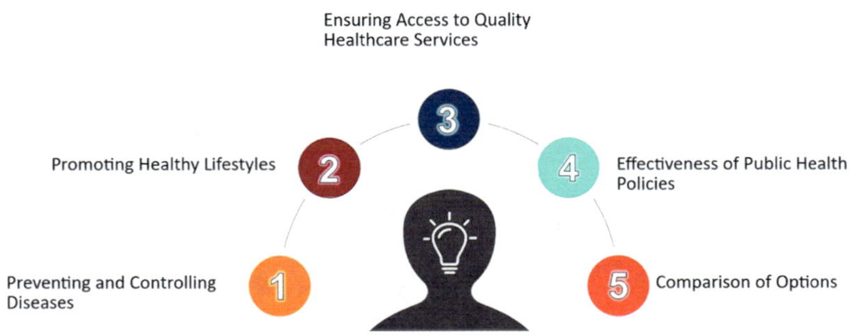

Figure 3.11. Public health policy development.

Source: FasterCapital. (n.d.). *Thriving Nations: The Role of Health Economics in Development & the Role of Public Health Policies in Development.*

Tools such as the UNECE Convention on Long-range Transboundary Air Pollution are a good case of science and policy collaboration, whereby policy traditionally leads and science provides guidelines and becomes an integral part, usually with significant reductions in harmful emissions and some pleasant ecological benefits. Overall, these instances serve as a reminder that consistent research and ongoing surveillance are crucial in making changes to health policy over time, reaffirming the principle of all being interconnected as presented in that Epidemiological Triangle. Secondly, having various groups collaborate most definitely makes a difference when it comes to public health strategies. When you blend in diverse perspectives – from grassroots health organizations to community health groups and other stakeholders – policies turn out to address a variety of health issues that vary between people. At times, building broad frameworks involves engaging these local stakeholders to more closely tailor interventions. See, as the concept of acid rain critical loads brought stakeholders around a common purpose, teamwork demonstrates that when people come together for a common cause, public health efforts become more successful. Ultimately, such collaborations assist decision-makers in untangling the mess of health concerns, utilizing the interrelated factors outlined in the Epidemiological Triangle to create communities that can manage health issues more effectively (Figure 3.11).

3.6.3. Research and Surveillance Methods

Epidemiology is always this delicate waltz that requires pretty cutting-edge methodologies to sift through the messy mechanisms of how diseases get around. It is all about understanding how hosts, agents and environments blend together—basically the nub of what people call the Epidemiological Triangle. One nifty approach is applying Geographic Information Systems (GIS) to chart where diseases emerge. Consider, for instance, a Colombian coffee triangle study published looking at Hepatitis A; it caught subtle, near-invisible trends in case rates between various municipalities. Analysis such as this, with all its nuance, not only increases our total knowledge but enables us to guide public health actions so resources can be targeted precisely where they are required (Atehortua-Otero et al., 2019). And then, of course, there is molecular epidemiology, which is particularly useful when tackling stubborn infections such as multidrug-resistant tuberculosis (MDR-TB). Through the application of technology such as MIRU-VNTR typing (a name that reads much more daunting than it is), scientists can construct transmission maps way beyond what normal contact tracing does. In the majority of instances, a UK national TB surveillance project even reported that a small segment of MDR-TB cases resulted from local spread—yet included that being UK born and injecting drug use had a key role to play. This finding, in broad terms, illustrates just how important molecular data can be in guiding intelligent public health measures (Abubakar et al., 2014). Ultimately, research and monitoring must be adaptive, evidence-based and prepared to pivot as the Epidemiological Triangle brings new obstacles into play. Merging various approaches such as GIS mapping with molecular profiling provides public health staff hints that are practical and insightful. If you combine those in-the-field geographic glimpses with in-laboratory molecular information, you not only identify the hotspots but also capture a richer image of what's igniting outbreaks. Overall, such combined methods assist policymakers in designing more detailed public health strategies to curb the spread of infection at its origin while getting at the root causes (Abubakar et al., 2014; Atehortua-Otero et al., 2019).

CLOSER LOOK

Epidemiological Triangle

The Epidemiological Triangle is an epidemiological model that describes the way diseases are transmitted. It emphasizes the relationship between three entities: the agent, the host, and the environment. It explains how a disease can develop, persist, and be spread from one person to another.

Here is a closer look at each component

- **Agent:** This is the causative agent of the disease, which may be a microorganism (such as bacteria, viruses, fungi, or parasites), a chemical, or a physical force.
- **Host:** This is the organism that carries the disease, which can be human or animal.
- **Environment:** This includes the external conditions affecting the interaction between the host and the agent, ranging from physical and biological to social.

How the Triangle works

The Epidemiological Triangle proposes that disease transmission takes place when all three elements are present and act interactively in a manner that enables the agent to infect the host. For instance, in a respiratory infection, the agent could be a virus, the host would be an individual vulnerable to the infection, and the environment may be the situations under which the virus is transmissible (e.g., crowdedness, poor airflow).

Through knowledge of how these factors interact, public health professionals can plan interventions to avert and manage disease transmission. Interventions, for example, may aim at the agent (e.g., vaccination), the host (e.g., enhancing immune status), or the environment (e.g., hygiene, sanitation).

SUMMARY

The Epidemiological Triangle is not some abstract book idea—it demonstrates how the host, agent, and environment all blend together in ways that immediately impact how disease spreads. This concept has been pretty influential in public health for many scenarios: it's counterintuitively insightful about how these three pieces come together and change the quantities of disease we observe. Consider, for instance, research such as the CARDIA study (Zhao et al., 2024) which suggests a downward trend between exercise and conditions including coronary heart disease and hypertension. In general terms, as we press for physical activity, not only do we nudge behaviors at the level of the individual but also bump up against broader environmental and societal determinants in which the enabling conditions for disease to take its course are constructed. These findings, in general, serve to inform the way we design public health interventions to reduce risk among more vulnerable groups. Examining in closer detail how personal and environmental factors interact, we also gain a richer understanding of health inequities. Investigations in stunting-haunted areas, for example, identify such things as maternal knowledge and even exclusive breastfeeding as the primary factors shaping children's health outcomes (Ummah et al., 2023). Such findings—as not always uncomplicated—guide us to a call for an expanded paradigm within public health that does not only key into disease causation biology but also attends to socio-economic and education-based influences. The adaptive shape of the Epidemiological Triangle allows us to fold in such complexities, giving us a more complete, near-holistic view of what counts for successful health interventions. Such an approach to relating disparate factors can assist professionals to more readily identify and address the systemic inequities that so often keep disease susceptibility simmering in various communities. In the end, what we learn from the Epidemiological Triangle is far more than mere theory—it has implications for future research and policy as well. Further excavation into the dynamics of how hosts, agents, and their environments interact may very well hone our strategies for disease prevention and quantify how effective our efforts are. Given recent evidence, such as the protective effects of exercise against some age-related problems and the large role maternal influences have in child health, there is an evident, urgent need for policymakers to allocate resources more effectively. This change, in turn, facilitates the creation of environments that promote health equity and reduce the total disease burden. The model here not only assists us in identifying risk factors, but it provides a bit of a foundation for broad interventions that account for the dirty, complicated interplay of factors impinging on population health.

Agents, hosts, and the environments in which they reside all combine in ways that matter most to public health. Rather than keeping everything clear and separate, sometimes you will discover that a messy examination of how the pieces fit together uncovers hidden clues, such as how particulates floating in the air in crowded US cities have been shown to contribute to additional respiratory problems. Scientists have observed, for example, that an increase in toxic pollutants is accompanied by additional health issues in individuals, demonstrating that our environment can make us susceptible. Examining disease in this way, by essentially a three-component model called the Epidemiological Triangle, provides an innovative means to recognize patterns and determine interventions that can safeguard communities. Now, the triangle is not confined to human health. Its influence carries over into learning about zoonotic diseases, also. Let us consider research on Border Disease Virus (BDV) in Pyrenean chamois—this research (often traced back through domestic sheep) uncovers a tale of viral evolution and transmission that is not immediately apparent. With techniques such as phylogenetic analysis, researchers have followed transmission patterns that appear to classify isolates by host species, with what animal is involved having the potential to alter the entire picture. These factors—hosts together with changing environmental conditions—provide key clues in the majority of instances on how disease leaps from one species to another (Cabezón et al., 2016). In the end, the Epidemiological Triangle does not merely exist as a clear intellectual concept, but as something that policymakers find themselves employing in actual cases. When politicians approach health issues arising from both nature and biology, they usually end up using this model as a sort of handbook for interpreting the causes of diseases. Think about how, through protracted debates over particulate matter regulation, careful examination of scientific evidence—even in the context of political intrigue—can inform improved standards for health. It appears that untangling the interplay among agent, host and environment is more than abstract; it is a step toward more effective decision-making that can prevent outbreaks and improve overall health.

KEY TERMS FROM THIS CHAPTER

- Epidemiological Triangle
- Environment
- Virus
- Parasite
- Immunity
- Nutrition
- Climate
- Reservoir
- Agent
- Bacteria
- Fungus
- Susceptibility
- Genetics
- Socioeconomic status
- Sanitation
- Intervention

REFERENCES

1. Aboda, C. (2012). An assessment of the impact of climate variability on malaria in Uganda: A study from Mount Elgon region of Bududa district. https://core.ac.uk/download/646175138.pdf (accessed on 6 May 2025).
2. Abubakar, I., Anderson, L. F., Brown, T., Mullarkey, et al. (2014). Transmission of multidrug-resistant tuberculosis in the UK: A cross-sectional molecular and epidemiological study of clustering and contact tracing. *Lancet Infectious Diseases, 14*, 406–415. https://core.ac.uk/download/29416292.pdf (accessed on 6 May 2025).
3. Adler, A., Adler, A., Al Zabadi, A., Alexeeff, A. S., Lewis, A., Bacigalupe, B., Barzyk, et al. (2011). Non-chemical stressors and cumulative risk assessment: An overview of current initiatives and potential air pollutant interactions. *International Journal of Environmental Research and Public Health, 8*(6), 2020–2033. https://doi.org/10.3390/ijerph8062020.
4. Anderson, R. M., Dickinson, K. L., Fowler, V. G., Kramer, et al. (2009). Using decision analysis to improve malaria control policy making. *Health Policy, 92*, 133–140. https://core.ac.uk/download/62565298.pdf (accessed on 6 May 2025).
5. Armand, T., Souquet, M., Pichon, E., & Jacquot, E. (2024). Impact of susceptible wheat cultivars on epidemiological parameters involved in the introduction and spread of wheat dwarf disease. *Plant Pathology*. Retrieved from: https://www.semanticscholar.org/paper/92e7cf55654bf917d242a18529085e68f668aa1d (accessed on 6 May 2025).
6. Atehortua-Otero, M. A., Calvache-Benavides, C. E., Cortes-Madroñero, D. F., Henao, et al. (2019). Medical geography in the study of hepatitis A, in the Coffee-triangle region, Colombia, 2007–2011. https://core.ac.uk/download/299842874.pdf.
7. Batengana, B., Chacha, M., Emidi, B., Kabula, et al. (2011). Detection and monitoring of insecticide resistance in malaria vectors in Tanzania mainland. https://core.ac.uk/download/pdf/11307282.pdf (accessed on 6 May 2025).
8. Battiston, F., Cencetti, G., Iacopini, I., Latora, V., Lucas, M., Patania, A., Young, J. G., et al. (2020). Networks beyond pairwise interactions: Structure and dynamics. *Physics Reports, 874*, 1–92. https://doi.org/10.1016/j.physrep.2020.05.004.
9. Luzzago C, Ebranati E, Cabezón O, Fernández-Sirera L, Lavín S, Rosell R, et al. (2016) Spatial and Temporal Phylogeny of Border Disease Virus in Pyrenean Chamois (*Rupicapra p. pyrenaica*). PLoS ONE 11(12): e0168232. https://doi.org/10.1371/journal.pone.0168232(accessed on 6 May 2025).
10. Culbert, C., Holden, T., Loftin, K. C., Ly, et al. (1993). The application of integrated knowledge-based systems for the biomedical risk assessment intelligent network (BRAIN). https://core.ac.uk/download/pdf/10448038.pdf (accessed on 6 May 2025).
11. Deeb, R., & Eid, S. (2012). The environmental causes of cancer distribution in Syria. 6th International Congress on Environmental Modelling and Software - Leipzig, Germany - July 2012; https://core.ac.uk/download/55777028.pdf (accessed on 6 May 2025).
12. Dobson, A., Donnelly, A., Fitter, A., MacLeod, A., Rytkönen, A., Woods, A., Zocca, A., et al. (2012). Impacts of climate change on plant diseases–opinions and trends. https://core.ac.uk/download/10932891.pdf (accessed on 6 May 2025).

13. Tzoulaki, I., Elliott, P., Kontis, V., & Ezzati, M. (2016). Worldwide Exposures to Cardiovascular Risk Factors and Associated Health Effects: Current Knowledge and Data Gaps. *Circulation, 133*(23), 2314–2333. https://doi.org/10.1161/CIRCULATIONAHA.115.008718 (accessed on 6 May 2025).
14. Fedele, G., González-Domínguez, E., Rossi, V., Salinari, F., et al. (2020). A general model for the effect of crop management on plant disease epidemics at different scales of complexity. *Agronomy, 10*(4), 462. https://core.ac.uk/download/604620243.pdf (accessed on 6 May 2025).
15. Goldsmith, C. F., Medford, A. J., Peterson, A. A., Rose, et al. (2020). Heterogeneity in susceptibility dictates the order of epidemiological models. http://arxiv.org/abs/2005.04704 (accessed on 6 May 2025).
16. Grennfelt, P., Engleryd, A., Forsius, M., Hov, Ø., Rodhe, H., & Cowling, E. B. (2019). Acid rain and air pollution: 50 years of progress in environmental science and policy. *AMBIO, 49*, 849–864. https://doi.org/10.1007/s13280-019-01244-4.
17. Hampson, K., Haydon, D. T., le Roux, K., Mollentze, N., et al. (2014). A Bayesian approach for inferring the dynamics of partially observed endemic infectious diseases from space-time-genetic data. *Proceedings of the Royal Society B: Biological Sciences, 281*(1782), 20133251. https://core.ac.uk/download/20480131.pdf (accessed on 6 May 2025).
18. Illiano, P., Brambilla, R., & Parolini, C. (2020). The mutual interplay of gut microbiota, diet, and human disease. *FEBS Journal, 287*, 833–855. https://doi.org/10.1111/febs.15217.
19. Islami, F., Sauer, A. G., Miller, K. D., Siegel, R. L., Fedewa, S. A., Jacobs, E. J., McCullough, M. L., et al. (2017). Proportion and number of cancer cases and deaths attributable to potentially modifiable risk factors in the United States. *CA: A Cancer Journal for Clinicians, 68*, 31–54. https://doi.org/10.3322/caac.21440.
20. Keeling, M. J., Hollingsworth, T. D., & Read, J. M. (2020). Efficacy of contact tracing for the containment of the 2019 novel coronavirus (COVID-19). *Journal of Epidemiology & Community Health, 74*, 861–866. https://doi.org/10.1136/jech-2020-214051.
21. Kerr, C. C., Stuart, R. M., Mistry, D., Abeysuriya, R., Rosenfeld, K., Hart, G. R., Núñez, R. C., et al. (2021). Covasim: An agent-based model of COVID-19 dynamics and interventions. *PLOS Computational Biology, 17*, e1009149. https://doi.org/10.1371/journal.pcbi.1009149.
22. Lestari, R., & Setyawan, F. E. B. (2021). Holistic-comprehensive approaches to improve nutritional status of children under five years. *Journal of Public Health Research, 10*, 218. https://core.ac.uk/download/401623990.pdf (accessed on 6 May 2025).
23. Mavaddat, N., Michailidou, K., Dennis, J., Lush, M., Fachal, L., Lee, A., Tyrer, J. P., et al. (2018). Polygenic risk scores for prediction of breast cancer and breast cancer subtypes. *The American Journal of Human Genetics, 104*, 21–34. https://doi.org/10.1016/j.ajhg.2018.11.002.
24. Muscillo, A., Pin, P., & Razzolini, T. (2018). Spreading of an infectious disease between different locations. http://arxiv.org/abs/1812.07827 (accessed on 6 May 2025).
25. Ralph, R., Lew, J., Zeng, T., Francis, M. E., Xue, B., Roux, M., Ostadgavahi, A. T., et al. (2020). 2019-nCoV (Wuhan virus), a novel Coronavirus: Human-to-human transmission, travel-related cases, and vaccine readiness. *The Journal of Infection in Developing Countries, 14*, 3–17. https://doi.org/10.3855/jidc.12425.

26. Semianiv, L., Todoriko, Y., & Vyklyuk, D. (2024). Application of geospatial multi-agent system for simulation of different aspects of tuberculosis transmission. *Infusion & Chemotherapy*. Retrieved from: https://www.semanticscholar.org/paper/880d259d2e070b175c7f5ce1fdab6f9ceafe7cd9 (accessed on 6 May 2025).

27. Wurtzer, S., Marechal, V., Mouchel, J. M., Maday, Y., Teyssou, R., Richard, E., Almayrac, J. L., & Moulin, L. (2020). Evaluation of lockdown effect on SARS-CoV-2 dynamics through viral genome quantification in waste water, Greater Paris, France, 5 March to 23 April 2020. *Euro surveillance : bulletin Europeen sur les maladies transmissibles = European communicable disease bulletin*, *25*(50), 2000776. https://doi.org/10.2807/1560-7917.ES.2020.25.50.2000776Xu, G., Walker, D. H., Jupiter, D. C., Melby, P. C., & Arcari, C. M. (2017). A review of the global epidemiology of scrub typhus. *PLoS Neglected Tropical Diseases, 11*, e0006062. https://doi.org/10.1371/journal.pntd.0006062.

28. Zavaleta-Cortijo, C., Ford, J. D., Galappaththi, E. K., Namanya, D. B., Nkwinti, N., George, B., Togarepi, C., et al. (2023). Indigenous knowledge, community resilience, and health emergency preparedness. *The Lancet Planetary Health, 7*, e641–e643. https://doi.org/10.1016/s2542-5196(23)00140-7.

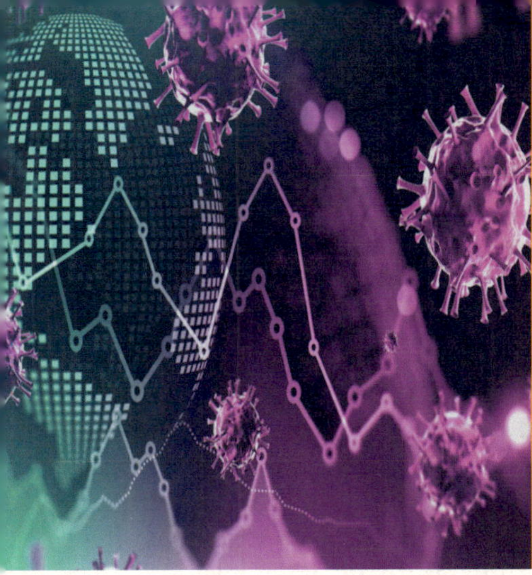

Chapter 4

MATHEMATICAL FOUNDATIONS FOR DISEASE MODELING

Contents

Introduction

Disease dynamics drive public health, guiding how communities respond to outbreaks and distribute resources. Mathematical modeling comes in as a useful ally—it allows scientists to simulate how infections are transmitted and test various intervention strategies. You can observe its value when it comes to difficult diseases such as Ebola or cholera, where it's important to be able to get a handle on transmission. Models not only place a figure on what interventions could ultimately achieve, but they also enable officials to receive a pre-warning about where an epidemic could next be heading. These numerical pointers, arrived at by using analytical models and some number-work, then shape policy and resource decisions that in most situations can soften the grip of a health crisis. At its core, this strategy is intended to put healthcare steps first and protect the public combating contagious diseases. As a model of the transmission of disease, R0—the basic reproduction number—is fairly crucial. This measurement essentially indicates whether or not an infection is going to catch on in a population or wither away; in most instances, if R0 is below one, the disease decays, but if more than one, you are looking at an instance where the infection becomes established. Differential equations and stability analyses assist us in pinning down such numbers and making sense of the state of disease-free equilibrium vs. endemic spread. To illustrate, if you look at Ebola or cholera, you realize quickly that transmission and recovery rates play a crucial role in fine-tuning R0. This sort of simple, but vital, insight enables one to create interventions that not only slow illness but also improve public health communications—keeping the people attentive and prepared. Strong disease modeling does not remain within a single discipline; it intertwines mathematics, biology, and public health. Mixing these areas of study, investigators plunge into intricate situations—from changing population behaviors to the practical impacts of immunization and public outreach. Take cholera for instance: some models investigate how vaccination and better sanitation, as well as daily practices, can redirect disease pathways in unexpected ways. Computational simulations commonly accompany theoretical work, providing a means to visualize possible outbreak patterns in real time—even if the visualization is not always perfectly clear. In the end, these mathematical building blocks not only hold the potential to clarify our current knowledge but also to prepare us for those that lie ahead, even if projections occasionally introduce a little doubt.

Definition of Disease Modeling

Math and epidemiology blend together in a fashion that lies very much at the core of disease modeling—it is all about breaking how infections pass on. We apply math-based simulations to simulate disease transmission through populations, which most of the time provides us with valuable clues regarding transmission patterns and means of curbing outbreaks. A good model will toss variables such as infection rates, speed of recovery, and even the population density of a location into the mix to give experts a sense of direction in which an outbreak will proceed. Models aren't static; they must be able to keep up with new data and shifting circumstances—a glimpse into how inexact real life is. This has to change comes through particularly when emerging diseases strike, as quick changes in the figures can influence public health actions in a significant manner. Finally, what results from these models informs vaccination and quarantine decisions, and where resources are allocated. How to comprehend disease modeling can truly enhance public health work. Take COVID-19, for instance—it forced scientists to change their methods overnight when nothing was normal anymore. Humans soon realized that human behavior has a tremendous role in disease spreading; after all, how we behave can significantly alter transmission rates. It is for this reason that models progressed beyond simple compartment arrangements to more sophisticated, sophisticated models that incorporate behavior patterns and even the dynamics of social networks. Such innovation tends to highlight the value of continuous innovation, ensuring our approaches are as up-to-date as possible. As our understanding of disease dynamics improves, so does the multi-layered intricacy of the models designed to examine them—demonstrating that a solid foundation in the mathematics underlying these systems is absolutely essential for scientists and policymakers attempting to mitigate the impact of outbreaks. Combining disparate theoretical perspectives in disease modeling truly enriches the landscape, paving the way for better predictions and improved interventions. The latest COVID-19 challenge demonstrated the way that models from SEIR (Susceptible-Exposed-Infectious-Recovered) configurations to agent-based models each contributed to crisis management. Which model you wind up utilizing generally hinges on the disease's idiosyncrasies and the exact nature of the outbreak. And drawing upon data from everywhere—whether that's hospitals, official health reports, or even social media discussion—helps make models more robust and responsive. This mixture of diverse data feeds gives close-to-real-time insights into the movement of diseases, resulting in projections that are apt to be on the money. To summarize, the interaction between mathematics and epidemiology not only enriches insights into illnesses but also enables informed decision-making during epidemic outbreaks, once more demonstrating why the firm mathematical underpinnings are so crucial in disease modeling.

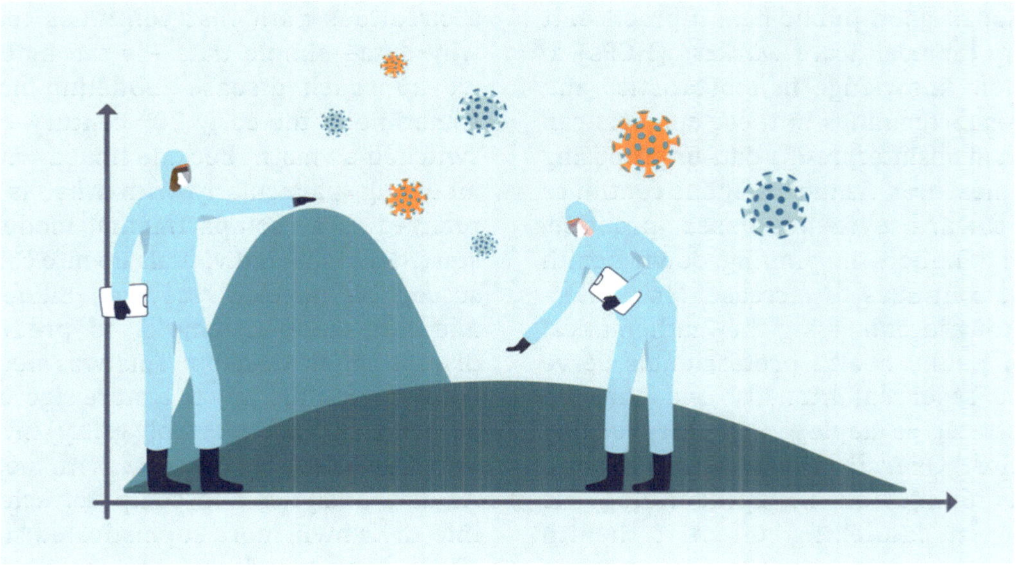

Source: https://caltechsites-prod.s3.amazonaws.com/scienceexchange/images/Modeling-lower-res.2e16d0ba.fill-933x525-c100.png

Importance of Mathematics in Epidemiology

Epidemiology illustrates how mathematics and public health intersect in surprising ways. It relies on simple number tools to understand the spread of disease through populations. Models such as the SIR (Susceptible-Infected-Recovered) model commonly serve as go-to maps, allowing officials to draw out what could occur with various interventions. This type of foresight assists in not only developing where resources can be directed, but also coming up with measures to maintain the spread of disease in control. Biostatistics, being but a specialized study of statistics, also demonstrates how number-crunching can unveil definite information about how prevalent illness is and how much danger it poses. Without a strong math foundation, studies could easily go off track and spend effort and money on methods that lack sufficient support from actual data (Lee et al., 2019). New health threats—whether it is an unexpected pandemic or increasing antibiotic resistance—make it even more apparent that mathematics has an even larger part to play today. In most instances, sophisticated computer methods and massive data analytics have turned the tide, allowing researchers to solve issues that previously only appeared too daunting. By analyzing massive amounts of data from various healthcare sources, these algorithms cut the precision of predictions and models. A firm grasp of statistics and how it can bridge cause and risk allows epidemiologists to chart through the murky waters of uncertainty, making their conclusions feel as natural as they are trustworthy. Altogether, this mathematical core not only underpins major studies but also inspires the development of original solutions to public health emergencies (Dunjko et al., 2018). Without precise models, our attempts at combating contemporary outbreaks could readily fail. At the core of it all, hiding math deep in the work of epidemiology builds a critical pillar of good public health practice. It is necessary for healthcare workers (HCPs) to develop their knowledge in biostatistics and modeling—shortcomings in these subjects can easily result in misinterpreting data or proposing ineffective measures. As the discipline continues to move toward evidence-based practice, the role of numbers in pinning down health results just continues to increase. Most often, measures toward enhancing the mathematical abilities of public health professionals serve to increase research intensity and sharpen practical strategies deployed in safeguarding communities. Overall, establishing a solid numerical foundation in epidemiology is imperative in launching effective health initiatives that reduce disease and increase overall community welfare (Lee et al., 2019).

4.1. Historical Context of Disease Modeling

Disease modeling dates back to when individuals first began employing rudimentary number-crunching to comprehend how illness was transmitted. At that time, a few early minds, such as John Snow, whom many refer to as the father of modern epidemiology—experimented with collecting data and hand-drawing maps to identify the cholera epidemic in London during the 19th century. His meticulous case mapping, not at all lacking a dash of intuitive sense, showed that where individuals resided tended to be connected with where the illness emerged. Subsequently, employing instruments such as regression analysis (you know, the sort that introduces many variables into play) permitted scientists to construct models that grew increasingly complex with time. Years passed, and those original approaches evolved into potent means of determining just how diseases were transmitted through populations, which in a vast majority led to more pointed public health responses. It is a circuitous path that continues to highlight why data—simple data—is the blood of how we approach disease modeling now. Then, sometime in the early 20th century, everything switched as math became linked with disease modeling, particularly with what is currently referred to as compartmental models. People started dividing individuals up into categories—susceptible, infected, recovered (SIR for short)—and this made it simpler to predict how a disease might develop. This was not merely a theory; it led the way to a more rigorous (albeit occasionally uncomfortably gritty) investigation into how diseases interact with populations. As data analytics and computer science came into their own, more sophisticated simulations with clever algorithms became de rigueur in outbreak planning, allowing experts to test out various scenarios to see what could occur. One could argue that this constant development in mathematical modeling is a testament to our continued quest to better understand diseases, even as the world becomes slightly more interconnected. Disease modeling today is married to new technology and innovative methods that blend traditional concepts with entirely new ones. Consider the Digital Twin idea, for example—a technology that, in most instances, provides real-time simulations that replicate physical processes in our health systems. Sure, the Digital Twin means different things in different circles, but its usefulness in modeling disease dynamics is becoming hard to ignore. Its 13 identified characteristics, for example, create a rather robust framework to explore how the tangible and virtual worlds intersect during a health crisis. While the whole terrain of disease modeling continues to change, there is definite need for further research cutting across boundaries and a little willingness to admit to uncertainties—making sure that future models are not only founded on firm theory but can also balance the grubby niceties of real life (Jones et al., 2020; Najjar, 2023) (Figure 4.1).

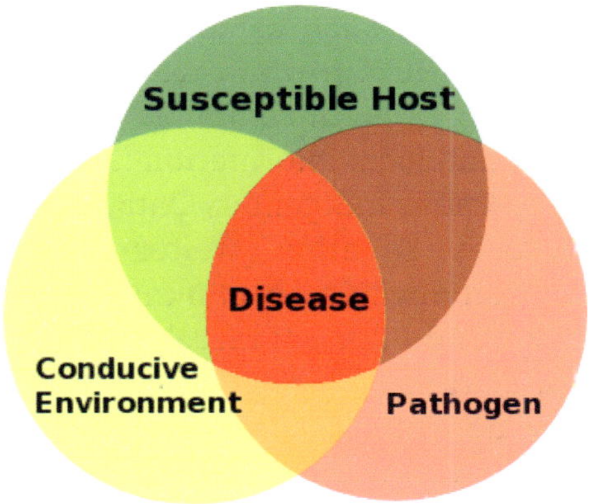

Figure 4.1. Historical context of disease modeling.

Source: By Earlycj5 - Own work, CC BY-SA 3.0, https://commons.wikimedia.org/w/index.php?curid=3674648

4.1.1. Early Models and Their Impact

In the early times, disease modeling started with simple mathematics that attempted to quantify the transmission of infections across communities. The initial concepts, while fairly simple about what we currently have, still managed to illustrate how contagion functions to summarize. Take the SIR model—Susceptible, Infected, recovered—as one reliable example; it connects different population groups and even predicts an outbreak's trajectory. This type of groundwork provided public health leaders with a means of formulating plans to stem infections and more effectively control scarce resources. Over time, as our understanding of both biological complexities and daily human dynamics increased, these models developed organically, underscoring their continued relevance in contemporary epidemiological studies (Adhikari et al., 2020). Individuals from other fields contributed to refining those early models, demonstrating that combining expertise truly makes a difference when it comes to tracing disease transmission. Biostatistics, for instance, is more than simply working with numbers; it provides actionable ways to wade through and interpret epidemic data, making a model's prediction more reliable. When crises like the COVID-19 pandemic came along, the necessity for more sophisticated approaches became painfully obvious. By combining knowledge of behavior, the environment, and traditional medicine, these collaborative projects enabled the development of models that were flexible and better attuned to actual conditions. In the majority of instances, the incorporation of biostatistical knowledge into initial disease models represented a major leap in the battle against infections (Lee et al., 2019).

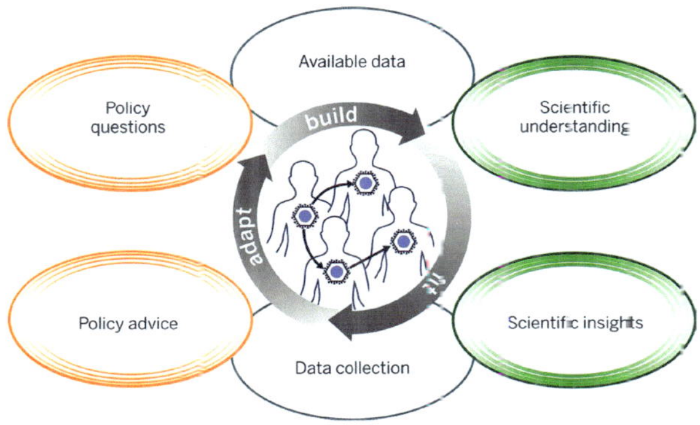

Figure 4.2. Early models and their impact.

Source: American Association for the Advancement of Science. (2015). A new approach to the study of the molecular basis of the immune response. *Science, 347*, 347.

In retrospect, the history of early disease models has a rather fascinating story to tell regarding public health and infection control. Improvements in computing power and the deluge of data available moved things from crude math to sophisticated simulations that can now capture the messy, multifaceted reality of outbreaks. Contemporary methods rely on massive datasets to hone predictions and fill in gaps observed in their earlier, simpler versions. In times of crisis, such as the recent pandemic, the demand for rapid, trustworthy models has never been clearer. Overall, this development—from simple equations to complex simulations—is a testament to the importance of solid disease modeling in protecting public health (Adhikari et al., 2020) (Figure 4.2).

4.1.2. Key Figures in the Development of Mathematical Epidemiology

Looking back over the history of using math to study diseases, a few names stand out. Ronald Ross, working in the early 1900s on malaria, did some surprisingly straightforward work that set the stage for how we see infections today. He figured out a way to link mosquito numbers to malaria cases, showing us that nature's uniqueness matter when you try to predict disease behavior. His initial concepts enabled him to bring math together with the imperfect reality of nature—concepts that, for the most part, provided policymakers with a clearer idea of how to fight off outbreaks. If not for Ross's combination of calculation and gut, our responses to epidemics may have appeared radically different. Next is George MacDonald, who sort of did the opposite by centering numbers up front. He combined day-to-day statistics with sound biological knowledge (occasionally even with a dash of on-the-scene observation) to describe how diseases like malaria would spread. MacDonald added the concept that we today refer to as the basic reproduction number, R0, a measure that enabled scientists to quantify just how infectious diseases were. Through the integration of information from clinical trials and field observations into his models, he provided a new perspective on the linkage between theory and practice—a linkage that continues to direct intervention efforts today, even if sometimes with the additional steps and slight tabulations. Now, the insights from those early visionaries still reappear as the debates about global health issues rage on. For instance, in the case of concerns such as antimicrobial resistance (AMR), research, such as that mentioned in Coque et al. (2023)—indicates that a solid understanding of math combined with culture, economics, and local information is imperative. Examining where Indigenous Data Sovereignty comes into the equation (Walter et al., 2020) indicates that engaging communities in health data stewardship doesn't merely incorporate a social spin but in fact, refines the models upon which we depend. The majority of the time, getting all of those factors to work together is a matter of having responses to disease that are not just about numbers but also honor the actual-world necessities of individuals, even if the process isn't always neatly clean.

4.1.3. Evolution of Models Through the 20th Century

Revolutionary developments in mathematics modeling in the 20th century truly rattled our perception of biology. In the beginning, models made fixed numbers and linear relations when considering something like simple population trends. These simple methods gave us a handle on disease transmission, even though they were rather basic. But as we pushed further into the sloppy details of living systems, it was apparent that more sophisticated methods were required. That is when models that accommodate randomness began to emerge, dealing with the natural variability in biological data better than their strict ancestors. This shift from being so overly simplistic in our approaches to ones that are capable of tolerating a little bit of randomness has become an ongoing effort to better our projections and catch what is happening in disease dynamics. Around the same time, toward the close of the century, computers started revolutionizing the construction and validation of these models. AI began infiltrating medicine, particularly with respect to how we examine disease. Instead of depending exclusively on numbers by hand and elementary theories, specialists started applying algorithms that were capable of processing gigantic sets of numbers. As stated in Najjar (2023), machine learning and deep learning unveiled new avenues for close-up image analysis and even enabled predictions for results in radiology. These new technologies not only more accurately diagnosed but also enabled treatment plans to be individualized for every person. The union of powerful algorithms with fundamental concepts from epidemiology reveals the extent to which computational power and conventional mathematics can collaborate in addressing health problems. At the same time, as technology became smarter and theories became deeper, individuals began fretting about the moral side of all this modeling stuff. With increasing dependence on such complex algorithms—occasionally regarded as impenetrable black boxes—issues regarding data quality, bias, and fairness soon arose. The issue that some models do not precisely demonstrate how they function can cause serious issues about accountability. One finds the suggestion that solutions to these challenges come from cooperating—math specialists, clinicians, and AI coders must cooperate together to use technology in sensible ways. Fighting through these issues is not simply about improving models; it is also about our ethical standards keeping up with innovation, ultimately leading to policies that connect sound mathematical concepts to actual health impacts in a manner that simply makes sense (Najjar, 2023) (Figure 4.3).

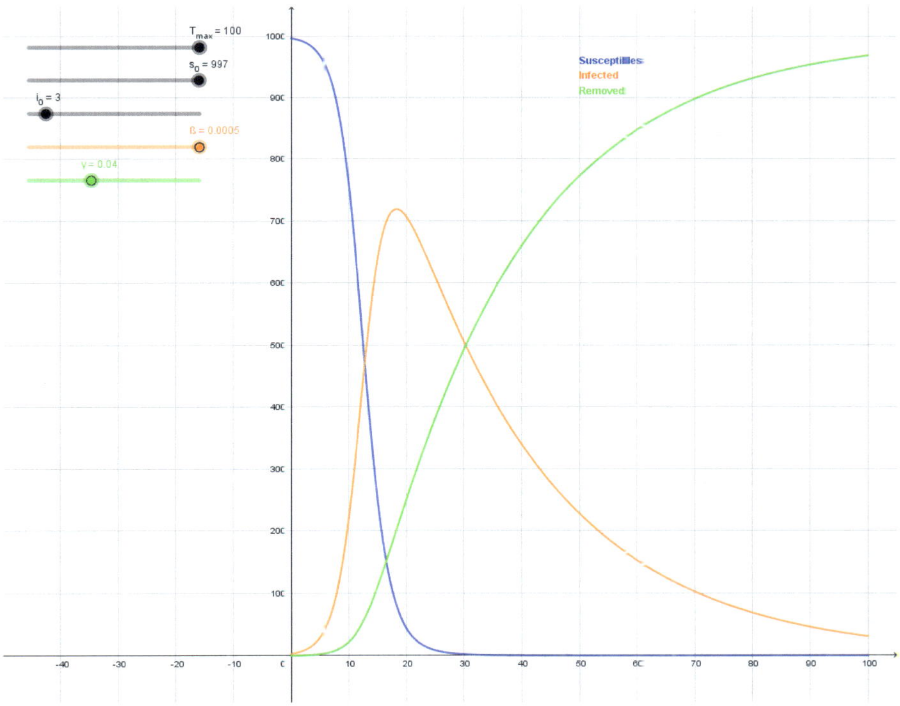

Figure 4.3. Evolution of models through the 20th century.

Source: https://en.wikipedia.org/wiki/Mathematical_modelling_of_infectious_diseases#/media/File:SIR_model_anim.gif https://media.springernature.com/lw1200/springer-static/image/art%3A10.1007%2Fs40139-020-00213-x/MediaObjects/40139_2020_213_Fig1_HTML.png

4.2. Basic Mathematical Concepts in Epidemiology

Math provides the basis for epidemiology—it is what allows us to model how diseases spread among populations and experiment with potential control strategies. The central concepts—rates, ratios, and proportions—appear as common-sense tools for interpreting how disease acts. Rates, for instance, allow researchers to determine how frequently a disease manifests over time, whereas ratios and proportions simplify comparisons across groups. In a sense, these straightforward constructs identify which populations may be at increased risk and pave the way for intervention when an outbreak occurs. Accurately getting those numbers involves relying heavily on sound statistical thinking. For this role, biostatistics—a combination of math and statistics—comes to the forefront, extracting useful meaning from health data. In general, being able to see is most important, particularly when dealing with new diseases where hiccups in biostatistical processes have sometimes resulted in muddled data analysis and public health misjudgments (Lee et al., 2019). The more the norm becomes for big data and sophisticated disease models, the more a plunge into higher mathematics is necessary. Models such as the SIR (Susceptible-Infected-Recovered) model reveal the interdependence of population dynamics and disease spread. This framework—and its many modifications—illuminates how factors such as contact rates and recovery times influence the course of an infection within a population. Quantitative techniques, when used judiciously, enable predictions of the effects of interventions such as vaccination or quarantine. In the majority of instances, as research becomes increasingly sophisticated, there is an increasingly evident demand for individuals who can manage both rigorous statistical analysis and innovative computational methods. This focus on biostatistics not only keeps methods in line but also intensifies the understanding discovered in epidemiological research (Dunjko et al., 2018). At the end of the day, a strong understanding of mathematical concepts is imperative for anyone looking to make a difference in public health. The disease modeling landscape is shifting quickly—older methods must adapt to address issues such as genomic data and the complex interactions within communities. Training programs must devote additional resources to biostatistics and mathematics to enable future health workers to navigate the data maze and derive meaningful insights. A solid foundation in these topics also steers clear of the booby traps of "cargo-cult statistics," that crafty menace that can invalidate good scientific work. With an actual dedication to sound biostatistical education, the discipline can avoid systematic errors, enhance study quality, and, in the end, enhance medical outcomes globally (Lee et al., 2019) (Figure 4.4).

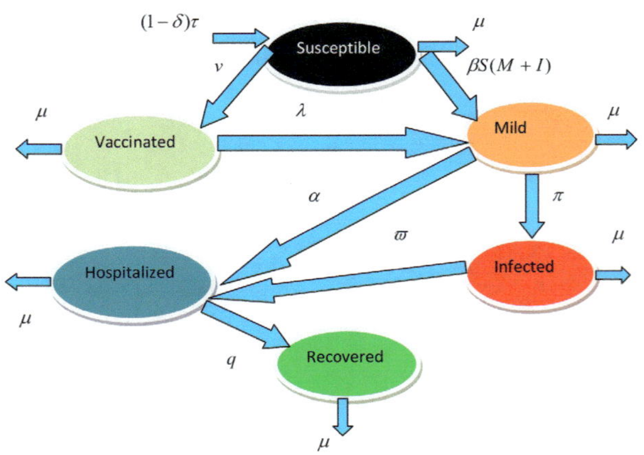

Figure 4.4. Basic mathematical concepts in epidemiology.

Source: Haq IU, Ullah N, Ali N, Nisar KS. A New Mathematical Model of COVID-19 with Quarantine and Vaccination. Mathematics. 2023; 11(1):142. https://doi.org/10.3390/math11010142

4.2.1. Differential Equations and Their Applications

It's not easy to deal with disease transmission; that's why people resort to differential equations. These mathematical tools provide us with a good means of simulating how various components of an outbreak interact in the real world. Scientists apply them to take a glimpse at how fast a disease can spread, what impact control measures can make, and what can happen to entire populations over time. Consider the SIR model, for instance—it distinguishes populations into Susceptible, Infected, and Recovered categories, allowing us to measure infection and recovery rates over time. This is not merely a matter of getting a grasp on the short-term effect of an illness; it also enables us to more accurately project future outbreaks and compare which interventions are most effective. With healthcare issues evolving nearly day by day, fine-tuning these models is well-nigh a necessity for targeted, efficient action. Artificial intelligence (AI) is filling the gap too, giving a new spin to our traditional math approaches. AI algorithms now assist in strengthening differential equation models so that they become more intelligent when they consider the intricate details of biological systems. In the majority of instances, chucking enormous amounts of data into the equation allows AI to unearth subtle trends that more conventional means may readily overlook.

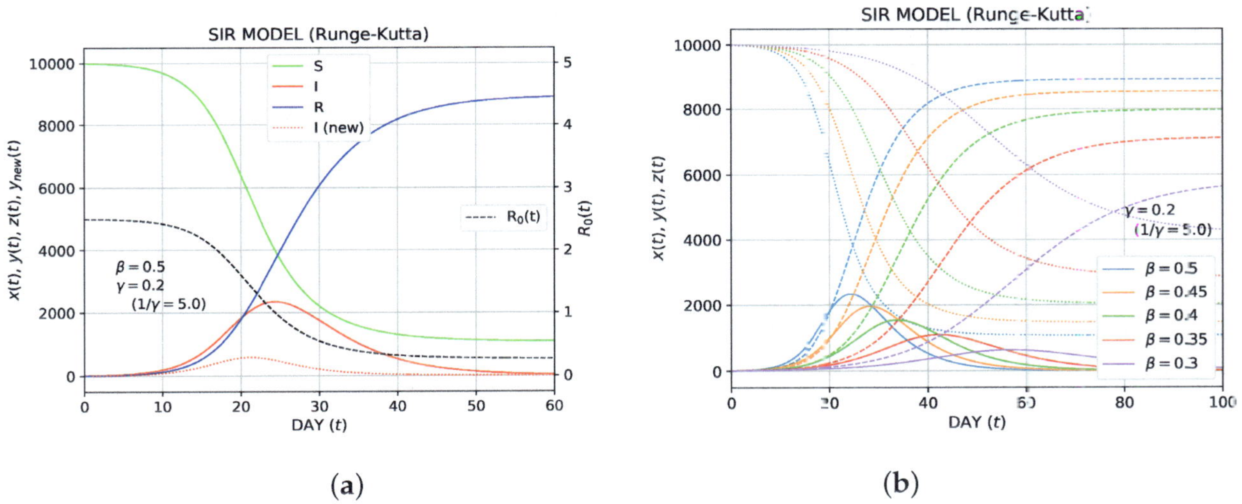

Figure 4.5. Differential equations and their applications.

Source: Okabe Y, Shudo A. A Mathematical Model of Epidemics—A Tutorial for Students. Mathematics. 2020; 8(7):1174. https://doi.org/10.3390/math8071174

By mending hard facts with the gritty complexity of biology, AI does not just aid in quicker diagnostics of challenges but also flattens decision-making for public health interventions. This type of collaboration between differential equations and AI revs up the accuracy of our disease spread predicts and makes plans for intervention somewhat clearer as a whole (Ezanno et al., 2021). Outside of the world of healthcare, these equations extend into economics as well. A fairly recent framework even incorporates theories of disease dynamics and wealth flow models to explain how pandemics can destabilize economic systems. Through kinetic equations, scientists investigate how gain and loss change as diseases unfold—discovering that an epidemic does more than play havoc with health; it can also undermine the distribution of wealth among various groups in society.

In general, although disease models prefer to concentrate on health outcomes, they end up demonstrating to us that socioeconomic factors usually get caught in the crossfire, sometimes even exacerbating already present inequalities. By examining such multifaceted relationships with differential equations, researchers can understand the whole scenario of health as well as economic repercussions in a better manner, which is conducive to greater, more equal policy solutions toward reducing pandemic effects (Dimarco et al., 2020) (Figure 4.5).

4.2.2. Probability Theory in Disease Spread

Probability theory is a large part of it when you consider the way diseases are transmitted—it is not purely theoretical math. Statistical techniques allow us to estimate how frequently an outbreak would occur, and that data provides public health officials with the ammunition to intervene. A nice trick is applying Bayesian MCMC to determine estimates for stuff such as infection and cure rates, which are important in monitoring disease transmission. Surprisingly, these concepts are not trapped in one box; they have also been applied by researchers to monitor how buzz is transmitted on Twitter, similar to how an infection spreads through a crowd (Skaza et al., 2015). This blend of live data with mathematics, it turns out, tells us that sometimes, numbers can be the magic ingredient in addressing health emergencies and unraveling complicated webs. Disease spread models aren't quite the same anymore. Previously, individuals tended to employ compartment models that examined only simple measures such as infection, recovery, and immunity, a pretty simplistic approach, in general. But it's been a decade, and models have changed; new models draw inspiration from graph theory and network dynamics, attempting to get at the messy way people interact. These adjustments have provided us with a greater sense of how our social connections drive infections around, and the predictions have become significantly sharper. Today, models even account for varying modes of transmission and how carriers act, which is rather crucial in our interconnected world. This combination of probability and network analysis has ignited new research into the messy intricacies of epidemics (Kuperman et al., 2013). Probability theory is not just about crunching numbers—it sets the stage for smart disease control. When officials get a grip on what might happen, they can zero in on strategies that cut down spread. For example, digging into probability patterns helps decide who should get vaccines first based on how likely they are to get sick and pass it on. Modeling alternative outbreak situations also allows individuals to prepare for anything, increasing the overall resilience of our health infrastructures. The interplay between mathematics and real-world modeling continues to refine our ability to predict and curb disease transmission. As things continue to evolve, more studies and new math methods will always be pivotal in battling emerging health risks in our globalized world (Kuperman et al., 2013; Skaza et al., 2015).

4.2.3. Statistical Methods for Data Analysis

Strong statistical methods are the foundation upon which disease modeling is built—it's difficult to emphasize this enough. Scientists mining health data must employ a combination of techniques instead of trusting the standard figures. Simple measures such as accuracy and F1 scores read well on paper, but fall flat when datasets are skewed; you cannot always rely on them. Take the Matthews correlation coefficient (MCC): it monitors all categories in a confusion matrix, providing a more holistic picture of model performance. This is generally an enhancing force for the validity of binary classification tasks and allows scientists to extract insights that matter, which is quite important in biomedical research and public health programs (Chicco & Jurman, 2020). Data analysis in biostatistics is not as straightforward as selecting the appropriate metric; it is more a matter of interweaving a larger framework, particularly with the era of big data in full bloom. Statistical thinking—essentially a convenient toolkit—allows researchers to uncover meaning from messy and uncertain data. In areas like epidemiology and bioinformatics, these techniques underpin advances in research—they inform everything from study design to the making of sound conclusions from clinical trials. In general terms, combining contemporary statistical methods into disease modeling doesn't only respond to current health issues; it opens the door for changing methods that are both reliable and accurate (Lee et al., 2019). The dance between theory and practice is one of the primary drivers in developing disease modeling. Biostatistical training is critical; it does not merely increase your math crunching ability but also enhances your understanding of the underlying math. Many reviews suggest when training is suboptimal, researchers tend to misinterpret data, resulting in unforeseen consequences for public health initiatives. Closing that gap between theoretical knowledge and its application creates a more nimble scientific community, one able to navigate the intricacies of contemporary health information. Ultimately, investment in both education and research in biostatistics not only fortifies the general quality of health research but also ensures that the research outputs benefit public health policy and everyday practice tangibly (Lee et al., 2019) (Figure 4.6).

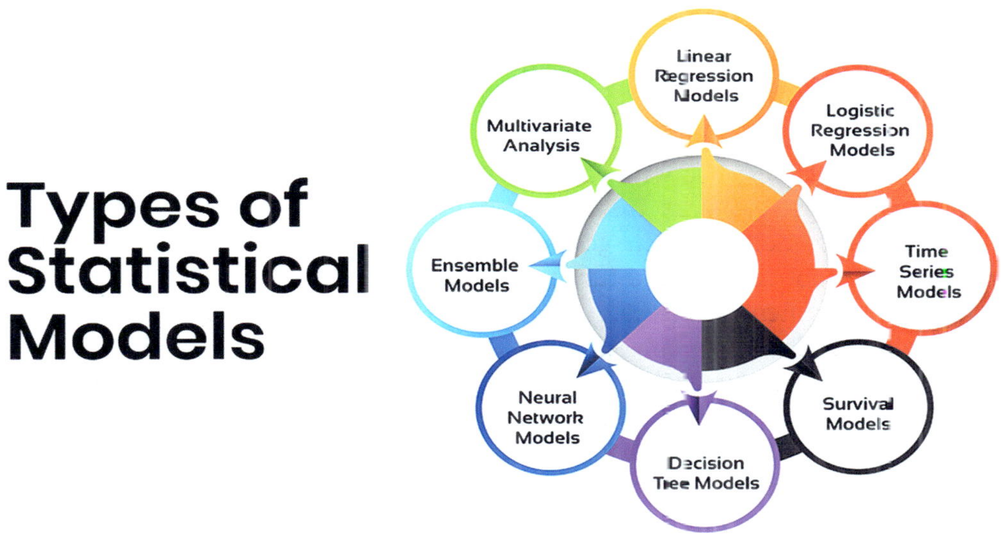

Figure 4.6. Statistical methods for data analysis.

Source: Data Science Council of America (DASCA). (n.d.). *Types of Statistical Models.*

4.3. Types of Disease Models

Disease dynamics don't come with a clear recipe—instead, they challenge us to divide up modeling into compartments that address various research problems and public health challenges. Compartmental models, for example, are ubiquitous in epidemiology; they divide up a population into pieces such as susceptible, infected, and recovered, and this allows us to follow the course of infections over time. These models rely on ordinary differential equations to demonstrate, very simply, how fluctuations in transmission or recovery rates destabilize disease spread. In the majority of instances, when diseases such as COVID-19 are in the equation, understanding how these groups interact is crucial for informing intervention strategies and public health policy (Adhikari et al., 2020). Plus, their ability to mimic everything from steady endemic situations to full-blown epidemics makes them useful in a range of contexts. Switching gears a bit, stochastic models offer a livelier view of disease spread. Unlike those deterministic models that always churn out the same results from fixed starting points, stochastic approaches throw in a dose of randomness and variability to capture the messy unpredictability inherent in biology. This increased randomness makes a big difference when individual actions and interactions are highly variable. For instance, when you consider outbreaks, a stochastic model can suggest a range of possible outcomes, allowing public health people to estimate risks associated with various intervention approaches. In most instances, such models enter into action when general parameters simply do not capture the turns of nonlinear disease dynamics, particularly now that personalized medicine is gaining traction (Lee et al., 2019). Agent-based models, however, get down to the nitty-gritty by modeling each individual's behavior within a population. They allow researchers to incorporate quotidian details such as age, geography, and even offbeat social habits into models, adding greater texture to models of disease transmission. The appeal here is to watch a whole variety of individual behaviors tilt the overall view in aggregate. Consider modeling vaccination distribution: several people holding out may just edge out herd immunity. As one tries out different strategies, these models bring forth possibilities that are difficult to reproduce in the real world. Generally, as our knowledge about public health continues to expand and embrace the combination of numerous small variables, these simulations become indispensable to develop informed responses (Adhikari et al., 2020).

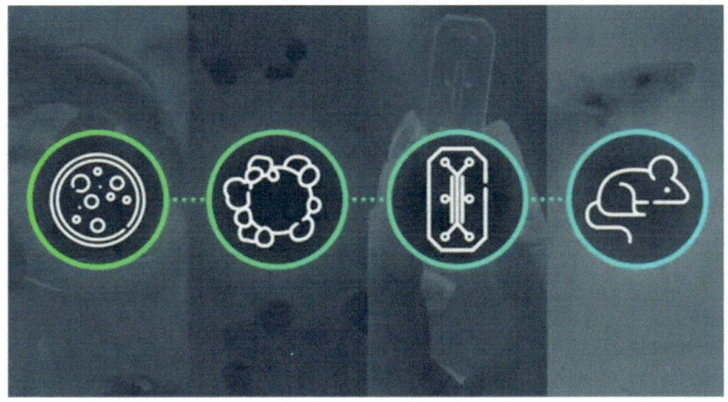

Source: https://images.contentstack.io/v3/assets/blte41c17d7f8dda379/blt23a7faf2c72da751/64e5089404539b87f05ab3b6/BlogHeader_A.png?format=pjpg&quality=70&auto=webp&width=560

4.3.1. Deterministic Models and Their Characteristics

Deterministic models are at the center of disease modeling—they provide a clear system for working out how diseases get around. They are based on set parameters and initial conditions, so you come out with conclusions that are relatively easy to predict, which is very helpful in terms of planning public health interventions. Compared to stochastic models—those that throw in randomness and variability—deterministic ones provide a simple, near-mathematical image of how an infection could spread through a population. They rely on assumptions such as constant transmission rates and that everybody mixes in the same manner, allowing specialists to formulate certain equations relating to different factors; this, in turn, enables them to develop intervention plans tailored to specific health situations. Major characteristics of such models come into action every time they are applied to analyze disease dynamics. For instance, differential equations are usually applied to chart how the numbers of susceptible, infected, and recovered individuals evolve over time. This rigorous mathematical underpinning provides scientists with an opportunity to test various strategies—perhaps adjusting parameters to understand how vaccination or social distancing would perform in reality. Sure, assuming a uniformly mixed population does not always line up with reality, but the clarity of these models still offers valuable insights into how control measures might affect an outbreak. That clear-cut depiction makes it easier to share risk assessments and outcomes with decision-makers like public health officials and policymakers, generally speaking. While deterministic models do have some very attractive advantages, they do have some drawbacks one cannot discount. Their dependence on static parameters may ultimately reduce complex, heterogeneous populations to simplistic levels. Factors such as environmental factors, changing individual behaviors, and the intricacies of social networks tend to introduce variability that these models may not account for. Therefore, while they perform a great service in pointing out some trends and possible effects in disease transmission, employing them alone may not provide the whole picture; sometimes it is better to combine them with stochastic models. In the majority of instances, additional investigation is required—investigating enhancements to deterministic techniques and even combining them with sophisticated instruments such as machine learning—to make more precise predictions and handle the ominous realities of real-world epidemiology better (Dunjko et al., 2018; Hussain et al., 2020).

4.3.2. Stochastic Models and Their Significance

Biological systems are nothing if not full of surprises, and disease dynamics don't adhere to some clear rulebook. What we require are models that can keep up with the surprise turns such systems often throw at us; hence, stochastic models step into the frame, adding random variables into the equation to reflect the randomness of how diseases transmit, mutate, and sometimes just disappear. These methods allow us to simulate a variety of "what if" situations illustrating varied outcomes in shifting scenarios. By accepting randomness, scientists gain better control over outbreak risks and can experiment with which intervention moves will be most effective. Consequently, these findings end up being quite important for public health planning—they are suggestions about the type of resources and hospital configurations that may be needed when epidemics, or even pandemics, strike. Consider how stochastic models have become absolutely essential when working with real-time data during outbreaks of infectious diseases. When the COVID-19 crisis hit, researchers reached for these techniques to predict anything from new case numbers to death tolls each day for different time ranges in the future. As a general rule, even predicting results a matter of only a few days in the future has been an actual game-changer when it comes to resource distribution and public reaction; it is a combination of history with a little bit of luck. Deep learning technologies, including LSTM and GRU, have also been married into the process, putting their own spin on infection trend predictions, while their stochastic versions assist in smoothing out the unclear uncertainties of raw data. By combining older datasets with new random information, policymakers discovered a potent tool to combat outbreaks like COVID-19. It's not only a matter of predicting where a disease is going next—there is much to discover about what's going on beneath the surface. Running a range of 'what if' scenarios, such models highlight who could be particularly at risk, identify possible super-spreader events, and even show how modest adjustments to our daily routines can impact the spread. As modeling paradigms change and begin to incorporate new developments in data analysis and AI, it becomes more and more crucial that we can communicate these intricate outputs in simple terms. Explainable artificial intelligence (XAI) techniques, for example, serve to narrow the gap by making sure that decision-makers and experts alike can understand how all of these stochastic predicts aggregate together. This sort of openness—though having some rough edges along the way—establishes the trust basis for good judgment amid health emergencies (Ayoobi et al., 2021; Dwivedi et al., 2022) (Figure 4.7).

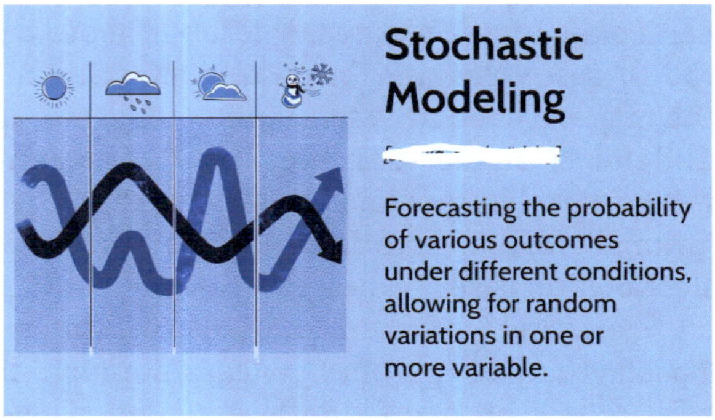

Figure 4.7. Stochastic models and their significance.

Source: Investopedia. (n.d.). *Stochastic Modeling.*

4.3.3. Agent-Based Models and Their Applications

Infection spread is complicated and messy, and cookie-cutter models just can't capture its turns. Agent-based models—abbreviated as ABMs—are what step in instead, assigning each "agent" its own personality and habits. You see how small, daily choices accumulate to create big picture consequences in the course of the disease. This additional information not only assists us in working out the nuances of an outbreak but also identifies spots where an urgent intervention could truly make a difference.

For instance, in times of outbreaks, ABMs have been employed to monitor how disease makes its way through communities, allowing decision-makers to observe the potential ripple impact of various containment strategies. During a period where quick responses are required to ward off new public health threats, these models hold their own (Jones et al., 2020). Once you get into epidemiological research, ABMs aren't merely simulating disease transmission—they are more like an experimental ground for hypotheses regarding the way diseases spread. Old-fashioned models tend to model everyone the same, but real life ain't that neat; how we interact, our habits, and even the social networks we are part of make a huge difference. Scientists can incorporate things like age, levels of income, and the way people get around their day, and they can all shift the story of the spread of a disease. And as you can watch how specifically targeted interventions—a vaccination campaign, for instance, or a period of mandatory social distancing—are applied to selected communities, that support a high degree of policy decisions in public health (Hussain et al., 2020).

And there's the complete data aspect, I suppose. With the contemporary technologies such as the Internet of Things, those algorithms get the real-time minutiae regarding whereabouts of individuals and where they are concerning their physical state—at times in true time. This continuous flow of information forms a kind of feedback loop where subtle adjustments in the model are reflected instantaneously in the results we observe. And now, with machine learning and AI being added to the equation, ABMs are becoming increasingly adept at identifying potential epidemics and adjusting strategies to prevent them. It's not simply about being able to foretell events more precisely; it's about being able to respond to a wide range of health issues, whether that's chronic disease management or abrupt, sudden outbreaks. Mixing proven mathematics with cutting-edge technology showcases the way malleable methods can be our greatest friends in the battle against disease (Jones et al., 2020).

4.4. Key Mathematical Models in Disease Dynamics

Math models are now at the forefront of unraveling the way infections spread. Scientists tend to model the spread of disease through populations to catch the important clues about transmission. You find methods such as the SIR model (Susceptible, Infected, Recovered) and its companion SEIR (Susceptible, Exposed, Infected, Recovered) which map the course from health to illness and vice versa. Such simulation assists in tracing outbreaks, and it also provides public health professionals with a good foundation for making decisions on interventions. For instance, when handling vaccine-preventable illnesses, such models emphasize why one should be vaccinated on time and prioritize high-risk zones (Shankar et al., 2024).

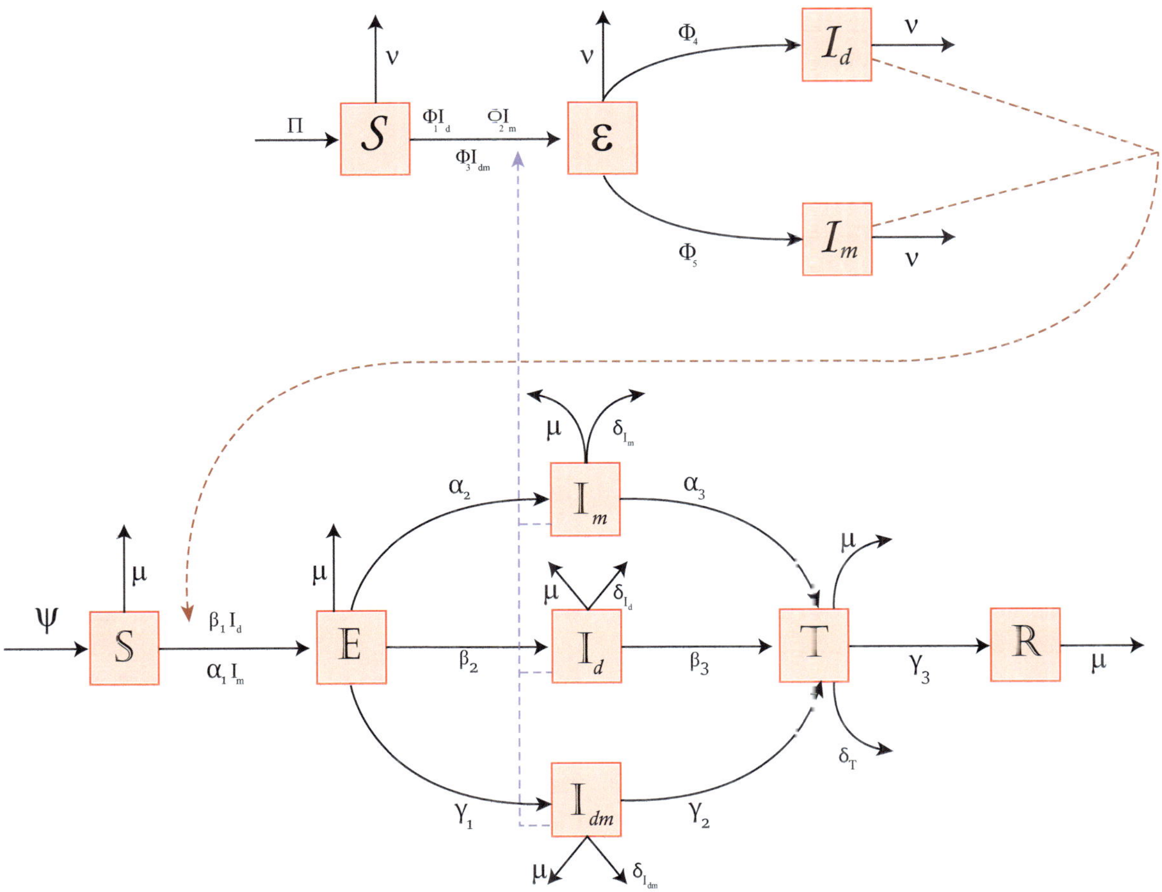

Figure 4.8. Key mathematical models in disease dynamics.

Source: Butt AIK, Imran M, McKinney BA, Batool S, Aftab H. Mathematical and Stability Analysis of Dengue–Malaria Co-Infection with Disease Control Strategies. Mathematics. 2023; 11(22):4600. https://doi.org/10.3390/math11224600

Whenever emerging threats such as COVID-19 emerge, determining the primary drivers of transmission is a priority. Current research tends toward the notion that the presence of a large viral load in the upper airway is a key driving factor in how infection spreads. By incorporating information about viral load into their equations, researchers can more effectively disentangle the mechanisms of transmission and, in most instances, make educated guesses at what will follow. This type of understanding not only directs treatment and vaccine approaches but also, in combination with research from molecular analysis, reveals correlations between our immunological responses and viral levels, focusing on public health initiatives overall (Marjaneh et al., 2023). Not all concerning disease modeling goes smoothly, however. Their accuracy relies a great deal on how good and comprehensive the underlying data is—a small error in inaccurate or tardy reports could contaminate the entire picture. There are many complicating factors: varying ways in which individuals act, varied geographic locations, and a complex network of social interactions all contribute to the challenge. Previous outbreaks have, quite obviously, demonstrated that improved data gathering and a little more collaboration between disciplines can make a significant impact. Recognizing these failures and advocating for more open dialogue between modelers and decision-makers can improve how we apply math models to inform public health interventions (Shankar et al., 2024) (Figure 4.8).

4.4.1. SIR (Susceptible, Infected, Recovered) Model

Infectious diseases are unpredictable and messy, but you can model their behavior with a mathematical trick such as the SIR model. It cuts people into three groups: those at risk (Susceptible), those who are currently ill (Infected), and those who have recovered. Seeing how people transition between these groups over time gives a good indication of how a disease could spread. This basic methodology provides a glimpse into transmission dynamics and indicates how various elements can push the outbreak in various directions. As a case in point, modifying the SIR arrangement by incorporating awareness moves—concepts even adopted from Yoga practice—has been observed to redistribute both vulnerability and recovery in rather fascinating ways (Bhatta et al., 2024). Varying the mix even more can serve to make the SIR snapshot clearer. Sometimes splitting the infected crowd into folks who are in the know versus those who are not—like in some Ebola studies—helps tailor public health responses a bit better. Adding an extra compartment, say for hospital visits, gives a more honest look at how healthcare resources get used and which safety measures work best. Stability analysis has its role as well; in the broad sense, it assists in establishing the thresholds that determine whether a disease will gain momentum or implode. One crucial metric in this case is what we refer to as the basic reproductive number, R0. When R0 falls below one, the disease tends to dwindle, but an R0 greater than one tends to signal the presence of a sustained, endemic condition. Such division directs essential policy decisions and intervention strategies (Ullah et al., 2024). Sensitivity tests in this model introduce another dimension of understanding. Even subtle alterations in factors such as transmission rate or recovery time can alter R0 quite a bit, calling for adaptable health policies. Raising awareness and education may reduce how quickly the infection spreads from one person to another, thereby reducing overall risk. Essentially, relying on these mathematical models provides a convenient toolkit for predicting disease dynamics, installing control measures, and allocating resources wisely. The SIR model—in particular when we add in new compartments or spin it slightly—remains a foundation of contemporary disease research, driving public health policy and even influencing day-to-day actions in the battle against infection (Bhatta et al., 2024).

4.4.2. SEIR (Susceptible, Exposed, Infected, Recovered) Model

The SEIR model provides a handy methodology to deconstruct how disease spreads. Individuals are initially vulnerable, then exposed—i.e., they have acquired the bug but are not yet infecting others—before they become actively contagious and, lastly, recover. This deconstruction allows specialists to visualize the entire process within a timescale, which picks up small changes that count along the way. It is not merely the general concept similar to the SIR model; by separating exposed from infecting, it provides greater specificity. In most cases, such additional focus on every stage assists in the customization of public health activities, particularly when various populations act differently (Biron-Lattes et al., 2020). Employing this model involves going into some fairly complex math. Differential equations generally express how people transfer from one category to the other—e.g., from being susceptible to becoming exposed—and whether or not it happens can, for example, depend on the frequency with which people mingle and what policy considerations may be present. For a large majority, these computations, as unclear as they do at times, are crucial if one is operating in populations in which small fluctuations in behavior matter because they tilt the scales. Recent research, in fact, has shown how flexible and responsive this model can be in actual outbreaks such as COVID-19 (Baez et al., 2022). On the computational side, even the SEIR model comes into its own in simulations. Scientists employ pieces of software that enable them to create stock and flow diagrams, breaking down such moves into images that make the underlying mathematics more understandable—albeit not always perfectly—that much easier. This interactive approach allows them to add in additional layers of complexity, like adding spices to a dish, so that several aspects of disease transmission are taken into account. Such flexibility not only enhances its predictive capacity but also aids in developing focused health policies, ultimately leading to improved results when combating infectious diseases (Biron-Lattes et al., 2020; Baez et al., 2022) (Figure 4.9).

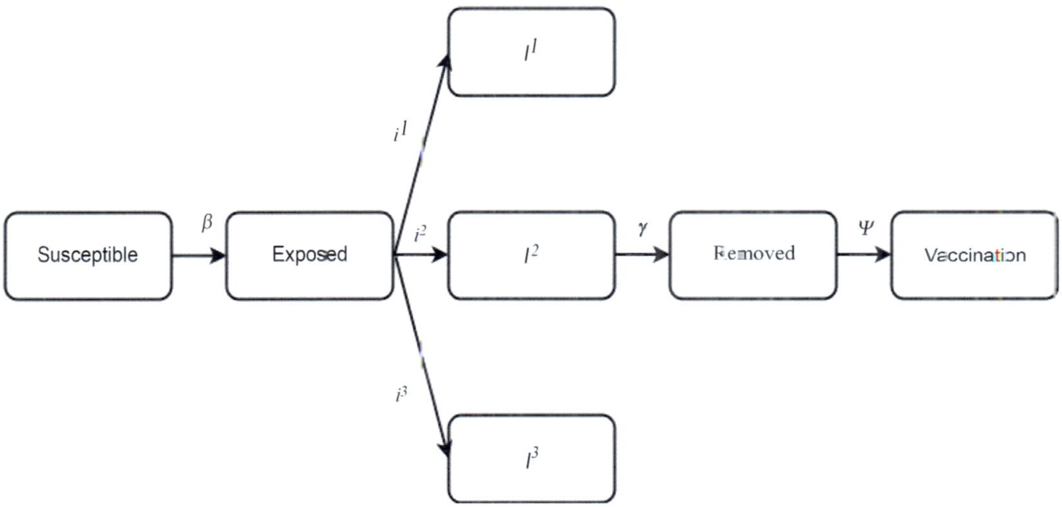

Figure 4.9. The SEIR model offers a useful way to break down how diseases spread.

Source: Poonia RC, Saudagar AKJ, Altameem A, Alkhathami M, Khan MB, Hasanat MHA. An Enhanced SEIR Model for Prediction of COVID-19 with Vaccination Effect. Life. 2022; 12(5):647. https://doi.org/10.3390/life12050647

4.4.3. Network Models and Their Relevance

Disease transmission is quite murky, but if you try to get a grip on it by mapping out the ways that we all interact with one another, what you're essentially doing is creating a little dot for each person with lines radiating out to everybody they touch. This basic concept makes us understand where a virus could leap from one individual to another, and it makes us understand which locations are that little bit more crucial—if you isolate or shield an essential dot, the entire chain reaction can be hindered. Public health strategies tend to focus on those critical spots in particular when there is limited to share. Recently, novel computer techniques have improved the ability to catch latent patterns in such networks and provide us with a better sense of how an outbreak could spread. Our daily connections, both real and online, also influence disease spread in our contemporary world. Most times, individuals cite studies demonstrating increased use of AI in medicine to assist us in screening both in-person contacts and online interactions (Secinaro et al., 2021). How we post things—whether they are accurate information or not—can significantly influence the actions of individuals during an epidemic. Network models burrow into various levels of connectivity, extracting small clusters that inform policymakers which groups may require a unique strategy. When disinformation begins spreading like an infodemic, it just reinforces the importance of getting our communication strategies correct (Tangcharoensathien et al., 2020). Combining concepts from various disciplines brings a new perspective to comprehending health challenges. Mixing social studies with what we already know about disease reveals that our health truly is a team effort. It's not simply germs and biology; it's also how we behave and interact. Gathering together everyone from researchers and doctors to community leaders and regular people helps make the big picture more understandable. As we learn to gather data in smarter ways, these network models can continue to improve, adding new pieces and parts that make their predictions more precise. Ultimately, understanding how people and their connections operate is the key to making smart public health moves and being prepared for whatever comes next.

4.5. Parameter Estimation and Model Fitting

When we construct models of disease patterns, it's important to get the numbers correct. Selecting the correct parameters is a big deal—it determines a model's opportunity to reflect actual behavior. Scientists tend to rely on methods such as maximum likelihood or Bayesian inference (in most instances) to draw numbers directly from observed data, and, to be honest, the method used can alter how robust the model feels. Occasionally, combining high-level computer technology assists as well; for example, machine learning can select top models of number sets, providing the overall model with a more "fit." In artificial intelligence, being aware of these tricks is central to producing trustworthy disease predictions; a mix of simple mathematics and cutting-edge computing. Fitting a model to the reality of what you truly observe from the data is just as critical. Frequently, methods such as least squares or even generalized additive models are used to narrow the gap between the predicted and observed. Such fit not only supports the model theory but also guides actual public health measures. You will occasionally monitor a model's performance with goodness-of-fit statistics; measures such as the Akaike Information Criterion (AIC) or Bayesian Information Criterion (BIC) assist in balancing the pros and cons between simplicity and complexity. Getting that balance right is important—models that are too complex may overfit and then simply collapse when you apply them to actual use. But of course, it's all about the fancy maths—parameter selection and model fitting are more complicated than it seems. The scientists have to fight with data that may be noisy or incomplete, concealing the real patterns of disease spread. Overcoming these glitches involves occasionally turning to robust statistical techniques that can survive data variation. Recently, explainable AI (XAI) is gaining prominence, because people desire models that can explain why they are making the predictions they do. In medicine, this sort of transparency assists in establishing trust and informing wise policy decisions. Whereas our conventional methods provide a good foundation, the sheer speed of real-world data implies new approaches must keep pace—highlighting the continued need for research and innovation in disease modeling (Hussain et al., 2020; Dwivedi et al., 2022).

4.5.1. Techniques for Estimating Model Parameters

Advanced disease modeling requires robust means of parameter estimation, and estimates wind up having a very important bearing on the accuracy of our projections in epidemiological contexts. Gradually, a combination of methodologies has emerged—traditional statistical approaches nowadays frequently married to computational gimmicks—in forms that are not always fixed. One such promising idea, Compressive Big Data Analytics (CBDA), provides an extensible mechanism for parameter estimation even when confronted with gigantic, jumbled sets of data. By repeatedly taking random subsamples, CBDA maintains the typical noise and disorder of large data in line, enhancing both the precision and reliability of its estimates via bootstrapping techniques, which in numerous situations allow researchers to draw meaningful conclusions from potentially incomplete or simply askew data (Marino et al., 2018). All things being equal, CBDA's malleability makes it a go-to instrument for managing the complexities of epidemiological modeling. Recently, as disease modeling continues to advance, genetic approaches to pinning down model parameters have begun to receive a lot of attention. Early geneticists such as Fisher created rudimentary statistical tools that essentially laid the groundwork for grasping how genes affect disease prevalence. Those early approaches have expanded from simple genetics into advanced models that incorporate environmental and behavioral variables as well. For instance, more recent advances in quantitative genetics allow us to observe how several genes interact—adjusting the horizon of parameter estimation to encompass such things as epistatic effects and gene – environment interactions. In general terms, this type of multi-perspective approach widens our analytic perspective and addresses the complexities that previous models tend to overlook, leading to sharper and more pertinent disease predictions (Álvarez-Castro et al., 2014). Combining new methods into disease modeling involves pursuing an interdisciplinary route combining insights from statistical genetics and computational science. As high-throughput data pours in and more intelligent algorithms process it, scientists now cut through intricate datasets more quickly than ever. Increased application of machine learning for parameter estimation makes it possible for models to fine-tune adaptively, as algorithms progressively refine estimates according to new data trends. This adaptability is particularly convenient in disease modeling, where parameters might change rapidly with varying epidemiological conditions. Ultimately, by drawing on many estimation methods, scientists are developing models that are both specific and statistically sound—even if the process at times seems a little scatterbrained, it is all with the goal of enhancing public health interventions and responses (Álvarez-Castro et al., 2014; Marino et al., 2018) (Figure 4.10).

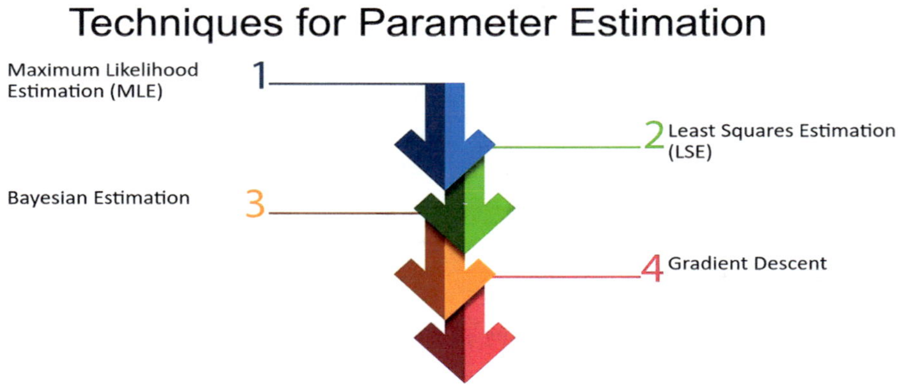

Figure 4.10. Techniques for estimating model parameters.

Source: FasterCapital. (n.d.). Nonlinear regression models for advanced data analysis: Techniques for parameter estimation. *FasterCapital*.

4.5.2. Importance of Data Quality in Model Accuracy

Input quality takes center stage in constructing any model. In disease modeling in particular, the fundamental assumptions directly come from data sets that chart out how diseases transmit, how individuals interact, and what types of control measures are deployed. If that foundation data proves to be incorrect—perhaps measurements are incorrect, some information is incomplete, or sources fail to match—the model then becomes unusable and can lead us astray toward bad conclusions. A study on cocoa black pod disease, for example, indicates that a sensitivity test is quite important; it highlights the fact that even slight changes in data can alter disease management practices and points toward the necessity of spot-on, full data entry (Ezekiel et al., 2025). Quality of data is not merely a technical challenge—it also raises very serious ethical issues. Dependence on poor-quality information in AI-based health models will exacerbate current public health disparities, particularly among groups with varying socioeconomic status. In medicine, if policies are based on models developed from low-quality data, the actions taken may fall short for most diverse populations. In most instances, a closer inspection informs us that the balancing of data source trustworthiness and the understanding of the implications of inaccurate predictions are as significant as the figures themselves, as evident in comparisons between such locations as the USA and Africa (Ohalete et al., 2024). Addressing the dangers posed by poor data requires an effort of cooperation from researchers, policymakers, and data scientists. With robust methods to collect information, establishing clear criteria for verifying that data, and promoting collaboration between disciplines, we can enhance how much we believe the numbers. Staying current with regular assessments allows models to evolve as public health environments change. Ultimately, good disease modeling is more than math—it begins with solid-as-a-rock data. Through quality coming first, experts may support disease control approaches and government health policy using firmly grounded evidence-based suggestions (Ohalete et al., 2024; Ezekiel et al., 2025).

4.5.3. Challenges in Fitting Models to Real-World Data

Disease modeling is not as simple as we might imagine. Biological systems can act in unclear ways – natural variability easily spoils clean model predictions. Consider chronic lymphocytic leukemia (CLL) as an example; split responses to therapy are common among patients, and specifics such as lymphocyte kinetics matter more than we sometimes like to think. Mathematical models, when constructed from averaged cohorts instead of individual profiles, tend to lose track of those finer details. Therefore, predictions can become less accurate, in general, and that is why the demand for new methods that catch the idiosyncratic character of biology without abandoning serious analysis is more than justified. Availability of data also turns out to be a big hurdle. In most instances, researchers hit significant boundaries when attempting to gather high-quality, long-term data that are essential for robust models. For example, a mathematical examination of the Nipah virus has revealed—more or less—that actual-world data assist in revealing main transmission dynamics. However, without sufficient robust datasets, models end up relying on weak assumptions or partial information, which damages their credibility. This is a challenge that requires better data collection methods and more cooperative research settings where data sharing is valued so that closing the data gap can result in significantly improved predictions for public health initiatives. A final barrier is the interpretability of these complex models. New approaches, such as combining deep learning with conventional epidemiological practice, tend to offer greater accuracy but at a cost: a lack of transparency. It becomes increasingly difficult for public health professionals to understand the implications hidden in the numbers. When working on studies related to CLL or the Nipah virus, aligning model complexity with meaningful, actionable insight is critical. Techniques that make the mathematics more transparent without diminishing the robust predictive advantage are crucial if we are going to translate those numbers into effective health policies. In most cases, the resolution of these issues is essential for disease modeling to continue to be a reliable instrument in public health planning.

4.6. Applications of Mathematical Models in Public Health

Math models are today an essential instrument in public health, allowing us to track the path of infections and shift—albeit sometimes a little rough around the edges. They basically simulate the spread of a disease, allowing us to grasp trends which, in general terms, is crucial for preparing against outbreaks. Take the COVID-19 days, for example researchers in Pakistan wedded an SEIR model (you know, the one split into Susceptible, Exposed, Infected, and Recovered) with some pretty new fractional operators to mirror the virus's quick spread based on real infection numbers. This pair not only illuminated the fundamental reproduction number—suggesting the virus was spreading at a rapid pace—but also initiated a wider debate on applying math models to inform resource allocation decisions, policy measures, and health interventions (Ahmad et al., 2020). Math modeling is not merely about finger-pointing for tomorrow's trends; it also burrows deep into analyzing the implications of public health actions. By throwing various scenarios into the equation, these models assist in speculating what will occur with changing health measures, which in most instances assists policymakers in making decisions on where to invest their money and time. For example, Liu et al. observed that mental health problems such as excessive anxiety and depression peaked in COVID-19—a reminder that crises are not just physical issues

(Zhou et al., 2020). Whereas models incorporate psychological effects, they tend to provide a wider, more integrated view of the chaos public health epidemics can be, ensuring we are also taking into account the emotional and social ramifications in addition to disease transmission. Meanwhile, the nature of math models is that they continually learn and change with new data coming in—yes, they do get iterative at times. With each new body of results, these models are refined, enabling improved predictions and, in turn, better intervention plans. COVID-19 made this eminently clear: You need to have models that can adapt to shifting patterns of infection, changing public behavior, and changing policy responses. For instance, constant fine-tuning of these mathematical models proved quite vital when verifying how well lockdowns, immunization campaigns, and public health campaigns were working in stamping out the outbreak at its onset. Essentially, this constantly evolving strategy wonderfully shows how math models can be more than mere reflective moments—they can help design wiser health policies and, in turn, bolster community health (Ahmad et al., 2020) (Figure 4.11).

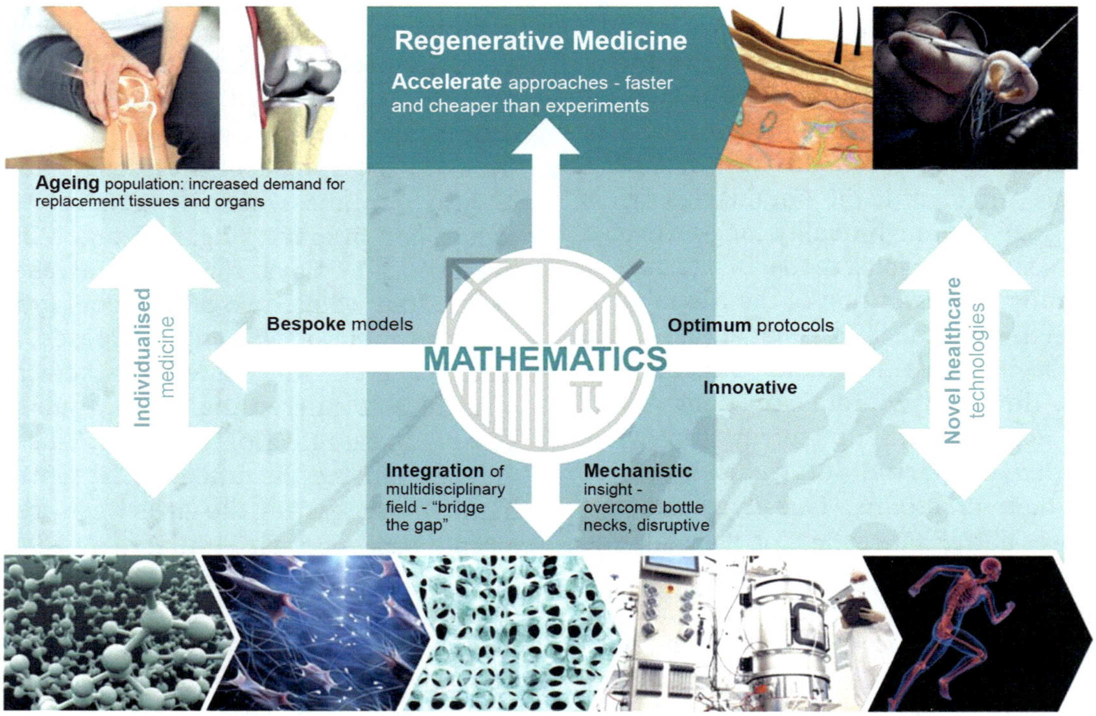

Figure 4.11. Applications of mathematical models in public health.

Waters, S. L., Schumacher, L. J., & El Haj, A. J. (2021). Regenerative medicine meets mathematical modelling: Developing symbiotic relationships. *Regenerative Medicine*, *6*. Article 24.

4.6.1. Predicting Disease Outbreaks and Trends

Predicting disease outbreaks now is no longer a matter of gut instincts—it's a matter of combining mathematical modeling with good data analysis. Scientists gather all sorts of information, such as raw epidemiologic records, population data, and even social media buzz, to identify possible threats. When some new infection begins to appear, having this predict on hand becomes particularly vital, as fast, accurate information can guide useful action. For example, the World Health Organization has, in most instances, emphasized establishing systems that not only address the health implications but also address the infodemic wave—what most refer to today as infodemics (Tangcharoensathien et al., 2020). In brief, by emphasizing numbers and patterns (yes, sometimes simply repeating what we already understand), scientists provide information about how diseases spread, which in turn influences where resources and strategies are best deployed. Furthermore, the success of these predictive models largely depends on the quality and quantity of data that go into them. You can have plain models that split populations into clear compartments, or very complex systems that attempt to model time-varying behavior and even introduce environmental variables. In the COVID-19 pandemic, for instance, an examination of approximately 65 research papers identified a significant increase in publications targeting prevention and control—obviously an indication that credible data were in great demand (Adhikari et al., 2020). In real-life applications, data flowing in from hospital records, reports on individual mobility, and even weather predicts all ultimately refine those model estimates. As models are calibrated to reflect real real-world dynamics, public health workers can then prepare more effectively for both existing needs and any incoming future crises. Predicting disease trends accurately is not only a matter of short-term response; it also feeds into long-term policy development and even into enhancing community resilience. Models that can identify groups at risk and geography-based hotspots enable targeted vaccination campaigns and intelligent distribution of critical resources. As with the current world response to COVID-19, when epidemiology and data science are combined, the resulting solutions can truly deliver in terms of overall health gains. In addition, with new challenges such as climate change and globalization putting increased pressure on their ability to anticipate and respond effectively, having valuable models becomes imperative to neutralize new health hazards. In short, combining new, innovative approaches and utilizing diverse disciplines keeps us better in the position to comprehend and react to epidemics (Adhikari et al., 2020; Tangcharoensathien et al., 2020).

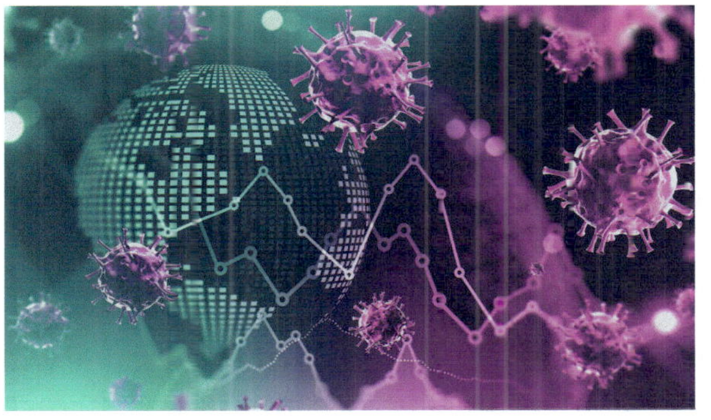

Source: European Molecular Biology Laboratory. (2020). Funding to predict the risk of infectious disease outbreaks. *EMBL*.

4.6.2. Evaluating Intervention Strategies

Assessing intervention strategies is more important than ever. Mathematical models allow scientists to simulate the spread of a disease and observe what occurs when you introduce vaccines, quarantine, or new public policy. This type of simulation demonstrates how these various efforts – sometimes even collaborating with each other – influence outcomes in a community. AI, upon being included within these models, focuses better how one would predict up-oncoming dangers and adapt to handle them. Modern research predominantly underscores that AI augments the rate of diagnosis, as well as optimizes care plans, with implications to meet the greater imperative for practitioners of various fields collaborating in an ever-tightening partnership (Secinaro et al., 2021).

Examining these measures isn't a clean, one-shot process; rather, it compels us to look both at raw epidemiological data as well as at the real operations of our health systems. When COVID-19 initially struck, researchers found that interventions such as social distancing, mask-wearing, and contact tracing did work to reduce transmission rates. Dissolving these approaches with numbers can not only display how effective they could be but also the burden they have on healthcare systems as a whole. Certainly, early observational studies are where it's at, but combining those findings with quantitative models gets longer-term effects. This layered method not only verifies that which we believe to be factual but also sketches out gaps, which aid in constructing intervention designs that are tailor-made to the individual requirements of various groups (Adhikari et al., 2020). Fundamentally, merging simple arithmetic with disease modeling provides health practitioners with a type of toolkit for making more intelligent choices. Assessing these methods isn't merely intellectual - it is vital to ensure that resources are allocated both effectively and in an ethically defensible manner. If decision-makers examine these data, they can more accurately predict results, maximize resource efficiency, and even compare alternative policy trade-offs, too. By drawing on such quantitative information, public health administrators leave the task a bit more secure when handling complex disease crises, which ideally results in more aggregate positives. For most situations, continuous studies on what does work continue to be fundamental for adapting to new patterns of diseases and constructing strength in readiness for the next adversity (Adhikari et al., 2020; Secinaro et al., 2021).

4.6.3. Informing Policy Decisions and Resource Allocation

Public health crises today require choices made on firm evidence. Governments, balancing everything from wobbly economies to concerning pandemics, are reaching into mathematical models as never before. These models don't simply paint pictures of what could be—rather, they inform how to distribute scarce resources when things get desperate. Consider a health emergency, say: through monitoring how a disease plays out, such number-crunching tools can influence policy on who receives healthcare or how vaccines could be distributed. This combination of number-crunching and policy-making becomes the foundation for utilizing limited resources wisely. In most instances, when choices are made based on evidence, not only are short-term problems addressed, but also longer-term concerns are kept in mind, allowing for the building of trust in meaningful ways.

Data-driven decisions are not only short-term solutions; they also reach out to solve larger, system-level enigmas such as the Sustainable Development Goals. Think about water management—it is a reminder that a lot of society's requirements are pieced together, and sometimes lessons from disciplines such as sociohydrology become relevant. Numbers allow policymakers to observe the interactions of human activities with nature in unforeseen ways. By delineating resource options under a single generic umbrella, leaders can, for the most part, avoid errors that occur when strategies become too fragmented.

This type of reasoning not only aligns with international demands for resilience and sustainability but also incorporates a buffer against future shocks. Essentially, incorporating math into policymaking ends up being a catalyst that sparks smarter, more equitable sharing of resources, addressing both immediate and sustained challenges (Baldassarre et al., 2019). As such number models evolve further, they continue to push for policy that can roll with changing social and environmental trends. Evidence-based actions appear more pressing than ever these days, particularly when disinformation and public discontent with governance is an ongoing concern. With guidance from these models, governments can typically fashion responses that feel more in line with what the people require, and occasionally even manage expectations slightly better. In this manner, people get the feeling that their voice counts when supported by careful, data-driven planning. Relying on the foundation of math is not all about responding in the moment; it also sets the stage for ideas that can adapt to the constantly shifting beat of society. In total, when mathematical insights are combined with policy design, it produces a foundation support for real and long-lasting advancement.

CLOSER LOOK

The Basic Reproduction Number (R_0) in Infectious Disease

The reproductive number (R0) is a mathematical definition used to define how infectious an infective disease is. It is the number of new infections caused by a single infectious individual in a fully susceptible population. A fully susceptible population is an abstract concept where anyone would be able to become infected, and there are no preventive interventions.

It is essential to know that R0 is a constant property of every pathogen within a given population. Just like a car has a top speed rating with ideal conditions (empty road, ideal weather), a pathogen possesses an R0 indicating how many individuals it might infect under perfect conditions for spread – before any vaccines, masks, or other public health interventions kick in.

How is R0 calculated?

R0 is determined by many major factors, each having a great impact on how an infectious disease will transmit throughout a population.

- **Duration of Infection:** A main contributing factor is the infectious period, which is the time frame in which an infected individual will be able to pass on the disease to others. The longer the infectious period, the more likely the disease will spread.
- **Contact Rate:** Contact rate, which is the number of individuals an infected individual meets during his infectious period, is another important element.
- Increased contact rates tend to enhance the probability of disease transmission. These variables can differ based on the infectious organism, population, and environmental parameters like climate and living conditions.
- **Mode of Transmission:** Mode of transmission is another major determinant. The diseases may be spread by many ways, for example, by respiratory droplets, by contact with contaminated surfaces, or by vectors such as mosquitoes. For example, respiratory illnesses such as influenza are spread through droplets when a patient who is infected coughs or sneezes, whereas illnesses such as malaria are spread through the bite of mosquitoes.

SUMMARY

Recent research that burrows into the mathematics of disease research illustrates just how important these methods may prove in solving health mysteries. A series of studies—even one that followed chronic kidney disease in type 2 diabetics—indicate these mathematical models have a role in unmasking the blend of clinical signals and patient outcomes. Scientists even looked at something referred to as the glomerular filtration drop and created test models that suggest why it appears that conditions such as age, body mass index, and treatment history influence the way that diseases progress. In the majority of instances, these findings support the notion that math models don't just predict fairly well, but also figure into day-to-day clinical decisions, paving the way for greater individualized treatment (Pervyshin, 2024). Combining machine learning methods puts another spin on the entire scenario. Certain research that investigates correlations between blood metal concentrations and CKD risk makes it apparent that our environment could be as much a factor as genetics. Methods such as Bayesian Kernel Machine Regression—yes, that one—assist in deconstructing a lot of interrelated variables, allowing us to gain a better idea of how factors such as serum potassium and sodium adjust kidney functions. This flexible way of modeling pretty much speaks for itself, showing that smarter, more modern analytics are needed today if we're to push personalized medicine into the mainstream (Wu et al., 2024). All things considered, looking back on these advances in math-driven disease research, it seems evident that such frameworks are not just extra bells and whistles but a real backbone in tackling chronic illnesses. The combination of medical information and computing methods has pushed the limits of what predictive analytics can accomplish, bringing early detection and highly specific treatments within reach. As continuous research continues refining these models, integrating them into routine clinical choices should improve patient outcomes. By coming together across disciplines—from math and medicine to epidemiology—we are laying the foundation for new thinking that can entirely transform how we treat and even prevent diseases in the years to come.

Mathematical modeling and infectious disease transmission are closely intertwined topics that appear in a range of case studies—frequently featuring real-world illustrations where these models demonstrate their relevance to public health. Soil-transmitted helminth infections provide one such illustration: in these, a form of deterministic compartmental method is employed to model transmission pathways that interweave human, animal, and environmental pathways. In the majority of instances, scientists calculate a rough reproduction number, an important number that highlights important intervention points and assists in increasing control activities. It is noteworthy to consider how sensitivity analyses, by consistently highlighting factors such as frequency of ingestion and the rate of disease progression, underscore the fact that a multi-faceted strategy is necessary to address STH issues in endemic regions (Imoro et al., 2025). Dengue fever modeling also provides another glimpse at why flexibility is important in disease pattern research. A model that consolidates both human and mosquito populations ultimately captures the fine details of how viruses transmit. By adjusting the model and focusing on essentials such as the basic reproduction number, researchers can simulate realistic cases that inform possible interventions. Historical records in Nepal—even with a few minor glitches in its recording—serve to back up these simulations, giving the entire method strong credibility and hints about where the disease may be going, and eventually supporting data-based public health decision-making (Gholami et al., 2025). Beyond all of these isolated examples, mathematical constructs provide a foundation for cross-disciplinary collaboration, erasing the distinctions among human, animal, and environmental health. The idea behind One Health comes alive in studies of STH infections, where the conversation about cross-species transmission naturally overlaps with broader concerns in both public and veterinary health. A similar story unfolds in analyses of different dengue fever models—their comparisons not only reveal the varying strengths of each method but also underscore how essential it is to keep refining our mathematical tools. When such models begin integrating socio-economic variables, the image becomes richer and more complex, assisting researchers in formulating healthcare strategies that not only address the biology but also accommodate the social realities of disease control (Gholami et al., 2025; Imoro et al., 2025).

KEY TERMS FROM THIS CHAPTER

- Compartmental models
- SEIR model
- Infectious
- Transmission rate (β)
- Basic reproduction number (R_0)
- Latency period
- Stochastic models
- SIR model
- Susceptible
- Recovered
- Recovery rate (γ)
- Effective reproduction number (R_e)
- Infectious period
- Equilibrium

REFERENCES

1. Ezekiel, Adegbite Bamidele, Adeniran Adebayo, and Idris Mutiu Amosa. 2025. "Mathematical Modeling and Optimal Control of Cocoa Black Pod Disease in Osun State, Nigeria". *Asian Journal of Mathematics and Computer Research* 32 (3):15-39. https://doi.org/10.56557/ajomcor/2025/v32i39234. (accessed on 6 May 2025).

2. Adhikari, S. P., Sha, M., Wu, Y. J., Mao, Y. P., Ye, R. X., Wang, Q. Z., Sun, C., et al. (2020). Epidemiology, causes, clinical manifestation and diagnosis, prevention and control of coronavirus disease (COVID-19) during the early outbreak period: A scoping review. *Infectious Diseases of Poverty, 9*. https://doi.org/10.1186/s40249-020-00646-x.

3. Ahmad, Z., Arif, M., Ali, F., Khan, I., & Nisar, K. S. (2020). A report on COVID-19 epidemic in Pakistan using SEIR fractional model. *Scientific Reports, 10*. https://doi.org/10.1038/s41598-020-79405-9.

4. Ayoobi, N., Sharifrazi, D., Alizadehsani, R., Shoeibi, A., Górriz, J. M., Moosaei, H., Khosravi, A., et al. (2021). Time series predicting of new cases and new deaths rate for COVID-19 using deep learning methods. *Results in Physics, 27*, 104495. https://doi.org/10.1016/j.rinp.2021.104495.

5. Baez, J., Li, X., Libkind, S., Osgood, et al. (2022). An algebraic framework for stock & flow diagrams and dynamical systems using category theory. https://arxiv.org/abs/2211.01290 (accessed on 6 May 2025).

6. Bhatta, R. B., Shrestha, S., Panthi, D., & Bhatta, C. R. (2024). Impact of yoga awareness on transmission dynamics of communicable diseases: SIR model analysis. *Communications on Applied Nonlinear Analysis*. https://www.semanticscholar.org/paper/eca1ca44ac4f5078b000208dfd0b7c12b87cd36c (accessed on 6 May 2025).

7. Biron-Lattes, J. P., Contreras, S., Medina-Ortiz, D., Olivera-Nappa, et al. (2020). A multi-group SEIRA model for the spread of COVID-19 among heterogeneous populations. *Chaos, Solitons & Fractals, 136*, 109925. https://doi.org/10.1016/j.chaos.2020.109925.

8. Cadot, S., Audebert, C., Dion, C., Ken, S., Dupré, L., Largeaud, L., Laurent, C., et al. (2024). New pharmacodynamic parameters linked with ibrutinib responses in chronic lymphocytic leukemia: Prospective study in real-world patients and mathematical modeling. *PLOS Medicine, 21*. https://www.semanticscholar.org/paper/4cd2ab988350dab0341c6f3652106621039d8349 (accessed on 6 May 2025).

9. Chicco, D., Jurman, G. The advantages of the Matthews correlation coefficient (MCC) over F1 score and accuracy in binary classification evaluation. *BMC Genomics* **21**, 6 (2020). https://doi.org/10.1186/s12864-019-6413-7

10. Coque, T. M., Cantón, R., Pérez-Cobas, A. E., Fernández-de-Bobadilla, M. D., & Baquero, F. (2023). Antimicrobial resistance in the global health network: Known unknowns and challenges for efficient responses in the 21st century. *Microorganisms, 11*(4), 1050. https://doi.org/10.3390/microorganisms11041050.

11. Di Baldassarre, G., Sivapalan, M., Rusca, M., Cudennec, C., Garcia, M., Kreibich, H., Konar, M., et al. (2019). Sociohydrology: Scientific challenges in addressing the sustainable development goals. *Water Resources Research, 55*, 6327–6355. https://doi.org/10.1029/2018wr023901.

12. Dimarco, G., Pareschi, L., Toscani, G., & Zanella, M. (2020). Wealth distribution under the spread of infectious diseases. *Physical Review E, 102*. https://doi.org/10.1103/physreve.102.022303.

13. Dwivedi, R., Dave, D., Naik, H., Singhal, S., Rana, O., Patel, P., Qian, B., et al. (2022). Explainable AI (XAI): Core ideas, techniques, and solutions. *ACM Computing Surveys, 55*, 1–33. https://doi.org/10.1145/3561048.

14. Ezanno, P., Picault, S., Beaunée, G., Bailly, X., Muñoz, F., Duboz, R., Monod, H., et al. (2021). Research perspectives on animal health in the era of artificial intelligence. *Veterinary Research, 52*. https://doi.org/10.1186/s13567-021-00902-4.

15. Jones, D., Snider, C., Nassehi, A., Yon, J., & Hicks, B. (2020). Characterizing the digital twin: A systematic literature review. *CIRP Journal of Manufacturing Science and Technology, 29*, 36–52. https://doi.org/10.1016/j.cirpj.2020.02.002.

16. Kuperman, M. N. (2013). Invited review: Epidemics on social networks. *Papers in Physics, 5*, Article 050003. https://core.ac.uk/download/129476376.pdf (accessed on 6 May 2025).

17. Lee, K. J., Moreno-Betancur, M., Kasza, J., Marschner, I. C., Barnett, A., & Carlin, J. B. (2019). Biostatistics: A fundamental discipline at the core of modern health data science. *The Medical Journal of Australia, 211*, 444–444. https://doi.org/10.5694/mja2.50372.

18. Marino, S., Xu, J., Zhao, Y., Zhou, N., Zhou, Y., & Dinov, I. (2018). Controlled feature selection and compressive big data analytics: Applications to biomedical and health studies. *PLoS ONE, 13*. https://www.semanticscholar.org/paper/29b05eb6f43fed510d2888cbe74e8a38669d94f7 (accessed on 6 May 2025).

19. Secinaro, S., Calandra, D., Secinaro, A., Muthurangu, V., & Biancone, P. (2021). The role of artificial intelligence in healthcare: A structured literature review. *BMC Medical Informatics and Decision Making, 21*. https://doi.org/10.1186/s12911-021-01488-9.

20. Skaza, J. S. (2015). Mathematical modeling of trending topics on Twitter. https://core.ac.uk/download/56736688.pdf (accessed on 6 May 2025).

21. Tangcharoensathien, V., Calleja, N., Nguyen, T., Purnat, T. D., D'Agostino, M., García-Saisó, S., Landry, M., et al. (2020). Framework for managing the COVID-19 infodemic: Methods and results of an online, crowdsourced WHO technical consultation. *Journal of Medical Internet Research, 22*, e19659. https://doi.org/10.2196/19659.

22. Walter, M., Kukutai, T., Russo Carroll, S., & Rodriguez-Lonebear, D. (2020). Indigenous data sovereignty and policy. *Routledge eBooks*. https://doi.org/10.4324/9780429273957.

23. Wu, M., Hou, W., Qin, R., Wang, G., Sun, D., Geng, Y., & Du, Y. (2024). Comparative mathematical modeling of causal association between metal exposure and development of chronic kidney disease. *Frontiers in Endocrinology, 15*. https://www.semanticscholar.org/paper/b1ca5ebdf0256a96242c64d10f0d54328a280d32 (accessed on 6 May 2025).

24. Zhou, J., Liu, L., Xue, P., Yang, X., & Tang, X. (2020). Mental health response to the COVID-19 outbreak in China. *American Journal of Psychiatry, 177*, 574–575. https://doi.org/10.1176/appi.ajp.2020.20030304.

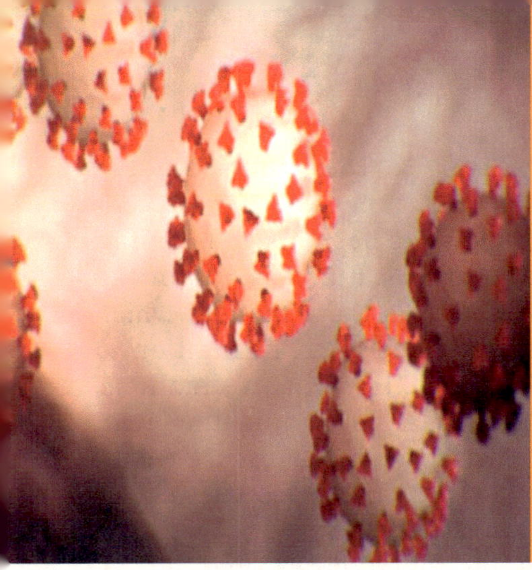

Chapter 5

COMPARTMENTAL MODELS OF TRANSMISSION (SIR, SEIR, ETC.)

Contents

Introduction

Over the past few years, infectious illnesses have truly gotten everyone's attention, particularly with such emergencies as COVID-19 and even the resurgence of diseases like mpox. Being able to get a handle on how such diseases act is fairly crucial to making plans for public health strategies, and, more often than not, a lot of that planning relies on clever modeling strategies. Consider this: models such as SIR (Susceptible – Infectious – Recovered) or its somewhat more complex cousin, SEIR (Susceptible – Exposed – Infectious – Recovered), segment individuals into various categories. Rather than a clear, predictable trajectory, these models indicate how people progress from being susceptible to becoming ill, and ultimately recovering. Researchers, meanwhile, look into these flows and, through number crunching and transition tracking, attempt to determine outbreak potential and intervention effects—helping to disentangle some fairly knotty epidemiological problems. Consider the SEIR model, for instance; it's a twist to include an "exposed" group—individuals in the incubation period who already acquired the infection but are not yet transmitting it. This additional step provides a softer perspective on spreading time delays, which has been noted by many recent studies. For example, how sexual activity contributes to mpox contagion has been instrumental in informing predictions for public health cases (Cordeiro et al., 2024). Public health workers, for the most part, are refining their plans according to what they have learned from these models, which are not only data instruments but also do-it-yourself manuals in making decisions. In addition to chiseling out where diseases travel, compartmental models allow planners to test what-if situations, such as vaccinating campaigns or behavior change within risk groups. By experimenting with varied intervention strategies, stakeholders can sense what would work and when a disease would settle in or be chased away for good (Agyingi et al., 2019). As infectious challenges continually change, these models need to be fine-tuned constantly as an ongoing, necessary yet sometimes grimy aspect of navigating the epidemiology world and protecting our communities (Figure 5.1).

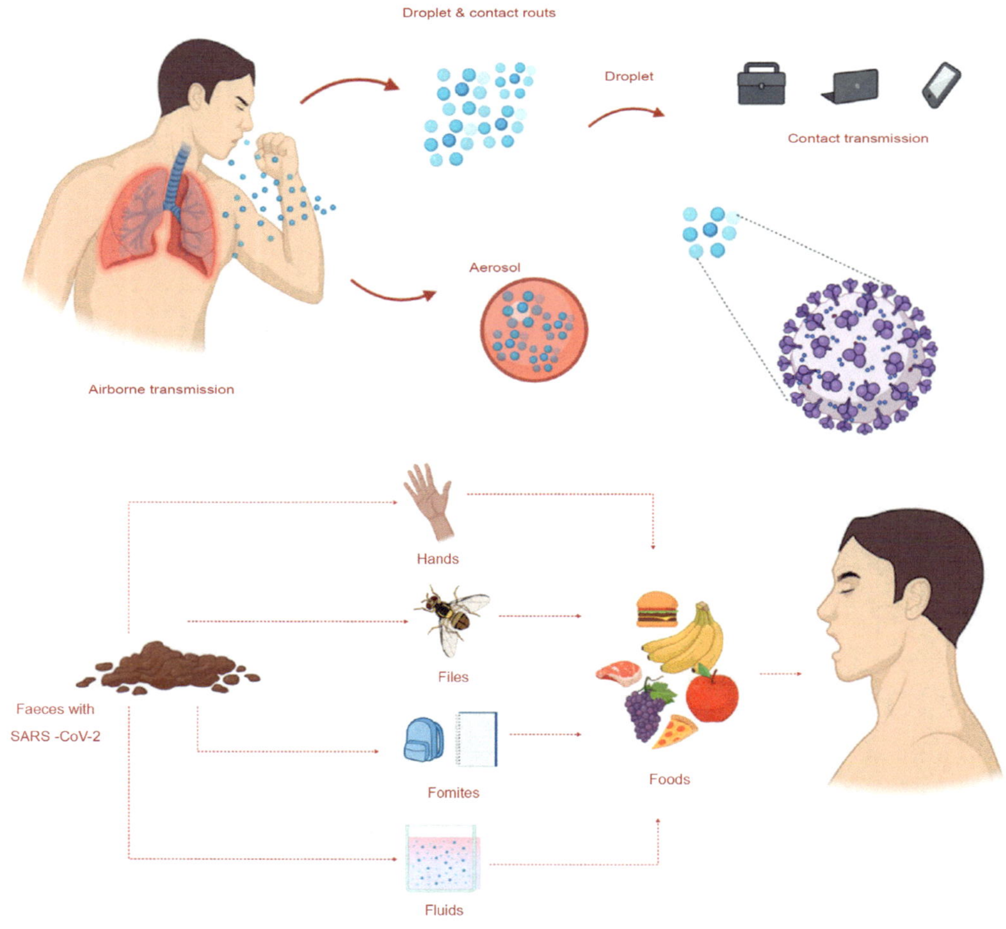

Figure 5.1. Infectious diseases have grabbed attention—especially with crises like COVID-19 and even the comeback of illnesses such as mpox.

Source: Ramasamy, A. (2021). Mathematical modeling and optimization of complex biological systems. *Biologics*, *1*, 17–38. https://doi.org/10.3390/biologics1010002.

Definition of Compartmental Models

Compartmental models are one of the most important tools in epidemiology. They're used by researchers to divide disease transmission into categories by putting individuals into buckets such as susceptible, infected, or recovered—rendering it a wee bit simpler to disentangle the way diseases like influenza or dengue spread through a population. Differential equations illustrate how people transition between groups, providing a qualitative snapshot that can be adjusted according to the peculiarities of the disease, like how long a person remains ill or whether there is a silent, latent period. In most instances, choosing between models, e.g., SIR vs. SEIR, ultimately boils down to the particular characteristics of the disease under investigation. As time went by, how we work with these models changed quite a lot. Newer methods now combine some sophisticated computational methods that refine predictions and accuracy. For instance, Bayesian Integrated Nested Laplace Approximation (INLA) has been applied with models such as SIR-SI when scientists examine dengue hemorrhagic fever data to identify parameters much more quickly than former Markov Chain Monte Carlo procedures. This mix of new methods even sometimes feeds into early warning systems that enable public health teams to respond quicker, so interventions can be tailored to fit each specific outbreak—sometimes with surprising ease. What strengthens these models even further is how they're able to hop between various diseases and allow scientists to compare results in various settings. A recent influenza study even re-calibrated SIR, SEIR/SLIR and SLAIR models based on Valencian Community 2016–2017 data. The study suggested that a significant portion of the population could transition into the recovered category due to previous immunizations, highlighting the models' ability to cope with complex immune responses. They went on to predict how probable it is that infected individuals will seek care—information that truly supports public health initiatives. All things considered, these calibration efforts do more than describe disease dynamics; they help solve current epidemiological mysteries in diseases as diverse as dengue and influenza.

Importance of Modeling in Epidemiology

Examining how infectious diseases develop; compartment models have become very trendy—they're a nice way to dissect what's happening within a complicated biological system. Rather than getting bogged down in infinite details, these models categorize populations into categories such as those who can become sick, those who already are, and those who've recovered. Consider the SEIR model, for instance; it even isolates individuals who have been exposed but not infectious yet, which adds a little more spice to the understanding of the transmission of disease. All this information serves to inform public health people about where things could go to take proper measures. In models of the French COVID-19 epidemic, for example, it is quite evident from the SEIR model that variation in social behavior can significantly influence the way an epidemic outbreak (Dolbeault et al., 2020). It isn't only the ability to deconstruct disease spread that these models have; they are also quite useful in determining what can occur with various health interventions. By simulating different scenarios, epidemiologists can observe how social distancing and isolation, for instance, appear to influence the rate of infection. A modified version of the SEIR model implemented in Croatia, for instance, was able to predict how the disease evolved under tight control measures. This allowed local health officials to make informed decisions about the effects of quarantines and other precautions, even as the predictions remain less than ideal. For the most part, these predictions are invaluable in assisting in quick decisions during outbreaks, and they take our knowledge of transmission dynamics and turn it into something that can be applied during public health emergencies. No model is perfect, however, and that is why there is always the potential to improve our methodology. Accuracy largely relies on the quality of input data as well as the accuracy of the assumptions made. See that very same SEIR model again—it illustrates just how much effect the adherence to health measures can have on the outcome. In most instances, being able to capture these small subtleties is important to minimizing error when estimating valuable indicators such as the reproduction number. As scientists continue refining such models and incorporating the messy realities of daily life (yes, even minute data imperfections), their contribution to creating effective responses for future outbreaks is that much more crucial.

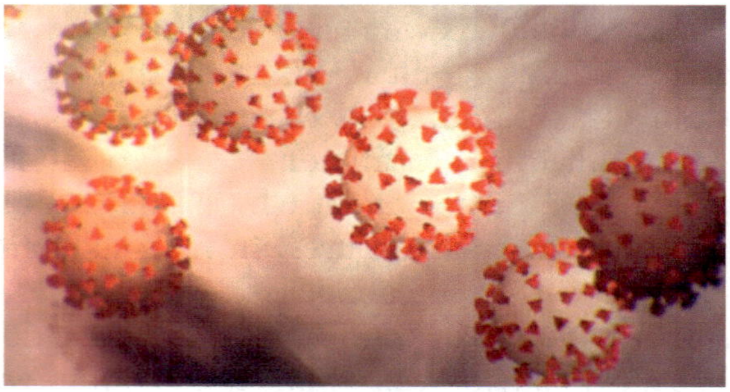

Source: https://journalistsresource.org/wp-content/uploads/2020/05/200303-A-TC012-005-860x466.jpg

5.1. Historical Background of Compartmental Models

Years ago in the early 1900s, concerns about contagious diseases prompted a combination of mathematicians and disease fighters to begin assembling methods for comprehending the spread of illness. Individuals started testing models that, in a very straightforward way, divided the population into categories – individuals who might get sick, those who had it, and those who had recovered. Years earlier, in 1927, Kermack and McKendrick implemented this concept as the SIR model. It was not complex – merely three simple categories – but it laid the ground for subsequent variations by demonstrating, in a simple manner, how these groups behaved over time. That model also informed thinking about strategies such as vaccination and quarantine, and before long it was quite apparent that splitting things up like this enhanced our understanding of disease transmission. Before long, it became clear that the initial SIR methodology was lacking a twist. There was this entire time when someone was infected but not infectious yet, a phase that could not be overlooked. So, the SEIR model emerged, introducing an "exposed" group to account for that incubation period. For most diseases, this modification did the trick in explaining diseases, such as influenza and, more recently, COVID-19—where people can infect others before exhibiting a symptom of illness. During the pandemic, the SEIR model was very handy when authorities were frantically trying to adopt policies such as social distancing and vaccination campaigns; its utility was even mentioned in policy circles (Fisher et al., 2023). In other words, it provided public health professionals with a more detailed picture to work from when things were changing rapidly. These days, the models have become more complex – incorporating such factors as vaccination impact and how immunity may wane with the passage of time. Scientists have begun to merge these traditional concepts with artificial intelligence (AI) to pin down prediction specifics and tighten up intervention strategies. For instance, one of the creative twists on the SEIR model now takes hospitalizations and mortality rates into account, illustrating how these actual results can influence disease spread (Shuvo et al., 2024). They are not abstract formulas; they are what health officials use to catch a glimpse of how outbreaks could unfold and guide decisions on where to deploy scarce resources. Overall, it has become evident that what started as a simple way to group people has grown into a vital tool for both immediate responses and long-term strategies to tackle future pandemics.

5.1.1. Early Models and Their Limitations

Initially, individuals relied on simple compartment models such as SIR and SEIR to comprehend the spread of disease. These models were a good beginning, but as the COVID-19 experience demonstrated, they had some significant blind spots. They made assumptions that conditions remained static and were not able to effectively capture the fluctuations in vaccination behavior, hospital bed capacity, or changing public health responses. For example, a traditional SIR model equates public attitude toward vaccination as if it were fixed—even though it can easily switch sides—and that discrepancy caused projections about hospitalization and deaths more and more inaccurate, which made healthcare and resource planning a true challenge (Bui et al., 2024). And then there was the problem of keeping pace with the times. Dependence on historical data caused these initial models to consistently fail at capturing what was occurring in real-time. Retrospective analysis of data from the Italian pandemic, for instance, was able to demonstrate just how difficult it was to date these models during periods of extreme uncertainty. The failure of these predictions highlighted an undeniable demand for more adaptable frameworks, frameworks that could adapt to abrupt changes in transmission dynamics. When models attempted to identify such critical thresholds as the peak of the epidemic with measures like the Mean Absolute Error (MAE) and the Mean Absolute Percentage Error (MAPE), such measures occasionally resulted in major errors, thereby making it even more difficult to cope with rapidly evolving outbreak conditions (Acar et al., 2023). To address these shortcomings, experts started incorporating additional factors into the models. They began modifying the classic SEIR configurations by introducing such things as vaccination rates, public health interventions, and even healthcare system capacity. At times, the reality that vaccination hesitancy has a significant influence on the way an outbreak develops resulted in completely new approaches to modeling public attitudes and their impact. In most instances, such minor adjustments underscored the importance of relying on models that could process nascent data to inform timely response approaches. With COVID-19 so vividly demonstrating, it is not only a plus to transform into a more responsive and inclusive model—it is entirely necessary to make effective public health planning as well as minimize deaths during existing and impending epidemics (Bui et al., 2024) (Figure 5.2).

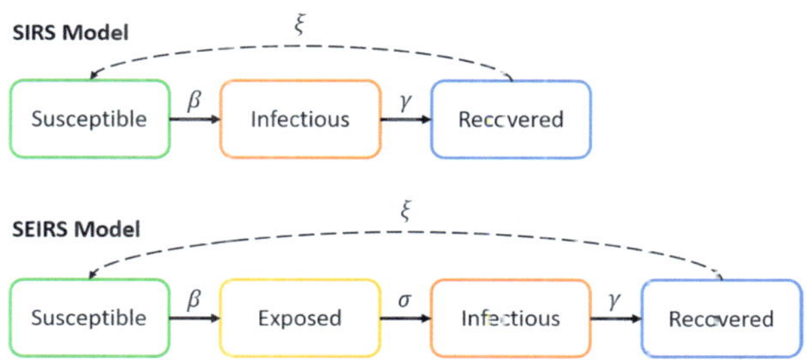

Figure 5.2. Early models and their limitations.

Source: Kaur M., & Singh, D. (2020). Image depicting the SIRS and SEIRS epidemiological models. *Sensors*, *20*, 4967.

5.1.2. Development of the SIR Model

Epidemic modeling begins with a handle on the way diseases behave. Early on, people invented what came to be called compartment models—consider the SIR model, for instance, which divides people into compartments such as Susceptible, Infected, and Recovered. Thought up, loosely speaking, in the early 20th century, this strategy is straightforward but unexpectedly robust at modeling outbreaks. It does this by placing people in various "buckets," allowing researchers and public health professionals to model disease transmission under different conditions and, in the majority of instances, inform decision-making in health emergencies. Over time, as our conception of public health evolved, the utility of these models continued to increase, living up to expectations when it came to planning and reducing transmission rates. Things eventually became more complicated. The original SIR model, good as it was, needed to be changed to deal with the messy nature of disease transmission. Variants such as the SEIR model—even though it is merely an extension where "Exposed" enters the picture to deal with incubation periods and silent, asymptomatic spreading—demonstrate that the world does not accommodate neatly. Researchers started incorporating more advanced statistical techniques and even machine learning techniques, which, to be honest, better capture the idiosyncrasies of human behavior and social interactions. With these sophisticated algorithms working for you, the predictions tend to turn out better and provide insights you can take action on. This gradual evolution highlights the need for models that can learn as our world evolves. If you glance at the current scene, predicting epidemics computationally is not quite as easy anymore. Rather, the trend now is to combine sophisticated computational methods, such as deep learning—with those classic compartment models. For instance, hybrid configurations like the residual leaky network (LeakyNet) take what has happened in the past and outline what will happen next, and they perform better than the older, more linear models. This type of creative reasoning addresses the standard pitfalls of simple methods, particularly when they are disrupted by the unpredictable, on-the-ground nature of real conditions. Finally, moving from the simple SIR framework to more sophisticated systems—like the vulnerable–contaminated–immuned (VCI) model—is a crucial advance in contemporary epidemiology to provide timely and effective interventions in response to public health crises (Raychaudhuri et al., 2023; Youssef et al., 2024).

5.1.3. Introduction of the SEIR Model

The SEIR model expands the outdated SIR concept by throwing in a twist—a compartment for individuals who've been exposed to a virus but aren't infecting others at the moment yet. This additional "Exposed" compartment provides us with a glimpse into diseases that incubate over time; most times, people may unknowingly transmit the disease during that interval. By including this lag between contact and contagion, the model will better predict outbreaks – a particularly useful asset in high-case-number regions where solutions are required to act fast (Marzouk et al., 2022). In practice, scientists and health professionals have used SEIR in a range of contexts to inform policy. For example, in one such case at a college, the model was employed to simulate SARS-CoV-2 transmission among the students and faculty so that efficient control steps could be initiated. It happens that even making subtle changes in the frequency of how frequently individuals are screened—say weekly versus monthly—can significantly impact reducing the total number of infections. These findings point out how adaptable the SEIR method is; it is not only a thought experiment, but one that has real data to inform significant decisions (Lopman et al., 2021). Another clear observation is how the model's sophistication allows it to blend in a lot of varying components, such as vaccination rates with other public health measures. When varying scenarios are simulated—variance vaccines or other interventions—the findings tend to indicate which strategy may best allocate resources in the event of a pandemic. Given that some non-pharmaceutical interventions at times don't prove as effective for all, adding vaccination tactics into the equation becomes quite important. Overall, the SEIR model ultimately acts not just as an explanation of the spread of diseases but also as a useful tool for policy-making spontaneously(Marzouk et al., 2022).

5.2. The SIR Model Explained

Learning about disease dynamics tends to begin with compartmental models, and a very simple tool in these cases is the SIR model. It divides people into three crude categories: those who can get infected (Susceptible), those who have the infection (Infected), and those who recover with immunity (Recovered). Individuals get infected when they encounter an infected person—a process that is usually explained by the transmission rate of a virus. In most instances, when an individual becomes ill, he or she recovers and develops a degree of immunity, so that fewer susceptible individuals can become infected. Differential equations, although they may sound too technical-sounding, trace out how the numbers in each category change over time, providing analysts with a glimpse of where an outbreak is likely to go and providing a direction for public health interventions. Looking a bit deeper, the SIR model turns out to be quite handy when exploring different epidemic situations. It is not just about dividing folks up neatly; it also shows how factors such as vaccination, everyday social habits, and various intervention efforts play into disease spread.

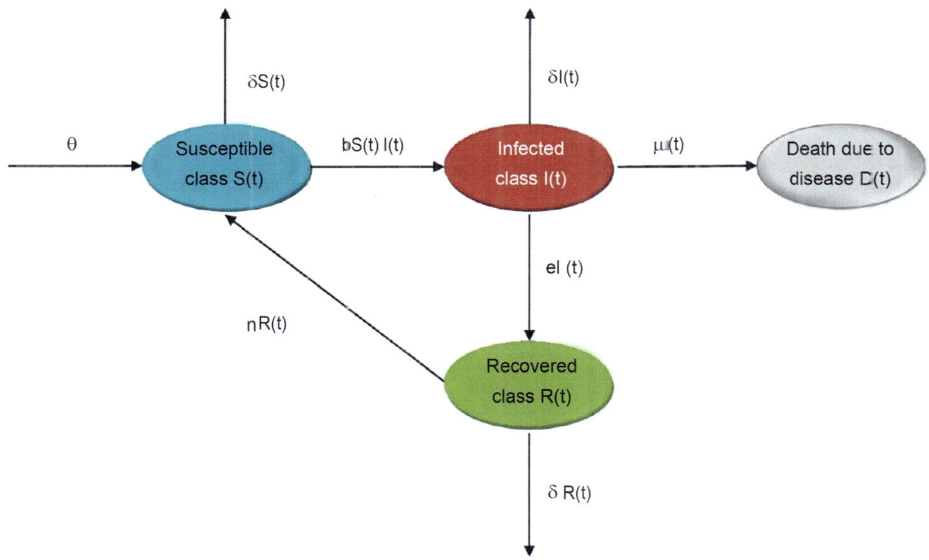

Figure 5.3. The SIR model explained.

Source: Djenina N, Ouannas A, Batiha IM, Grassi G, Oussaeif T-E, Momani S. A Novel Fractional-Order Discrete SIR Model for Predicting COVID-19 Behavior. Mathematics. 2022; 10(13):2224 https://doi.org/10.3390/math10132224

For example, a drop in the transmission rate via public health initiatives can change how an outbreak unfolds. The model even allows for run-throughs of many what-if scenarios, allowing policymakers and health officials to sift through possible outcomes (Sanz et al., 2023). Overall, though, studies suggest that this simple SIR strategy at times fails to capture the complete messiness of actual disease transmission, particularly when multiple variants arise or when individuals express varying levels of susceptibility or immunity. Despite these limitations, most still consider the SIR model as the foundation for more complex models such as the SEIR model, with an additional "Exposed" group representing those infected but not infectious. These modifications serve to better indicate the clumsy biological realities a little more clearly and result in better predicting when other factors, such as differing interaction rates between different strains of the pathogen—are brought into play (Ghimire, 2021). For the most part, as new techniques become available, a firm understanding of the simple SIR model is still paramount; it forms the basis for developing more advanced mathematical techniques although we continue to run up against the problem of modeling realistic, real-world outbreaks. Ultimately, learning and refining the SIR model is important for researchers looking to refine their analyses and open the door to improved public health policy (Figure 5.3).

5.2.1. Components of the SIR Model: Susceptible, Infected, Recovered

SIR makes us view disease transmission in terms less of clear equations and more of the dynamics of human interaction. Rather than rigid categories, imagine individuals broken down into three approximate groups: those who are vulnerable (the Susceptible), those who are presently engulfed by the disease (Infected), and those who survive (Recovered). It is not complicated —when people who have not yet been infected mingle with the infected, things begin to happen very quickly. Population density, how people intersect, and even pure chance all come into play. In most instances, monitoring how many individuals are still just on the brink of infection can seriously mitigate an outbreak; that concept is a major reason why this paradigm continues to resonate with community health planning. When an individual becomes sick, it's more than just a label change—it represents a critical transition into the Infected category. Things such as how infectious a person is and for how long become the issue. When these infected people encounter people who have yet to be exposed, the numbers spike in an almost exponential manner. Simple public health measures, such as quarantining the sick or finding their recent contacts—can make a significant impact on that growth. In general, the mathematics of such transitions gives policymakers an indication of just how quickly they may need to intervene to get the situation under control (Benterki et al., 2023). There is, of course, the point at which a person recovers. Recovery does not simply imply a feeling of improvement—it typically brings some measure of immunity, effectively putting the individual into the Recovered category. This change has a cascading effect on the overall balance in society, with an influence on how the disease progresses. The combination of having too many vulnerable individuals and an increasingly recovered population creates a sort of natural immunity, a buffer, so to speak, for others who are still at risk. What we notice here is a dance among various groups, each influencing the other's destiny, and this phenomenon plays a significant role in planning long-term health strategies. In the majority of instances, the observations from the SIR approach still influence our understanding of how to construct community resilience against future outbreaks (Hunter et al., 2022).

5.2.2. Mathematical Formulation of the SIR Model

Consider a way that follows the spread of an illness within a society—this is what the SIR model accomplishes with differential equations. The concept starts by dividing all people into three categories: those who would catch the sickness (the susceptible), those who have contracted it (infected), and individuals who recovered (recovered). Instead of making things too complicated, it depends on a few important parameters such as how rapidly the disease spreads and how rapidly people recover. In most instances, these values determine the direction and magnitude of the outbreak. By connecting these groups with a straightforward set of ordinary differential equations (ODEs), scientists can investigate what occurs when normal behaviors change, new vaccines are introduced, or treatments improve. There's beauty in its simplicity—it provides straightforward glimpses into how diseases may develop under various conditions. However, the model relies on some rigid assumptions that can overlook the messy nature of disease spread. It assumes that individuals mix homogeneously and infection and recovery rates never change. In reality, individuals don't mix the same way everywhere; the rate of contact differs between groups, and that can disrupt predicts. Also, by not allowing for spatial variations or specific vaccination campaigns, the model may miss the more complex patterns that we observe currently. Often, researchers have discovered that including additional terms, such as spatial terms that bear some resemblance to chemotaxis—is helpful to the model to better simulate spread in the real world. On the whole, these limitations encourage continued refinements in the SIR model to make it a better predictor of outbreaks. Recently, new mathematical tools have truly given us a better understanding of how illness works. Methods such as the Laplace-Adomian Decomposition sound weighty, but they've given researchers access to solving more intricate variations of the SIR model—ones that include simultaneous multiple infections or time-dependent capacities for treatment. These innovations enable specialists to take a closer examination of how interventions shift the game when diseases spread. When these improved models are calibrated against real-world data, they provide more realistic estimates of important parameters, opening the door to public health strategies that are more adapted to real conditions. Overall, this additional analytical thrust not only supports the core SIR strategy but also highlights the necessity for ongoing refinements in light of new infectious threats (Acheneje et al., 2024; Colli et al., 2024).

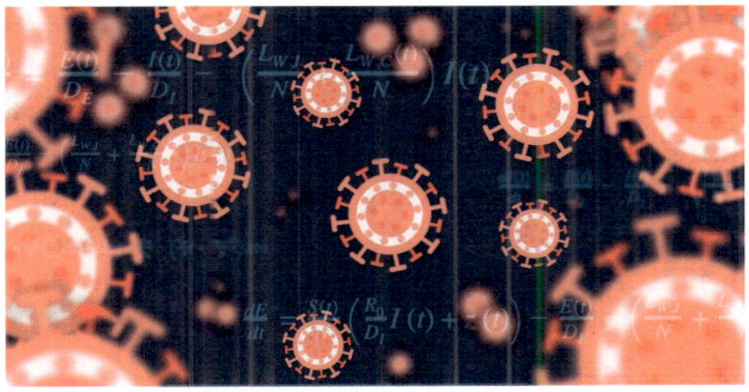

Author unknown. (n.d.). Virus illustration with mathematical modeling equations. *Medium*.

5.2.3. Applications of the SIR Model in Real-World Scenarios

Public health professionals have noticed the SIR model take center stage recently, particularly as they struggle with outbreaks worldwide. It breaks up the chaotic spread of illness into three simple categories—Susceptible, Infected and Recovered—which tends to make it simpler to take a glimpse at future trends and imagine plans. Consider COVID-19 as an example; at that point, several governments operated extensions of the model to gain a grasp of various infection pathways and estimate healthcare capacity. This action positioned the model squarely in the middle of difficult choices—assisting officials in making decisions regarding such steps as social distancing and lockdowns while approximating fairly well how well they were likely to succeed. And then adding tricks such as agent-based modeling, the entire SIR framework becomes slightly more sophisticated in illustrating how populations interact (Shuvo et al., 2024). Basically, it's not purely an academic exercise but an applied technique for actual health interventions. What's fascinating is that the SIR model is not merely limited to massive pandemics—it truly excels in smaller, local-scale outbreaks as well. In most cities, local authorities combine dense, on-the-ground data with the model to observe transmission progress nearly in real-time. Experts tweak the model according to local idiosyncrasies such as population density, daily social routines, and the healthcare infrastructure available. For instance, some have calibrated the SIR model to track COVID-19 in Canada, providing detailed hints regarding infection curves and hospital burdens (Shuvo et al., 2024). This type of personalized analysis is very important as it allows policymakers to weigh public security against the economic demands of their locality by concentrating on the individual specifics of their region. We also cannot overlook the way fresh computational concepts have improved the model overall. Methods like machine learning and deep reinforcement learning have been incorporated into the classic compartment model, developing more holistic frameworks for making choices. One neat twist is using agent-based methods that zoom in on individual behaviors to see how even a partial lockdown might change the epidemic's progression. Such approaches not only hand over sharper insights into which interventions might work best, but they also remind us that the world of disease modeling is constantly evolving. Through an appeal to these new concepts, the SIR model remains precisely at the leading edge, guiding researchers and public health professionals through the constantly evolving maze of disease transmission and reaction.

5.3. The SEIR Model Explained

The SEIR model isn't merely an additional layer over the traditional SIR method—it includes an entire additional step for individuals who have been exposed but aren't yet transmitting the illness. For many diseases, particularly those with a defined incubation period, this additional point of detail makes a big difference because it illustrates the small lag time between exposure and being infectious. You have a split into those who are still at risk, then those exposed, then those who are ill, and then the recovered. This added spin puts the projections much more in line with what is occurring in real life, particularly when every minute matters in severing an outbreak. SEIR has something else quite cool to it: its flexibility. For the most part, it deals with changing rates of transmission and recovery pretty effectively—important when disease goes skipping from place to place in varying modes and causes communities to respond with all kinds of reactions. Public health interventions and changes in behavior happen sometimes simply because of how things are moving in the general public, and the model can be adjusted to reflect that. Policymakers frequently appreciate that kind of ability when attempting to determine which strategies would be best. As newer data are input into the model, its predictions continue to sharpen, which does the natural good of enabling decision-makers to act more rapidly and intelligently in the face of an epidemic. In recent times, with global health issues changing so rapidly, the SEIR method has become even more critical. Recent studies indicate that it not only captures how illnesses spread but also provides a glimpse at what could happen next under different intervention regimes. For instance, phenomena such as repeat infections and vaccine-induced immunity have prompted researchers to add complexity to the simple SEIR concept. More recent models—think of the AEIHD model—have been extending the old framework to include these new complexities, hence increasing accuracy in predictions. Mixing mathematical observations with actual public health requirements, the SEIR model remains an essential instrument in the ongoing battle against infectious diseases (Mukherjee et al., 2024; Shi et al., 2025).

5.3.1. Components of the SEIR Model: Susceptible, Exposed, Infected, Recovered

Infectious diseases generally spread through populations in non-neat but definable groups;

consider the SEIR method, for instance. Essentially, what this model does is divide people into some states—although it may appear as if it is a neat list, it gets into the nitty-gritty of who may contract the disease. One of the central groups is those who yet to fall victim to it, the so-called Susceptible individuals; they are vulnerable, and how many there are can tip the balance toward an epidemic. Health officials usually attempt to reduce these numbers with vaccines and awareness campaigns. Understanding how many individuals remain uninfected and in danger, the majority of the time provides professionals with an indication of where an outbreak is potentially going, and it reminds us all why the discussion of risk is important (Phaijoo et al., 2025). Before long, a few of those high-risk individuals move into a less vocal, less observable category—the Exposed category. This is not the time they begin passing the disease around; rather, it is a phase more like an incubation period, in which you have the microbe but can't yet pass it on. In most instances, this stage ultimately becomes very important because it is that quiet time when things are fermenting below the surface. Researchers tend to monitor how long that latent period takes because that can determine how high the eventual peak in cases will be. Rapid testing and contact tracing during these times can occasionally disrupt the chain of infection before it builds up (Paneva et al., 2024). Then, once a person is fully in the Infected stage, things begin to happen quickly—this is when the individual becomes a disease vector, and case numbers can suddenly spike unexpectedly. Health officials, of course, spring into action, keeping a close eye on the situation and responding as new cases emerge with little notice. Eventually, most individuals find their way into the Recovered state, either through successful treatment or naturally acquired immunity, and this transition contributes to developing what some would refer to as herd immunity. As more people recover, fewer are in that at-risk group, which decelerates how rapidly the disease spreads throughout the community. Ultimately, how these populations interface determines not only the emergence but also the eventual dissipation of an outbreak; modelings based on scenarios such as influenza or dengue have been instrumental in refining methods to combat disease outbreaks more efficiently (Paneva et al., 2024; Phaijoo et al., 2025) (Figure 5.4).

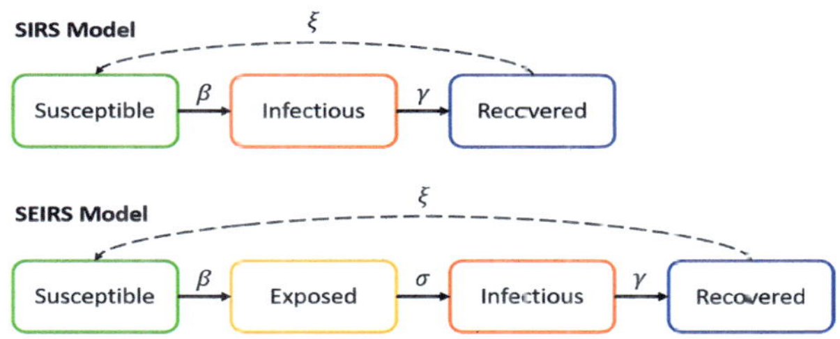

Figure 5.4. Components of the SEIR model.

Source: Ancerez DO, Kanjo E, Pogrebna G, Kaiwartya O, Johnson SD, Hunt JA. A COVID-19-Based Modified Epidemiological Model and Technological Approaches to Help Vulnerable Individuals Emerge from the Lockdown in the UK. Sensors. 2020; 20(17):4967. https://doi.org/10.3390/s20174967

5.3.2. Differences Between SIR and SEIR Models

Looking at the ways diseases transmit reveals a crazy collection of facts you need to know transmission patterns. The SIR model divides individuals into three categories—Susceptible, Infected, and Recovered—and does so by assuming everyone mixes equally, a simplification that is a math shortcut but one that occasionally glosses over important idiosyncrasies in actual illness patterns. And then of course there is the SEIR approach, that adds a fourth group for people who are Exposed; that additional phase does the incubation period, which allows one to get a more realistic snapshot if there is the lag between exposure and actual infection. Both methods account for public health, but both bring varying methodologies to managing outbreaks. The SEIR model, by highlighting that additional Exposed group, provides a more nuanced view of when individuals get ill. For illnesses such as measles or COVID-19—where a considerable wait may go between an exposure and an onset—it captures information that the straightforward SIR method may not. For example, when it comes to predicting the peak of infection waves or hospital overload, SEIR performs better, allowing epidemiologists to target interventions on specific outbreak stages. In most scenarios, the decision between these models depends on the duration of the exposed phase, a fact that can influence the entire strategy. Adding additional layers to these models can sometimes confuse the results quite a bit. More recently, agent-based methods have emerged that model individual interactions rather than bundling everybody together; this allows us to visualize a range of mixing patterns that ordinary compartment models may overlook. When people compare results from these individual-to-individual simulations to the SEIR's predictions, they tend to find shifts in peak times and even peak magnitudes. For instance, one paper demonstrated that after accounting for scheduled movements, the results differed significantly from traditional SEIR projections (Hunter et al., 2022). Overall, increasing model complexity step by step serves to emphasize the extent to which our initial assumptions are capable of influencing the reliability and general character of any prediction in the real world (Sanz et al., 2023).

5.3.3. Use Cases for the SEIR Model in Disease Outbreaks

The SEIR model provides us with a richer perspective on how illness spreads, particularly when infections contain that strange latent period—when one has been exposed but isn't yet contagious. It comes into its own with outbreaks like COVID-19, where becoming susceptible, then exposed, then infectious, then recovering can make all the difference. Other researchers even experimented with a revised SEIR method to monitor COVID-19's trajectory across various areas, which, in the majority of instances, assisted in informing local containment strategies. By examining such as infection and recovery rates, the model allows us to visualize how interventions could influence the course of the outbreak, providing a path to personalized control measures that respond to actual-world data and public action (Ramalingam et al., 2025).

Combining vaccination tactics into the SEIR framework has also brought new possibilities, particularly when combating vaccine reluctance, a giant obstacle to hindering disease spread. Simulations, tuned using real compliance data, show that adjusting vaccination rates and existing safety protocols can significantly alter results. In general, there is an emphasis on how immunity, whether gained from an illness or through an injection, pushes disease susceptibility in the long run. And considering how individuals behave once they get vaccinated, it makes the model seem much closer to the unglamorous reality of newly emerging variants and changing social mores (Tanwar et al., 2024). Another clear aspect is the model's ability to work with various outbreak scenarios. Epidemiologists tend to modify its composition depending on the particular microbe, local population, or even bizarre environmental conditions. Consider measles, say, as the disease sweeps through a population, to fit the model with emphasis on the size and interconnection of the susceptible group to highlight its predictive capability. All this flexibility makes the SEIR model not only a predicting tool but also a policy guide by relying on empirical evidence in a crisis, resulting in more intelligent health interventions and more efficient use of resources (Ramalingam et al., 2025) (Figure 5.5).

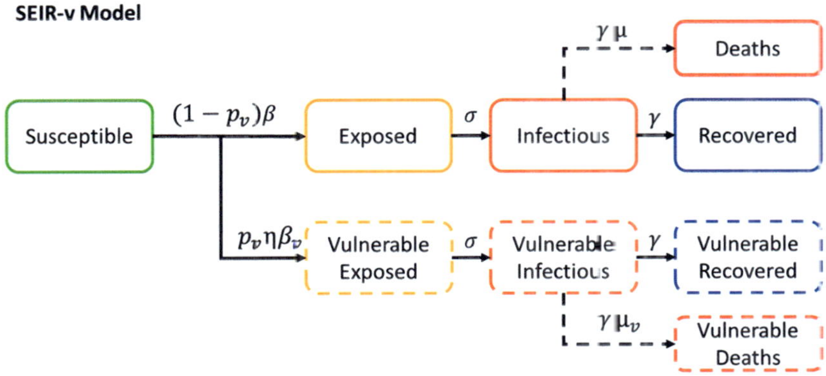

Figure 5.5. Use cases for the SEIR model in disease outbreaks.

Source: Anderez DO, Kanjo E, Pogrebna G, Kaiwartya O, Johnson SD, Hunt JA. A COVID-19-Based Modified Epidemiological Model and Technological Approaches to Help Vulnerable Individuals Emerge from the Lockdown in the UK. Sensors. 2020; 20(17):4967. https://doi.org/10.3390/s20174967

5.4. Extensions and Variations of Compartmental Models

Epidemiological modeling has changed. Old models such as SIR and SEIR are now a thing of the past, replaced by strategies that attempt to model the messy, real-world variables we currently encounter. Outbreaks—consider Ebola or H1N1—have truly demonstrated that the clear, idealistic concepts of yesteryear simply do not apply any longer. In most instances, these occurrences remind us that things such as how organizations react and those unanticipated, unexpected bumps in the road must be incorporated into our models. When you add these unforeseen elements into the mix, the models necessarily become more complex and, quite frankly, require more strenuous computations. Occasionally, you may even have to resort to sneaky pre-processing stunts that make the technicalities of analysis simple without compromising essential insights into epidemic control. All this extra work matters if we're going to construct foolproof schemes to counter novel infectious dangers because it addresses both biology and response logistics (Brown et al., 2017). And then there is the twist of introducing environmental elements into the equation. A couple of recent studies have essentially demonstrated that you can model airborne disease transmission by combining old-fashioned compartment concepts with quanta conservation-based equations. It does this by connecting, say, the rate at which quanta are created and how rapidly indoor air will dilute them—with time eventually showing how an outbreak could unfold. It is a departure from the traditional, nearly reductionist steady-state concepts to one that provides a richer, more complex picture of what is going on within an enclosure. It not only reinforces the epidemiological predicts but also sort of uncovers new doors for public health interventions, allowing specialists to speculate on the severity of outbreaks across various scenarios (Burridge et al , 2023). Last but not least, there's the emergence of hybrid models that combine deterministic rules with a pinch of randomness. This mix appears to more effectively cope with the uncertainties inherent in the way diseases spread in the real world. By closing the gap between traditional, rule-based models and the unpredictable idiosyncrasies observed in outbreaks, these hybrid models provide us with a more complete view of disease dynamics. They even account for interpersonal variation in the likelihood of illness or transmission of an infection, allowing for more customized public health reactions. With infection interactions becoming ever more sophisticated, it is now apparent, on the whole, that adaptable models are a requirement. Future studies should, in general, aim at sophisticating these hybrid models so that we can improve our projections and design improved public health interventions (Brown et al., 2017).

5.4.1. Introduction to the SIRS and SEIRS Models

Research in infectious diseases frequently relies on models that enable us to grasp how diseases spread and how they heal. SIRS and SEIRS, for instance, diverge from the normal SIR method by illustrating that immunity will not always last forever. Instead of a direct pass from vulnerable to infected to recovered, the SIRS model allows immunity to decline over time—which is fairly applicable to something like the flu, where defenses slowly decrease and reinfections happen. The SEIRS version takes it a bit further by including an exposed category for people who are not yet infectious; this small adjustment adds an additional layer of depth when considering diseases that have a longer incubation period, something that counts a great deal in the current epidemiological environment, particularly in outbreaks of vector-borne illnesses (VBDs) (Mukherjee et al., 2024). Adding in that additional exposed category alters things subtly. It addresses the difficult timing of when an individual begins to spread the disease, and in most instances, this accounts for why undetected, asymptomatic periods can prolong the life of an outbreak in a population. You can visualize people transitioning from being at risk to bumped up into an exposed state, becoming infected, and ultimately recovering, which in turn illuminates crucial measures such as the basic reproduction number (R0) that public health officials use. When these concepts are used to study challenges such as the COVID-19 pandemic, scientists discover that fine-tuning, such as adding vaccination or other social interventions—can change the direction of the disease. Even some studies indicate that these dynamic models provide wide-ranging advantages, especially in regions where socioeconomic dynamics also add an additional layer of complexity to the everyday spread of disease (Madaki et al., 2024). As diseases remain dynamic and continue to evolve, the convenient flexibility of models such as SIRS and SEIRS becomes increasingly vital. Frequently, specialists modify such frameworks to include various speeds of transmission or unique characteristics from different groups influencing both susceptibility and recovery. Consider vector-borne diseases; scientists have married these models with behavior and environment to reveal fresh depths of knowledge regarding disease spread. In the broad scheme of things, this flexibility is paramount now that new and unfamiliar pathogens are emerging all the time. Through the employment of SIRS and SEIRS models, government health departments will be able to improve their preparedness, custom-fit solutions according to specific challenges in regions, and ultimately mitigate the burden infectious diseases place upon various populations (Mukherjee et al., 2024).

5.4.2. Role of Vaccination in Modified Models

Models that incorporate vaccination have been found to have an improvement in how well they predict outbreaks and contribute to real-world public health concerns. Simple frameworks such as SIR and SEIR are now being combined with vaccination measures – this adjustment provides us with a clearer image of how disease travels within groups. It is not merely about reversing who is at risk; vaccination also influences how rapidly a disease spreads and how strong herd immunity becomes. In other words, some research (Gabriela et al., 2022) indicates that vaccine programs can, in most situations, slightly increase overall herd immunity, particularly when individuals already have some natural immunity. These findings, as a rule, can inform leaders as they construct interventions that attempt to achieve better health results while minimizing economic damage. When new models are assembled, looking more closely at differences among individuals in exposure and susceptibility enables a more realistic model. A model such as the multi-risk SIR (MR-SIR) disaggregates by age and other risk factors, allowing us to target vaccine strategies in novel manners. In most cases, the notion is that the most efficient vaccination strategies target certain groups to achieve improved health outcomes without overwhelming budgets. An example is prioritizing older people to significantly reduce death rates—even exempting lower-risk individuals from having to endure widespread lockdowns (Whinston et al., 2020).

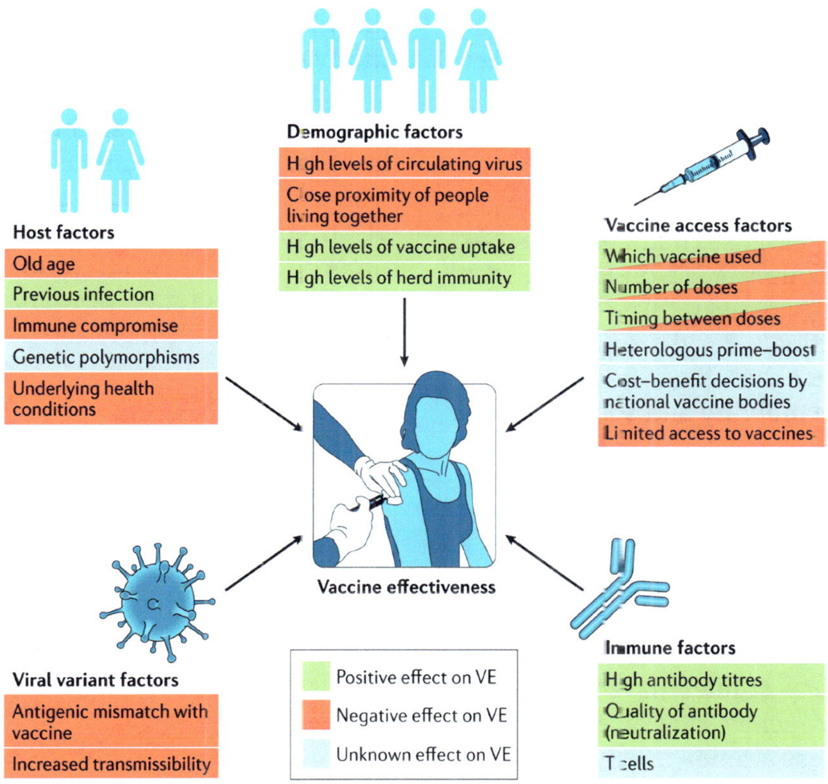

Figure 5.6. Role of vaccination in modified models.

Source: Sette, A., & Crotty, S. (2021). Immune responses to SARS-CoV-2 infection and vaccination. *Nature Reviews Immunology*.

This type of targeted approach is, to summarize, crucial for reducing the broad impact of pandemics and reveals how central vaccination is to shaping epidemic trajectories. Vaccines, meanwhile, do more than simply contain the transmission of disease in the short term in these upgraded models; they ripple out to have wider social impacts. Intelligent vaccination campaigns can take pressure off hospitals by reducing severe cases and hospitalization, which in turn increases resilience for the next outbreak. The linkage between the number of people receiving injections and how well people adhere to other health protocols continues to be a key—if occasionally tricky—

component of the overall situation. When the models include vaccination, they can even suggest outbreak potential as a result of the unexpected changes in people's behavior and uptake of the vaccine. In short, incorporating vaccines into these compartmental models solidifies their role within public health planning and the role they have in influencing how we react as a society (Gabriela et al., 2022) (Figure 5.6).

5.4.3. Incorporation of Spatial Dynamics in Compartmental Models

Compartmental models perform much better when you begin to consider space. Rather than adhering to the traditional SIR and SEIR methods that presume everyone mixes homogeneously—a concept that frequently fails in the real world—introducing spatial information reveals how where individuals reside and travel can influence disease transmission. In a pandemic, differences in local mobility and social contacts can alter how rapidly an outbreak is initiated and transmitted. Recent research, for example, indicates that observing where individuals are can provide a better understanding of epidemic behavior, which is useful when making public health moves and allocating resources. Since the traditional models sometimes ignore local idiosyncrasies, many studies have resorted to agent-based approaches that accept spatial variation. With these frameworks, researchers can model individual behavior and patterns of movement in a variety of environments, providing a new perspective on the way diseases spread. For instance, when you tinker with the way agents interact in a particular environment, you may find that small outbreaks percolate up—even in areas where everyone tends to follow health regulations. This type of trial has demonstrated that even small breakdowns in adherence can increase the transmission of a disease, since some recent work on social heterogeneity under lockdown conditions shows (Dolbeault et al., 2020). It certainly makes you wonder if the default compartment models may require a rethink. In a wider context, these findings have enormous implications for informing public health policy. By incorporating spatial dynamics into the equation, compartment models can be calibrated to take into account variables such as network links or varying mobility patterns. When you compare models, the ones that include these factors tend to make predictions that vary, particularly with regard to the timing and magnitude of epidemic peaks and the overall effect. Studies contrasting basic SEIR models and agent-based simulations repeatedly demonstrate that a slight increase in realism in modeling how humans act will frequently lead to a more gradual, yet controllable, course of an epidemic (Hunter et al., 2022). Overall, incorporating spatial information not only enhances predictive precision but also steers us toward more flexible and precise intervention measures.

5.5. Limitations of Compartmental Models

Compartment models such as the SIR and SEIR configurations rely on simple concepts that usually don't cut it when you consider the actual world. They appear to believe that everyone interacts equally, so each has an equal opportunity to run into anyone else. That perspective neglects the messy realities of our social existence—for example, where you reside, your age, or even how you act have a role. This type of oversimplification can readily distort projections of how disease spreads and what control will be effective. More and more, scientists are committed to combining with network analysis to more accurately capture the messy, day-to-day social networks among individuals; this marriage attempts to combine the virtues of both methods while mitigating their weaknesses (Mendes et al., 2024). Time is another twist of fate with these models. Frequently, they commit to set parameters as if things never change, yet events such as public interventions or behavioral changes can disrupt disease progress quite significantly. That sort of inflexibility can make predictions that miss the mark, particularly in situations where conditions rapidly change. To add to that, outside forces, such as unforeseen weather fluctuations or economic change—tend to be swept aside, giving us only a moment's snapshot of an epidemic that is too frozen. In most instances, experts now advocate for models that incorporate real-time data and adjust spontaneously to better capture these changes (Mukherjee et al., 2024). Then there is the hitch with simplified compartmental frameworks failing to catch the stratified character of diseases transmitted through vectors. The mathematics that underlies these models may gloss over the effect of asymptomatic carriers, varying degrees of infectiveness, or the unclear effect of co-infections. They may also fail to catch key transitional phases that arise in more complex systems. For example, when it comes to vector-transmitted illnesses, analytical expressions remain pretty underexplored because the focus usually stays on classic models like the Kermack – McKendrick approach. Neglecting these little details can end up giving us a half-baked picture of an outbreak, ultimately getting in the way of sound planning and response strategies (Mukherjee et al., 2024).

5.5.1. Assumptions Made in Compartmental Models

Compartment models for the simulation of disease transmission frequently get into difficulties since they rely on simplifying assumptions about reality. One is that all individuals within a group are alike, i.e., that each has the same risk and probability of infection. But, as we observe in life, people are not alike—a combination of age, behavior, and local conditions truly mixes things up. This clear-as-a-pin perception can result in exaggerated reports of an outbreak, such as occurred with H1N1-2009 and COVID-19, where the classical models were likely to project a bigger pandemic than materialized (Mukherjee et al., 2024). A second glitch arises from holding onto constant transition rates between groups, without considering that circumstances do change over time. Most models make steady-state assumptions with individuals traveling from one compartment to another, ignoring variables such as new intervention approaches or changes in public behavior. Such constant assumptions sometimes limit the flexibility of models when outbreaks change. You can easily visualize the issue with VBDs with transmission rates going wildly with such variables as weather or changes in the vector population. Even methodologies like SEIR models—adjusted with treatment or carrier phases—need to blend in these variable dynamics to truly reflect the disease's effect (Mukherjee et al., 2024). Being overly reliant on a few compartments can also overcompress conclusions regarding disease control. Although models such as SIR and SEIR allow to pin down simple reproduction numbers, they tend to leave out the sordid specifics of transmission routes, particularly in situations with a mixture of populations and host – vector interactions. At other times, incorporating additional compartments—those accounting for lost immunity, vaccination, or treatment—can cut down on inaccuracies. Adding real-world elements such as mobility patterns and natural diversity in the population gives us insights that are more aligned with what's seen in reality (Jiang et al., 2024). Briefly put, reconsidering these fundamental assumptions and refining the models can improve our capacity to predict outbreaks in a more realistic way.

5.5.2. Challenges in Parameter Estimation

Compartmental models bring plenty of challenges, especially when it comes to working out key numbers. Think of models like SIR or SEIR: they lean heavily on data, but that data sometimes does not capture every twist in how diseases spread. Uncertainty in the figures, natural variability, and incomplete records make it hard to nail down things like the basic reproduction number (R0) or the rate at which diseases transmit. Such unpredictability can result in inaccurate predictions that then impact public health interventions. Occasionally, when long-span detailed datasets are unavailable, such as in countries with less developed health infrastructures—the entire process of calibration becomes more challenging. All this explains, broadly speaking, why we need improved means of collecting accurate data, as researchers have demonstrated through AI methods (Shuvo et al., 2024). On top of that, one also cannot deny the extent to which socio-economic factors confuse the issue even further. Populations, healthcare access, and cultural patterns are all variables that can alter disease dynamics in unpredictable manners. In populations such as Sub-Saharan Africa, where there is a lack of healthcare facilities and stigma may cause underreporting, gathering the appropriate data is an actual nightmare. For example, the SEIR deterministic model, which includes variables such as latent periods and even vertical transmission, makes it obvious that local, detailed data is essential. And when attempting to quantify how effective interventions are, you've got to base it on good, region-specific estimates—something research on hepatitis B in Ghana has highlighted, with the implication that various regions may require their own specific numbers (Awuah-Mensah et al., 2018).

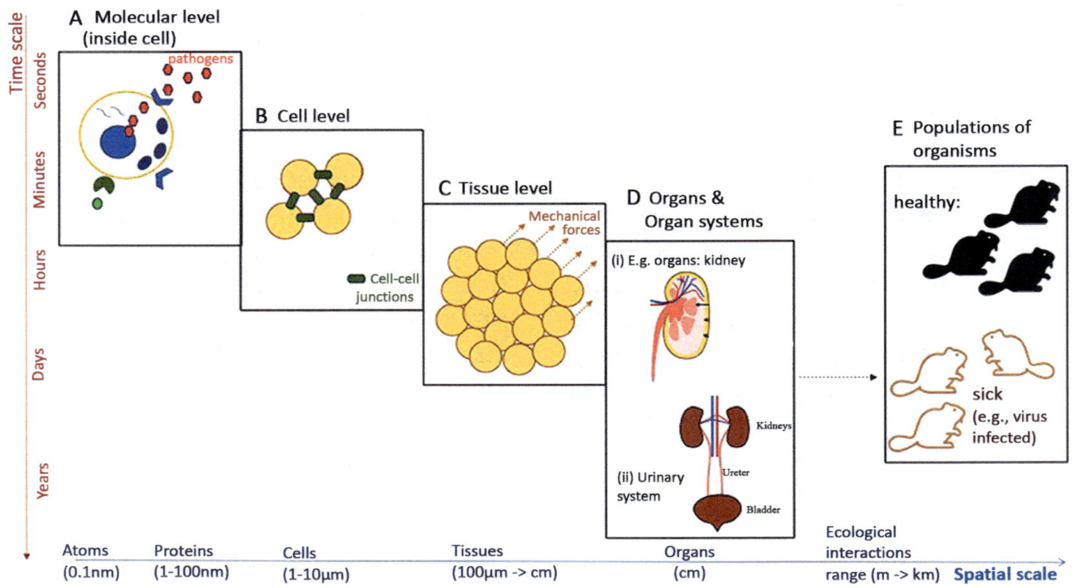

Figure 5.7. Challenges in parameter estimation.

Source: Eftimie R (2022) Grand challenges in mathematical biology: Integrating multi-scale modeling and data. Front. Appl. Math. Stat. 8:1010622. doi: 10.3389/fams.2022.1010622

And then there's the entire computational aspect of it—all another complication to the narrative. The processes we employ, such as iterative algorithms (a combination of hybrid nonlinear least squares, genetic algorithms, and Levenberg-Marquardt in many cases), can be rather sensitive to their initial values. Omitting even the smallest detail about such sensitivities may result in sums that do not work out, particularly where parameters interact with one another non-linearly and in some ways unpredictably. With how high the stakes are in predicting outbreaks and informing public health interventions, it is precisely essential to hone these computational methods. In the majority of instances, breaking these problems will take sophisticated tools and a healthy dose of interdisciplinary collaboration, making our compartmental models more reliable across a variety of situations (Shuvo et al., 2024) (Figure 5.7).

5.5.3. Impact of Heterogeneity in Populations

Populations do not interact in a perfectly uniform manner, which fundamentally alters disease transmission. Rather than taking it for granted that everyone mixes the same, as most SIR or SEIR models do, reality teaches us that individuals engage in very different ways. For instance, certain individuals—consider healthcare workers (HCPs) or critical workers—find themselves in contact with far more individuals than the majority, triggering tiny, concentrated clusters even when more general social distancing is occurring. What we find, however, is that applying simple averages conceals a lot of variation in the transmission rates, and therefore it's reasonable to take more notice of these variations when constructing models and designing public health measures (Dolbeault et al., 2020). It has been found that if you account for these variations, even the simple compartment models will change their behavior considerably. In general, when the reproduction number is greater than one, adjusting models with a negative binomial type to simulate changing contact rates makes results resemble the results of traditional models if the variations are small. However, as the difference between them expands, the results can become pretty far off from those traditional predictions. In general, individuals combine in cohorts determined by age, profession, and everyday routines—factors that simple models often overlook, particularly when a couple of super-spreading events enter the scene. By combining this type of heterogeneous mixing into the model, scientists are left with projections that more closely match actual patterns and assist in creating more intelligent intervention strategies (Kong et al., 2016). How people interact also influences the way we understand disease control measures. Consider COVID-19, for instance: even in populations largely adhering to lockdown, a few individuals with high-contact lifestyles were able to keep the virus circulating. Some scientists even indicated that even with overall compliance, this small percentage of the population kept the spread going, so infection rates did not decline as rapidly as anticipated during lockdown periods. Such observations, in which representative numbers can cover up significant particulars, remind us that we also have to look at the rough edges. Sensing these variations opens the way for tactics not only responding to an outbreak but also expecting the idiosyncrasies of population diversity—to better stem subsequent surges in the future (Dolbeault et al., 2020).

5.6. Case Studies of Compartmental Models in Action

Compartment models have long enabled us to gain a handle on disease dynamics. Consider the Zika virus in Brazil: scientists used SIR-type techniques to observe how the disease unfolded in various areas. They incorporated previously published epidemiological information to support their results—demonstrating that such critical values as the basic reproduction number (R0) aligned relatively well with others who had observed it elsewhere. It so happens that monitoring both human hosts and mosquito vectors is rather important if you desire a model that reflects reality. Ultimately, these findings provide a firm nudge toward applying compartmental models to public health policy in the event of viral outbreaks (Boret et al., 2017). The same occurred with COVID-19, with altered SEIR models providing new insight into the ways the virus spreads. For example, scientists focusing on Croatia drew upon official tallies of confirmed cases and fatalities, adjusting their model to predict where the pandemic would go under different health precautions. Overall, things such as social distancing and quarantines proved their value when the model picked up on dramatic changes in infection rates. Especially, that basic reproduction number that was derived acted as a sanity check on the model's assumptions itself, highlighting how such tools can be central in planning and response when things turn weird. Therefore, the SEIR method led health authorities in the right direction at the right time. These studies also highlight something more general: compartmental models are quite flexible. You can observe it in the contrast between the Zika model, which focused on the complicated interaction between people and vectors, and the COVID-19 model that paid closer attention to direct human-to-human interaction and the impact of external interventions. Each model, in its own manner, demonstrates that it can be reconfigured to capture the idiosyncrasies of various epidemics—thus being applicable across various contexts. The aspect that researchers continue to update these models using new data not only enhances their capacity to predict what is to happen next but also underscores the extent to which math-based modeling has taken center stage in contemporary epidemiology, truly emphasizing such methods in public health management (Boret et al., 2017).

5.6.1. Analysis of the COVID-19 Pandemic Using SIR and SEIR Models

It isn't always a simple process of disease spread. Folks tend to decompose this with compartment models such as SIR and SEIR; they divide up a population into groups depending on whether or not an individual is exposed, infected, or recovering. The SEIR variation even sets aside an "exposed" category—so you have individuals who have become infected but aren't yet infecting others. This additional step, in most instances, provides a more nuanced view of how infections roam about—a point of note when browsing actual-world outbreaks. Scientists make various public health maneuvers through these models to observe what could go right or wrong; in places with diverse healthcare responses, such insights can guide local control efforts. In practice, numerous studies have relied on the SEIR configuration to follow the course of COVID-19. For instance, studies conducted on areas such as Tamil Nadu, Maharashtra, and Andhra Pradesh adopted a modified SEIR framework in plotting the path of the pandemic. Data from May 1 to May 31, 2020, presented variations in the basic reproduction number; these presented a picture of variations in the effectiveness of health measures that was not even but rather fluctuated from one location to another. This frequent exploration of the most important epidemiological factors—factors that mattered most in this type of modeling—contributed to constructing a richer, though disorderly, image of COVID-19 transmission dynamics. Compartment models, it seems, have a significant influence on crafting strategies that correspond to local public health performances, informing resource allocation and intervention strategies. Control strategies that are incorporated into such models only add to their out-of-the-classroom appeal. One particular study, for example, did not merely adhere to infection dynamics; it included optimal control problems that were engineered to suppress infections via drugs as well as non-drug means. Drawing on concepts such as Pontryagin's maximal principle, the researchers examined everything from vaccination campaigns to quarantine policies. Their equilibrium analysis revealed that, in general, targeted approaches can hold good public health responses fairly well. In brief, application of SIR and SEIR models during COVID-19 shows how mathematical models, however theoretical they might be, are capable of influencing decisions and improving health outcomes in the presence of infectious diseases (Muniyandi et al., 2024; Ramalingam et al., 2025) (Figure 5.8).

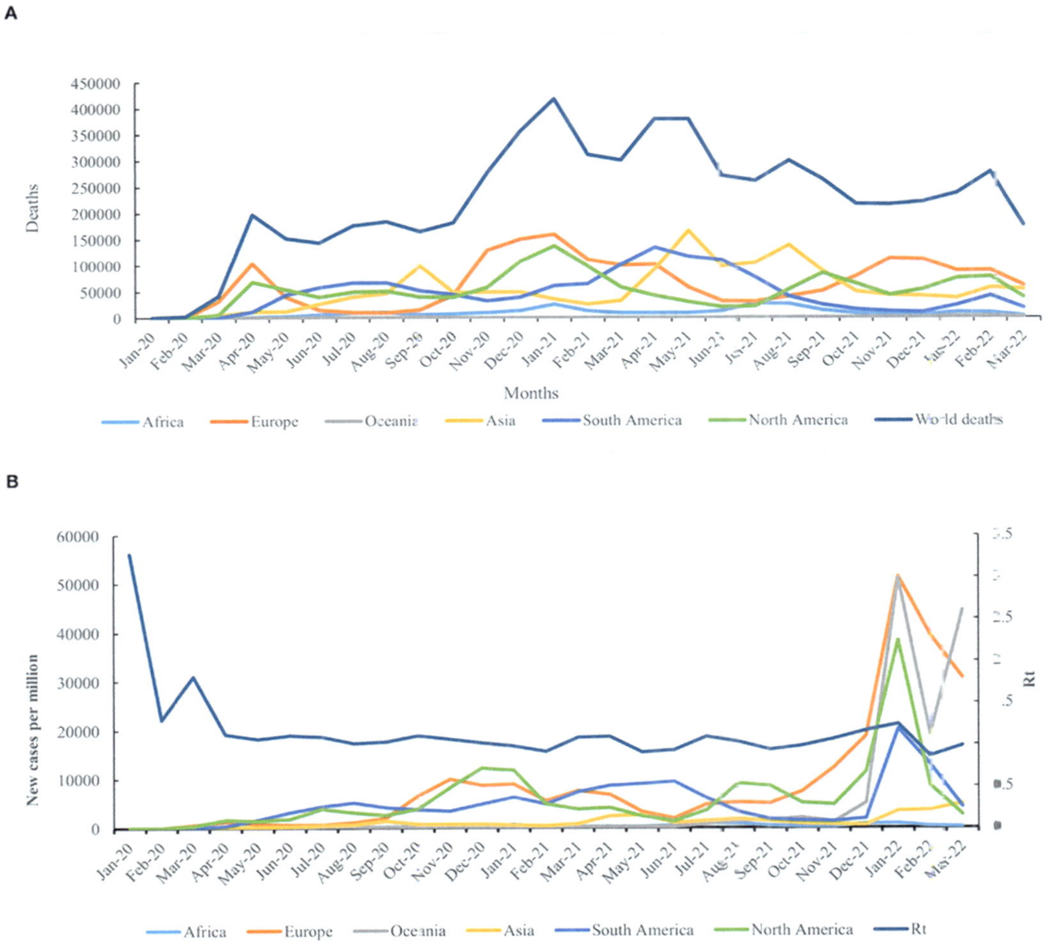

Figure 5.8. Analysis of the COVID-19 pandemic using SIR and SEIR models.

Source: Gao L, Zheng C, Shi Q, Xiao K, Wang L, Liu Z, Li Z and Dong X (2022) Evolving trend change during the COVID-19 pandemic. Front. Public Health 10:957265. doi: 10.3389/fpubh.2022.957265

5.6.2. Historical Case Studies: Measles and Influenza

Epidemics are not statistics on a graph—epidemics are histories. Consider measles and flu; if you go back into case histories, you find out a lot about the way these diseases spread. San Francisco in 1918 saw the flu burst in crowded residential areas, an almost uncontrolled, exponential flame.

The chaotic combination of human action, public health changes, and social configurations has a gigantic role to play in these trends. That is why, in the majority of instances, scientists rely on models such as SIR and SEIR—they assist in connecting observed outbreaks to the theories that inform public health actions. Even if they seem geeky, these models are just devices to predict how diseases unfold and what the best interventions may be. Referring to older epidemic data, you can observe directly the crazy heterogeneity in how diseases spread from person to person. Consider measles, for instance; its high infectiousness tends to unleash a quick chain of infections within populations that haven't yet established defenses.

Research tends to emphasize that it is important to pin down the initial growth phase—such a phase is responsible for identifying major figures such as the basic reproduction number. When previous outbreaks come under examination by way of statistical analysis, the findings tend to inform compartmental models that incorporate aspects such as generation time and daily contact patterns. Okay, perhaps it does sound a bit nerdy, but these models provide us with a more complete picture of measles dynamics and, most importantly, set the stage for intelligent vaccination and control policy today. Both influenza and measles strongly reinforce the message that mathematical models are crucial when trying to understand infectious diseases. Dusty records are not simply dusty relics; they offer essential hints regarding a disease's potential for transmission and help lay the ground for planning in the future. Take, for example, new methods of researching historic influenza outbreaks, which illustrate that we require models keen enough to detect the constantly shifting ballet of an epidemic. They illustrate how factors, such as who is talking to whom, small changes in behavior, and different intervention strategies—can rearrange the deck in epidemic situations. Scientists have even observed that outbreak growth differs significantly based on geography or social configuration, suggesting the messy, patchy nature of our world. Overall, incorporating historical information into these models appears to be quite an effective measure for enhancing our preparedness to respond to future epidemics (Chowell & Nishiura, 2007).

5.6.3. Lessons Learned from Model Predictions and Real Outcomes

Early in an outbreak, things are usually unclear, and it's hard to nail down reliable predictions. Under COVID-19, a variety of compartmental models got added into the equation and, surprisingly, the Generalized Additive Model (GAM) tended to excel in predicting new case numbers—while exponential or Poisson models strangely performed better for cumulative totals. Data in those initial days was everywhere, and therefore predictions of peak epidemics tended to be wrong. This comes through, in most instances, that even though such models may provide useful insights, the unreliable character of initial data requires a prudent interpretation and an openness to changing policies (Acar et al., 2023). Infectious disease modeling itself has evolved a great deal over time - lessons were not only drawn from the successes but also from the failures.

Historically, models relied on idealized assumptions that don't always align when an outbreak occurs. Recent experience, in general, suggests that the loop behind controlling epidemics has its own sort of unpredictable friction embedded right within public health systems. Stretching typical models to fit messy, real-world complications might appear to add both structural and computational burdens, but it also pushes us toward new ways of managing epidemics more intelligently. Overall, a layered approach might just be what public health authorities need to prepare them more adequately for future threats (Brown et al., 2017). What we discover through balancing model predictions against actual outcomes has huge implications for how we prepare for the future. COVID-19 taught us predictive models can spew out wildly varying numbers based on the parameters and data sets employed. In many instances, receiving immediate feedback from actual cases tends to modify and improve those models in real-time, a process that, in most instances, leads to more informed decision-making. Including strong measures along with risk assessments into our framework not only raises our game in decision-making but also, when combined with close monitoring for gaps in predictions, helps improve further. Ultimately, cultivating a habit of ongoing learning out of these prediction glitches ought to help construct a more resilient public health system equipped to handle the gritty realities of future epidemics (Acar et al., 2023).

CLOSER LOOK

The SEIR Model

The SEIR model is a commonly applied epidemiological model that can explain and predict the spread of infectious diseases in a population. SEIR is an acronym for Susceptible, Exposed, Infectious, and Recovered, which are the four main stages that individuals go through during an outbreak.

1. **Susceptible (S):** These are the people who have not yet been infected but can contract the disease.
2. **Exposed (E):** Individuals who have contracted the infection but are not infectious yet fall into this category. This is the incubation phase, during which the pathogen is within the body but the symptoms have not yet shown up.
3. **Infectious (I):** Individuals in this category are capable of infecting others with the disease. This is the stage where symptoms usually manifest, though there are some infections that can be transmitted by asymptomatic carriers.
4. **Recovered (R):** These patients have recovered from the illness and are usually assumed to have developed immunity, lowering their risk of reinfection.

The SEIR model extends to more basic models such as SIR by including the Exposed phase, and it is particularly helpful for illnesses with a latent (incubation) period, including COVID-19 or measles. By representing shifts among these phases, public health authorities can make predictions about how quickly an illness will spread and assess the effect of interventions such as quarantine or vaccination.

SUMMARY

Disease spread models such as SIR and SEIR have truly revolutionized the way we view infections. These allow public health individuals and scientists to quantify the extent of an outbreak and consider trial interventions practically. At times, introducing a little additional step, such as the exposed category in SEIR—can refine our projections for actual cases. New spins, such as the SEIR-HVQD model (Oyelade et al., 2022), keep emerging and show that ideas in disease modeling keep evolving as our understanding deepens. Better tech and improved ways of gathering data only boost these methods' role in shaping health policies that work. Recent global health crises have made it clear that these compartmental models are more than academic puzzles. Broadly speaking, employing targeted lockdowns—locking up high-risk segments while leaving lower-risk people to live more freely—is seen to raise public health and economic results alike (Acemoğlu et al., 2020).

Lockdowns, for instance, are targeted specifically at older groups; they serve to bring infection rates down considerably without restraining younger groups too much. This combination-and-mix strategy of dealing with diverse populations demonstrates that models may be applied as hands-on tools instead of being purely theoretical exercises. In all but a handful of instances, how these frameworks are evolving is the key to future policies that restrict how severely infections affect us. Overall, the ongoing fine-tuning of these models commingles mathematical concepts with practical health practice. With challenges such as COVID-19 turning up unforeseen surprises in how illness spreads, models must continue to evolve—adjusting their algorithms to function with new data and emerging understanding of behavior. Others are even pushing the boundaries by adding sophisticated methods, such as the Ebola Optimization Search Algorithm (Oyelade et al., 2022), to enhance predictive capability. This type of flexibility is paramount in the face of the numerous layers of infectious disease, ensuring that health responses are as pragmatic as they are scientific. The constant development of these models, with a few rough edges along the way, truly serves to emphasize their usefulness in safeguarding global health.

Compartmental models such as SIR and SEIR provide us with a glimpse of how infections spread in terms that may not be immediately obvious to the naked eye. If you compare these models to empirical data, particularly what transpired during COVID-19—you can see that they have their strengths and weaknesses. In a study that examined various epidemic response strategies, it was found that the SEIR-QD and SEIR-PO versions tended to surpass the traditional SIR method. This improved demonstration of performance tends to be related to getting the right balance between introducing a little complexity and fitting the data, so the predictions regarding infections become a bit more acute. Evidently, during outbreaks that quicken rapidly, initial predictions tend to fall short until the models are further refined, as in the case of Yang et al. (2021).

Contemporary computational devices, such as those through machine learning, have also assisted these compartmental models to get a level-up. Deep Learning, for instance, has quietly become a central character in predicting disease trends by managing massive amounts of data and extracting time-based patterns. Researchers now employ Natural Language Processing and data mining in unforeseen manners to elicit important pieces of information that previous frameworks may have missed. This union of sophisticated methods not only provides new avenues to address problems such as a lack of definition or challenges with generalization in the earlier models, but it also smoothes over some of the usual criticisms – a fact pointed out in Shorten et al. (2021).

Interweaving these compartmental models with modern data analysis techniques appears to hold out hope for a better future for public health approaches. As diseases evolve and mutate, having models updated with constant fine-tuning becomes nearly inevitable to make the correct decisions fast. The relatively mixed bag experienced under COVID-19, particularly near those inflection points, indicates that there is much more to learn and get better at. Looking to the future, combining the old-school epidemiological method with new, innovative technology is not only beneficial—it is necessary for addressing today's issues as well as tomorrow's public health emergencies. This general combination provides a good foundation for a robust framework in infectious disease study.

KEY TERMS FROM THIS CHAPTER

- Force of infection
- Herd immunity threshold
- infectious illnesses
- Integrated Nested Laplace Approximation (INLA)
- Contact rate
- Model parameters
- intervention strategies
- Valencian Community

REFERENCES

1. Acar, A. S., Azzolina, D., Berchialla, P., Comoretto, R. I., Corciulo, M. A., Gregori, D., Lanera, C., et al. (2023). Fitting early phases of the COVID-19 outbreak: A comparison of the performances of used models. *Healthcare, 11*(17), 2363. https://core.ac.uk/download/590393326.pdf (accessed on 6 May 2025).
2. Acemoğlu, D., Chernozhukov, V., Werning, I., & Whinston, M. D. (2021). Optimal targeted lockdowns in a multi-group SIR model. *American Economic Review: Insights, 3*(4), 487–502. https://doi.org/10.3386/w27102.
3. Acheneje, G. O., Omale, D., Agbata, B. C., Atokolo, W., Shior, M. M., & Bolarinwa, B. E. (2024). Approximate Solution of the Fractional Order Mathematical Model on the Transmission Dynamics on The Co-Infection of COVID-19 and Monkeypox Using the Laplace-Adomian Decomposition Method, International Journal of Mathematics and Statistics Studies, 12 (3), 17-51 (accessed on 6 May 2025).
4. Altun, K., Altuntaş, S., & Dereli, T. (2021). An interaction-oriented multi-agent SIR model to assess the spread of SARS-CoV-2. *Hachette Journal of Mathematics and Statistics, 50*(5), 1548–1559. https://core.ac.uk/download/491582195.pdf (accessed on 6 May 2025).
5. Awuah-Mensah, K. A. (2018). *Epidemiological Model of the Transmission and Spread of Hepatitis B Pandemic in Ghana*. https://core.ac.uk/download/210551722.pdf (accessed on 6 May 2025).
6. Benterki, A., Brar, M., Chishtie, F. A., Drozd, et al. (2023). Modelling of COVID-19 using fractional differential equations. https://core.ac.uk/download/588591626.pdf (accessed on 6 May 2025).
7. Boret, S. E. B., Buitrago, R., Escalante, R., & Villasana, M. (2017). Mathematical modelling of Zika virus in Brazil. http://arxiv.org/abs/1708.01280 (accessed on 6 May 2025).
8. Bui, H., Eksioglu, S., & Proano, R. (2024). Evaluating the impact of vaccine hesitancy on the allocation of vital resources during the COVID-19 pandemic. http://arxiv.org/abs/2403.07971 (accessed on 6 May 2025).
9. Burridge, H., Craske, J., & Wood, S. (2023). Relating quanta conservation and compartmental epidemiological models of airborne disease outbreaks in buildings. *Scientific Reports, 13*, Article 17335. https://core.ac.uk/download/590242376.pdf (accessed on 6 May 2025).
10. Kong, L., Wang, J., Han, W., & Cao, Z. (2016). Modeling Heterogeneity in Direct Infectious Disease Transmission in a Compartmental Model. *International journal of environmental research and public health, 13*(3), 253. https://doi.org/10.3390/ijerph13030253
11. Chowell, G., & Nishiura, H. (2007). Quantifying the transmission potential of pandemic influenza. http://arxiv.org/abs/0711.3088 (accessed on 6 May 2025).
12. Chowell, G., Simonsen, L., & Viboud, C. (2016). A generalized-growth model to characterize the early ascending phase of infectious disease outbreaks. *Epidemics, 15*, 27–37. https://doi.org/10.1016/j.epidem.2016.01.002.
13. Colli, P., Marinoschi, G., Rocca, E., & Viguerie, A. (2024). Chemotaxis-inspired PDE model for airborne infectious disease transmission: Analysis and simulations. *Journal of Nonlinear Science, 35*(28). https://www.semanticscholar.org/paper/308a892a3a73be4b888813bd08eb8fe1f6e901e6 (accessed on 6 May 2025).

14. Dolbeault, J., & Turinici, G. (2020). Heterogeneous social interactions and the COVID-19 lockdown outcome in a multi-group SEIR model. http://arxiv.org/abs/2005.00049 (accessed on 6 May 2025).

15. Fisher, A. (2023). Mathematical modeling, analysis and simulation of COVID-19 dynamics. A dissertation submitted in partial fulfillment of the requirements for the degree of DOCTOR OF PHILOSOPHY WASHINGTON STATE UNIVERSITY Department of Mathematics and Statistics DECEMBER 2023 https://core.ac.uk/download/603337256.pdf (accessed on 6 May 2025).

16. Gomes, M. G. M., Ferreira, M. U., Corder, R. M., King, J. G., Souto-Maior, C., Penha-Gonçalves, C., Gonçalves, G., et al. (2022). Individual variation in susceptibility or exposure to SARS-CoV-2 lowers the herd immunity threshold. *Journal of Theoretical Biology, 540*, 111063. https://doi.org/10.1016/j.jtbi.2022.111063.

17. Lopman, B., Liu, C. Y., Le Guillou, A., Handel, A., Lash, T. L., Isakov, A. P., & Jenness, S. M. (2021). A modeling study to inform screening and testing interventions for the control of SARS-CoV-2 on university campuses. *Scientific Reports, 11*, 85252. https://doi.org/10.1038/s41598-021-85252-z.

18. Oyelade, O. N., Ezugwu, A. E., Mohamed, T. I. A., & Abualigah, L. (2022). Ebola optimization search algorithm: A new nature-inspired metaheuristic optimization algorithm. *IEEE Access, 10*, 16150–16177. https://doi.org/10.1109/ACCESS.2022.3147821.

19. Phaijoo, G. R., & Gurung, D. B. (2025). Sensitivity analysis of SEIR SEI model of dengue disease. https://www.semanticscholar.org/paper/5416eff668a6bdb67212b000703624d000dcbbb0 (accessed on 6 May 2025).

20. Ramalingam, R., Gnanaprakasam, A., & Boulaaras, S. (2025). Stability and control analysis of COVID-19 spread in India using SEIR model. *Scientific Reports, 15*. https://www.semanticscholar.org/paper/b3bb988a2d47995f00d3093f146dc70731707800 (accessed on 6 May 2025).

21. Raychaudhuri, S. J., & Babu, C. (2023). Recursive stacked Leaky Net-based compartmental model for analysis of COVID-19 transmission dynamics. *Journal of Information & Knowledge Management, 22*, 2350020:1–2350020:23. https://www.semanticscholar.org/paper/7cfa7296b41513bcdfa2cc9ad652a37e77fdd18e (accessed on 6 May 2025).

22. Shi Y, Zhu X, Zhu X, Cheng B, Zhong Y. Kalman Filter-Based Epidemiological Model for Post-COVID-19 Era Surveillance and Prediction. Sensors. 2025; 25(8):2507. https://doi.org/10.3390/s25082507 (accessed on 6 May 2025).

23. Shorten, C., Khoshgoftaar, T. M., & Furht, B. (2021). Deep learning applications for COVID-19. *Journal of Big Data, 8*. https://doi.org/10.1186/s40537-020-00392-9.

24. Tenriawaru, A., Wibawa, G. A., Abapihi, B., Ahmad, S. W., & Sudayasa, I. P. (2025). Bayesian stochastic INLA application to the SIR-SI model for investigating dengue transmission dynamics. *Intelligent Automation & Soft Computing*. https://www.semanticscholar.org/paper/98e095353e00861029358662768ec20b2bcd35ef (accessed on 6 May 2025).

25. Usán Sanz, P. (2023). *Mathematical Modelling of The Epidemic Dynamics Due to Viral Interference*. https://core.ac.uk/download/613973620.pdf (accessed on 6 May 2025).

26. Whinston, M. D., Werning, I., Chernozhukov, V., & Acemoğlu, D. (2020). *A Multi-Risk SIR Model with Optimally Targeted Lockdown* (CEMMAP Working Paper No. 14/20). https://doi.org/10.1920/wp.cem.2020.1420.

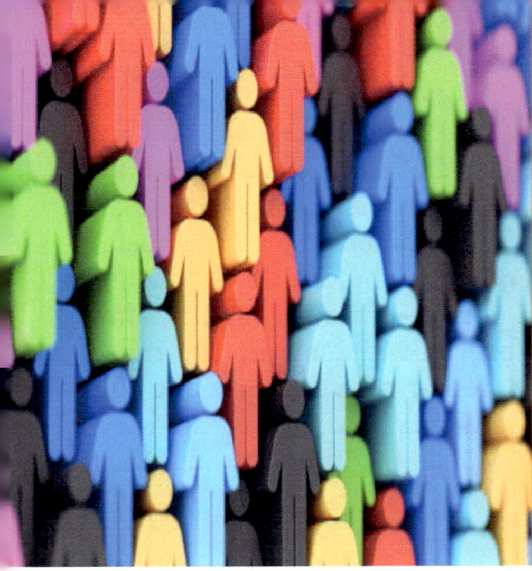

Chapter 6

HETEROGENEITIES IN POPULATIONS

Contents

Introduction

Populations in the wild can be quite surprising. They show up in so many ways—one moment it is about their genes, the next it is how they act or look. This mix-up of behaviors, body shapes, and even how they interact fuels the changes we see in nature. In many cases, these differences matter when it comes to bouncing back from tough times or sharing resources, and scientists often stumble upon hidden patterns that hint at deeper biological secrets. It is almost like the more you peer into these features, the more you uncover, setting the stage for all kinds of future research. Sometimes, where you look and when you look changes the picture entirely. Dynamic differences, for example, can spring up because of stress in the environment or even a scramble for resources. One study—focused on, say, those non-ergodic states tied to attractive colloidal glasses—shows that the timing counts. Short waiting periods can make particles zip around more freely, while longer waits tend to leave things looking uniform as if the particles have settled into a predictable pattern. Generally speaking, these findings suggest that variability is not a fixed trait but something that shifts with conditions (Puertas et al., 2006). When it comes to infectious diseases, these uneven traits among hosts play a huge role. Take *Leishmania infantum* parasites: they seem to accumulate differently across hosts, with higher numbers in some, especially in skin tissues, which then boosts the chance of passing the microbe on to sandflies. This uneven spread is not just a trivial detail—it has big implications for how we manage diseases and target control measures for those individuals who are most infectious. To summarize, watching how parasite numbers clump together offers a peek into the complex dance between a host's own features and disease spread, reinforcing why studying these differences is so important in both health and ecological research (Mohammadiha et al., 2013).

Definition of Heterogeneity in Populations

Diversity is evident in a lot of forms in population studies—it is not simply a matter of numbers but actual differences that border on social, health, and environmental concerns. This mix, which can be referred to as heterogeneity, encapsulates the different differences that we observe among groups, ranging from geography and culture to age and background. These differences, which are replicated again and again in the data, make a difference when attempting to understand phenomena such as infertility. For instance, it has been suggested by some studies that the lifetime risk of infertility can wildly vary from one place to another, which implies that how things are measured can have results that do not entirely correlate. It is a difficult task to define and quantify infertility, and that difficulty reflects the larger one of adapting to heterogeneous populations. More often than not, it's all about gaining a good understanding of these subtleties to develop interventions that respond to each group's respective needs (Cox et al., 2022). Differences in method, it turns out, matter a great deal, particularly in health-based studies. Consider comparing studies that examine records from the past with those observing time-to-pregnancy results; these varying methods have a way of influencing the numbers we derive.

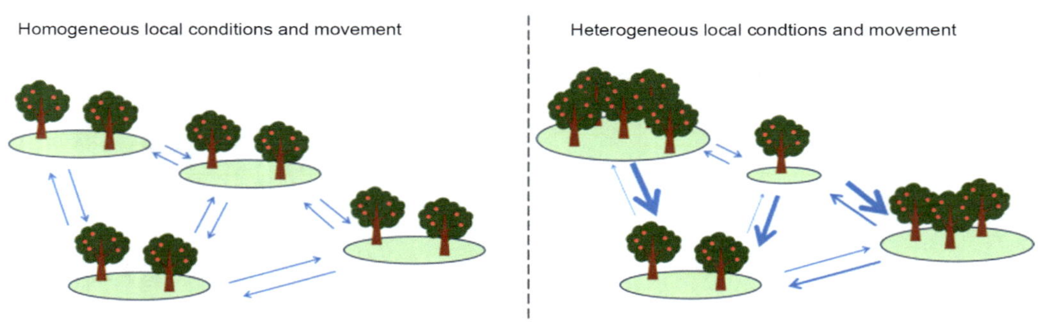

Figure 6.1. Definition of heterogeneity in populations.

Source: Okinawa Institute of Science and Technology. (2024). *Contrast Between Idealized Homogeneous and Heterogeneous Local Conditions and Movement.*

Occasionally, the meta-analyses demonstrate that despite attempts to iron out variation in definitions, the confusion with measures leaves considerable heterogeneity in estimates of prevalence. Thus, despite the apparent face of overall frequencies of conditions such as infertility being quite alarming, the sloppy undertow of variation in methods smudges the image. For the most part, having one uniform method of gathering the data would resolve these discrepancies and allow us to compare populations with greater assurance (Page et al., 2021). Ultimately, these varied patterns in populations don't remain on paper—they influence real-world public health and policy decisions. A close examination of how diversity comes into play in health outcomes can inform strategies for addressing the issues that various groups experience. Consider it similar to designing school programs or organizing healthcare services that suit the real needs of communities with high infertility rates. By taking into consideration, the uneven allocation of traits among populations, policymakers can design interventions that are effective as well as equitable, directing resources precisely where they are required. This method not only enhances the effectiveness of health programs but also constructs a more inclusive conversation on population health, which is, of course, critical to solving such multifaceted problems (Page et al., 2021; Cox et al., 2022) (Figure 6.1).

Importance of Studying Population Heterogeneities

Population variations count for a great deal when it comes to controlling infectious disease—a point not always self-evident. Glance more closely and you notice that immunity is not distributed evenly; rather, it is influenced by a combination of age, social behavior, and geography. Scientists now tend to employ serological surveys directly to measure immunity in different groups, and such tests can reveal underlying layers of resistance and vulnerability, which are critical when predicting outbreak behavior. In many cases, establishing something like a World Serology Bank might boost how precisely we capture these trends and, in turn, refine vaccination plans for specific groups, thereby aiding in disease control and deepening our grasp of immunity landscapes (Page et al., 2021). Looking beyond mere infection control, studying these population differences touches on why some communities face tougher environmental and social health challenges. Reflect on how the framework of planetary boundaries shows that when humans push nature beyond its limits, the health consequences are not equally distributed across all groups. Policymakers can better identify and focus on the communities most affected by climate change and other ecological disturbances by noting these differences. This knowledge becomes essential in devising interventions that address immediate health emergencies as well as longer-term sustainability challenges. In the end, such customized approaches can foster resilience, enabling communities to adapt and even flourish in the face of environmental adversity (Steffen et al., 2015). At the end of the day, delving into how populations vary is a foundation of work that bridges health science, environmental research, and social policy. Identifying that various groups experience vulnerability in their own way makes it possible for researchers and decision-makers, in general, to design more equitable interventions and sustainability efforts. Doing so not only yields rapid gains in public health but also helps us better understand how social and environmental settings influence well-being. A close examination of these differences is not only helpful—it is necessary for furthering scientific understanding and advancing social justice in our health and environmental policy discussions (Page et al., 2021).

6.1. Types of Heterogeneities

Populations are not homogeneous; they inherently exhibit traits of variation that can be seen throughout biology and social life. Consider how our genes are not the same as one individual. The variation within can influence everything from susceptibility to disease to treatment mechanisms, even overall health. With personalized medicine increasingly becoming the norm, it's become fairly evident that understanding this genetic information is important when it comes to individualizing therapies based on one's needs. For the majority of instances, when you combine personalized medicine with concepts in network pharmacology, it happens that a one-size-fits-all principle simply doesn't cut it. Accepting the fact that there is genetic diversity drives us toward more intelligent approaches in drug discovery and treatment design, ultimately allowing us to better cope with the variety of responses observed in various groups (Marsh et al., 2010). Changing gears, how we look or act also matters a great deal—that is what we refer to as phenotypic heterogeneity. Environmental pressures, individual habits, and social contexts all contribute to the formation of characteristics that can differ broadly even within one population. In ecology, for instance, shifting landscapes can push populations to evolve in unexpected ways, and those variations tend to instigate changes in how humans relate as well. Occasionally, characteristics such as strong personality traits will alter group behavior—altering cooperation, access to resources, and even simple habits. Overall, immersing ourselves in these tangible traits provides us with great insight into evolution and the dynamics of communities, illustrating that adaptive traits could well be an inevitable response to continually evolving socio-environmental pressures (Delgado-Serrano et al., 2009).

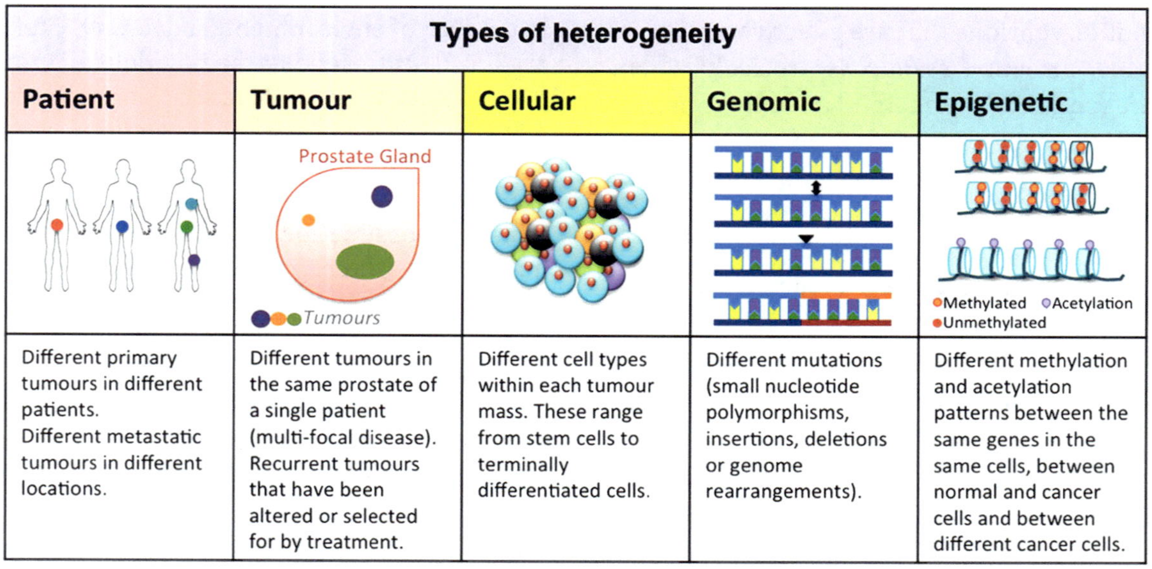

Figure 6.2. Types of heterogeneities.

Source: Brennan, P. A., & Thomas, G. J. (2021). Multiple types of heterogeneity require consideration when treating cancer patients. *ResearchGate*.

Time also has its trick. Temporal heterogeneity—that is, how groups change as time elapses—closely mirrors changes instigated by both intrinsic forces and external pressures such as changing resources or social shifts. Observing how a population changes over time allows scholars to catch trends of transformation or stability, providing a window into resilience and adaptability. Seeing that our historical context does have an impact allowed us to observe how those past environmental influences contribute to the structures of today's groups. To illustrate, think about how galaxies have changed over billions of years—those stark contrasts between ancient and modern structures underscore these processes. Generally, responding to these time-dependent changes is important when planning effective conservation measures and controlling ecosystems to enhance long-term resilience (Delgado-Serrano et al., 2009) (Figure 6.2).

6.1.1. Genetic Heterogeneity

Genetic differences emerge in many unexpected ways among people, which makes it tricky to pin down why illnesses show up and react differently. It is a reminder that, in most cases, we need clear-cut methods to deduce these various variations. Current research, for example, proposes breaking these differences down into categories such as feature, outcome, or associative variation – a rough map that illuminates everything from the display of traits to the ways genes mix and mingle in heterogeneous groups. Every cut of this puzzle points to its own genetic idiosyncrasies, and catching them allows scientists to adjust their strategies so that neat-by-the-numbers models do not mislead us (Woodward et al., 2022). Rare genetic variants throw even more complexity into the mix. Classic statistics models most often assume that gene effects are uniform across the board, a possibility that can hide significant information about how people vary. This is where the gap exists and why new concepts are called for. One clear solution, a conditional autoregressive model, handles these genetic influences as if they simply appear at random – a trick that increases our odds of selecting out subtle, heterogeneous effects, particularly when rare variants contribute significantly to disease. For the most part, this approach provides a little more heft in identifying those subtle differences, allowing researchers to get a better sense for how diseases truly function and tease out smarter, more individualized treatments (Shen et al., 2021). Genetic disparities are not simply an intellectual challenge – they hit close to home in public health and routine medical practice. If we examine the wide combination of gene patterns across individuals, it's easy to see that medicine can be tailored to accommodate various communities. Consider, for instance, how distinctive genetic markers of disease risk could inform novel screening concepts or treatment strategies that cater to specific group requirements. The challenging bit is still how best to characterize and research all these turns, frequently having to mash together massive pieces of genomics and other omics data. This turned-around interaction between our genes and the environment, put together, can assist in constructing a healthcare system that is more equitable and aligned with the genetic profile of each group (Woodward et al., 2022) (Figure 6.3).

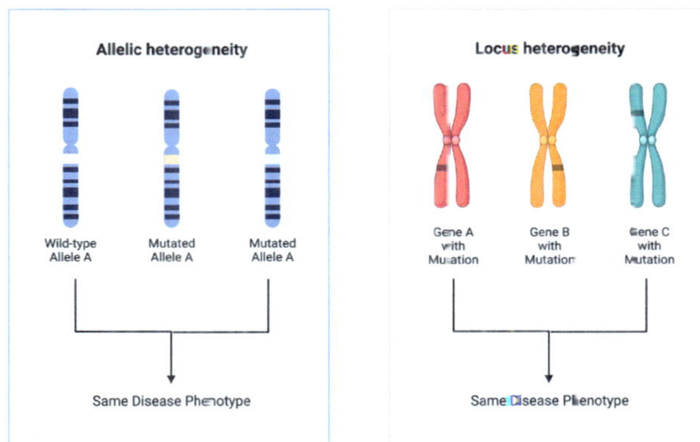

Figure 6.3. Genetic heterogeneity.

Source: BioRender. (n.d.). Allelic heterogeneity and locus heterogeneity. *Wikimedia Commons.*

6.1.2. Phenotypic Heterogeneity

Phenotypic variation plays a central part in cracking the code of how biological communities function. Even when it's members within the same species, differences emerge everywhere—sometimes disguised in genes and sometimes obvious in appearance or behavior. Consider cancer cells evolving under stress; in acute myeloid leukemia (AML), for instance, scientists typically identified four distinct cell groups that are resistant to venetoclax. Every group demonstrates its own combination of characteristics, genetic idiosyncrasies, and drug reactions. All of these differences, in most instances, render treatments that much more difficult, i.e., a one-size-fits-all solution just will not work (Mohanty et al., 2024). Even outside the world of cancer, the array of differences that can be observed even extends to microbial life. A research study of the *Klebsiella pneumoniae* species complex, for example, revealed an unexpectedly varied array of isolates. Some remain the traditional type, some tend toward what you could term hypervirulent, and even some that act as if they are hypermucoviscous. It happens that these classifications are not merely names—there are huge implications. Hypervirulent strains, for example, exhibit stark differences in their infective factors and how they resist antibiotics, which can subsequently produce quite different clinical presentations. All of these subtleties highlight how evolution can mix things up and make us reconsider infection control and public health measures (Níguez-Medina et al., 2024). Taking a step back, it is evident that grasping these turns and twists of phenotypic variation requires an interdisciplinary response combining the insights of molecular biology, ecology, and public health. When you look at the mechanism of resistance across cancer cells and bacteria, you begin to notice some common strategies. For instance, AML treatment regimens may inadvertently privilege some cell states and enhance diversity within a tumor. Likewise, the identification of multiple clonal groups in *K. pneumoniae* highlights the evolutionary forces that influence their drug resistance and virulence. As a general point, this twofold dimension of variation not only educates us in terms of our cancer treatments and uses of antibiotics but also indicates the importance of the ongoing study to continue addressing these evolving systems (Mohanty et al., 2024; Níguez-Medina et al., 2024).

6.1.3. Environmental Heterogeneity

Complex ecosystems transform with changing environments—the combination of conditions determines who's present and how populations act. Environmental heterogeneity, as some term it, is central to initiating biodiversity and general resilience. Consider forests: varying patches of habitat here allow an entire collection of species, each attuned to its own conditions, a chance. Natural disturbance-based management (or NDBM) relies on understanding why nature's own combination—its form and makeup following disturbances such as fires or floods—is important. For the most part, by keeping ecological processes diverse (and yes, biodiversity is responsible for much of that diversity), NDBM attempts to sidestep a bland, homogeneous landscape that might be inordinately susceptible to large, abrupt changes (Andren et al., 2006). In short, caring for that natural mix not only protects today's species but also creates a sort of insurance plan for tomorrow's shifts in ecosystems. Soil diversity is also a giant contributor to this overall mix, even though it may be out of sight. See how soils support a wacky variety of microorganisms and tiny animals that fuel nutrient cycles and support overall ecosystem health. More recent research, such as from the UK Soil Biodiversity Program—has demonstrated an astonishingly diverse range of soil dwellers hard at work on things like carbon and nitrogen cycling (Finlay et al., 2005). It appears that, beyond what we can see above ground, the small, subterranean populations quite literally make or break how an ecosystem functions. One might say, in a sense, by cultivating more fertile soil life, land managers could potentially enable terrestrial systems to recover more vigorously following perturbation, laying the groundwork for a more vigorous response to environmental change. Additionally, having a range of conditions entails that species ultimately adopt varying survival strategies. Nature's unevenness provides niches, allowing different species to define their own niches and relaxing the competition pressure—a dynamic that usually results in improved coexistence. The concept resonates with resilience theory, which typically posits that if a system is diverse, its constituent parts will absorb shocks in different ways, so the entire system is less likely to crash simultaneously. As we are making plans for landscapes in an age of changing climates, it absolutely pays to be thinking not only about how variable the environment is, but about how that variation fosters flexibility and affects relationships between species. Overall, staying tuned into these subtleties of environmental heterogeneity provides keys to framing conservation management that maintains biodiversity thriving and ecosystems stable while the world is still changing (Figure 6.4).

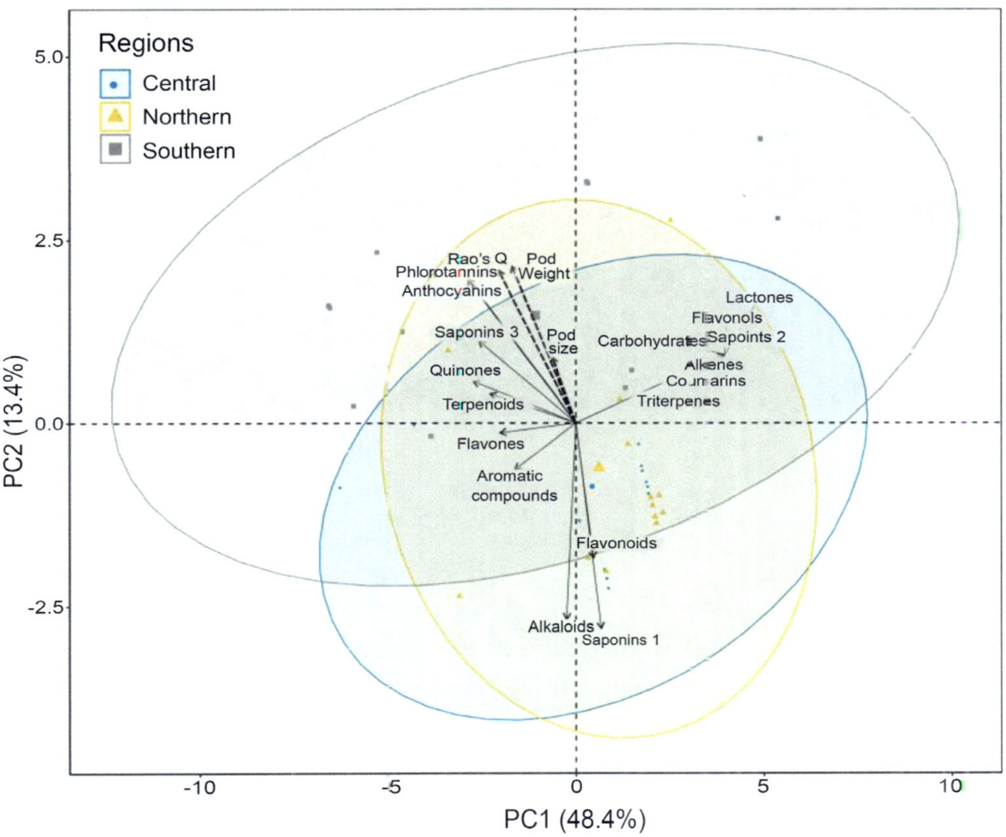

Figure 6.4. Environmental heterogeneity.

Source: Esparza-Orozco A, Carranza-Becerra L, Delgadillo-Ruiz L, Bollaín y Goytia JJ, Gaytán-Saldaña NA, Mandujano-García CD, Delgadillo-Ruiz E, Michel-López CY, Huerta-García J, Valladares-Carranza B, et al. Environmental Heterogeneity Drives Secondary Metabolite Diversity from Mesquite Pods in Semiarid Regions. *Ecologies*. 2025; 6(1):19. https://doi.org/10.3390/ecologies6010019

6.2. Causes of Heterogeneities

Populations are an assortment of influences—ecological context, social behavior, and geography all get tangled up in ways that are not necessarily clear. Human things, however, do not take a back seat; they are capable of altering the entire landscape. Consider rabies in household dogs:

following its transmission requires observing how human movements and cultural practices get confused with the spatial organization, and determining how quickly viruses hop around and persist. Identifying these human-influenced landscape adjustments is significant, particularly where people and their animals get close to one another (Anderson et al., 2012).

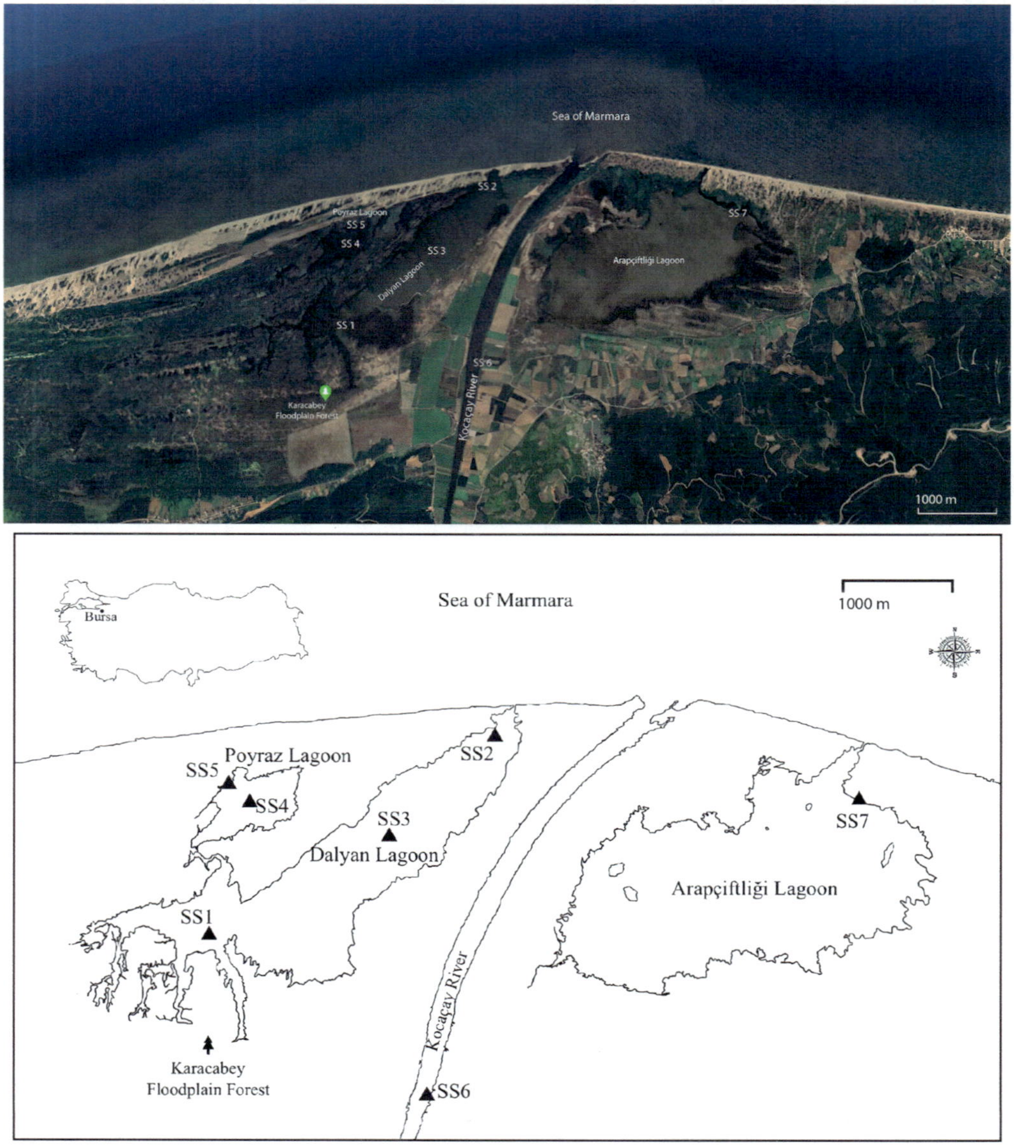

Dalkıran N, Zünbülgil-Ünsal B. Environmental Heterogeneity and Salinity Gradient Impacted the Alpha and Beta Diversities of Diatom Assemblages in a Coastal Delta Wetland. *Water*. 2023; 15(19):3414. https://doi.org/10.3390/w15193414

In the majority of instances, these interrelated factors account for why variations arise between groups. Biological idiosyncrasies come into play as well. At the cellular level, the tale of lipid bilayers illustrates just how diverse things can become. Coarse-grained molecular dynamics simulations demonstrate that mixtures of lipids at times appear mixed evenly, while at other times create identifiable pockets or phases—again, depending on the system's size. This information—that size is critical—is an important detail when attempting to explain what happens in minute systems and shows us the same in larger social groups as well (He et al., 2018).

Internal forces and external pressures, all mixed together, yield a complicated, if not random, result. Genes play their part as well by creating discord among populations. Even minute genetic differences have the power to ignite changes in bodily characteristics, viability, and robustness—occasionally allowing some members to cope with adverse conditions more effectively than others. Tools such as landscape genetics assist us in unraveling this interaction through the consideration of migration routes, use of resources, and risk of disease, all via the prism of genetic diversity. Combining that which we understand about genes with environmental observations presents a rich, multi-layered picture of how variable a population might be. Overall, this requires a combination of genetic research and ecological understanding to develop wiser, customized conservation and management strategies (Anderson et al., 2012) (Figure 6.5).

6.2.1. Evolutionary Processes

Evolution appears in so many layers of nature—it powers the diversity we observe in living organisms day by day. One of the earliest things to observe is that small adjustments within a species—what most refer to as microevolution—occur progressively over generations. Consider minute changes in gene types; these modifications, powered by natural selection, drift, and gene flow, assist organisms in fitting more comfortably into their immediate environments. There follows a wider sweep of change, sometimes referred to as macroevolution, where large changes do indeed create new species via occurrences such as speciation or even extinction. In most instances, it is this intricate combination of small and large changes that forms the genetic tapestry of life. Adaptation, incidentally, is not a linear, uncluttered progress; rather, it's an uneven dance between various forces that shape groups with time. A dramatic change in the environment may press a species into adapting abruptly, sometimes bifurcating a population or even producing discrete branches—subclades—that split in unforeseen directions. You see this complex branching in cancer as well: tumors, for instance, display a tangle of clonal varieties responding to both tiny local changes and therapies. Recent research even suggests that these evolutionary pathways are not clean at all, further supporting the notion that evolution is a combination of various, unreliable mechanisms.

In short, putting ecological, genetic, and evolutionary perspectives together can unlock our understanding of how so diverse populations are. Recent genomics research has, in a sense, opened the door to an in-depth examination of these evolutionary enigmas. Next-generation sequencing now allowed scientists to reveal sweeping vistas of mutations—uncovering complex histories embedded in the DNA of organisms. Techniques such as comparative genomics and even molecular evolution analyses (such as the MEGA software, for example, estimates times of divergence) are remodeling how we map these routes. These technological advances are not so much cool laboratory tools; they are essential to solving real-world problems in cancer therapy and conservation biology. When classical evolutionary concepts meet modern technology, scientists can outline plans to enhance genetic well-being and strength, preparing us for whatever turns nature has up its sleeve.

6.2.2. Ecological Factors

Ecological and population forces combine in complicated ways. Occasionally, species and their environment find themselves in a sort of improvisational dance—consider *Fontainea*, for example. This species of plant, occurring in diverse habitats, appears with conspicuous changes in its genetics that inform us greatly about the ability of local conditions to influence evolution. Regional environments and landscapes tend to create peculiar adjustments in how species adapt; they don't merely survive; they succeed in surviving and even thriving within their own niche in the world. In most instances, obstacles such as extreme weather or difficult terrain hinder gene exchange, which in a circuitous manner accumulates unique genetic characteristics and initiates the emergence of local variants (Brunton et al., 2024). If you consider ecological sensitivity, it happens that this term is quite central to comprehending how populations adapt in various landscapes, particularly when human activities impose additional stress. The West Qinling Mountains, for instance, show how increases and decreases in population density and local economic conditions can tip an area's susceptibility. The terrain appears to whisper tales of changing sensitivity over the years; you may observe that between 2000 and 2020 the overall indicator of sensitivity has stumbled a little bit, possibly indicating some environmental relaxing.

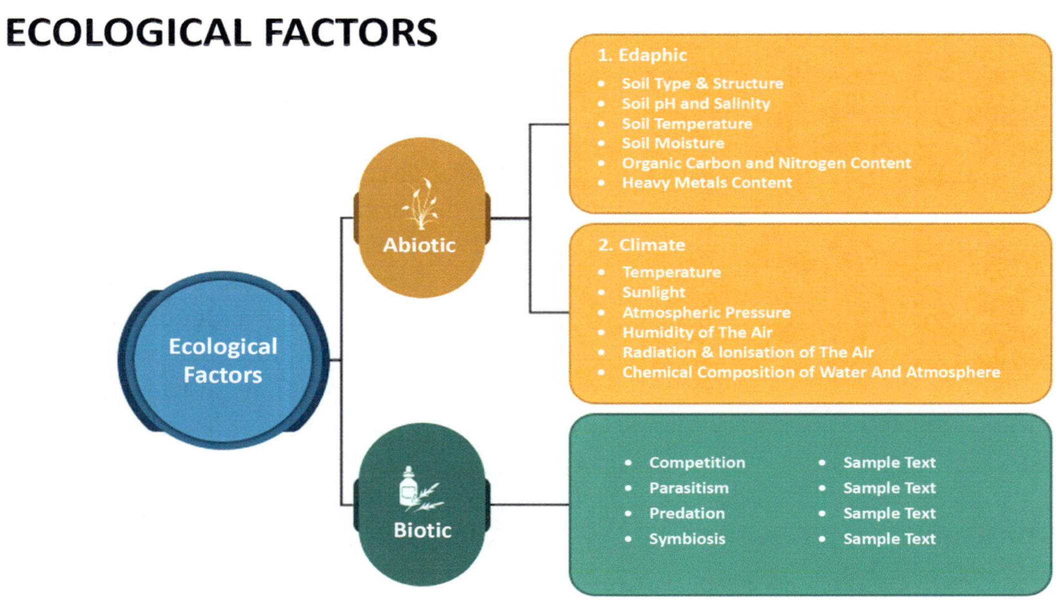

Figure 6.6. Ecological factors.

Source: Collidu. (n.d.). *Ecological Factors*.

In general, these changes require periodic check-ins on what's evolving and assist us in identifying regional variations and inform informed conservation actions against human threats (Zhao et al., 2024). It ultimately boils down to understanding how all these ecological drivers interact with population characteristics being fairly important to informing conservation planning. Consider

Fontainea once more—how its adaptations emerge highlights because we require customized protection strategies that take into account the distinctive environmental and genetic context. In the same way that recognizing ecological sensitivity is not uniform across regions can guide us toward more sophisticated strategies for habitat restoration and management. In most instances, addressing these issues requires a mix — taking ecological knowledge, genetic information, and even socioeconomic considerations — and bringing these together to create a framework that truly captures the big picture. Finally, enhancing resilience of populations involves initiating intelligent, well-crafted measures that honor the complicated, interconnected character of ecological factors, under the conditions of sudden environmental change (Brunton et al., 2024; Zhao et al., 2024) (Figure 6.6).

6.2.3. Social and Cultural Influences

Populations tell you so much when you view them in the context of shared traditions and day-to-day habits. Traditions and community ways define what people become and how groups coalesce, not only by creating rudimentary social conventions but by mapping out hierarchies as well. Oftentimes, simple concepts such as family ties, education, or even deeply rooted religious beliefs direct who ascends the social scale or achieves economic success. These cultural factors frequently build unconventional paths for people, and one ends up with a diverse array of reactions to policies and community customs. You may even find yourself observing that stances on authority, learning, or new ideas among people stick society together or knock it off course—as communities navigate their dreams and everyday realities, so planning for the future is even more knotted up. Matters of money also have an enormous, under-acknowledged influence on how culture and social energies combine. Economic conditions, in most cases, become entwined with cultural identities to determine who gets access to opportunities such as education, employment, or essential resources. Where there are large wealth disparities, the superimposition of culture becomes quite obvious and manages to fuel social tensions. For instance, in those communities that are hard-struck by poverty, there is commonly a strong tendency toward communal aid—even if, in the process, it strengthens economic divisions. These remind us, in the main, that any glance at culture or social conduct must have a glimpse of how economic influences enter into it.

Therefore, when considering development strategies, it is necessary to observe how economic and social factors combine to reinforce or erode cultural identities in diverse populations, eventually determining overall outcomes. The combination of social, cultural, and economic forces overflows into global linkages that confuse localized narratives. Globalization tends to pour in foreign cultural forces, which frequently undermine traditional values and push individuals into changing their social arrangements. Such changes may introduce fresh cultural diversity or ignite conflict as societies struggle with contemporary pressures. At the same time, a flood of external ideas, habits, and economic structures tends to exacerbate inequalities—sometimes helping some groups at the expense of others. For the most part, it is prudent to look a little closer at how those outside influences meld with native customs. As those groups accommodate these changes, they construct new identities but still sometimes hold on to what used to be, creating a rich, if somewhat complicated, tapestry of human experience that enriches our conversation about cultural diversity in a globalized world.

6.3. Impacts on Population Dynamics

Population patterns become influenced by a combination of things, with each adding a small twist to the way various species act. Availability of resources and regional climate—pretty simple things, as it turns out—usually provide the basis for how rapidly a species may expand or dwindle. For instance, when you observe certain species filling up special niches, you know that they react differently to environmental stressors, resulting in irregular growth spurts. In most instances, knowledge of such changes not only provides us with clues on how species interact but also informs us on where next to expect populations to migrate to; it is akin to discovering the essence of biodiversity. This type of knowledge, as a general rule, is important in the establishment of protocols for safeguarding vulnerable species and maintaining eco-system equilibrium (Sharpee et al., 2016). The interplay between genetics and observable traits puts another layer into the entire picture. Differences in genetics allow species to adapt when their environment changes, typically making them more resistant to diseases and random fluctuations in resources. Obviously, the physical characteristics—derived from both what they have written in their genes and what life throws their way—impact everything from how successfully an animal breeds to how it exploits what is present. This natural combination of characteristics sometimes provides certain species an advantage in accessing particular niches, sometimes outpacing their rivals. So, essentially, understanding the interaction of genetic idiosyncrasies and measurable traits is almost a prerequisite for someone to explore the intricacies of natural populations (Sharpee et al., 2016). Likewise, human activity is now adding its own random element that interferes with the natural balance of these groups. Habit loss, increasing pollution levels, and climate changes are reshaping the habitats most species inhabit, resulting in declining populations and increased competition among the survivors. These human-induced pressures often cascade through ecosystems, at times triggering sudden and unexpected changes in population patterns. For proper management and rehabilitation, it is necessary—if not downright crucial—to know precisely how our activities mix with the natural processes themselves, opening the doors to sustainable operations aimed at mitigating harmful effects on biodiversity (Sharpee et al., 2016).

6.3.1. Effects on Reproduction and Survival

Population dynamics rely on environmental signals that influence both how species reproduce and how long they live. Temperature fluctuations, for instance, can truly shake things up—changing everything from egg viability to adult longevity in mosquitoes. Consider species like *Culex pipiens*, *Culex quinquefasciatus*, and *Culex tarsalis*: warmer temperatures generally correlate with faster development, but survival and egg stability tend to follow a more nonlinear, less predictable trajectory. This is no clear academic quirk; it has practical significance when predicting disease spread, particularly as climate change presents new challenges our way. Identifying such species-specific nuances can inform the recalibration of public health programs and the design of intervention efforts to minimize threats from vector-borne diseases (Moser et al., 2023). Mast seeding is yet another fascinating element of the ecological jigsaw, highlighting how resource availability and population dynamics are interlinked in a close relationship. Take the case of wild boars—acorn yield here is no small variable at all; it has a significant influence on survival, growth, and even reproduction. When there are plenty of acorns, more females breed and even the smaller females appear to enhance their growth, collectively pushing the population higher. But these results are not everywhere uniform; where there are rich resources, animals take advantage of the present plenty, but when resources are meager, sometimes they change tactics by tapping stored resources from past years. Results like these, viewed from differing perspectives within and among populations, underscore ecological heterogeneity (Gamelon et al., 2021). If you pull back, the scene is even more complex. The ripple effects of these patterns extend far beyond individual species, showing a range of behavioral and reproductive adaptations across ecosystems. Some species, for example, may increase reproduction when resources are abundant, while others adopt a more conservative, nearly reserved strategy—reflecting what some refer to as a capital - income breeding balance. This process not only affects individual fitness but also shapes community structures and ecosystem interactions. Through exploration of these frequently-complicated relationships, scientists are more effectively able to develop conservation strategies that defend both species and habitat. In the majority of instances, examining these reproductive and survival consequences in the face of population disparity is integral in predicting long-term ecological patterns and addressing significant issues such as biodiversity decline and adaptation to climate change (Gamelon et al., 2021; Moser et al., 2023) (Figure 6.7).

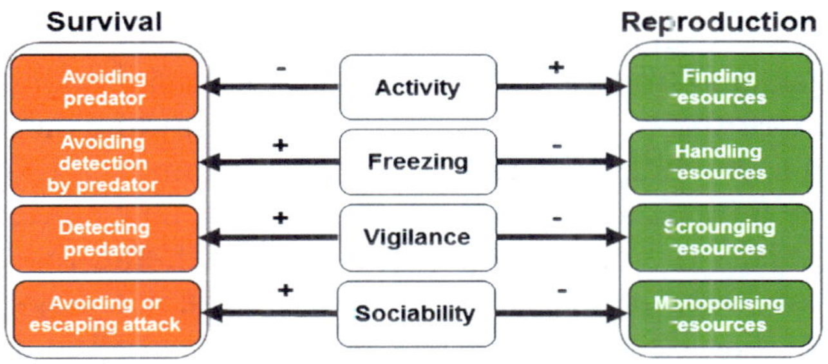

Figure 6.7. Effects on reproduction and survival.

Source: Montiglio, P.-O., Dammhahn, M., Dubuc Messier, G., & Réale, D. (2018). Behaviors mediate the trade-off between current and future reproduction through their effects on various components of resource acquisition and risk of predation. In *the Pace-of-Life Syndrome Revisited: The Role of Ecological Conditions and Natural History on the Slow–Fast Continuum.*

6.3.2. Influence on Population Growth Rates

Cities are full of human activity, and that daily hustle truly influences the way populations act, particularly in those crowded urban areas. Human behavior mixes with nature in strange ways; when a lot of people's masses congregate, it doesn't only alter how people live but plays around with local ecosystems as well. You can observe it when highly different species end up interacting, sometimes creating new diseases. In most instances, when people, wild animals, and livestock become too comfortable with each other, diseases can transfer from one to another. Deciphering this complicated interaction provides insight into threats we may encounter and suggestions about how continuous population growth unravels our natural world. And, as more people spill into city areas, the breaking up of green spaces tends to shrink biodiversity, which then changes how germs spread among these mixed groups (Hassell et al., 2016). It is not just cities that matter either—money matters and life conditions stir these changes further. Unequal provision of good medicine, clean water, or even just a good environment means that some communities take the brunt of infections more than others.

Local examples abound, such as a patchwork neighborhood's layout of buildings and services causing actual disparity in the spread of disease, just because the economic and infrastructure gaps are so extreme. This tends to make life more difficult in densely populated, informal settlements, where high densities and patchy sanitation prevail. Even more worrying, perhaps, is that climate change appears to amplify such difficulties, tipping local conditions and social positions into a mix that incites entirely novel health threats. All these interrelated impacts drive us to consider approaches widely, to ensure everyone remains safe (LaDeau et al., 2015). There is the entire issue of how our environment interferes with population growth, particularly when disease-carrying insects and microbes are included. Urban heat islands—that is, those small areas in the city where the temperature is significantly higher than surrounding areas—can alter everything about how these animals live, from how long they persist to how quickly they grow. Small temperature fluctuations could change how these vectors manage to live or even how hungry they are to bite, scattering their numbers unevenly across the urban landscape. This can increase the risk of disease, especially in communities that cannot afford to protect themselves. In most instances, recognizing such subtle, dynamic interactions is essential to understanding and controlling possible outbreaks in high-density city areas. Examining closely the cooperation of social and natural forces is crucial if we are to understand the new public health issues on our doorstep (Hassell et al., 2016).

6.3.3. Role in Species Interactions and Community Structure

Species interactions are at the core of community life; each animal appears to do more than merely survive. Characteristics such as how an animal hunts for food or breeds evoke a combination of relationships—competition, predation, even unlikely partnerships—that alter the balance of the community. In areas where resources are unequally distributed, these differences in traits drive species into creating novel niches, a process that increases biodiversity and introduces an element of resilience. Occasionally, as these differences shake things up, they escalate competitive forces while also initiating positive feedback that fosters a variety of life, a connection that is most important for maintaining stability in larger ecosystems (Sharpee et al., 2016). Have a look at predator – prey relationships; they are quite a mixed lot that determines the way populations peak and trough. When predators are absent or in excess, the ripples can flip the numbers of both mid-tier and base species in ways that resonate throughout the entire community. Keystone species, Overall, end up bearing much of the weight in maintaining habitats. Environmental changes fine-tune these pressures of predation, shifting community combinations and suggesting the natural unevenness between habitats. This natural push-and-pull not just points out how species adapt fly-by-fly but also shows how ecosystems can be very fragile under human influence. It all serves to inform ecologists to make better predictions of what is going to occur next, which informs wiser conservation actions (Sharpee et al., 2016). Ultimately, the complicated web of species connection constructs the very infrastructure of communities, and in doing so shows us that imbalanced environmental bits count. Such connections impact not only where and how many critters loiter but can influence their evolutionary trajectories. If species form up in co-mutualities, this allows diverse life forms to establish adjacent to each other, something which tends to improve overall productivity as well as ecosystem resilience. As climate change and habitat destruction continue to disrupt ancient ecological balances, observing these interactions becomes increasingly important. By identifying this complicated web, scientists can design management practices that work to maintain biodiversity in a rapidly changing world (Sharpee et al., 2016) (Figure 6.8).

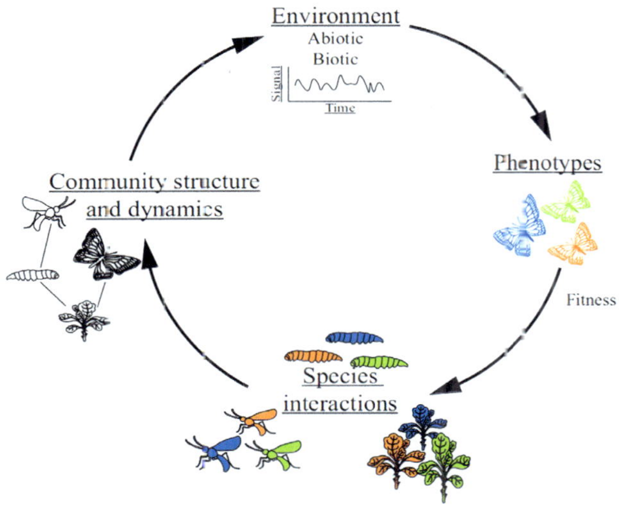

Figure 6.8. Role in species interactions and community structure.

Source: Costaz, T. P. M., de Jong, P. W., van Loon, J. J. A., & Dicke, M. (2023). Overview of Section: Consequences of fluctuating thermal regimes for species interactions and community structure. In It is about time: Effects of thermal fluctuations resulting from climate change on trophic interactions with a focus on host–parasitoid interactions. *Evolutionary Ecology.*

6.4. Measurement and Analysis

Biological populations exhibit lots of variation, and scientists sometimes have to have quite clever methods of measuring these differences, particularly when attempting to figure out how they influence the spread of disease and pathogen behavior. *Leishmania infantum* infections, for example, may be counted in different hosts to establish latent patterns of infectiousness that simple observation may overlook. Research has indicated that parasite load checks in sites such as bone marrow or even ear skin provide valuable hints regarding transmission risks from asymptomatic carriers. In most instances, elevated parasite loads in the skin correlate with increased likelihood of infectivity, which suggests a definitive connection between population variation and disease spread and control (Mohammadiha et al., 2013). Incorporating cutting-edge analytical techniques has become the secret to plunging into the microscopic operations of microbes and cells. Tools such as flow cytometry enable researchers to perform a high-speed screening on the behavior of individual cells—even within varied cell populations—which picks up on things that are otherwise missed. The technique plays a significant role in fine-tuning bioprocesses by demonstrating how cell-to-cell idiosyncrasies make up the overall efficiency. Through the combination of general population balance with cell level modeling, scientists receive more complete insight into causes of variability, and this ensures that designs for bioprocesses are sound as well as scalable (González-Cabaleiro et al., 2017). As for experimentation with population differences in cases involving disease or bioprocess use, having reliable measurements and analysis is just too crucial to ignore.

More sophisticated frameworks that weave together experimental information and math-rich modeling are unlocking promising avenues to observe novel population phenomena. Using these new techniques, one can move beyond mere description to constructing models that realistically predict future directions and guide intelligent interventions. For infectious disease, associating a host's characteristics with transmission patterns is central to designing tailored control strategies. Ultimately, this mix of exact measurement, systematic analysis, and a dash of natural randomness appears to be the key to unraveling the messy complexity of diverse biological populations and producing improved results for both public health and business (Mohammadiha et al., 2013; González-Cabaleiro et al., 2017).

6.4.1. Statistical Methods for Assessing Heterogeneity

Researchers have to excavate the grubby specifics of heterogeneity if they wish to mix results from various studies with success. Statistics become involved big time in this case – consider meta-analyses, for example – since tiny differences could entirely distort our perceptions. In the vast majority, these appear to confer from variations of who was under study, what was applied as a control or intervention, or even the method of how things were done. The Q statistic, for instance, examines whether the differences in effect sizes are beyond what is possible to be explained by chance, while the I^2 statistic provides an approximate estimate of the proportion of the entire spread contributed by these differences. Overall, employing these instruments ensures that when studies are combined, the conclusions are as reliable and unshakeable as possible (Ilmawan, 2024). Exploring the origins of heterogeneity is not merely a matter of performing some quick tests – it's diving deep into variability of clinical trials and interventions. Researchers tend to rely on subgroup analyses and meta-regression as means of identifying precisely where those differences originate. On occasion, taking the data apart by age, gender, or even certain health issues can tease out some subtle point that may otherwise be buried in the numbers. Not only does this help to clarify what the aggregated data may be indicating, but it can also suggest how interventions could more effectively be designed for specific populations. , this closer examination of the nitty-gritty has proven its value in fields such as critical care studies, in which patient condition and reactions can differ fairly considerably (Harhay et al., 2020). In terms of interpreting heterogeneity, the decision to use fixed- versus random-effects models is a genuine balancing act. Fixed-effects models are based on the assumption that each study is observing the same underlying true effect, sometimes masking crucial differences between study groups. In contrast, random-effects models recognize that studies can differ and therefore allow researchers to drill down into a richer, more textured representation of the outcomes. Researchers also add in techniques such as the Hedges technique every now and then to temper the blow of any outliers that could bias the effect size. Of course, there are still issues – consider residual heterogeneity, publication bias, and the fact that study quality is not always high. By combining a combination of statistical methods, researchers can address these messy differences more effectively, eventually constructing a more trustworthy overall image (Ilmawan, 2024).

6.4.2. Use of Genetic Markers

Learning about how populations vary can be almost a treasure hunt, and genetic markers come into their own with this. They're like little flags wafting in the breeze, indicating differences within one group and between distinct ones. Let's take research on *Rhaponticum carthamoides*, for instance—scientists uncovered a surprising diversity of variation from one environment to another. With ISSR markers (these are instruments that screen for easy repeating DNA pieces), researchers surprisingly discovered that plants from many cenopopulations grouped into different clusters, indicating that environmental factors could be causing the mix-up. This approach, in the majority of instances, not only aids in the organization of conservation plans but also informs the choice of seed samples with a high concentration of genes for breeding programs, eventually contributing to the conservation of distinctive characteristics of rare species (Zhmud et al., 2023). Genetic markers don't simply inform us of which species is which; they allow us to look into the genetic blueprint of our crops and observe how these characteristics may mix when plants are crossed. Take sugar beet (*Beta vulgaris* L.)—scientists accessed SSR markers and wound up discovering a lot of various alleles that had plenty of variation even within similar lines. It so happens that selecting the correct markers for identifying progenitor lines with good potential is no small matter in the quest for high-yielding hybrids. Such genetic foresight allows the breeder to select parent pairs according to how genes differ between them—a procedure that naturally sets the stage for populations with more desirable characteristics. In a sense, this use of genetic markers extends far beyond identification, serving a vital role in driving farming practices forward and helping to overcome food security issues (Amangeldiyeva et al., 2023). When you explore how populations differ, genetic markers essentially disentangle the complex web of gene associations. By quantifying genetic distances and variances, researchers learn about the organization of populations—how genes move or cling to their own kind. For example, research on *Rhaponticum carthamoides* indicates geographic isolation may produce significant genetic differences, as if environment has a strong voice as to whom combines genes with whom. Similarly, research on sugar beet has shown that the majority of genetic variation appears between isolated groups and not within each group, a circumstance that would logically guide breeding practice. Overall, employing genetic markers gives us a glimpse of the intricate interplay between and within populations, furthering our understanding of biodiversity and directing the routes we pursue in conservation as well as selective breeding programs (Amangeldiyeva et al., 2023) (Figure 6.9).

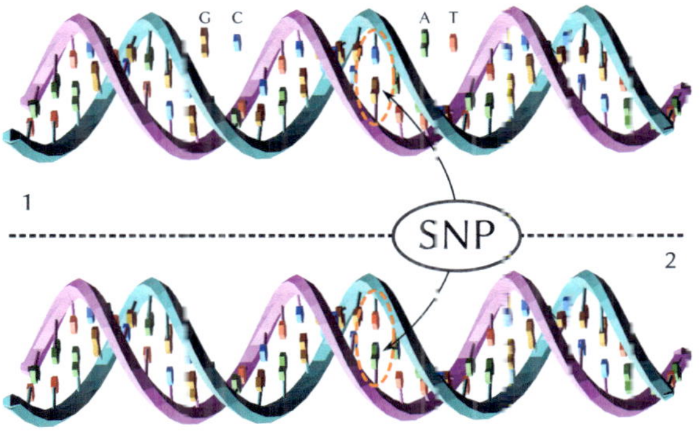

Figure 6.9. Use of genetic markers.

Source: By SNP model by David Eccles (gringer), CC BY 4.0, https://commons.wikimedia.org/w/index.php?curid=2355125

6.4.3. Ecological Modeling Approaches

Ecosystems are complex—many things are going on simultaneously. Sophisticated models, for example, attempt to reproduce those unexpected turns in species interactions without necessarily mapping out a clear design. Studies indicate that when urbanization or intensive agriculture enter the picture, species interactions and population dynamics change in ways we are still attempting to define. In most instances, integrating concepts from both nature observations and human activity shows how much our activities disrupt the natural order. Models involving different hosts, reservoirs, and changing environment factors highlight that disease transmission is not an easy tale, but one interwoven with complexities. These strategies suggest not just the dangers associated with zoonotic disease, but also how to step in and mitigate those dangers (Hassell et al., 2016). Recently, the concept of planetary boundaries has emerged as a method of considering our challenges to sustainability. Essentially, this concept identifies safe boundaries for Earth's systems if we are to prevent global catastrophe. Steffen et al.'s revised work—broadly speaking—reminds us that these limits are interconnected, so a change in one area (e.g., climate change) can get the others in a twist such as biodiversity. Examining these limitations at a more local level allows scientists to view how day-to-day population dynamics are influenced by sweeping, global changes, explaining why certain species evolve and others struggle (Steffen et al., 2015). Meanwhile new technologies in information collection and speed of computation continue to challenge scientists to construct increasingly sophisticated ecological models. These models, taking into consideration such variables as genetic idiosyncrasies, fragmented habitats, and daily species interactions, allow scientists to make all sorts of simulations that indicate how populations may respond to natural change and human stress. At times, these models even predict how species might do when confronted with temperature fluctuations or alterations to their habitats—emphasizing, in the majority of instances, that population dynamics are central to addressing our increasingly dynamic world. In the end, these modeling exercises are pragmatic bases for developing conservation plans designed to maintain biodiversity in the face of increasing uncertainties (Hassell et al., 2016).

6.5. Case Studies

Case studies provide a hands-on means of exploring the gritty particulars that make every group different. By taking a close-up view of a certain segment of the population, researchers can identify trends, pitfalls, and even silent opportunities that sweep surveys might not catch. The review of HIV drug resistance in priority groups across sub-Saharan Africa, for instance, tends to illustrate how domestic factors accumulate to shape aggregate rates of HIV transmission. This type of research isn't merely counting numbers—it also attempts to unravel why interventions at times fail, paving the way for more adapted interventions and future research guided by the local situation. In doing this, these targeted examinations help researchers and practitioners adapt their techniques to the nuances each group carries. Changing tack, regional research is more likely to expose disparities that can literally rock policy and program planning. When scholars compare the demographic and economic differences between

Lombardy and Campania in Italy, they discover that local circumstances tend to influence the experiences of immigrant workers in ways that are not necessarily expected. By employing a multi-level analysis, the research demonstrates that labor markets can appear completely different based on the geographic location—even in a nation that may appear homogeneous at first glance. Such reports, in the majority of instances, highlight the necessity of region-specific interventions rather than applying a one-size-fits-all approach (Benassi et al., 2024). Consequently, continued case studies continue to fill the void between general theory and actual detail. Ultimately, the combination of the analysis of extensive case studies with the broader population trends creates a fairly convoluted picture of how society functions. While big surveys give us a general picture, it is those detailed up-close looks which reveal the hidden nuances and local voices within the numbers. Systematic reviews and local stories—whether of health or labor trends—combine to paint a richer picture of what is at stake. This combination of targeted and regional research propels progress by basing policy on hard evidence as well as on the commonplace experiences (Benassi et al., 2024). In the end, these methods remind us that behind each statistic lies a human experience that one number simply cannot convey.

6.5.1. Heterogeneity in Human Populations

Human population studies remind us that our health is determined by a combination of biological characteristics and environments in which we live—a myriad of factors exist. Individuals do not all inhabit the same environment; economic situation, cultural practice, and geographic location come into the picture differently. When you are working with infectious diseases, you can truly observe how those differences have an enormous effect on the way diseases spread. For instance, by closely examining differences in how hosts become infected, you can gain valuable information for the control of disease. Measuring how contagious various groups could be makes it possible to achieve well-targeted interventions to prevent outbreaks, which is the reason why it matters to look at both individual vulnerabilities and the big picture of disease patterns (Mohammadiha et al., 2013). On the other hand, the way human-induced changes mix with the natural world plays a significant role in determining population patterns. Although genetic studies once centered primarily on biology, more recent studies in landscape epidemiology have directed interest toward our behaviors and mobility. By combining the day-to-day cultural specifics with spatial models, we have a richer understanding of how diseases could be spreading in unexpected manners across communities. Consider, for example, the impact of migration on rabies—this type of research shows that cultural traditions and natural barriers can adjust the path that an epidemic will follow. In the majority of instances, this type of information is vital when planning public health interventions, ensuring that the appropriate resources reach the appropriate areas (Anderson et al., 2012). It is just as significant to note that not everyone is identical when developing health policies and disease control initiatives. Health initiatives must cross beyond the biological aspect of outbreaks and penetrate into socio-political environments as well. After all, issues such as healthcare access, education deficits, and economic struggles can complicate the way diseases spread through populations. An intelligent public health reaction must consider such turns, frequently combining in local interventions that resonant with the community's distinctive culture and social atmosphere-even to the point of revisiting fundamental concepts in slightly different form. Overall, by remembering that human diversity is multi-layered and complex, health programs can be designed more precisely to the needs of various groups, ultimately enhancing both their fairness and effectiveness (Mohammadiha et al., 2013) (Figure 6.10).

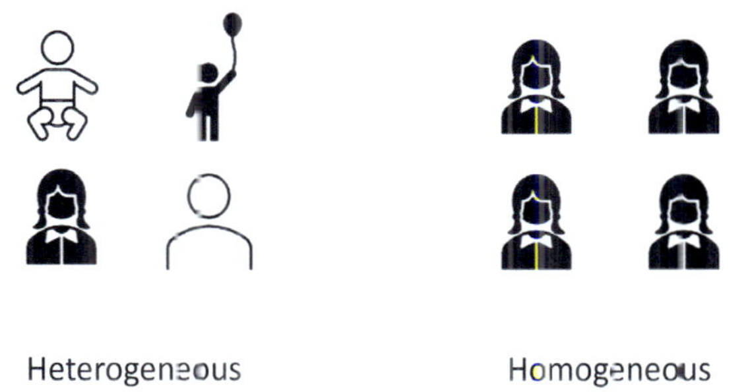

Figure 6.10. Heterogeneity in human populations

Source: Statistics How To. (2023). *Homogeneous and Heterogeneous Groups of People.*

6.5.2. Heterogeneity in Animal Populations

Animal populations are a lot more secretly complex when you examine the variation between individual animals—what many refer to as heterogeneity. One piece of research on *Leishmania infantum* looked at parasite burdens in reservoir and non-reservoir hosts, and the scientists saw some surprising relationships between the number of parasites that animals carry and how infectious they may be. They discovered that the number of parasites in the skin is a fairly reliable indicator of a host's capacity to transmit the disease. Furthermore, this figure ranges widely not only between species but even within an individual animal. All in all, it points to the idea that targeting those with high parasite loads—say, domestic dogs with their extra potential for high transmission—could make a difference (Mohammadiha et al., 2013). Wildlife, on the other hand, is not just about the numbers on the animal side; the environment plays a big role too. Genetic variation combines with the terrain in ways that alter the pattern of diseases, a notion that has become central to landscape epidemiology. As examples, the epidemics of rabies in domestic dogs are a reminder that humans' impact on the environment needs to be understood to tackle disease transmission. In general terms, the incorporation of methods such as molecular analysis with spatial mapping and even a consideration of local cultural influences can contribute to enhanced disease control measures. By incorporating all these irregular factors, researchers have begun to construct metapopulation models that reflect the sloppy, real-world interactions—aiding in guiding interventions where needed most (Anderson et al., 2012). The awareness of these differences also allows for more adaptable management programs. Because how hosts cluster and act can vary so much, implementing targeted vaccination campaigns or surveillance activities requires you to get a sense of the idiosyncrasies of each environment. This process allows you to identify areas where infections could burst out more quickly due to high population density, changing human mobility, or local socio-cultural practices. In the majority of instances, as researchers borrow concepts from landscape genetics and elaborate on epidemiological models, public health responses improve in managing the peculiar challenges presented by such heterogeneous populations, toward more sustainable responses to epidemic diseases (Anderson et al., 2012).

6.5.3. Heterogeneity in Plant Populations

Plant evolution might be a roller coaster ride, tending to create a combination of genetic variations that do not fall into any clear pattern. Habitual factors, such as changing climates, diverse soils, and the day-to-day jostle with other organisms—incrementally affect these blueprints of genetics. Mostly, you observe changes in allele frequencies since natural selection comes to favor features which are best suited in a given environment. Consider crop studies, for instance; farmers growing organically compared to conventionally end up with groups that have significantly different genetic compositions. Overall, this type of diversity counts a great deal—not only in terms of how ecosystems heal, but also in terms of maintaining farming productive and sustainable. Check out one study on a spring barley hybrid that came out to be quite diverse. Scientists developed a population by crossing wild barley with an elite cultivar and allowed nature to take its own course in organic and conventional environments for almost 20 years without any intentional human adjustment (Schneider et al., 2024). The organic population became more genetically diverse through generations, demonstrating that various farming practices can change allele frequencies in unexpected ways. In all but a few instances, these lessons make us remember the profound connections between plant architecture and farming methods, providing hints at breeding tactics that increase crop strength as well as productivity. And with global warming hurling more curveballs each day, relying on this built-in genetic hybrid appears more crucial than ever. In the end, the role of genetic diversity in plants goes way beyond immediate harvest outcomes—it touches on broader ecological issues that deserve our attention. When plants can adapt in just a few generations, it becomes clear that keeping a diverse genetic pool is crucial. For example, those wild alleles that assist with pest resistance and determine root structure turn out to be a blessing in disguise for developing harder, stronger crops (Schneider et al., 2024). That these changes can occur so rapidly indicate a critical need for breeding programs that are inclined toward organic farming, so that plants are not only high-yielding but also equipped to withstand environmental stress. Basically, to get to the root of plant natural variability is the solution to improved agriculture and the conservation of biodiversity in a world that is constantly changing.

6.6. Implications for Conservation

Populations vary in ways that count. Differences appear in everything from their genes to the way they act and what roles they play in the natural world. When the climate shifts, not all groups respond to stressors, such as warming trends, in an identical fashion. Freshwater macroinvertebrates, for instance, exhibit a variety of thermal responses—some appear more responsive to warmer temperatures, which can, in turn, influence their growth, reproduction, and community assembly. Knowing these variations is paramount; knowing each group's idiosyncrasies allows conservation strategies to be adjusted to the particular requirements of these animals (Bonacina et al., 2022). Considering disease dynamics within these composite populations puts another spin on things. Populations that have diverse social structures may exhibit erratic patterns of disease transmission. Infections sometimes spread in ways that can create precipitous drops, particularly when environmental pressures are involved. More often than not, studies conclude that including not only behaviors but also demographic information provide a more accurate picture of the risk. Social networks can influence how diseases pass through populations, so it is only logical that conservation strategies target not only how densely things become but also how much people interact. By incorporating a bit of epidemiological understanding, managers can develop tactics that more proactively manage the effect of disease on at-risk wildlife populations (Silk et al., 2019). With more than just short-term solutions in mind, recognizing these differences has significant ramifications for long-term restoration and management. For restoration to be effective, it is frequently important to maintain or even increase genetic diversity; a more diverse set of characteristics allows populations to better withstand environmental fluctuations. Knowledge of how various species interact across an heterogeneous landscape can also inform habitat management, maintaining ecosystems both functional and resilient. Conservation, after all, has to take into account that perturbations in one group have the potential to ripple out and impact others. A sweeping, fairly intuitive strategy that accepts these natural fluctuations could very well be the key to developing plans that protect not just individual species but the stability and robustness of entire systems (Bonacina et al., 2022).

6.6.1. Importance of Genetic Diversity

Genetic variation is one of the key forces behind why populations vary so extensively. It plays a significant role in how groups cope with changing circumstances and disease challenges. For example, groups with a broad array of genes tend to cope well with changes in their environments—whether it's an unforeseen climate turn or a shift in local ecosystems. Conversely, small populations with little genetic diversity tend to get into difficulties, lacking the qualities to live in difficult situations. Grasping these impacts is central to planning intelligent conservation strategies, particularly for species facing habitat fragmentation and human-induced ecological changes. For the most part, simply incorporating some genetic diversity elements into management can ensure ecosystems remain resilient under stressors such as urban growth and intensive farming (Hassell et al., 2016). When genetic diversity falls, the consequences ripple far beyond individual populations and begin disrupting whole ecosystems and the services they provide. Less variety can leave fewer backup possibilities when stressors, such as disease or invasive species—strike. Occasionally, species lose their specific functions, disrupting natural equilibrium and even minor discontinuities in gene types can disrupt predator – prey relations and nutrient cycles. In general terms, a broad gene pool is essential for an ecosystem to be able to recover from adversity. This close connection between genetic composition and general ecological health reminds us that it is necessary to study them in conjunction with each other, informing strategies that seek to conserve biodiversity and maintain nature functioning properly in the face of human stresses (Singer et al., 2016). In the context of zoonotic disease, genetic diversity has a double function. It can serve as a protective shield, providing individuals with diverse immune responses which strengthen a group's overall resistance. However, once uniformity arrives, it can also accelerate how rapidly diseases progress in a population. Urbanization—placing wildlife and humans closer to one another—adds even greater complexity to this scenario. Too often, mixed genetic ancestry leads to diverse reactions that retard the spread of disease, while excessive similarity allows doors to open to pathogens. By monitoring these genetic variations, scientists and public health professionals can identify and control better the risks of zoonotic spillover. Overall, paying proper heed to genetic specificity is an essential aspect of formulating effective, well-balanced health policies in our globalized world (Hassell et al., 2016) (Figure 6.11).

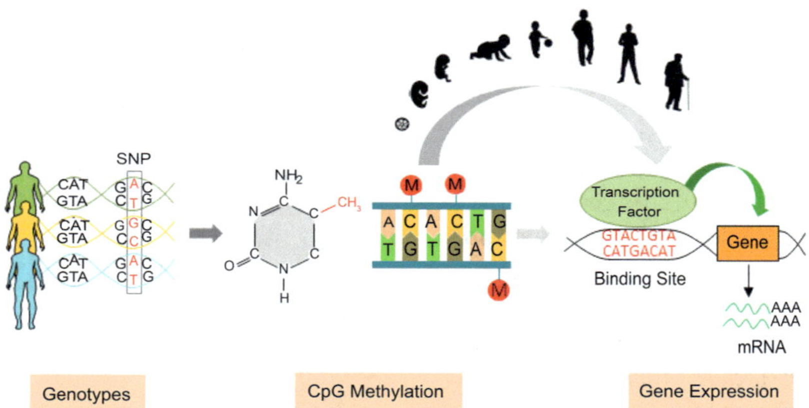

Figure 6.11. Importance of genetic diversity.

Source: By Anke Hoffmann, Michael Ziller and Dietmar Spengler * - https://doi.org/10.3390/genes7120104, CC BY-SA 4.0, https://commons.wikimedia.org/w/index.php?curid=128128531

6.6.2. Strategies for Preserving Heterogeneity

Populations flourish when there is a hybrid of various traits—a diversity that will serve them well in facing surprise environmental changes and challenges. A nice way to preserve that variety is by constructing casual networks where people exchange resources and ideas. With these groups, every individual contributes his or her own individual type that gives rise to new innovation and sets the stage for long-term sustainability. How effort, resource sharing, and working together play off each other not only streamlines the mundane but also multiplies the rewards of having such a mix. Models that examine how individuals invest their resources in social and economic environments reinforce the message: that maintaining diversity intact typically involves making intelligent investments and coordinating efforts among all stakeholders so that everyone can adapt as circumstances shift (Cabrales et al., 2007). Another strategy is to implement systems that take into account how behavior affects everything from sharing resources to making decisions. Consider animal health surveillance, for instance—it happens that knowing how behavior influences such systems is central to saving money while managing the disease. When you begin prodding the dynamic between resource investment, how diseases change, and what drives those changes, you can design surveillance systems that aren't merely effective but also attentive to the differing needs and routines around. Employing a model that burrows deep into these interconnections, it is easier to determine how to maintain a good balance while monitoring upcoming challenges. In most instances, this approach illustrates how crucial it is to incorporate behavioral understanding when crafting systems intended to safeguard diversity, such that various points of view have an equal voice in making decisions (Denwood et al., 2013). Policy actions that promote inclusive practices are also a significant contributor to keeping this mix intact. Rather than a cookie-cutter approach, these policies should ensure that all have an equal opportunity for resources and access, regardless of background. That gives room for a variety of identities and experiences to soar. More often than not, when individuals from all walks of life are involved, not only is there more emphasis on the specific needs of every group but also more varied input. Education, health, and economic-advancement policies are important to creating an environment that accommodates differences. And when communities have input into these policies, there develops a sense of ownership, increasing the likelihood that these regulations remain in place. Ultimately, frameworks based on inclusivity are a primary measure in protecting the rich, diverse fabric of our populations from forces that would otherwise seek to impose sameness.

6.6.3. Challenges in Managing Heterogeneous Populations

Diverse populations give rise to both unexpected opportunities and some pretty knotty problems when it comes to management. Take farming, for example—mixing different kinds of plants can sometimes make crops tougher against unpredictable weather and pathogens. In the case of common beans, local changes and shifting weather patterns mean that breeding is not just a straight-line process but more like a careful balancing act that pays attention to each plant's unique traits. It is odd, because even though these mixed crops can often ward off diseases and bump up yields when the climate changes, rules usually push for plants that all look alike. This insistence on sameness can clip the wings of the natural strengths hidden in genetic variety, leaving both farmers and policy folks scratching their heads. Striking this balance, generally speaking, is a tough nut to crack for anyone managing such agricultural systems (Plestenjak et al., 2024). Public health, on the other hand, has its own messy mix of issues when dealing with a varied population. People's behaviors and their health outcomes weave together into a tapestry that shifts a lot from one group to the next. Think about trying to chip away at cancer risks by tweaking everyday habits; here, different cultural or economic backgrounds show up with their own distinct routines, making one-size-fits-all solutions nearly impossible. The challenge is pretty layered—figuring out what works requires a close look at many overlapping factors; sometimes even using biomarkers to flag high-risk individuals can help, though teams often run into bumps when sifting through data. In most cases, you would need some solid statistical methods that handle all these convolutions to design strategies that cut the risk among diverse groups (Lee et al., 2024). Then there is the real-world side of managing diverse groups, which goes well beyond theory. In schools, for instance, teachers find themselves juggling a mix of students with different backgrounds, learning styles, and abilities, and the old "one-model-fits-all" approach just does not fly. That natural diversity calls for teachers to keep adjusting their methods, even if it gets a bit messy sometimes. Similarly, community projects trying to bring people together have to reckon with varying cultural perspectives and social needs—not an easy task by any means, yet absolutely vital for real inclusion. Celebrating these differences while also handling the extra complications they bring is key. Approaches that lean on inclusivity and flexible strategies seem, in most cases, the best bet for navigating such ever-changing, dynamic environments (Plestenjak et al., 2024).

CLOSER LOOK

Immunity

Immunity refers to the body's innate defense mechanism against harmful pathogens such as bacteria, viruses, fungi, and parasites. It guards us against infections and aids in our recovery when we fall ill. Immunity can either be innate (naturally occurring) or adaptive (acquired) and functions together to maintain the body in good health. Innate immunity is the initial line of defense and consists of physical barriers (such as skin), chemical barriers (such as stomach acid), and immune cells that react rapidly to invaders. This form of immunity is non-specific, as it attacks a wide variety of pathogens.

Adaptive immunity, however, is developed over a period of time and is very specific to the pathogens that the body has encountered in the past. It includes lymphocytes like B cells and T cells. The B cells make antibodies, whereas the T cells kill infected cells. After the adaptive system has reacted to an infection, it creates a memory, thus allowing for a quicker and more powerful response when the same pathogen comes back.

Immunity can also be divided into active (vaccination or infection) or passive (transplacental from mother to child or antibody therapy). It is important to understand immunity to develop vaccines, treat infections, and control public health. A healthy immune system is crucial for long-term well-being and freedom from illness.

SUMMARY

Populations are heterogeneous and slightly unclear, so it is worth paying attention to the way that health problems and social effects operate differently. Different research indicates that medical conditions can quite markedly vary from one group to another. For example, when you consider oropharyngeal dysphagia (OD), its common prevalence compels us to consider health policies that are not necessarily one-size-fits-all. In general, systematic reviews indicate a rate of about 43.8%, but for people with dementia, the figure increases to 72.4% (Rajati et al., 2022).

This significant disparity pushes us to think that adapting interventions to groups could be more effective than using the same solutions for all. The psychological aspect is not much different, particularly under pressure from incidents such as the COVID-19 pandemic. Evidence from the COVID-19 Psychological Research Consortium tends to suggest that although overall levels of anxiety-depression appeared to remain stable, the trajectories individuals followed were everywhere (Shevlin et al., 2021). Some individuals demonstrated a resilient recovery while others declined. Such mixed findings emphasize that mental health reactions are as diverse as the people themselves, and that a tailored approach could make a real difference in support services. Putting it all together, exploring these differences individually is crucial for both healthcare professionals and policymakers. Large numbers in diseases such as OD and the broad spectrum of responses to stress inform us that wide statistics can at times conceal vital details. As the planet struggles with a range of health issues, examining these nuances more closely can result in more sharply focused, potent strategies. Going forward, gathering and analyzing more granular, disaggregated data is necessary—not just to design improved interventions but also to advance a more equitable outcome in public health, even if the journey is not always a straight line.

Disease transmission is not a neat business—there is a whole lot occurring that makes a huge difference about the way things are spread between people. Biology is involved, but the environments we live in and patterns of human activity also influence these outcomes. Studies of dog rabies, say, indicate that the addition of human movement and cultural variables to natural factors can transform the scene entirely. In a majority of the instances, knowing where individuals go and how they are engaged with nature assists with deciding the correct manner in which to allocate resources, so that strategies of control will strike the right note (Anderson et al., 2012). And then, of course, there is the landscape itself. Rivers and roads can be either obstacles or stepping stones for a virus to travel through an area—sort of like nature's own double-edged sword. Certain studies highlight that examining local transmission independently of these wider eco-influences is significant.

Scientists even employ Bayesian phylogeographic models to disentangle how these landscape idiosyncrasies influence disease routes at varying scales. By merging epidemiological information with environmental and genetic indicators, it is less complicated to identify the most influential drivers of how a disease circulates in different environments (Biek et al., 2018). At the end of the day, incorporating a broad array of factors into our models of disease is essential if we are to fully understand how populations are impacted. Consider rabies in the Serengeti—it illustrates that the one-size-fits-all public health solution can overlook significant local specifics, such as how dogs influence the route of the spread. Obviously, site-specific intervention is necessary when local considerations play such a significant role. This general perspective on spatial processes forces us to look further at what metrics perform well for intervention, enabling researchers and policymakers to formulate control measures that suit the particular demands of disease control in heterogeneous populations (Anderson et al., 2012; Biek et al., 2018).

KEY TERMS FROM THIS CHAPTER

- Demographic variation
- Spatial heterogeneity
- Age structure
- Social structure
- Behavioral variation
- Contact patterns
- Risk groups
- Heterogeneous transmission
- Mobility patterns
- Genetic diversity
- Temporal heterogeneity
- Sex ratio
- Resource distribution
- Susceptibility differences
- Mixing patterns
- Population stratification
- Subpopulations
- Network structure

REFERENCES

1. Anderson, C., Cross, P. C., Cullingham, C. I., Horton, D. L., Dietzschold, B., Eng, C., Brunker, K., et al. (2012). Integrating the landscape epidemiology and genetics of RNA viruses: Rabies in domestic dogs as a model. *Parasitology, 139*(14), 1899–1913. https://core.ac.uk/download/9651666.pdf (accessed on 6 May 2025).
2. Andrén, H., Angelstam, P. K., Attiwill, P. M., Aubry, K. B., Augustine, D. J., Banner, A., Baskerville, G. L., et al. (2006). Can forest management based on natural disturbances maintain ecological resilience? *Canadian Journal of Forest Research, 36*(9), 2280–2295. https://core.ac.uk/download/pdf/9538149.pdf (accessed on 6 May 2025).
3. Biek, R., Brunker, K., Fooks, A. R., Hampson, K., et al. (2018). Landscape attributes governing local transmission of an endemic zoonosis: Rabies virus in domestic dogs. *Molecular Ecology, 27*, 773–788. https://core.ac.uk/download/150598912.pdf (accessed on 6 May 2025).
4. Bonacina, L., Fasano, F., Mezzanotte, V., & Fornaroli, R. (2022). Effects of water temperature on freshwater macroinvertebrates: A systematic review. *Biological Reviews, 98*(1), 191–221. https://doi.org/10.1111/brv.12903.
5. Cabrales, A., Calvó-Armengol, A., & Zenou, Y. (2007). *Effort and Synergies in Network Formation.* Working Paper 07-21 Departamento de Economía Economic Series 11 https://core.ac.uk/download/29398337.pdf (accessed on 6 May 2025).
6. Computational and Mathematical Methods in Medicine. (2023). Retracted: Genetic relationship and evolution analysis among *Malus* Mill plant populations based on SCoT molecular markers. *Computational and Mathematical Methods in Medicine, 2023*. https://www.semanticscholar.org/paper/5ba874d8f28fc84ca5e5cb9d710a6b6745f7e133 (accessed on 6 May 2025).
7. Cox, C. M., Thoma, M. E., Tchangalova, N., Mburu, G., Bornstein, M. J., Johnson, C. L., & Kiarie, J. (2022). Infertility prevalence and the methods of estimation from 1990 to 2021: a systematic review and meta-analysis. *Human reproduction open, 2022*(4), hoac051. https://doi.org/10.1093/hropen/hoac051
8. Delgado-Serrano, R., Flores, H., Hammer, F., Puech, M., et al. (2009). *How was the Hubble Sequence 6 Gyrs Ago?* https://core.ac.uk/download/268933167.pdf (accessed on 6 May 2025).
9. Denwood, M. J., Gunn, G. J., Mellor, D. J., Reid, S. W. J., et al. (2013). Systems approach to animal disease surveillance and resource allocation: Methodological frameworks for behavioral analysis. *PLoS ONE, 8*(11), e82019. https://core.ac.uk/download/16457252.pdf (accessed on 6 May 2025).
10. Finlay, B. J., Finlay, B. J., Groombridge, B., Kowalchuk, G. A., Liu, W. T., Manefield, M., Meselson, M., et al. (2005). Biodiversity and ecosystem function in soil. *Nature, 434*(7033), 206–209. https://core.ac.uk/download/58969.pdf (accessed on 6 May 2025).
11. Gamelon, M., Touzot, L., Baubet, E., Cachelou, J., Focardi, S., Franzetti, B., Nivois, É., et al. (2021). Effects of pulsed resources on the dynamics of seed consumer populations: A comparative demographic study in wild boar. *Ecosphere, 12*(4), e03395. https://doi.org/10.1002/ecs2.3395.
12. González-Cabaleiro, R., Mitchell, A. M., Ofiţeru, I. D., Smith, et al. (2017). Heterogeneity in pure microbial systems: Experimental measurements and modeling. *Scientific Reports, 7*(1), 42185. https://core.ac.uk/download/161514075.pdf (accessed on 6 May 2025).

13. He, S., & Maibaum, L. (2018). Identifying the onset of phase separation in quaternary lipid bilayer systems from coarse-grained simulations. *Journal of Physical Chemistry B, 122*(14), 3961–3969. http://arxiv.org/abs/1801.05495 (accessed on 6 May 2025).

14. Ilmawan, M. (2024). Navigating heterogeneity in meta-analysis: Methods for identification and management. *Deka in Medicine, 12*(1), 42–55. https://www.semanticscholar.org/paper/093b495864e5e8fc69f4f588224353822e846667 (accessed on 6 May 2025).

15. LaDeau, S. L., Allan, B. F., Leisnham, P. T., & Levy, M. Z. (2015). The ecological foundations of transmission potential and vector-borne disease in urban landscapes. *Functional Ecology, 29*(7), 889–901. https://doi.org/10.1111/1365-2435.12487.

16. Marsh, A., Singer, D. R. J., Taylor, P. C., Watkins, et al. (2010). Personalized medicine: The impact on chemistry. *Nature Chemistry*, 2(10), 862–865. https://core.ac.uk/download/45676.pdf (accessed on 6 May 2025).

17. Metcalf, J. E., Farrar, J., Cutts, F., Basta, N. E., Graham, A. L., Lessler, J., Ferguson, N. M., et al. (2016). Use of serological surveys to generate key insights into the changing global landscape of infectious disease. *The Lancet, 388*(10041), 728–730. https://doi.org/10.1016/s0140-6736(16)30164-7.

18. Mohammadiha, A., Mohammadiha, A., Maia-Elkhoury, A. N. S., da Costa-Val, A. P., Galvani, A. P., Travi, B. L., Vercosa, B. L. A., et al. (2013). Heterogeneities in *Leishmania infantum* infection: Using skin parasite burdens to identify highly infectious dogs. *PLoS Neglected Tropical Diseases, 8*(1), e2583. https://core.ac.uk/download/19444084.pdf (accessed on 6 May 2025).

19. Moser, S. K., Barnard, M., Frantz, R. M., Spencer, J. A., Rodarte, K. A., Crooker, I., Bartlow, A. W., et al. (2023). Scoping review of Culex mosquito life history trait heterogeneity in response to temperature. *Parasites & Vectors, 16*(1), 1–15. https://doi.org/10.1186/s13071-023-05792-3.

20. Page, M. J., Moher, D., Bossuyt, P. M., Boutron, I., Hoffmann, T., Mulrow, C. D., Shamseer, L., et al. (2021). PRISMA 2020 explanation and elaboration: Updated guidance and exemplars for reporting systematic reviews. *BMJ, 372*, n160. https://doi.org/10.1136/bmj.n160.

21. Plestenjak, E., Meglič, V., Sinkovič, L., & Pipan, B. (2024). Factors influencing the emergence of heterogeneous populations of common bean (*Phaseolus vulgaris* L.) and their potential for intercropping. *Plants, 13*. https://www.semanticscholar.org/paper/854ae0635d752c2e104634b597c1c189b3dcab69 (accessed on 6 May 2025).

22. Puertas, A. M., Asakura, K., Berthier, L., Doliwa, B., Donati, C., Flenner, E., et al. (2006). *Dynamical Heterogeneities in an Attraction Driven Colloidal Glass*. http://arxiv.org/abs/cond-mat/0510443 (accessed on 6 May 2025).

23. Rajati, F., Ahmadi, N., Naghibzadeh, Z. A., & Kazeminia, M. (2022). The global prevalence of oropharyngeal dysphagia in different populations: a systematic review and meta-analysis. *Journal of translational medicine, 20*(1), 175. https://doi.org/10.1186/s12967-022-03380-0 (accessed on 6 May 2025).

24. Schneider, M., Ballvora, A., & Léon, J. (2024). Deep genotyping reveals specific adaptation footprints of conventional and organic farming in barley populations—An evolutionary plant breeding approach. *Agronomy for Sustainable Development, 44*(1), 1–10. https://www.semanticscholar.org/paper/f9b6cbd3b39f7a20ab56a3771bb6bfdac0876efa (accessed on 6 May 2025).

25. Sharpee, T., Destexhe, A., Kawato, M., Sekulić, V., Skinner, F., Wójcik, D., Chintaluri, C., et al. (2016). 25th Annual Computational Neuroscience Meeting: CNS-2016. *BMC Neuroscience, 17*(1), 1–10. https://www.semanticscholar.org/paper/50920b36cca05c524a658a453fd5484e1498b898 (accessed on 6 May 2025).
26. Shen, X., Wen, Y., Cui, Y., & Lu, Q. (2021). A conditional autoregressive model for genetic association analysis accounting for genetic heterogeneity. *Statistics in Medicine, 41*(4), 517–542. https://www.semanticscholar.org/paper/418a42149b2d5c1417e24f87b459de1ce3c5707c (accessed on 6 May 2025).
27. Silk, M. J., Hodgson, D. J., Rozins, C., Croft, D. P., Delahay, R. J., Boots, M., & McDonald, R. A. (2019). Integrating social behaviour, demography and disease dynamics in network models: Applications to disease management in declining wildlife populations. *Philosophical Transactions of the Royal Society B: Biological Sciences, 374*(1779), 20180211. https://doi.org/10.1098/rstb.2018.0211.
28. Singer, M., Deutschman, C. S., Seymour, C. W., Shankar-Hari, M., Annane, D., Bauer, M., Bellomo, R., et al. (2016). The Third International Consensus Definitions for Sepsis and Septic Shock (Sepsis-3). *JAMA, 315*(8), 801–810. https://doi.org/10.1001/jama.2016.0287.
29. Steffen, W., Richardson, K., Rockström, J., Cornell, S., Fetzer, I., Bennett, E. M., Biggs, R., et al. (2015). Planetary boundaries: Guiding human development on a changing planet. *Science, 347*(6223), 1259855. https://doi.org/10.1126/science.1259855.
30. Tamura, K., Stecher, G., & Kumar, S. (2021). MEGA11: Molecular evolutionary genetics analysis version 11. *Molecular Biology and Evolution, 38*(11), 3022–3027. https://doi.org/10.1093/molbev/msab120.
31. Vendramin, R., Litchfield, K., & Swanton, C. (2021). Cancer evolution: Darwin and beyond. *The EMBO Journal, 40*(6), 1–15. https://doi.org/10.15252/embj.2021108389.
32. Woodward, A. A., Urbanowicz, R., Naj, A., & Moore, J. H. (2022). Genetic heterogeneity: Challenges, impacts, and methods through an associative lens. *Genetic Epidemiology, 46*, 555–571. https://www.semanticscholar.org/paper/0ac69fcc563de139f19e2d03ac447575955bff9b (accessed on 6 May 2025).
33. Zhao, Q., Liu, X., Wu, Y., Liu, H., Qu, F., Zhang, M., & Li, X. (2024). Spatiotemporal variations and driving factors of ecological sensitivity in the West Qinling Mountains, China, under the optimal scale. *Sustainability, 16*(2), 1–20. https://www.semanticscholar.org/paper/d1236f14db4fd1d131b5affb0296b854167727ed (accessed on 6 May 2025).

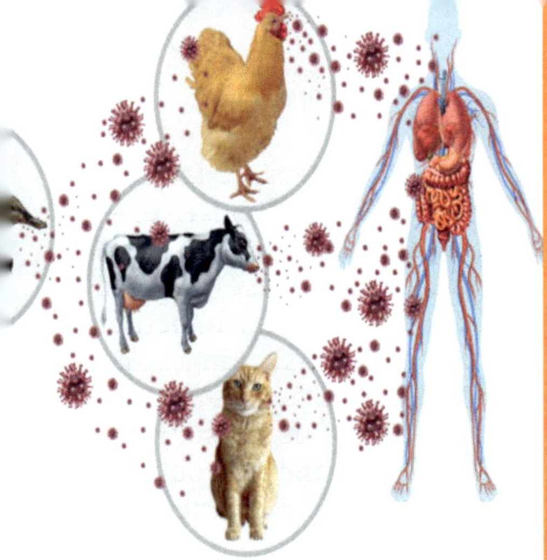

Chapter 7

VECTOR-BORNE AND ZOONOTIC DISEASE DYNAMICS

Contents

Introduction

Environmental issues and health hazards have become much more interrelated throughout the years. Urban places and other types of ecosystems exhibit their unique set of characteristics that influence the transmission of diseases caused by insects or transmitted from animals to humans. Wildlife encroaching too close to human territories, particularly where cities have expanded and altered the ecosystem—can accelerate the transmission of germs. One such study in some part of the Netherlands discovered that urban wild spots contained some other level of zoonotic pathogens than in non-urban areas. In most instances, being aware of these turns is everything to assembling public health plans that genuinely reduce risks. Not all people appear to have a similar awareness of these health problems, and that's a true concern. Consider dairy farmers, for example; many of them just do not have the complete picture regarding vector-borne diseases such as dengue and chikungunya. It is this confusion of unclear information that creates a gap that makes it harder to control diseases. A little more targeted training and education outreach to high-risk populations could encourage farmers to look for early warning signs and take action to safeguard both their animals and themselves—albeit at times with the message being repeated in various guises. Urban development combined with agricultural use ultimately creates a fairly complicated landscape in which these diseases can thrive. As cities expand and natural habitats shift, the disruption can drive the likelihood of pathogen transmission even further. Frequently, the connection between environmental changes and the way zoonotic diseases operate suggests that there is a need to collaborate across disciplines. Further studies in both congested cities and less disrupted natural sites appears to be the solution, assisting professionals in honing health strategies to more effectively address these problems. Expanding our general knowledge might lead the way toward more intelligent, efficient methods of mitigating the effects of these troublesome illnesses.

Definition of Vector-Borne Diseases

Vectors and the pathogens that they ride on are the key to how diseases are transmitted. Vectors such as mosquitoes, fleas, and ticks transmit germs that can have a serious effect on the health of humans, and they also determine the natural balance in their environments. It is not just a simple link – the way these tiny messengers work with their carried pathogens is complexed with environmental shifts, the way people live, and even changes in local ecosystems. Generally speaking, understanding these connections is key for tracking illnesses and planning control strategies, especially now that global travel and climate shifts are stirring up trouble in many regions.

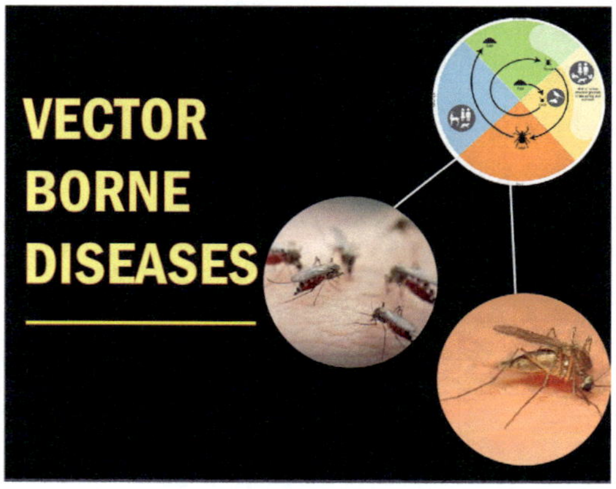

Source: Medical Dialogues. (2018). *Vector-Borne Diseases Infographic.*

The increase in vector-borne illnesses (VBDs) appears to be largely the result of human-induced changes. Changes in land use like deforestation and rapid urbanization can, for the most part, disrupt natural habitats sufficiently to allow pathogens to jump from animals to humans. New research suggests that such disruptions mess with the normal transmission pathways, leaving doors open for germs to enter areas previously considered secure. This combination of elements sends a strong message that addressing these health threats involves merging medical interventions with measures to preserve the environment and better manage our territories. Reducing the welcoming nature of habitats to vectors at times can decrease the rate at which the disease circulates, thereby safeguarding both vulnerable ecosystems as well as human lives. Climate change also has an increasing impact on these illnesses; unpredictable weather and temperature fluctuations are altering where vectors can thrive. Organisms that previously only survived in limited climates are now appearing to be venturing into new areas, occasionally initiating epidemics where no one anticipated them. As an example, if you look at infections sensitive to climate, it is clear that the activity of these pathogens closely interweaves with larger ecological shifts. This relationship between our emerging climate and disease dynamics is obvious in that full research and monitoring are required if we are to get the whole picture. Greater awareness and improved scientific cooperation are necessary if we are to come up with adaptive measures against the changing threat presented by these vectors (Omazic et al., 2019; Plowright et al., 2021).

Definition of Zoonotic Diseases

Humans, animals, and environments all get intertwined in ways that do matter when you're trying to solve diseases that leap from animals to humans. These diseases—which primarily occur through close contact, insects serving as carriers, or even contaminated environments—represent a significant health concern because they can result in all types of diseases and sometimes even kill. Sometimes you need to consider how small microbes and their hosts interact—and in general, that involves a fairly in-depth consideration of how nature and its minor details cooperate. Wildlife habitats are important, as disturbances to these spaces allow pathogens to spill over into human populations, which in turn agitate global public health issues (Kemp et al., 2022). Interdisciplinary thought simply cannot be ignored here. The swift transmission of diseases such as SARS-CoV-2 taught us, in most instances, that knowing the precipitators in nature is key to developing means to prevent outbreaks from spiraling out of control. Land use modifications, for instance, tend to go along with more opportunities for these diseases to find their way in—human activities sometimes compound the problem. It is truly important to investigate how these spillovers occur, not only to protect our health but also to maintain our natural world as resilient. As researchers struggle through the complex cascade from infection to shedding, spillover, and then spread, they begin to get clues about how our landscapes fare against these threats, and what conservation strategies can be effective (Plowright et al., 2021). To look at zoonotic diseases is not just to observe how infections transfer from animal to human but to make us think about the way these incidents disrupt entire ecosystems and the public health infrastructure we depend on. When they do occur, they can cause a lot of pressure on our healthcare systems, compelling us into emergency measures to attempt to prevent further outbreaks. It is the recurrent, sometimes volatile interaction between what humans do and the way wild places respond that continues to keep on our horizon the potential for zoonotic disease to break out. By understanding the messy, intersecting landscapes on which these things happen, health policy receives a shot of down-to-earth, evidence-based wisdom aimed at reducing risks. Besides, coping with the challenges of today is as much a matter of preparing for tomorrow as responding to the now—and maintaining nature in balance can be one of our best protections against global health.

Importance of Studying Disease Dynamics

It's important to understand disease complexity, particularly for diseases transmitted by vectors or those that leap from animals to humans. There's a great deal at stake here, ranging from the simple ecological blend to the minutiae of epidemiology. For example, studies in Pakistan show that ticks, like *Rhipicephalus microplus*, sometimes carry emerging microbes such as *Neoehrlichia mikurensis*; this finding (Hussain et al., 2024) reminds us that vectors, hosts and their environments are tightly interwoven in unexpected ways. Figuring out these dynamic relationships, in most cases, lets public health officials whip up targeted measures before things spiral into bigger crises. Climate change also increases the stakes in disease transmission, shaking things up by creating new hotspots in changing conditions. Zoonotic cutaneous leishmaniasis (ZCL) research in Iran illustrates how changed environments can ignite new sites for disease transmission. New geographic trends and even the emergence of new reservoirs indicate that it is becoming increasingly difficult to manage zoonotic diseases. One paper highlights the fact that climate change enhances ZCL dissemination through human adjustments to vector habitats such as wetlands and rodents – a minor change that requires flexible public health measures that can move in tandem with shifting disease ecosystems. Lastly, integrating work across sectors—what most refer to as One Health frameworks—drives home the relevance of human, animal, and environmental health in their interconnectedness. This communal risk focus invites scholars to develop multi-level intervention strategies, particularly where there is high risk, by investigating the complex network of dynamics underlying diseases such as ZCL and other tick-borne illnesses. It is evident that the comprehension of these connected dynamics not only informs local health policy but also constructs a more globally oriented public health workforce capable of responding to evolving danger (Hussain et al., 2024).

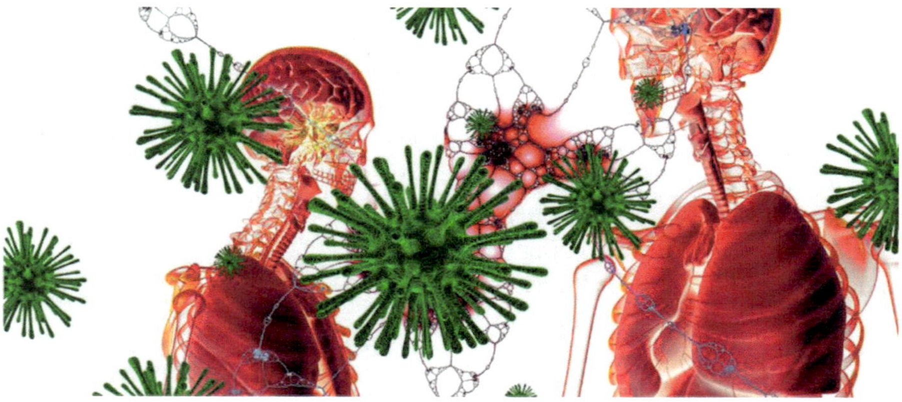

Source: Edinburgh Infectious Diseases. (n.d.). *Coronavirus Lungs.*

7.1. Historical Context

Agriculture's ancient history with disease overflows into our daily health. In the past, when humans traded their hunter-gatherer lifestyle for farming, they started running into wildlife much more—and this shift allowed animal germs to creep into human populations. A review once cited that as farms increased in size and the environment changed, the likelihood of these animal-originated microbes crossing species increased, particularly when our populations continued to rise. It is safe to say that our growing population, with changing lifestyles and all, has amplified these dangers even more. Examining the knotted connections between the way we produce food and our environment appears necessary if we are to anticipate future disease trends and create improved public health practices (Jones et al., 2013). History also dishes up lessons regarding disease complexity. Consider visceral leishmaniasis (VL), for example—it is commonly held up as an exemplar of the problems faced by the so-called neglected tropical diseases. Even the World Health Organization (WHO) established a lofty goal to knock VL out as a public health problem by 2017, a goal that serves to illustrate just how difficult it can be to combat such diseases. Surprisingly, despite math models being regarded as valuable vehicles for grasping the behavior of VL, there are not yet sufficient numbers of them in circulation. In most instances, a shortage of hard data and comprehensive analysis has held back intelligent intervention planning. Understanding precisely how infectious each step of the disease continues to be a central, yet still elusive, piece of information for reaching elimination goals (Adams et al., 2015). When we look back, even with some rough edges in the record, we can start to see patterns that inform improved interventions today. Looking at past outbreaks in conjunction with changes in farming practices and changing environments, researchers pick up on clues to the dangers we are facing today. Lessons from VL reiterated in history and repeated in present thought, indicate the necessity of approaches that synthesize human behavior, ecological trends, and pathogen patterns—no matter how often it requires repeating the same facts in alternate perspectives. And with climate change and urban sprawl driving us ever more toward possible new epidemics, relying on historical understanding is not only about patching up today's disaster; it is about establishing health systems that have a chance of surviving tomorrow's shock (Jones et al., 2013; Adams et al., 2015).

7.1.1. Major Outbreaks in History

Agriculture and the transmission of contagious diseases go hand in hand, and as it happens, this relationship is important to public health. Consider epidemics such as bird flu and swine flu—these illustrate how agricultural practices enhance the potential for diseases to make the leap from animals to humans. Industrial livestock operations, where animals are closely packed and antibiotics are applied frequently, provide environments that facilitate germs traveling. It's fascinating that studies show since the 1940s, more than a quarter of new infectious human diseases have origins linked to agriculture (Rohr et al., 2019). As farm sizes increase to feed our expanding global population, we can anticipate more such spillover occurrences unless we combine food production with robust health measures to keep outbreaks at bay. Seasonality also has a huge influence on how diseases, particularly those transmitted by microbes or animals, play out around the year. A lot of infections have their own seasonally driven cycles based on weather changes, the behavior of hosts, and even the germs' life cycles themselves. Take the flu, for instance. The flu typically peaks during the cold months, creating a kind of timeline for public health officials to work with (Martinez, 2018). And if you consider how other diseases such as chickenpox and polio peak in the spring and summer, respectively, you will understand that it is important to be aware of these cycles. This ebb-and-flow dynamic is one we must watch all year long by employing vaccination campaigns and intelligent resource allocation in anticipation of when infection rates are at their peak. History also has much to teach us regarding the evolving landscape of infectious diseases. The 1918 flu, for example, serves as a stark reminder of how rapidly a virus can spread through populations, particularly with troop movements worldwide stoking the flames during war. There is, of course, the West Nile virus outbreak in the United States, which demonstrated that when humans relocate into native habitats and the environment changes, mosquito-borne diseases can take hold. With agricultural practices continually evolving to suit our requirements, the combination of human endeavor, climate change, and disease outbreaks is only set to become more complex. Overcoming these challenges typically involves integrating initiatives in health care, agriculture, and environmental understanding—a policy that will be vital to preventing and managing disease in the years to come (Rohr et al., 2019).

7.1.2. Evolution of Vector-Borne and Zoonotic Diseases

Our daily behaviors appear entwined with the ways diseases transmitted by microbes or from animals make their way to us. Pressing agriculture harder to feed our growing numbers, for example, ultimately stirs the pot for such diseases. Deforestation or altering how we use land can provide ideal locations for insects and wildlife to commingle—with wild animals, then domesticated ones, and eventually humans. When wild and domesticated animals find themselves in the same location, the likelihood of becoming infected with a zoonotic microbe increases, reflecting the uncontrolled transformation of our environment and routines. Researchers are now stating, in broad terms, that we require research that connects how we use the land and how we mold nature to better predict and mitigate future epidemics (Jones et al., 2013). Other than how we farm, how we monitor these diseases is changing rapidly. In the past, people primarily responded once a spillover had occurred—not a viable way to manage things. Recently, virologists, ecologists, and computer-savvy biologists have met at workshops to discuss detecting potentially hazardous viruses before they jumped to humans. They are coming more and more to rely on genetic and natural clues to monitor which species may pass on the diseases. This early-warning strategy could potentially turn our entire strategy around since early detection of trouble could reduce its public health bite (Bush et al., 2012). Understanding how diseases are transmitted and evolve is not only important for the plans of today but also for tomorrow's science. With climatic changes tampering with habitats and where insects congregate, we are certain to witness new combinations between insects, animals, and humans that make things even more complicated. That is the reason why experts from various walks—ecology, biology, even social sciences—must join forces, although sometimes it makes for a mess of ideas. Pooling our efforts can make us better understand why these diseases get around and inform decisions that can reduce both their incidence and effects. By keeping our early-alerting tools honed (and perhaps a bit rough around the edges), we can prepare ourselves to meet the unpredictable surprises of disease transmission in a world that never stands still (Jones et al., 2013; Bush et al., 2012).

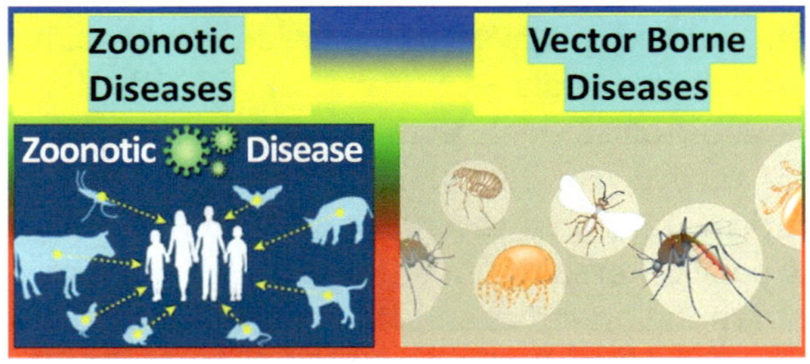

Source: Frank, T. (2018). *How to Learn Anything Faster – 5 Tips to Increase Your Learning Speed.*

7.1.3. Impact of Climate Change on Disease Emergence

Climate changes are upending the game for public health. Public health infrastructure now grapples with a blend of vector-borne and zoonotic diseases. Temperatures that fluctuate disrupt the traditional cycles of insects such as mosquitoes and ticks, which can increase how rapidly slimy pathogens propagate. Consider Rift Valley fever (RVF) for instance—this disease is encroaching into increasing areas of Africa, Rwanda not an exception, and its increasing spread indicates we need to seriously understand what is happening with how it spreads. In most instances, this implies reconsidering our public health actions, strengthening on-the-ground surveillance, and taking precautionary measures, particularly in regions where communities rely heavily on livestock. The pressure increases as more individuals get put at risk in these changing circumstances (Muvunyi et al., 2025). It's not only about increasing transmission levels; our warming climate also appears to be riling up diseases that we previously believed were in check. Consider the Arctic, for example. Warming, gentler winters now allow some pathogens and hosts to persist longer than they once did, and that can trigger a revival of some zoonotic diseases. You can get glimpses of danger from microbes such as Brucella spp. and Leptospira spp., and that's rather strongly indicative of the fact that we need to include climatic factors when anticipating future epidemics. Consequently, experts in local health could stand a better chance of identifying or even averting the next wave of infections once all these factors are in play. Unfortunately, these changes impact most harshly on marginalized communities, exacerbating global inequality regarding disease risk (Parkinson et al., 2014). The complex connections between a changing climate and emerging diseases demand a response that is far-reaching and practical. New technology, such as AI-driven surveillance and genomic information—is now in the arsenal that can assist in warning of vector-borne threats in advance and influence rapid, responsive defenses. In locations such as Rwanda, where both RVF and other zoonotic risks are a looming concern, a One Health approach could be just the ticket. This line of thinking doesn't just fuel initial warnings; it also connects the dots on how we approach problems on the human, animal, and environmental levels. As global warming continues to alter the behavior of disease, investing more research and money into creative solutions is merely a necessity for keeping people safe during these uncertain times (Muvunyi et al., 2025).

7.2. Mechanisms of Transmission

Ecological processes and host-pathogen relationships determine the pace at which vector-borne and zoonotic diseases are transmitted. The natural environment can facilitate the movement of pathogens or, in some cases, inhibit them—this concept rears its head in what is referred to as the dilution effect. Essentially, the more biodiversity there is, it appears that infections do not spread as readily among hosts because the web of interactions is more complex. However, it is not quite cut and dried; some vectors are quite finicky, altering the way disease is transmitted. In general terms, gaining a handle on these nuances is instrumental to predicting outbreaks and devising intelligent management strategies, particularly in areas where such zoonotic problems thrive. Geography and local environmental conditions create further subtleties in these transmission dynamics.

For example, outbreaks such as RVF in Africa demonstrate that environmental changes can turn up the threats. In Rwanda, the trend of RVF identifies gaps in what we currently understand about which vectors are up to the task and what factors pose a risk, suggesting the influence of changing climate and land use to foment disease transmission. As Muvunyi et al. (2025) point out, digging into such local modifications is essential if we wish to pin down prevention approaches based on improved diagnostics and surveillance—trying to catch new pathogens early, not running around after the fact. It's not all about nature or environment. How local hosts and communities are assembled is a major contributor to the transmission drama, too. A few studies indicate that when generalist vectors are in control, a richer diversity of species could result in fewer infections, which appears to support the dilution hypothesis. But occasionally, with specialist vectors, the results can turn out very differently—occasionally disease transmission is amplified, at others it is restrained. Occhibove et al. (2022) reveal that community composition effects on disease transmission are not uniform due to the complex natural dynamics involved. All of this indicates the necessity for models that combine these ecological findings together so that we can predict and control outbreaks more effectively in human and animal populations, opening the door to wiser public health and conservation actions.

7.2.1. Role of Vectors in Disease Spread

Vectors play a large role in how illnesses spread around, usually in less-than-obvious ways. Insects, ticks, and even mammals assist microbes in making that leap from one host to another. Take the West Nile virus, for instance—it illustrates how birds migrate and mosquitoes stir things up to force the virus past its initial boundaries. Birds that travel across continents not only migrate but also spread the virus, infecting both their own species and human beings. Their migration patterns allude to deep connections in our ecosystems and direct us to the points that will be under threat of outbreaks shortly, thus emphasizing the need for a combination of observation techniques and field-based vector control (García-Carrasco et al., 2023). Chagas disease adds another complicating factor to the equation. The existence of *Trypanosoma cruzi* is an intricate entwining of many triatomine microbe species found in various locations around the Americas. Rojas de Arias et al. even referred to the "practical impossibility" of fully preventing its transmission, primarily due to the fact that the disease is easily transmitted between animals and humans due to its extensive vectors. The reason why Chagas continues to resurface is that maintaining a close eye on these insect populations and the changes in their habitats is necessary. Even if control efforts knock back some populations, indigenous insects tend to rebound—highlighting that increasing insect monitoring and engaging communities is crucial to managing these complex issues (Gonçalves, 2022). Animal and human health are more entwined than perhaps we realize, and vectors are squarely in the middle of that overlap. These small carriers not only transport pathogens between wild animals, but typically span the gap to humans too, making control of disease difficult. Because of this dual purpose, we need to think holistically—a One Health approach that considers people, animals, and the environment together. Seeing the pattern of mobile animals and insect activity merge at times provides insights into potential outbreak hotspots and guides targeted preventive measures. Intersecting concepts from disparate disciplines—even though the process sometimes seems a tad unorthodox—is moving us closer to grasping the intricate disease dynamics and preparing us better for whatever emerging infections may arise (García-Carrasco et al., 2023).

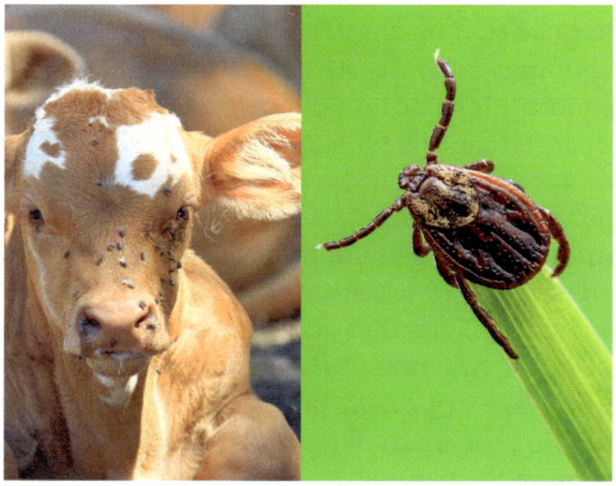

Source: Center for Food Security and Public Health. (2022). Cow Tick *(Rhipicephalus annulatus). The Livestock Project.*

7.2.2. Zoonotic Transmission Pathways

It's not necessarily as simple as it sounds to understand how illnesses are transmitted from animals to people. You have to examine a combination of things—biology, the environment, economics, even the way people think—to truly understand why these diseases spread so quickly. Studies typically find that it's not one factor; human behavior and changing environmental conditions are bound up together, and the whole mess is made rather complicated. This perspective, in the majority of instances, causes scientists to observe both purposeful behaviors and daily routines that sustain infections. As we explore these complicated interactions, our overall picture becomes more affluent though somewhat fragmented. In addition, wording it this way allows us not only to track where diseases may emerge but also to make more informed approaches in managing them in today's ever-complicated public health environment (Barnett et al., 2012). Unraveling how germs transmit among hosts in so many different ways—changing their tactics, even, based on the environment—is crucial if we're ever to deduce the Gordian knot of zoonotic disease. Most infectious agents appear to capitalize on alternative paths of transmission, even changing hosts or modes as circumstances evolve around them. This adaptability, in all honesty, makes the control of disease a headache in reality, and that is why we see the call so often for more comprehensive models—ones that encompass all these turns and detours. It is as if the continuously evolving dance between hosts and the transmission of things between them provokes us to examine more closely how even minor interventions can tip the balance. When you begin to peel away these layers and observe what is truly fueling the transmission, it opens the door to more targeted strategies for placing a lid on these outbreaks (Anderson et al., 2016). Gathering all different angles of research is one thing that simply needs to be near the head of the list in terms of knowing zoonotic pathways. As these diseases keep on going up across the world, including observations of community behavior, environmental changes, and hard biology is rather important to keep diseases in line. Interdisciplinary collaboration can guide stronger frameworks for anticipating and controlling outbreaks, even when the process is occasionally a little lopsided. Frequent cooperation in this open-ended format tends to push us toward perceiving that our natural systems are indeed interconnected—biology and environment are not separate entities. This combination of views typically ends up guiding policy decisions that try to mitigate the effects of these diseases, ultimately creating a healthier future (Barnett et al., 2012).

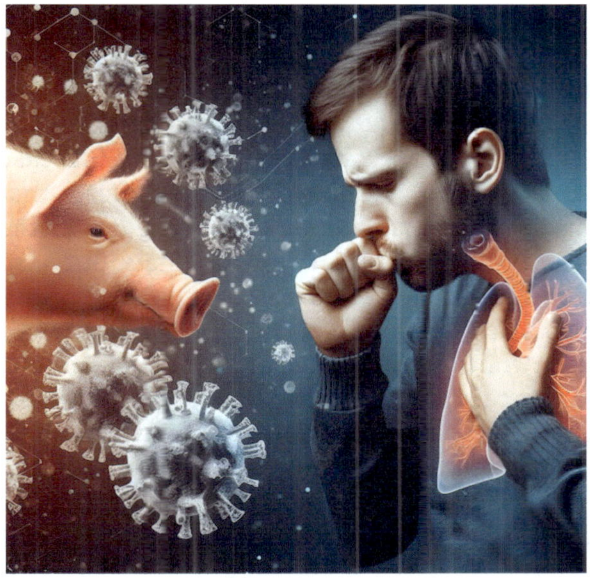

Source: Freepik. (n.d.). *Zoonotic Disease Transmission.*

7.2.3. Environmental Factors Influencing Transmission

External factors contribute a great deal to influencing how vector-borne and zoonotic diseases are transmitted. Sometimes in a given instance, weather conditions such as heat, humidity, and even rain can modify the life cycle of animals like mosquitoes and ticks—warmer weather, for instance, could prolong their breeding seasons so more of them are present, thus increasing the possibility of disease transmission. Consider Crimean-Congo Haemorrhagic Fever (CCHF): research has identified clusters of disease in southern France where local environmental idiosyncrasies appear to operate. One study even noted that regions which feature natural open countryside and coniferous woodland commonly go hand-in-hand with increased seropositivity in cattle; obviously, nature's impact on disease is subtle (Bernard et al., 2025). Urban expansion turns everything upside down, also by separating natural habitats and changing the way wildlife, insect vectors, and humans interact. When rural lands transform into urban sprawls, the likelihood of humans colliding with wildlife reservoirs increases—increasing spillover incidents. An example is in areas such as central rural Iran, where expanding urban footprint has been associated with an increase in ZCL case occurrences. The data in general indicate that this type of urbanization not only relocates the habitat of disease-carrying animals but also introduces new reservoirs of animals, further increasing the risk. While climate change is meanwhile rewriting the natural script—shifting ecological trends and sometimes pushing new disease hotspots into focus. As environments become increasingly welcoming to both vectors and their usual hosts, areas previously off the map for particular diseases can suddenly experience growing numbers.

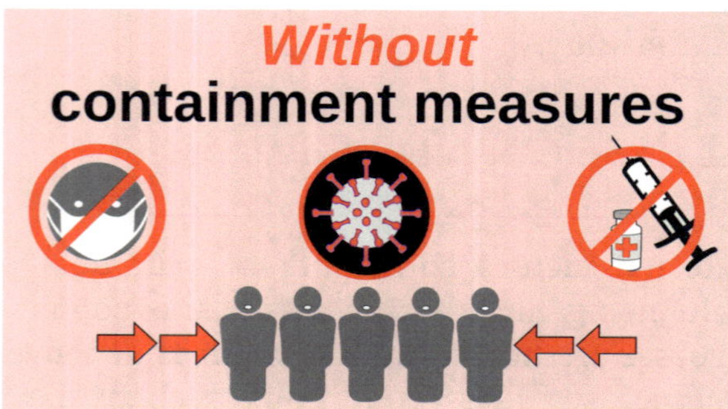

Source: By RCraig09 - Own work, CC BY-SA 4.0, https://commons.wikimedia.org/w/index.php?curid=91094938

The effect of climate on ZCL, for instance, suggests that conditions that favor vectors may even penetrate northwestern Iran. Preemptive, locally tailored interventions—i.e., to develop resilience in high-risk zones—can assist in anticipating and containing such emerging threats. Overall, the complicated interplay between our evolving world and disease transmission serves to indicate that controlling vector-borne diseases in this rapidly evolving world is far from simple.

7.3. Epidemiological Models

Vector-borne and zoonotic diseases are conditioned by both environmental and epidemiological factors. For most of these, comprehending the complicated dynamics involves employing models that disassemble the mechanisms of disease dissemination and even making estimates of when outbreaks will happen. Consider Shanghai, for instance—scientists there explored how air quality affects national infectious disease by employing a double-pollutant model that even considered exposure delays. They discovered that pollutant concentrations and reported disease fall into place in some interesting patterns (Lin et al., 2025). Overall, these sophisticated methods assist public health crews in cutting through the complex interconnections between our surroundings and disease transmission, providing them with a necessary advantage. Climate variables, added into the mix, can clarify trends we might otherwise overlook, particularly with diseases like dengue. A 23-year study in Peru revealed, rather amusingly, that variable climatic changes and urban expansion can increase populations of *Aedes aegypti*, the primary virus carrier. Interlacing time-based and geographic data, researchers identified obvious correlations between rainy-season rains and dengue outbreaks, to underscore the utility of models that adapt to shifting weather and city landscapes (Goche et al., 2025). In a sense, these findings not just shed light on today's public health enigmas but also facilitate more effective, more specific responses. The more complicated the overall picture of infectious diseases becomes, the more essential it is to assemble models that account for everything—the environmental pieces, socioeconomic information, even behavior trends. In such locations, for example, where dengue has struck hardest, issues such as poverty, sanitation, and the challenge of controlling insects all get combined in unforeseen combinations. Combining these ingredients into a single usable framework can refine projections and enable targeted interventions to reach those most at risk. In practice, while the public health systems struggle to reduce the effects of vector-borne and zoonotic illnesses, it is constantly pushing the models to evolve that is most important to adopting policies that prioritize community health—even when the specifics sometimes seem a little uncoordinated.

7.3.1. Basic Reproduction Number (R0)

Checking out the transmission of diseases is a matter of going into the nuts and bolts of numbers on transmission—those numbers that present, in a very literal sense, how infections spread from host to host. R0, that ubiquitous fundamental reproduction number, is a big part of it; it tells you, on average, how many new cases emerge from one infected individual in a completely vulnerable group. In vector-borne diseases, this figure is not merely another figure—it is embedded in the mathematical models which inform our control strategies. As a general rule, when R0 is one or less, the infection will dwindle, resulting in a sort of balance of disease-free state. But if R0 rises above one, then eventually you are facing an endemic scenario where the disease persists, basically requiring swift action to step in. There is more to R0 than initially meets the eye—it gets shaped by factors such as how people act, the way vectors travel, and even the general environment atmosphere. Certain research, for example, have understood the ways in which daily commutes and variations in vector migration can upset the apple cart, usually proving that under conditions in which hosts are not well-mixed, vector-borne diseases (VBDs) are more likely to persist. Typically, the models indicate that R0 is at its minimum when reservoir mixing is optimally well done, which highlights the importance of addressing the biological components as well as the ecological forces at play (Gao & Yuan, 2024).

At other times, such nuances are repeated, and it becomes clear that the relationship between nature and behavior is never linear. R0 also serves to map out means to battle against such nuisance VBDs. Recent research has made obvious connections between R0 and vector reproduction rates, such that adjusting the way we control these populations can have a direct effect on the rhythm of the disease. By prodding at equilibrium points in the models, researchers can extract stability thresholds that ultimately inform public health interventions (Diabat ABé et al., 2022). As a measure, R0 not only defines the disease dynamics but also inspires practical measures that can adapt to changing ecological conditions—and even host behaviors—over time. For the most part, this integration of theory with actual tactics brings us closer to controlling zoonotic diseases effectively.

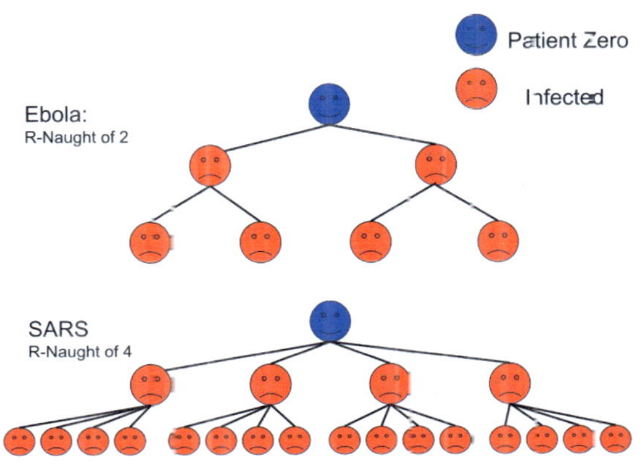

Source: Campbell, K. (2019). R naught Ebola and flu diagram. *Wikimedia Commons*.

7.3.2. SIR and SEIR Models

Infectious diseases follow a complex web of determinants—host behavior, environmental idiosyncrasies, and the cycles of vector populations all combine in unpredictable ways. Tools such as SIR (Susceptible-Infectious-Recovered) and SEIR (Susceptible-Exposed-Infectious-Recovered) divide individuals into various groups so scientists can understand how diseases spread through populations. The SEIR model, for instance, functions quite well when a disease takes a little while to get from being sick to being infectious—the model just puts those people into an "exposed" category. By adjusting the numbers in these models, researchers can simulate a variety of scenarios, which usually puts public health officials at an advantage when attempting to stem the tide. Dengue fever, for instance, illustrates how effective these methods can be. In most instances, combining the SEIR model with ensemble Kalman filtering (EnKF) techniques results in some remarkably accurate predictions across different areas. This real-time monitoring and planning can be particularly important when outbreaks appear to be imminent. The SEIR-SEI-EnKF combination does a much better job of capturing human and mosquito interactions than previous methods (Yi et al., 2021). That combination not only provides a sharper image of today's disease scenario but also sets the stage for how to address future threats from vector-borne diseases. Zoonotic problems put another twist into the narrative—consider zoonotic visceral leishmaniasis (ZVL) as an example. Some scientists use SIR models to probe how infection in a mother dog can be transmitted to her puppies, maintaining the reservoir of the disease. Knowing how the infected mother influences the offspring provides some additional leads on ZVL's broader patterns. It also reveals how such internally fueled groups can influence transmission among unexposed populations, especially when their destiny correlates with transmission via vectors (Ozanne et al., 2019). Simulation models, with some heuristic trial-and-error, gradually confirm that addressing both vertical and vector pathways can be crucial in developing effective health interventions in areas struggling with these endemic issues.

7.3.3. Importance of Modeling in Public Health

Environmental conditions and disease transmission are entwined in ways that require a more adaptive, less linear response than one would imagine. Climate change disrupts ecosystems constantly, and its byproduct is that pathogens such as mosquitoes begin to act – and spread – in unpredictable manners. Temperature, humidity, rain: these elements do not simply push diseases like malaria and dengue around in neat, predictable patterns; they set off a chain of events that is layered and, well, complicated. Using models to simulate these shifting conditions can help us get a rough idea of where outbreaks might emerge, which in most cases guides us to intervene faster. High-level case studies even suggest that when we add in accurate data, our preparedness for climate-sensitive disease in vulnerable populations becomes significantly enhanced (Alamri et al., 2024). Outside of environmental idiosyncrasies, advances in machine learning have truly married themselves with public health planning. The Multilayer Perceptron (MLP) and Support Vector Machine (SVM) models have started reshaping our expectations of VBD spread. Think about it – the MLP model, in one case, achieved an accuracy of 92% (which isn't too shabby if I do say so myself), whereas the SVM finds a balance between speed and accuracy at approximately 90.87%. These figures, quite frankly, highlight the value of selecting a model appropriate for the urgency and resource requirements of a particular scenario; quick decision-making can be the difference between life and death in a crisis (Tito et al., 2024). Predicting isn't all it's about, though – these models also act as templates for developing broader disease control plans. By mixing and matching datasets from climate records, socio-economic determinants, and health reports, public health researchers can map out possible risk areas. This type of multi-dimensional, occasionally messy, analysis makes us better understand how vulnerabilities intersect in given groups. Further, as the models get refined and revised over time, they assist adaptive management efforts geared toward stemming outbreaks. In short, integrating data-informed information with longstanding public health routines assists in unraveling the challenges presented by vector-borne and zoonotic diseases, particularly as our setting continues to change unpredictably.

7.4. Public Health Implications

People's everyday practices, the natural world, and how germs move around are all mixed together—forcing us to think in many different ways about public health. Environmental and biological issues, along with socio-economic pushes, now play a big role in how zoonotic diseases spread. There is not just one neat formula for it; insights from all kinds of fields end up overlapping. Consider, for instance, the way regular habits become married to environmental idiosyncrasies—this type of union can highlight the routes and natural refuges for such germs. Considering the entire picture pushes public health strategies to make a closer look at behavior, which can translate to improved means to prevent and manage infections that afflict both humans and animals (Barnett et al., 2012). Wildlife also comes into view as an obvious indicator of what is in jeopardy, particularly in the case of migrating animals. Certain wild birds that have been generally regarded as natural vectors are capable of going long distances carrying many microorganisms, which may ultimately become a human health problem. Of course, avian-to-human jumps are quite rare, but connections with diseases such as influenza A and West Nile virus are a reminder not to dismiss this. In most instances, as the climate change redistributes migratory routes, the threat scenario may alter in unanticipated manners. That is why it is crucial to monitor closely how animals relocate and interact to grasp how these diseases emerge and spread (Bauchinger et al., 2008). Addressing vector-borne and zoonotic issues is not merely a science issue—it requires community participation and new policy actions. Health projects ought to concentrate on educating neighborhoods about where these diseases originate and spread.

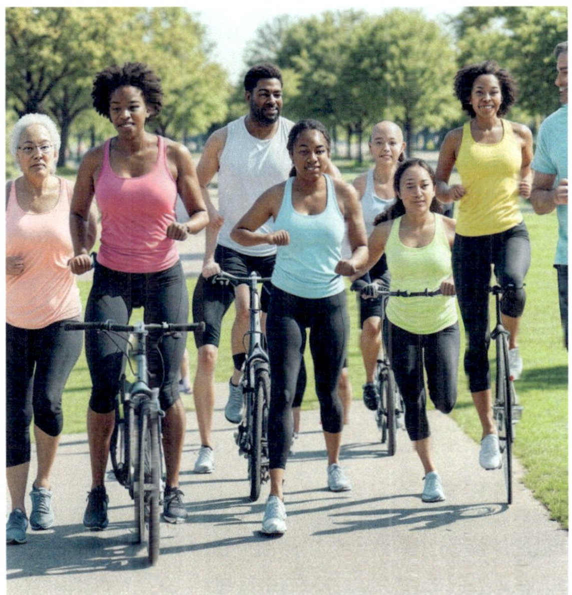

Source: https://external-content.duckduckgo.com/iu/?u=https%3A%2F%2Fgovtbenefits.org%2Fwp-content%2Fuploads%2F2023%2F11%2Fimg-PpMqog81G6gAA1ipLr4vi.jpg&f=1&nofb=1&ipt=23d24e38dc9c360890c7f4911ade2a48f5eca188d991395f5b46fa12336e82cc

Even more often, local populations possess indigenous knowledge that, when heard, enhances early warning systems for emerging threats. Additionally, partnerships between public health leaders, wildlife enthusiasts, and community members become crucial for developing intelligent, ground-level interventions. When local knowledge is mixed with scientific information, interventions can be tuned to the vagaries of every region, lightening the burden of these diseases while also assisting the environment and resilience of communities to stay resilient (Barnett et al., 2012; Bauchinger et al., 2008).

7.4.1. Surveillance and Monitoring Strategies

Determining the way infections get around is not an easy proposition. Diseases like those transmitted by insects or animals have a habit of appearing in strangely mixed circumstances, particularly when human alterations rock the boat. Rather than a clear equation, you find that you need an adaptable, pragmatic means of monitoring what is occurring. Public health people count on a sort of back-and-forth surveillance, detection of cases, balance of risks, then leaping into action when necessary. With modern technology and data software, it is simpler to match up bits of information, identify outbreak trends, and even influence policy. Combining information from all kinds of sources into one messy but effective framework sets the stage for rapid responses (Sun et al., 2025). Monitoring those disease-spreading critters is fairly important too, particularly as our environment changes in unforeseen ways. You learned not only where these microbes tend to congregate but how they move. Some recent research even suggests that combining precise, close-up environmental data with information about our own movements can enhance our tracking. Consider the case of *Culex pipiens*—when human activity adjusts our ecosystems, the typical footprint of these microbes can shift, increasing the risks of transmission. Models that add in variables such as weather, terrain, and human influence seem to pinpoint where these vectors will show up a whole lot more accurately. It is a message that our surveillance strategies must keep in mind our own tracks, guiding us toward more successful regulation of high-risk areas (Marcolin et al., 2025). On a general level, the explanations for the emergence of these vector-borne and animal-borne diseases necessitate a freer, but reflective, consideration of nature and its evolution. Urbanization, land-use change, and other modifications to our landscape alter how these vectors establish themselves and act—forces that can strongly influence disease patterns. Tracking mechanisms, therefore, need to remain flexible, merging insights from both nature and human society. A system that integrates real-time data with some anticipatory models can provide public health agencies with a timely warning about outbreaks. It is not only about being prepared; it is also about bringing ecologists, epidemiologists, and health officials together—even if the effort is a little unbalanced at times, to construct a response strong enough to slice the risks associated with these challenging diseases (Marcolin et al., 2025; Sun et al., 2025).

7.4.2. Vaccination and Prevention Measures

Vaccination is a game changer when battling infectious disease like that caused by vectors or transmitted from animals to humans. Humans, animals, and the environment are all caught up together in ways that compel us to consider prevention in several directions at once. Vaccination increases an individual's own protection and creates what could be thought of as a community shield—slowing the spread of diseases like RVF. In countries such as Rwanda, where RVF appears to be breaking out increasingly, launching vaccine programs that work for people and their animals becomes absolutely critical. This type of hands-on method can cut down on outbreaks as well as keep food supplies more consistent and help local economies for those who rely on animals (Muvunyi et al., 2025). In short, prioritizing vaccines in public health policy can significantly alter the disease control game. But it's not all about the shot in your arm; controlling diseases transmitted by insects or animals requires a combination of strategies.

Public health interventions that combine a little education, good care of the environment, and constant vigilance build a wide net to capture problems early. Mosquito control, for example—employing multiple methods in combination can reduce malaria and dengue illness significantly. Global surveillance systems tracking potential zoonotic threats are also needed; they allow us to leap into action when novel pathogens emerge. New technology—rapid testing, contact tracing, and genomic research—provides further knowledge on the way diseases travel (Piret et al., 2021). Overall, pairing vaccines with good prevention strategies makes a strong bulwark against the transmission of these sneaky diseases. New tech is now getting into the fray, amplifying the effect of both vaccines and overall prevention work. It's neat to watch AI-based drones monitoring obnoxious disease carriers, or genome-enhanced strategies assisting us to monitor what's going on in real-time as it happens. These technologies enable health teams to target trouble spots, ensuring that resources go exactly where they need to go. Similarly, discovering cheap means of delivering vaccines to arms, particularly in areas that could have problems with resources—will make a tremendous impact. Through a One Health approach, where human, animal, and environmental health are all considered, nations can establish more adaptable plans designed to catch problems early. This wide, sometimes unclear scheme not only addresses present problems but also keeps us alert for future outbreaks, building our defenses against vector-borne and zoonotic diseases (Muvunyi et al., 2025).

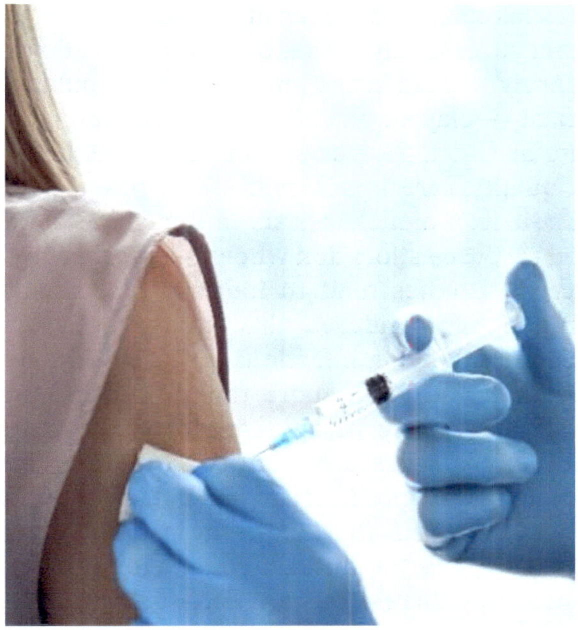

Source: https://cdcssl.ibsrv.net/cimg/www.officitecuratedcontent.smb/400x400_85/72/shutterstock-1859217856-722072.jpg

7.4.3. Role of Healthcare Systems in Managing Outbreaks

Vector-borne and zoonotic diseases are on the increase, and our healthcare systems today have to demonstrate nimble on their feet. It is not merely a matter of simply watching out for new dangers; there is a great deal more to it. A combination of careful surveillance, high-speed response, and an ability to fortify healthcare infrastructure are essential to detect issues before they get out of hand. For example, timely notification to communities will often prevent nascent outbreaks from developing into full-scale public health emergencies. With climate change and urbanization causing more frequent human – wildlife contact, coordinating human, animal, and environmental health initiatives becomes critical—even though it may sometimes seem like trying to juggle too many balls simultaneously. Around the world, as outbreaks of diseases worsen, healthcare systems come under even more pressure to quell them successfully. Social determinants, such as densely packed cities and growing population density—play a tremendous role in dictating the rate at which disease spreads and how access to quality care is achieved. Most often, using data-driven models assists in informing policy and resource allocation when it is most crucial. Overall, studies tend to indicate that climate change has rendered the environment less tolerant, allowing infectious disease outbreaks to occur and recur more freely. It is through the convergence of epidemiologists, doctors, and environmental scientists that one can develop strategies that address both short-term health concerns and long-term issues. We also cannot ignore the difficult connection between antimicrobial resistance (AMR) and outbreak control. As AMR rises globally, healthcare systems must navigate—excuse the typo—this complex issue while also managing zoonotic diseases. Lessons learned from the COVID-19 pandemic have pushed us to rethink how we use antibiotics, highlighting how closely human health and our environment are tied together. In most cases, addressing AMR demands a broad, systemic view that treats all parts of the health ecosystem as interconnected. Continuing research emphasizes the necessity of strong surveillance systems that can monitor both trends in infectious disease and patterns of resistance. When these factors are integrated, healthcare professionals are better positioned to anticipate, respond to, and control the various challenges posed by vector-borne and zoonotic diseases, ultimately enhancing public health and developing resilience in preparation for future outbreaks (Chala et al., 2021; Lio et al., 2023).

7.5. Socioeconomic Factors

Vector-borne and zoonotic diseases are agitated by socioeconomic factors. With the expansion of cities and population continuing to increase worldwide, boundaries between human settlements and wildlife habitats become blurred, increasing the likelihood of contracting infections. Mostly, these outbreaks trace their origins in the ordinary realities of poverty, land use changes, and how local infrastructure is established. Consider rural villages, for example – communities that are dependent on livestock tend to suffer from illnesses like RVF, which emphasizes so strongly the interdependence of health and economic well-being. Without good healthcare systems and sufficient medical resources, these areas can watch diseases intensify and persist longer than they need to. All these definitely direct us toward the necessity of resilience-building strategies and addressing the socioeconomic aspect of health emergencies (Muvunyi et al., 2025). Socioeconomic factors also influence how communities respond to threats such as West Nile virus. Crowding in the urban areas and the rapid rate of urban expansion usually create additional layers of complexity when responding to an outbreak. In many cases, research shows that spikes in West Nile cases are linked with gaps in public health policies – especially in densely packed urban settings. In these environments, limited access to healthcare, subpar mosquito control efforts, and a general lack of clear disease-prevention knowledge all combine to boost the risks from these pathogens. Observing how WNV infections rise and fall in places like Greece illustrates fairly well that integrating a more detailed examination of economic and social elements into health strategies can open the door to more targeted, community-centered measures (Kouroupis et al., 2023). Resilient socioeconomic environments play an important role in combating vector-borne and zoonotic illness. With the world changing at a breakneck pace—partly due to climate change, economic constraints, and social disparities—numerous communities are under increasing public health pressure. We need to invest in better diagnostics, vaccination outreach, and grassroots education efforts first if we're going to enhance outbreak response. In countries such as Rwanda, fixing social and political drivers of health disparities turns out to be just as important as leaping into novel scientific approaches. A balanced One Health strategy, that balances economic and environmental changes, is a requirement for sustainable success in public health. In the end, to reduce the burden of zoonotic infections, we need to focus socioeconomic perspectives in what and how we prepare and respond (Muvunyi et al., 2025).

7.5.1. Impact of Poverty on Disease Prevalence

Health and economic situation cut deep—consider vector-borne and zoonotic diseases as an example. People in more difficult financial situations often fail to receive the essentials, such as regular checkups, good sanitation, or even adequate health education. This shortage makes it easier for microbes and insect populations to thrive, thus increasing the number of illnesses. For instance, crumbling infrastructure in poor neighborhoods halts effective pest control in its tracks, allowing diseases like malaria and dengue fever to propagate freely. As cities expand, these underserved communities become hotspots for disease-carrying insects and animal-borne infections, further exacerbated by overcrowding and shoddy waste management. Obviously, this requires confronting economic inequality as part of any public health strategy (Chala et al., 2021). Zoonotic illnesses, in most instances, affect poor communities the most. Small farmers, hunters, and others who make a living off frequent contact with animals tend to put themselves at additional risks. These intimate contacts essentially provide an opportunity for germs to leap from animals to humans, increasing rates of infection in areas where people have little space to defend themselves. Economic strain at times compels families into unsafe habits, such as poaching or consuming wild animals—and this unwittingly opens up new channels for harmful microbes. On closer inspection, environmental degradation and animal trading, both poverty-linked and interconnected, determine how these diseases manage to spread. And then you have climate change coming along and putting another spin on it, changing the numbers of insects and the habitat of wildlife so that the worst people to deal with are hurt even more (Rahman et al., 2020).

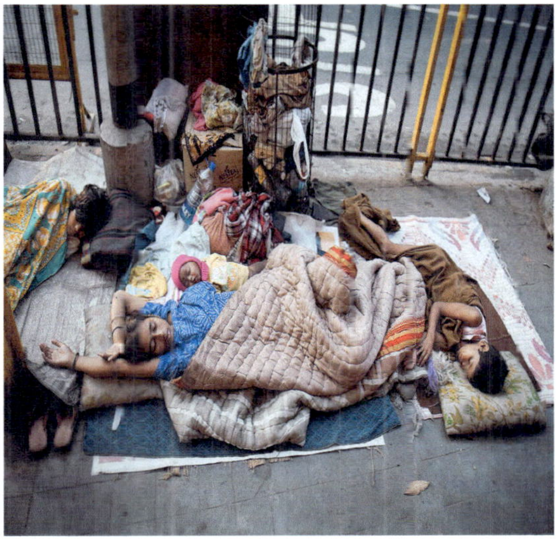

Source: By M M - flickr, CC BY-SA 2.0, https://commons.wikimedia.org/w/index.php?curid=40538730

If you're trying to reduce disease in poor communities, just repairing health services is not going to cut it. You need a combination of efforts that goes far beyond usual public health interventions. It involves shaking up economic growth, improved education, and better housing to reduce the risks to which these communities are exposed. Campaigns that engage locals and provide them with genuine opportunities to be heard can increase awareness and ignite measures that slow down how diseases are transmitted. Because poverty, insect infestation, and social ways of life allcombine, it is important to take a wide, inclusive approach. Through eliminating the root causes of poverty and encouraging sustainable economic growth, the vicious cycle of disease can be broken—resulting in improved health outcomes overall, as some recent research has indicated (Chala et al., 2021).

7.5.2. Urbanization and Its Effects on Disease Dynamics

Urban sprawl is transforming our daily lives and nature in general. Cities continue to balloon to accommodate ever-increasing populations, unwittingly influencing the environment in ways that can become disease-friendly for insects and animals. In zones near city outskirts—where natural environments gradually disappear—humans tend to mix with wildlife. In those areas, foreign species take up new residence and ordinary rodents become unintentional germ carriers. Consider Qatar, for instance; urban development there has been accompanied by an increase in rodent-borne diseases, with more than 50% of indigenous rodents carrying bacteria that are harmful to human health. Overall, observing such developments keenly is important if we do not wish to allow disease transmission in the speedily expanding areas (Islam et al., 2023). When cities expand into agricultural lands, even the rural open spaces do not remain untouched. As cities expand, previous agricultural landscapes transform in manners that occasionally increase the flow of pathogens. Trees are cut down and native wild patches split and fall, effectively reducing biodiversity, which in most instances translates into individuals colliding with wildlife increasingly often—usually in manners that can initiate zoonotic bargains. Agricultural shifts, such as mixed-species arrangements and poor farm security in Qatar, have been identified as being at the forefront of driving rodent-borne problems. Establishing strong surveillance systems and adopting a One Health strategy that connects our ecosystems, agricultural processes, and human health becomes important in controlling these new threats (Islam et al., 2023). Urban life also poses peculiar challenges to public health and disease control. High-density populations have the effect of stretching medical resources thin, at times leaving a system unprepared for surprise occurrences of vector-borne or zoonotic illness outbreaks. Past experience in the case of COVID-19 has demonstrated, quite vividly, how urban environments can drive disease transmission, highlighting the necessity for comprehensive, strong health initiatives. The combination of packed environments and the increase in spillovers of disease necessitates aggressive, new approaches, such as global disease surveillance systems monitoring how humans and animals engage with each other, and germs move about. Added to this, leverage breakthroughs in rapid diagnostics, contact tracing, and vaccine science can position us well to get ready for what comes next. While urban life forges ahead, an understanding of these changes in disease patterns is critical to maintaining our public health systems robust and our people secure.

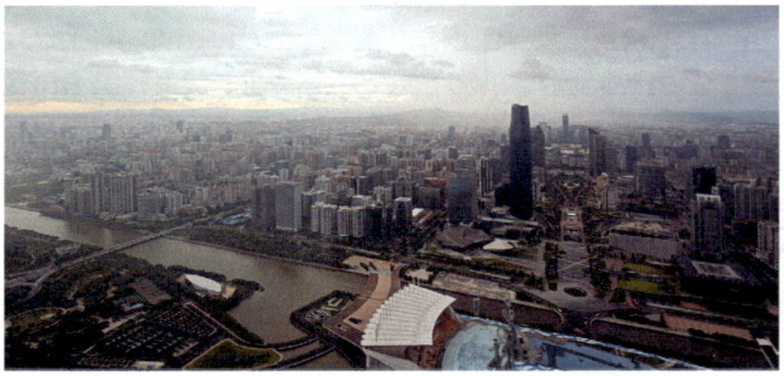

Source: By chensiyuan - Own work, CC BY-SA 4.0, https://commons.wikimedia.org/w/index.php?curid=15775341

7.5.3. Globalization and International Travel

Today's global connectivity has put human endeavors and environmental transformation into a knotted complex that is difficult to ignore. As populations spread and borders dissolve, nature's diverse ecosystems and humans find themselves bumping into one another more than ever before—frequently in unexpected ways that increase the threat of zoonotic disease. Urbanization, rolling out of new cropland, and expanding international commerce all tend to push wildlife, livestock, and people closer together, a combination that typically accelerates pathogen spillover. It has become evident that we require research that does not remain in one box but rather connects the way our landscapes function with public health measures. Certain collaborative work may even deduce the mysterious paths of infection transmission while igniting new inspiration for protection and enhancing what others refer to as "landscape immunity." Ultimately, these findings are fairly fundamental to figuring out policies that attempt to weigh economic development against keeping individuals healthy, particularly when global travel continues to rise and, honestly, making transmission of disease a greater concern (Plowright et al., 2021).

Cross-border travel—a clear indication of our globally interconnected times—can also create disruptions with vector-borne and zoonotic diseases. Frequently, disease-carrying microbes hitch a ride on travelers, migrating from regions where they are prevalent to regions with minimal exposure, at times creating sudden outbreaks. Just look back at COVID-19, which demonstrated so readily how a local outbreak is capable of rapidly expanding into a global health emergency, and how tightly travel and human health are intertwined. By business, pleasure, or going home to see family, individuals unwittingly serve as carriers for disease transmission. Public health measures such as travel warnings and screening checkpoints are fairly essential, in all but exceptional circumstances, for monitoring these dangers. In addition, speedy advancements in technology and surveillance equipment are imperative if we are to find and act promptly to any emerging threats that arise due to global travel (Piret et al., 2021). The impact of global interconnectedness on vector-borne and zoonotic diseases is not only a health concern—it also disrupts policy-making and governance. Today, health security must contend with the turns induced by global travel and commerce; this requires that governments cooperate in a response to the multi-layered threats represented by zoonotic pathogens. History teaches us that pandemics have tended to drive major changes in public health, from quarantine and isolation to more severe border controls, though those ancient methods may require a rethink in our contemporary, high-speed world. It is not only about quick diagnostic tests and vaccines but also requires inter-disciplinary collaboration to truly understand how ecosystems engage with disease. In general, refining international health governance is essential if we are to reduce the risks of global mobility and develop robust health systems that can withstand future epidemics (Plowright et al., 2021).

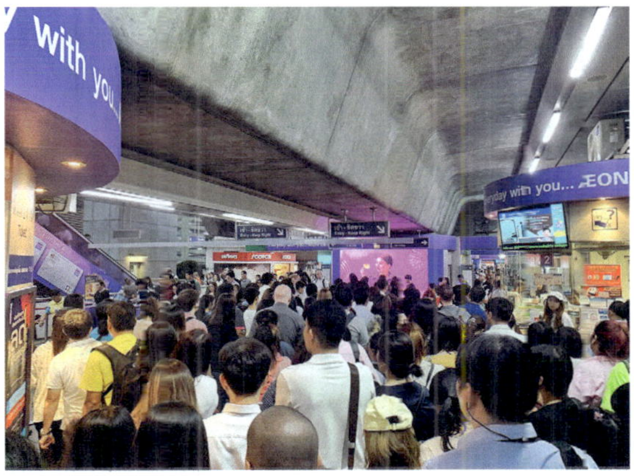

Source: By Chainwit. - Own work, CC BY-SA 4.0, https://commons.wikimedia.org/w/index.php?curid=89752753

https://external-content.duckduckgo.com/iu/?u=https%3A%2F%2Fstudy.com%2Fcimages%2Fvideopreview%2F8e5xxfke1b.jpg&f=1&nofb=1&ipt=b28880bb8a4b9d383b1fee366ddb6c0cdf0877ebc3ae33ac5d4da7f636f545c4

7.6. Case Studies

To trace the spread of vector-borne diseases depends heavily on uncovering in-depth case studies—actual snapshots in time that illustrate how both environmental changes and socio-economic pressures combine. These case studies are not presented in an orderly fashion; they at random expose how pressures such as changing weather and community health give rise to disease spread. Consider AVSim, say; this agent-based simulation simulates the spread of dengue through a population by utilizing realistic human motion and behavior trends, even adding in age-specific activities to approach realities closer. Not only does it outline the routes that disease takes but also leaves behind small, insightful details regarding how resources could be more efficiently distributed in our health systems, as established in Thennakoon et al. (2025). Climate change, however, has its own peculiar tendency for kicking the hornet's nest. As temperatures fluctuate erratically and the patterns of rainfall alter, the habitats and life cycles of vectors like *Aedes aegypti* and Anopheles mosquitoes evolve in ways that certainly affect disease transmission. Researchers tend to dive into ancient records, present-day statistics, and even projections of the future to draw out how temperature and precipitation adjustments can warp disease dynamics—something that crops up again in targeted case studies (Alamri et al., 2024). On a general note, these findings push us toward more integrated public health strategies and early warning systems, which, for the most part, are increasingly in need. And then there is the social aspect—places burdened with limited healthcare access, dubious sanitation, and overall socio-economic instability tend to have more severe outbreaks of disease like dengue or even the Zika virus. Thorough case studies tend to come full circle in explaining how these difficult social conditions blend with local ecology to make the entire scenario more complex than it initially appears. More often than not, disease transmission is a matter of viewing both the biological information and the human narrative behind it. Not only does such combined understanding make public health reactions more targeted but provides populations with an opportunity, even a push, to develop resilience—a truth that resonates with the results from analyses such as AVSim (Thennakoon et al., 2025).

7.6.1. Malaria and Its Global Impact

Environmental factors, quantifiable changing weather patterns, and the behavior of disease-carrying insects all become enmeshed in why malaria persists so tenaciously. Recently, there has been a visible increase in malaria and such diseases—urban transmission, climatic changes, and even forest depletion all appear to be involved. In 2020, for instance, the WHO estimated the numbers at around 627,000 deaths and some 241 million cases globally, which puts into perspective the public health blow this disease delivers. To add insult to injury, the malaria parasite is not particularly easy; it tends to and that its life cycle only serves to make vaccine or drug development more difficult. In most instances, that's precisely why measures such as insect sprays and growth regulators have come to become an integral line of defense against this constant threat (Anbalagan et al., 2025). Beyond being a health concern, malaria's impact extends into the very fiber of daily life, exacerbating economic hardship and further ingraining poverty in infected regions. Families are balancing significant medical expenses and lost income—repeatedly often—resulting in this undermining community resilience. On average, it is the most vulnerable individuals, such as young children and pregnant women, that bear it, further increasing the dire situation. When productivity among workers declines in these areas, economic growth is negatively impacted and overall well-being suffers. Although certain projects meant to increase healthcare and schooling show promise, consistent funding along with a wide, overarching strategy is still absolutely essential to address the socioeconomic ripple effects of the disease (Nafuna, 2024). Observing from the angle of our transformed world, it is difficult to disregard just how climate change disrupts malaria transmission. Temperature, rainfall, and even severe weather patterns have been changing the comfortable hideouts of the main carrier—the Anopheles mosquitoes. All these environmental adjustments have provided a habitat for more of them in areas that were once not suitable for them, thus increasing the danger for humans and wildlife in the area. Research in general indicates that warmer temperatures and modified precipitation play a role in the spread of the disease. That is why intertwining climate-resilience strategies with public health strategies is more pressing than ever. Enhancing disease surveillance, advocating for natural habitat rejuvenation, and engaging communities are all part of the cocktail that can reverse these looming dangers. By recognizing these interrelated challenges, decision-makers can better safeguard public health and, at the same time, maintain our ecosystems resilient (Anbalagan et al., 2025).

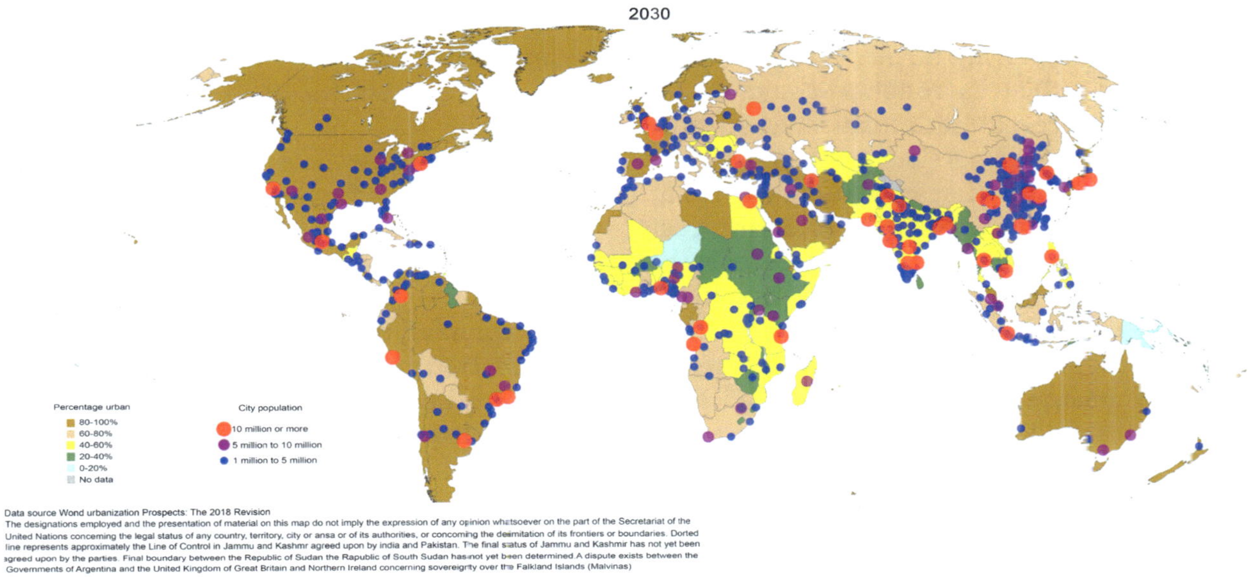

Source: By Nicxjo - Own work, CC BY-SA 4.0, https://commons.wikimedia.org/w/index.php?curid=93920149

7.6.2. Zika Virus Outbreak Analysis

Current trends indicate Zika is increasing as a significant threat among insect-borne diseases. It's not just how the insects themselves travel (particularly *Aedes aegypti*), but how our environment is changing and fitting into it. Urban sprawl and a warmer climate, in general, have provided breeding grounds for these mosquitoes more times than not, which increases the chances of outbreaks. Curiously, earlier studies even report that wild animals such as rodents occasionally appear to increase virus levels in man-made environments. All this suggests we shouldn't just monitor human cases but also the interaction between nature and our urban existence (Kesel et al., 2024). Travel and borders have a significant role to play in how Zika spreads. People on the move—tourists, migrants, you name it—can easily carry the virus into areas that normally would not see it, sparking small outbreaks in unexpected spots. If you look back, even during the late

19th century, there is evidence that *Aedes aegypti* got shuffled around by human hands; this old tale underscores how our movement influences where these disease carriers end up. Generally, these patterns require public health responses that combine an examination of both human behavior and environmental idiosyncrasies (Máttar et al., 2016). Combating this spread requires a combination of things. We require improved mosquito control and additional local education regarding the avoidance of the virus. Public health campaigns can, for the most part, get people, particularly those in highly populated cities—better acquainted with the dangers. Also, exploring further into how non-human hosts, such as rodents, could be in the mix could reveal additional mechanisms by which the virus persists and jumps into human lives. With diseases jumping from animals to humans increasingly occurring due to global changes and changing environments, unlocking these intricate dynamics is critical for intelligent interventions and policy-making. Overall, this type of forward-looking, as messy as it is, demonstrates that solving issues such as Zika involves pulling together a lot of different sectors (Kesel et al., 2024).

7.6.3. Lyme Disease and Its Ecological Implications

Lyme disease is increasing, a clear indication of the way our health intersects with nature changes. Global warming—thanks, in great part, to climate change—is making tick-hospitable areas expand into new territories, so humans are finding themselves more and more facing these insects than ever before. Urbanization and extensive deforestation are also disrupting the natural order, tending to create areas where ticks can thrive. In many instances, having a handle on such changing natural trends is central to risk management associated with such vector-borne diseases (Thomson and Stanberry, 2022). Wildlife does not merely paint our landscapes in color—it contributes significantly to the spread of Lyme disease as well. Deer mice and white-tailed deer are reservoirs for the bacteria, and when forests are cut down or land use changes in unexpected ways, their populations (and behaviors) may shift in astonishing directions. Climate changes do not just modify tick habitats but also fine-tune the relationships between hosts, ticks, and pathogens, frequently disrupting the balance that formerly rang true (Ortiz et al., 2021). The ripple effects of Lyme disease extend far beyond the individual case—the entire community and even the local economy are impacted. Added cases typically translate into more healthcare expenses, missed work hours, and public services strained to their limits. When communities are both subject to medical imposition as well as the expense of preventive action, things become all the more demanding, in some ways less than apparent. Generally speaking, a combination of ecosystem management, restoration of habitat, and careful planning of land seems the most viable path in creating resilience as well as a healthier future (Thomson and Stanberry, 2022).

A CLOSER LOOK

Zoonotic Disease

Zoonotic diseases are diseases that are transmitted between humans and animals. The diseases can be caused by bacteria, viruses, parasites, or fungi and form a high percentage of emerging infectious diseases worldwide. Some common examples include rabies, COVID-19, avian influenza, Ebola, and Lyme disease.

Zoonotic transmission can be through direct animal contact (e.g., bites or scratches), indirect animal contact (through contaminated surfaces or animal feces), vectors (e.g., ticks and mosquitoes), food (ingestion of undercooked meat or raw milk), or the environment (contact with contaminated soil or water). Wildlife, livestock, and household pets are all potential reservoirs for zoonotic disease-causing pathogens. Human behaviors like deforestation, agriculture, wildlife trade, and urbanization have increased human-animal contact, thereby elevating the chances of zoonotic spillover events.

Zoonoses may vary from mild diseases to major outbreaks with worldwide impacts, such as HIV/AIDS and COVID-19 pandemics. These diseases are best monitored, controlled, and prevented through a One Health approach that unites human, animal, and environmental health activities. Understanding zoonotic diseases is vital to avert future pandemics, protect food supplies, and ensure public and veterinary health.

SUMMARY

Environmental conditions, the actions of disease-vector animals, and the pathogens they carry combine together in combinations that have a significant effect on when and how vector-borne diseases emerge. Urbanization and changing climates—variables many studies have identified—are frequently the drivers that shove these disease mechanisms into high gear. When humans enter into wild habitats, it is not merely a matter of being near zoonotic reservoirs; the local balance of the ecosystem is disrupted, and the way is opened for such infections as ZCL to become epidemic. We simply must have a close examination of the particular vectors and reservoirs involved, particularly in hot-spot areas. Overall, preventing the spread of such diseases requires a strategy that connects ecological surveys and public health measures, protecting the most vulnerable ones. Non-human hosts also contribute in surprising ways to the transmission of arboviruses, illustrating the complex interconnections between wildlife, vectors, and humans.

Studies, in general, indicate that small mammals, particularly rodents—can be major amplifiers in human-altered environments, an aspect that falls through the gaps in usual disease modeling. Indeed, detection of antibodies to chikungunya and dengue viruses from these rodent groups suggests that they may have a role in initiating urban outbreaks (Kesel et al., 2024). This type of evidence encourages us to conduct research that crosses wildlife biology with epidemiology, so interventions are more effective at keeping pace with the specialized ecological contexts where disease arises and re-appears. Fundamentally, addressing vector-borne and zoonotic disease requires a unified, One Health strategy involving human, animal, and environmental health. Discoveries about ZCL, for example, emphasize—at least in the majority of instances—the importance of regional cooperation in regions such as the Middle East and North Africa to target tropical diseases that most severely impact rural populations. By incorporating adaptive management approaches that adapt to evolving ecological conditions, public health campaigns can be directed more specifically toward high-risk areas uncovered by ongoing research. As one integrated review describes, having this type of multi-layered knowledge available to health managers and policymakers not only aids in the provision of immediate responses but also fosters a certain type of resilience to future outbreaks, an important consideration in our time of ongoing environmental flux and change in social patterns.

Farm work and disease transmission are more knotted than they would at first appear. Individuals living or spending a lot of time near farms appear to have a greater chance of contracting diseases from insects and animals – so much so that a meta-analysis suggested that they are approximately 1.74 times more likely to become infected than others with no similar exposure. Oil palm or rubber plantations and even non-poultry livestock operations exhibit this trend quite evidently. Hookworm and malaria – these diseases spike in cases, as if farm practices inadvertently facilitate the spread of germs. It is difficult to dismiss these connections when our farm landscapes continuously change so rapidly (Shah et al., 2019). Emerging pathogens continue to emerge and, quite honestly, they throw giant challenges at global health systems. At its simplest, information processed cleverly in real-time is critical for rapid response when outbreaks happen. Outbreak analytics seeks to combine disparate data types so interventions may arrive on time. Distinct collection techniques begin to interact with each other in unplanned manners, and with some added sophisticated modeling, response teams can at times accelerate their preparedness and response times. On the whole, this adaptive blend of methods is proving to be a major resource for our battle against new diseases (Polonsky et al., 2019). Juggling viewpoints from agriculture, the environment, and epidemiology is what is needed when vector-borne and zoonotic diseases are involved. Land-use modification fueled by crop expansion can adjust where disease vectors such as wild animals or insects choose to congregate. That combination of wildlife behavior and human action creates a complicated landscape – more like scientists and policymakers must dance together than not. In most instances, it would appear sensible to incorporate health concerns directly into land planning to address the reasons that these outbreaks happen. Building tighter links between how we build our farms and how we address public health could very well enhance a community's capacity to deal with constantly evolving health challenges (Shah et al., 2019).

KEY TERMS FROM THIS CHAPTER

- Zoonosis
- Spillover
- Transmission cycle
- Incubation period
- Endemic
- Vector competence
- Pathogen
- Biodiversity dilution effect
- Reverse zoonosis (Zooanthroponosis)
- Bridge vector
- Biological transmission
- Climate sensitivity
- Reservoir host
- Amplifying host
- Host-pathogen interaction
- Extrinsic incubation period
- Epizootic
- Vector capacity
- Host range
- Anthropozoonosis
- Dead-end host
- Mechanical transmission
- Spatiotemporal dynamics
- Host density

REFERENCES

1. Adams, E. R., de Vlas, S. J., Hollingsworth, T. D., Le Rutte, E. A., Coffeng, L. E., & Medley, G. F. (2015). Uniting mathematics and biology for control of visceral leishmaniasis. *Trends in Parasitology, 31*(6), 251–259. https://core.ac.uk/download/77001793.pdf (accessed on 6 May 2025).
2. Anderson, R. M., Borlase, A., Beauvais, W., Disko, R., Dubey, J. P., Gage, K. L., Rudge, J. W., et al. (2016). Who acquires infection from whom and how? Disentangling multi-host and multi-mode transmission dynamics in the 'elimination' era. *Philosophical Transactions of the Royal Society B: Biological Sciences, 372*(1719), 20160091. https://core.ac.uk/download/45467936.pdf (accessed on 6 May 2025).
3. Jones, B. A., Grace, D., Kock, R., Alonso, S., Rushton, J., Said, M. Y., McKeever, D., Mutua, F., Young, J., McDermott, J., & Pfeiffer, D. U. (2013). Zoonosis emergence linked to agricultural intensification and environmental change. *Proceedings of the National Academy of Sciences of the United States of America, 110*(21), 8399–8404. https://doi.org/10.1073/pnas.1208059110 (accessed on 6 May 2025).
4. Bauchinger, U., Falagas, M. E., Kelesidis, I., & Kelesidis, T. (2008). Human infections associated with wild birds. *Journal of Infection, 56*(2), 83–98. https://doi.org/10.1016/j.jinf.2007.11.001.
5. Bernard, C., Apolloni, A., Grosbois, V., Peyraud, A., Saengram, P., Jori, F., Faure, E., et al. (2025). First detection of Crimean-Congo hemorrhagic fever antibodies in cattle and wild fauna of southern continental France: Investigation of explicative factors. *bioRxiv*. https://www.semanticscholar.org/paper/0b4d8d085cf3b255788812f5cbfe7f8001ff4060 (accessed on 6 May 2025).
6. Bose, B., & Kumar, S. S. (2024). Dairy Farmers' Awareness of Vector-Borne Zoonotic Diseases: A Pilot Study. *Vector borne and zoonotic diseases (Larchmont, N.Y.), 24*(9), 597–599. https://doi.org/10.1089/vbz.2023.0132 (accessed on 6 May 2025).
7. Bush, R. M., Cobey, S., Flanagan, M. L., & Glass, G. E. (2012). Anticipating the species jump: Surveillance for emerging viral threats. *Zoonoses and Public Health, 59*(3), 155–163. https://doi.org/10.1111/j.1863-2378.2011.01439.x.
8. de Cock, M. P., Baede, V. O., Esser, H. J., Fonville, M., de Vries, A., de Boer, W. F., Mehl, C., Ulrich, R. G., Schares, G., Hakze-van der Honing, R. W., van der Poel, W. H. M., Sprong, H., & Maas, M. (2024). T(r)icky Environments: Higher Prevalence of Tick-Borne Zoonotic Pathogens in Rodents from Natural Areas Compared with Urban Areas. *Vector borne and zoonotic diseases (Larchmont, N.Y.), 24*(8), 478–488. https://doi.org/10.1089/vbz.2023.0151 (accessed on 6 May 2025).
9. Gao, D., & Yuan, X. (2024). A hybrid Lagrangian-Eulerian model for vector-borne diseases. *Journal of mathematical biology, 89*(2), 16. https://doi.org/10.1007/s00285-024-02109-5 (accessed on 6 May 2025).
10. García-Carrasco, J. M., Muñoz, A.-R., Olivero, J., Figuerola, J., Fa, J. E., & Real, R. (2023). Gone (and spread) with the birds: Can chorotype analysis highlight the spread of West Nile virus within the Afro-Palaearctic flyway? *One Health, 17*, 100585. https://doi.org/10.1016/j.onehlt.2023.100585.
11. Gurgel-Gonçalves, R. (2022). Stronger control-surveillance systems for vector-borne

Chagas disease. *Memoria's do Instituto Oswaldo Cruz, 117*. https://doi.org/10.1590/0074-02760210130chgsb.

12. Islam, M. M., Farag, E., Hassan, M. M., Jaffrey, S. S., Atta, M., Al-Marri, A. M., Al-Zeyara, A. M., et al. (2023). Rodent-borne zoonoses in Qatar: A possible One Health framework for the intervention of future epidemic. *One Health, 16*, 100517. https://doi.org/10.1016/j.onehlt.2023.100517.
13. Kemp, L., Xu, C., Depledge, J., Ebi, K. L., Gibbins, G., Kohler, T. A., Rockström, J., et al. (2022). Climate endgame: Exploring catastrophic climate change scenarios. *Proceedings of the National Academy of Sciences, 119*, e2108146119. https://doi.org/10.1073/pnas.2108146119.
14. Magnano San Lio, R., Favara, G., Maugeri, A., Barchitta, M., & Agodi, A. (2023). How antimicrobial resistance is linked to climate change: An overview of two intertwined global challenges. *International Journal of Environmental Research and Public Health, 20*(3), 1681. https://doi.org/10.3390/ijerph20031681.
15. Marcolin, L., Zardini, A., Longo, E., Caputo, B., Poletti, P., & Di Marco, M. (2025). Mapping the habitat suitability of *Culex pipiens* in Europe using ensemble bioclimatic modelling. *bioRxiv*. https://www.semanticscholar.org/paper/e8d262c7e97db3a83b3ef2106dba41e141862f30 (accessed on 6 May 2025).
16. Martinez, M. E. (2018). The calendar of epidemics: Seasonal cycles of infectious diseases. *PLoS Pathogens, 14*(11), e1007327. https://doi.org/10.1371/journal.ppat.1007327.
17. Máttar, V. S., & MarcoGonzález, T. (2016). Adaptation de los vectors a los microorganisms o adaptation de los microorganisms a los vectors. *Revita MVZ Córdoba, 21*, 5477–5479. https://www.semanticscholar.org/paper/243418b65661b5dc3ef460d077a828667a818386 (accessed on 6 May 2025).
18. Muvunyi, C. M., Ngabonziza, J. C. S., Siddig, E. E., & Ahmed, A. (2025). Rift Valley fever in Rwanda is urging for enhancing global health security through multisectoral One Health strategy. *Microorganisms, 13*(1), 91. https://doi.org/10.3390/microorganisms13010091.
19. Nafuna, K. (2024). Impact of climate change on vector-borne diseases in wildlife. *Animal Health Journal*. https://www.semanticscholar.org/paper/c3a092a29296c0947552be5da42c44d39c1b96da (accessed on 6 May 2025).
20. Omazic, A., Bylund, H., Boqvist, S., Högberg, A., Björkman, C., Tryland, M., Evengård, B., et al. (2019). Identifying climate-sensitive infectious diseases in animals and humans in Northern regions. *Acta Veterinaria Scandinavica, 61*. https://doi.org/10.1186/s13028-019-0490-0.
21. Ortiz, D. I., Piche-Ovares, M., Romero, L., Wagman, J., & Troyo, A. (2021). The impact of deforestation, urbanization, and changing land use patterns on the ecology of mosquito and tick-borne diseases in Central America. *Insects, 13*, 20. https://doi.org/10.3390/insects13010020.
22. Polonsky, J. A., Baidjoe, A., Kamvar, Z. N., Cori, A., Durski, K., Edmunds, W. J., Eggo, R. M., et al. (2019). Outbreak analytics: A developing data science for informing the response to emerging pathogens. *Philosophical Transactions of the Royal Society B: Biological Sciences, 374*, 20180276. https://doi.org/10.1098/rstb.2018.0276.
23. Rohr, J. R., Barrett, C. B., Civitello, D. J., Craft, M. E., Delius, B. K., De Leo, G. A., Hudson, P. J., et al. (2019). Emerging human infectious diseases and the links to global food production. *Nature Sustainability, 2*, 445–456. https://doi.org/10.1038/s41893-019-0293-3.

24. Rufasto Goche, K. S., Lizarbe Castro, M. V., Lozano Zanelly, G. A., Lira Camargo, W. M., Ascayo Velasquez, E. Y., Murillo Carrasco, A. M., & Diaz-Obregón, D. (2025). Epidemiological dynamics of dengue in Peru: Temporal and spatial drivers between 2000 and 2022. *PLOS ONE, 20*. https://www.semanticscholar.org/paper/27a92464fa91b65b95882250ffa3b8998b6bf7ab (accessed on 6 May 2025).

25. Shah, H., Huxley, P., Elmes, J., & Murray, K. A. (2019). Agricultural land-uses consistently exacerbate infectious disease risks in Southeast Asia. *Nature Communications, 10*. https://doi.org/10.1038/s41467-019-12333-z.

26. Yinfu Sun, Dongliang Liu and Yufan Wu et al. Annual Summary of Global Infectious Diseases in 2024. *Zoonoses.* 2025. Vol. 5(1). DOI: 10.15212/ZOONOSES-2024-1006 (accessed on 6 May 2025).

27. Thomson, M. C., & Stanberry, L. R. (2022). Climate change and vector borne diseases. *New England Journal of Medicine, 387*, 1969–1978. https://doi.org/10.1056/nejmra2200092.

28. Tito, M. H., Jannat, M. H. E. ., Aktar, M. T. ., Saha, B. ., Das, P. ., Kawser, M. ., Hossain, M. A. ., Islam, M. N. ., Chohan , M. S. . . . ., & Khan, S. . (2024). Advancing vector-borne disease prediction through functional classifier integration: A novel approach for enhanced modeling: Machine learning tools and vector-borne disease prediction. *Letters In Animal Biology*, *4*(1), 17–22. https://doi.org/10.62310/liab.v4i1.135 (accessed on 6 May 2025).

29. Yi, C., Cohnstaedt, L., & Scoglio, C. M. (2021). SEIR-SEI-EnKF: A new model for estimating and predicting dengue outbreak dynamics. *IEEE Access, PP*, 1. https://www.semanticscholar.org/paper/623960e3e22a2232a7662443dde1a1058f6bbdd1 (accessed on 6 May 2025).

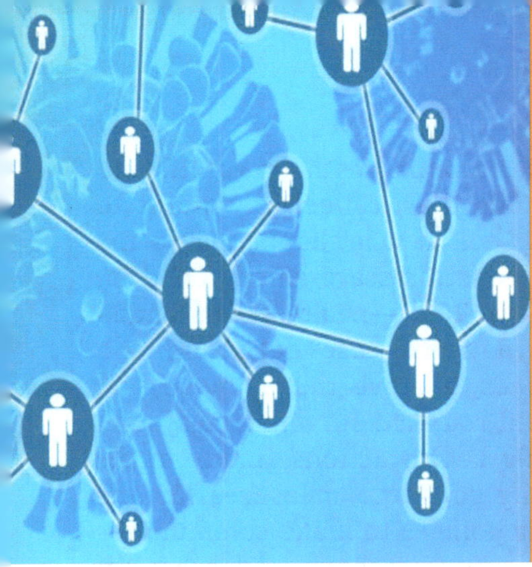

Chapter 8

DISEASE SURVEILLANCE AND OUTBREAK INVESTIGATION

Contents

Introduction

Quickly detecting and addressing outbreaks is important to public health – but it is not just human health. We also need to be watchful of animal health at all times, and sometimes the means we use to monitor diseases appear to overlap a lot of different approaches. SAVSNET, for instance, combined mathematical models with routine vet information in the UK to determine when canine diseases were more than mere random fluctuations. But there remains a clear omission: no one has quite perfected a tried-and-true method to declare that a statistical peak aligns with an authentic clinical problem before diving into complete investigations. It all comes down to being aware of what outbreak situations give vets sleepless nights; , knowing their preferences regarding outbreak thresholds can finally refine interventions and utilization of resources (Cuartero et al., 2024). Disease surveillance is no one-off trick relegated to the veterinary community–it has an equally important function in human health as well. Consider the Field Epidemiology Training Program (FETP) – Frontline, for example. Launched to equip local public health teams to respond during emergencies, the training program was able to enhance outbreak investigation expertise at the district level. Between 2016 and 2019, hundreds of front-line officers acquired the necessary skills, which in turn, for most, produced high-quality surveillance information and rapid response to outbreaks—whether for Zika, malaria, or other public health emergencies. In some way, concentrated training prepared communities with hands-on experience, building back health systems and preparing to tackle new challenges more efficiently (Camará et al., 2023). Establishing a robust surveillance system is central to all that comes next, and we can't overemphasize its role. Whether one is examining data from veterinary clinics or public health agencies, having solid, actionable information is what informs intervention policy. SAVSNET's efforts, taking into account veterinarians' actual-world perceptions of what appears to be an actual outbreak, paints a more earthy portrait of clinical significance. Similarly, the achievements of FETP – Frontline demonstrate, in general terms, that properly trained personnel can be a huge game changer in outbreak responses. Overall, by maintaining a wide, adaptable disease surveillance mindset, early issues can be detected and swift responses can be made—reducing the far-reaching effects of outbreaks and ultimately improving overall health outcomes in communities and across species (Camará et al., 2023; Cuartero et al., 2024).

Definition of Disease Surveillance

Public health management isn't always about crunching numbers; it's more like collecting little pieces of information—lab reports to day-to-day clinical notes—and connecting them together to identify where disease is spreading. It all begins with gathering, sorting, and distributing health information in a manner that sometimes appears a little mixed up rather than meticulously coordinated. You get clinical reports combining with lab results and population details that, collectively, point to disease trends. Look at what happened during a severe acute hepatitis scare among children in the UK back in 2022—health teams ended up drafting a national case definition and testing guidelines, a move that showed just how a strong, all-rounded surveillance system can steer public health actions (Liddy et al., 2025). By doing so, these measures lay the groundwork for policies to make communities safe. In the real world, disease surveillance is not a single-agency task; it requires a combination of organizations performing their portions in a loosely linked network. There is no rigid linear procedure here; rather, one segment may include establishing case criteria, another filling out data collection procedures, and another still occupying a slot to be concerned with careful reporting. All this converges when something out of the ordinary happens, such as the typhoid fever case in the Philippines in 2022. The system detected a remarkably high number of cases—over 200 were detected—but further scrutiny revealed that only a portion of them qualified as per the parameters laid out (Guzman et al., 2024). This type of hiccup truly highlights the necessity of adhering very closely to diagnostic standards, even if the process at times seems a little all over the map. At its core, disease surveillance far exceeds mere data gathering, but rather it is a proactive, constantly evolving process of finding and reducing health dangers. It encompasses a mixed bag of work, including determining risk factors, mapping how disease flows between communities, and determining if interventions do some good. It is not merely fast turnkey responses to epidemics; it is about establishing the foundation for long-term planning, resource allocation, and strategy. The combination of surveillance reports and public health interventions we had in the UK hepatitis episode and the typhoid overview in the Philippines (Guzman et al., 2024; Liddy et al., 2025) tells us how crucial it is to continually improve these systems. By strengthening the networks and mandating health agencies to collaborate, officials—apart from sporadic communication hiccups—can stay one step ahead of impending issues, resulting in healthier, better-resilient communities in the long term.

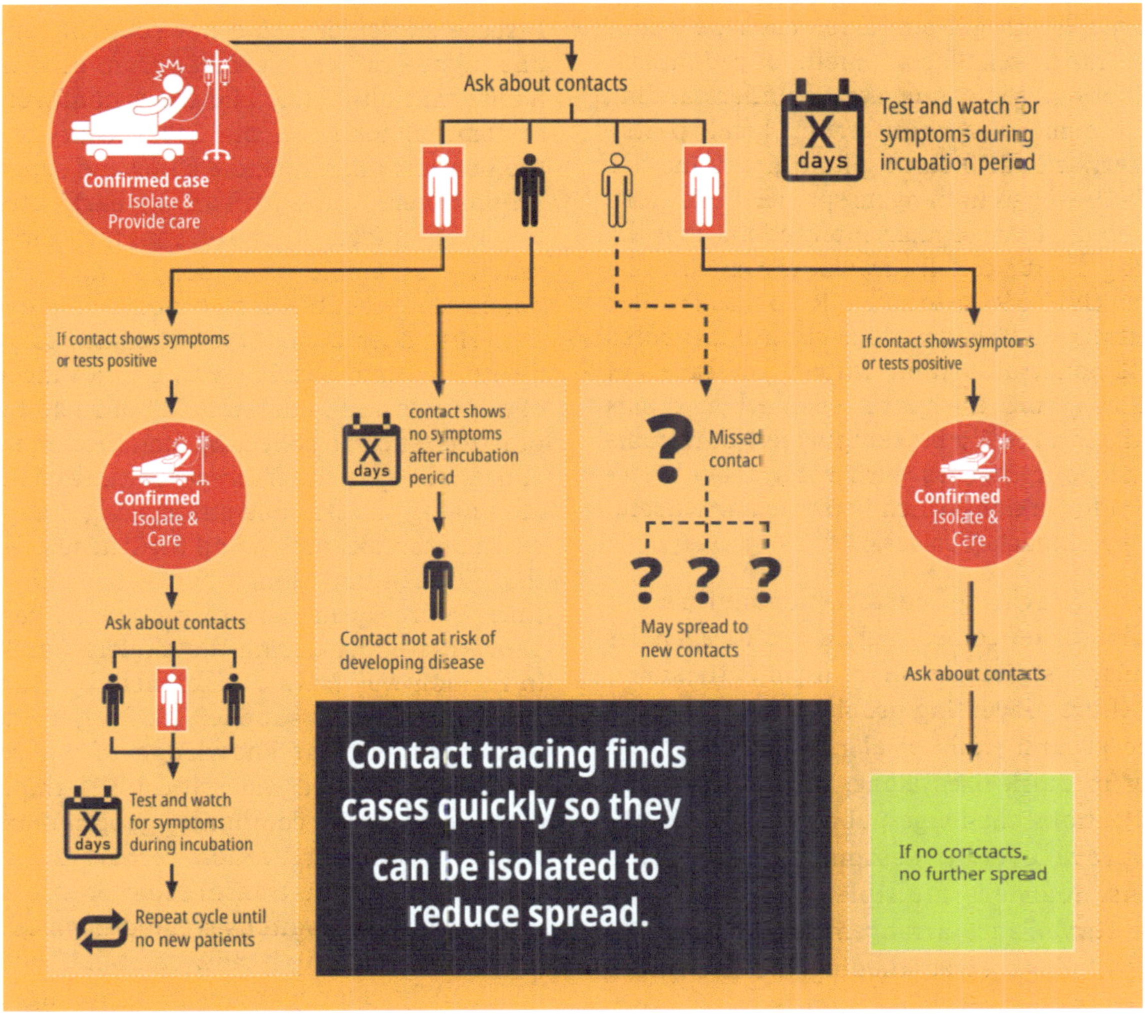

Source: By CFCF - Own work, CC BY-SA 4.0, https://commons.wikimedia.org/w/index.php?curid=88348237

Importance of Outbreak Investigation

Outbreak investigations define public health—much of what we do to help keep populations healthy starts with identifying and combating disease surges. They're not simply standard checks; these investigations probe possible trouble areas, methodically examining and slowing outbreaks before they spiral out of control. Health teams, for instance, rely on real-time surveillance systems that alert them to unusual trends almost in real time, suggesting fresh threats. Take the FETP, which has, in the majority of instances, fostered a team that is both swift and agile at filling gaps when necessary. We have witnessed its influence in situations ranging from containing Ebola to dealing with the recent COVID-19 debacle, demonstrating how a finely tuned game of investigation can be the difference between a contained situation and an enormous crisis (Martin et al., 2021). Epidemic investigations also teach us about how germs travel. Close, sometimes redundant, examinations yield nuggets of understanding that inform everything from local policy to international health planning. Consider COVID-19—by examining its spread, we're given hints about how regular interactions may be allowing a virus to fall through the cracks. The Oxford COVID-19 Government Response Tracker, for instance, dissects various control measures and demonstrates their impact on cases of infection across the globe, even when things sometimes appear a bit complicated. Such tools provide policymakers with robust, evidence-based information, which is particularly useful during unexpected crises.

By attaching certain behaviors to unequivocal outcomes, public health agencies can adapt strategies in real-time to spend more effort preventing problems from getting off the ground (Hale et al., 2021). It is not a matter of quick fixes alone, though. Outbreak investigations challenge public health systems to improve overall. Lessons learned—even lessons learned multiple times—inform leaner surveillance arrangements and quicker response plans, strengthening the healthcare infrastructure's resiliency. Consistent support for initiatives such as FETP constructs enduring know-how so that fresh threats can be addressed head-on; this is not merely a matter of crisis management. In a sense, a robust framework of investigation lies at the foundation of more resilient public health—a reality underscored by recent responses to animal-transmitted diseases and vaccine-preventable outbreaks. That sort of preparatory work is central to maintaining health security, shifting early interventions, and ultimately enhancing long-term results for all (Martin et al., 2021).

8.1. Historical Context of Disease Surveillance

Disease surveillance did not suddenly emerge one night—rather, it evolved from established habits that ultimately laid the groundwork for systems of today. In the 14th century, during the bubonic plague, whole ships and separated groups were walled off in an early attempt to isolate infection. Those attempts, largely a reactive scramble after danger had arrived, nonetheless identified that monitoring disease patterns does count when it comes to public health. As time passed, with the advancement of our tools and understanding of small things, practices such as collecting statistics on illness and death—yes, the figures—became central to identifying patterns and strategizing a response when outbreaks popped up their heads. During the 19th century, things began to change big time, courtesy in part to pioneers like John Snow. His effort during the cholera outbreaks in London was truly a watershed; by graphing cases along water supplies, he fairly evidently demonstrated that knowledge of where the infections occurred was critical. His empirical, data-based style, combining geographic data with mundane observation, recharted the way we understand the transmission of disease. In general, his observations created the model for how data gathering is now combined with in-depth analysis for contemporary investigations, abandoning the notion that a single vantage point will suffice to know an outbreak. Disease surveillance is a mix of outdated methods and new-fangled tools such as genomics and machine learning these days. Mathematical modeling often employed to model outbreaks provides public health officials with their necessary advantage—vaccine distribution and allocation of resources. Overall, research informs us these models are only effective when data input is solid as a rock, so the requirement for wide-ranging, accurate monitoring is ceaseless (Shankar et al., 2024). And with new and growing threats such as S.

enterica serovar Panama, it is apparent that the call for global collaboration in the identification and smothering of risks is more pressing than ever (Pulford et al., 2024).

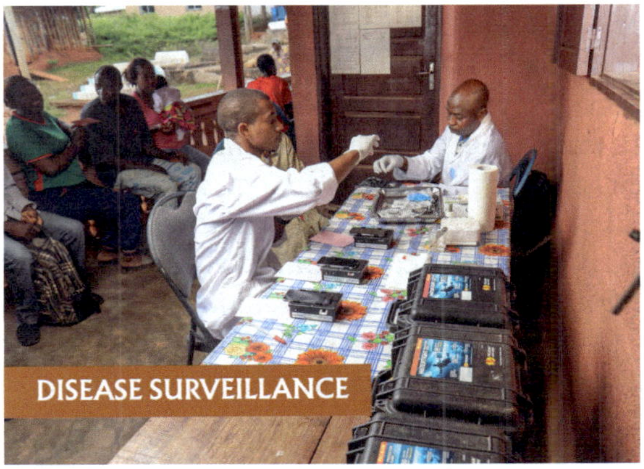

Source: Task Force for Global Health. (n.d.). *Our Areas of Work with Titles. https://www.taskforce.org/wp-content/uploads/2019/08/Our-areas-of-work-w-Titles_Images16-1024x768.png.*

8.1.1. Early Methods of Disease Tracking

Disease surveillance has developed a great deal, closely interconnected with our continued striving to comprehend, and combat infectious dangers. Before sophisticated technology entered the fray, individuals had to settle for observing strange patterns of symptoms and anecdotal evidence. Local doctors and community leaders would document or discuss anything unusual—strange illness, mysterious deaths—and warn neighboring regions by means at their disposal. This type of makeshift process, though short in space and time, ultimately paved the way for more systematic approaches. From elementary note-taking to a more systematic tracking system proved to be the turning point in identifying early symptoms of outbreaks and leading the way for systematic surveillance programs. The major leap forward was with syndromic surveillance, which, in broad terms, is concerned with capturing clinical signs and symptoms even prior to a definitive diagnosis. The process aids in accelerating responses by identifying potential problems early on. Consider EPIWATCH®: it employs artificial intelligence (AI) to track syndrome data—a technique that was quite used during the Marburg virus outbreak in Equatorial Guinea.

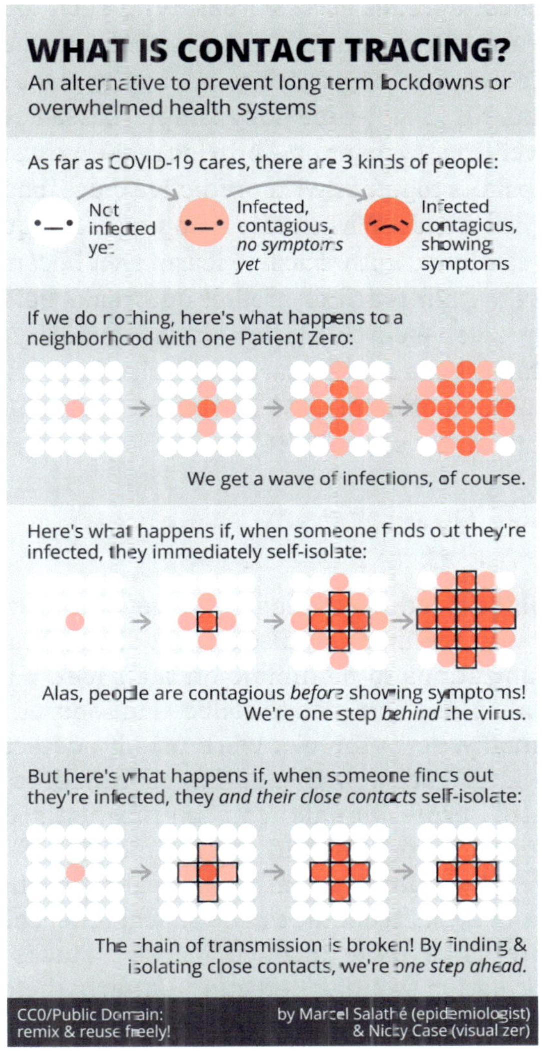

Source: By Epidemiologist @MarcelSalathe & Designer @NCasenmare - OneStepAhead https://blog.ncase.me/onestepahead/, CC0, https://commons.wikimedia.org/w/index.php?curid=88526423

It is a reminder that while live data can allow authorities to move quickly, local context is essential to get right in interpreting these signals (Zhang et al., 2025). Occasionally, even with the finest technology, missing the wood for the trees is a serious risk. GIS technology has also raised the bar by enabling us to see how sickness spreads across areas. With such tools, disease control authorities can look at where infections are congregating and modify plans for resources in real-time; for example, Lassa Fever surveillance systems now provide real-time visual snapshots together with predictive clues, based on past trends. When these mapping techniques are combined with machine learning, it becomes more within reach to predict outbreaks before they swell—emphasizing, in the majority of instances, the central part that technology takes in contemporary disease surveillance paradigms (Wattamwar et al., 2024).

8.1.2. Development of Modern Surveillance Systems

Sophisticated technology has revolutionized the way we monitor disease, requiring health organizations to be nimble on their feet. Early on, individuals needed to collect and report data manually, so outbreaks were usually detected too late. Today, with automated capabilities, health professionals can monitor disease patterns as they unfold – it's almost as if we have a live radar system. In general terms, new data analysis techniques and machine learning allow us to plow through massive stacks of information rapidly, detecting patterns before things spiral out of control. This new strategy not only enhances our situational awareness, but it also allows decision-makers to intervene before issues snowball. Maintaining the back-and-forth between medical professionals and technology specialists, even if it occasionally appears chaotic, is important to making these systems effective in the real world. Changing the subject somewhat, online discussion on social media has become part of disease surveillance as well. Platforms that allow information to travel at light speed have become an unexpected but critical component of detecting health threats. There is increasing buzz in research communities that social networks can be an early signal of public health trends – particularly when outbreaks create a combination of legitimate concern and out-of-control misinformation. By accessing social media insights, health teams can better understand community concerns and behaviors. This mix of online information can be combined to construct surveillance systems that are stronger and more agile. Some commentary on pandemic responses even emphasizes the necessity of refining methods to cull the trustworthy from the untrustworthy information (Salehinejad et al., 2021). We also cannot ignore the prickly matters of privacy and ethics in these emerging surveillance arrangements. With our technologies forging ahead, individuals are more and more uncomfortable about how their private health information is being vacuumed up and utilized. It is a delicate balancing act at all times: on the one hand, a need to sniff out outbreaks early, and on the other, one's right to privacy must be rigorously protected. Policymakers and public health chiefs need to ensure that any tracking remains within the law but at the same time maintains public trust – and that is easier said than done. There is a universal cry these days for improved public education on both the benefits and drawbacks of such surveillance so that transparency persists even in the event of a crisis. After all, during difficult times when advice is most needed, the system's trustworthiness can truly make or break how individuals respond (Klompas, 2020).

8.1.3. Key Historical Outbreaks and Their Impact

Good disease surveillance pays its dividends time and time again, particularly when previous outbreaks demonstrate just how vital it is to obtain proper information quickly. Years of outbreaks have taught us that taking the right information at the right moment is indeed a game-changer. Brazil is a case in point. A sudden rise in flu-like illness was picked up on by an Early Warning System that issued real-time alerts. Florentino et al. (2024) noted that constructing a Data Quality Index to verify whether the data was complete and timely served to hone these alerts. The steady stream of updates from various sectors was able to demonstrate that monitoring the situation, despite some overlap along the way, is the secret to managing infectious threats. Then there is Canada, where a significant method change transformed all of it. Rather than maintaining their adherence to pulsed-field gel electrophoresis, laboratories moved to whole genome sequencing (WGS) somewhere between 2015 and 2021.

This shift made it considerably easier to identify clusters of enteric illness. With this additional detail, officials would be able to rapidly track illnesses such as those caused by *Salmonella Enteritidis* to shared sources, such as the problems with frozen raw breaded chicken products. Morton et al. (2024) suggest that this more precise focus on connecting cases has much to do with the potential to slow disease transmission through newer methods of surveillance. In retrospect, it's obvious that the combination of intense data gathering, rigorous data verification, and intelligent policy gets to define how we respond to health risks. Think about how the rise of antibiotic-resistant strains—normally associated with finding errors in the system—demonstrates just how precarious this is. Clumsy data gathering, even slightly off in places, can slow our response times, exacerbating outbreaks. The experience with Brazil's system and Canada's deployment of WGS demonstrates that investing in innovative surveillance solutions not only improves early detection but also creates the adaptive public health strategies we require in an age where infectious diseases resurface repeatedly.

8.2. Types of Disease Surveillance

Public health begins with monitoring disease patterns in all conceivable ways. Older systems tend to rely on physicians and clinics to relay notifications whenever a case occurs—this passive surveillance reaches many at low expense, although it can fail to capture milder or even symptomless cases. At times, however, health teams become more active. Active surveillance, in which officials venture out seeking cases themselves, can detect subtle outbreaks; in the majority of instances, this is finding an emerging threat earlier. Employing passive and active methods simultaneously tends to result in a more complete picture overall, though the method is not necessarily well-balanced. Sentinel surveillance steps in when a targeted glance is desired. Instead of attempting to track everyone, this approach closely monitors chosen sites or populations, which can pick up on concealed trends in designated high-risk areas. For instance, a group of selected hospitals could continuously feed in flu information, allowing officials to detect outbreaks earlier and reallocate resources accordingly. In cases such as the sudden transmission of COVID-19, increased sentinel efforts typically were required; rapid data collection shaped decisions in real time, sometimes requiring action on preliminary leads before waiting for complete confirmation. And then there is syndromic surveillance, which values real-time signals. Through monitoring symptoms like fever and breathing difficulty reported in ERs, pharmacies, and other such locations, this strategy can suggest an outbreak even before test results are in. In the case of COVID-19, for example, recording clusters of typical symptoms enabled health authorities to leap in with prompt interventions—though, of course, deciphering all the data took robust analytics to separate out real warnings from noise. Combined with other surveillance methods in the majority of instances, syndromic checks assist us in staying one step ahead of developing threats, a reminder that an imperfect early warning can do some good (Augustine et al., 2020; Fan-Lan et al., 2020).

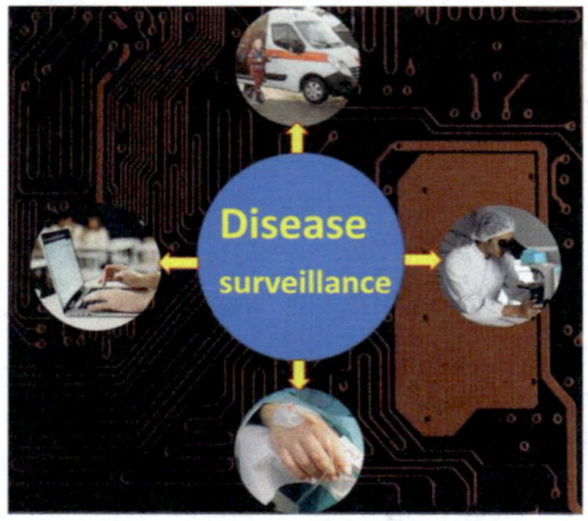

Source: https://external-content.duckduckgo.com/iu/?u= https%3A%2F%2 Fblogger.googleusercontent.com %2 Fimg%2Fb%2FR29vZ2xl%2 FAVvXsEgQdL6zDBEppKYQQMYkAkRkK0uQXLsVuuOcc3rATl3wm66b86fK20MeHkJ3mpG9gDyCNxpLQZeBFylA7lNP0002pmSR2oagY9n_vKaYgcMDPNtIoVxc6DWaty YSkFuGccupiMJG1eTuED7E__lrhKCxiIVzQH-VMvWxS8XkDm-s2TcPloO0e0wrS2hkog%2Fs548%2F12.jpg&f=1&nofb=1&ipt=401d6dfe427ee8503859b729d198bdf21ec6da003dc05903ce2516e4a0d931eb

8.2.1. Passive Surveillance

Passive monitoring is taking a significant role in disease tracking nowadays. It doesn't depend on those systems that sometimes take time to respond immediately; rather, it taps into information previously gathered from institutions such as hospitals and laboratories. This process, which works unobtrusively in the background, picks up trends in disease over time and provides insight into the spread of infections within various groups. For instance, it can uncover diseases that may not be commonly reported, providing us with a more complete picture of health issues. In most instances, such information results in wiser choices on where to concentrate resources and how policies ought to change. Merging new methods with this type of monitoring has provided us with greater insight into public health. Consider the SARS-CoV-2 pandemic – recall when wastewater monitoring became an unexpected weapon for monitoring viral trends without having to wait for symptoms to materialize? Passive samplers operating in near real-time assisted in demonstrating local surges in infection, as seen in case studies from the Rotterdam-Rijnmond region. It is a clear trick, particularly where standard surveillance could provide a distorted view due to restricted access or under-reporting. In most instances, as studies continue to reveal, it appears passive surveillance is being edged into tracking diseases such as monkeypox and potentially others, providing new avenues for the surveillance of public health. All the same, although the advantages are obvious, there are some practical and ethical concerns that require some careful consideration. In general terms, how individuals feel about these monitoring devices can impact just how effective they are, and research among healthcare professionals (HCPs) serves to emphasize this point again and again. When such tools as MAGPI, DHIS2, and SORMAS are employed, it is necessary to be aware of the pros and cons so that policymakers are guided to make decisions. Making these systems easy to utilize and ethical creates the trust that society must have to participate fully with public health initiatives. While passive surveillance grows to help battle fresh outbreaks, paying attention to user feedback will be crucial to refining these technologies to come.

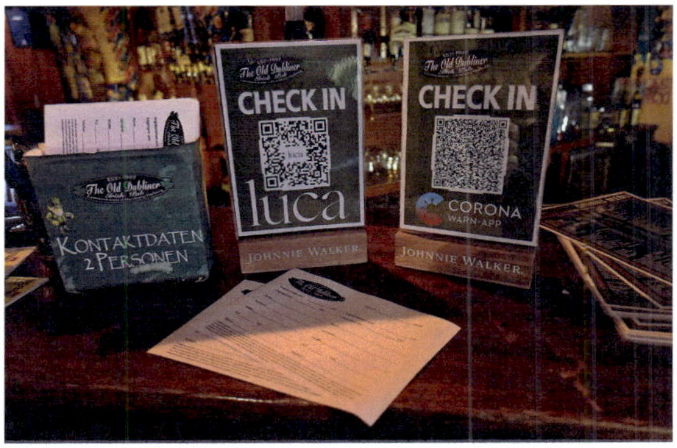

Source: By Hinnerk Rümenapf (Hinnerk R), https://hinnerk.ruemenapf.de - Own work, CC BY-SA 4.0, https://commons.wikimedia.org/w/index.php?curid=108016742

8.2.2. Active Surveillance

Monitoring for trends in disease is essential—we simply can't hazard a guess about how microbes will turn or evade our medications. Active surveillance dives right in; it reports on how frequently diseases strike, how prevalent they are, and how tough these microbes get. Health teams have a real-time view of outbreaks, allowing them to get on issues in a hurry. Take PubMLST, for example its database can deconstruct bacterial characteristics, detect genetic idiosyncrasies, and even map out physical characteristics. Everything combined serves to unravel the convoluted manners in which illnesses spread and persist, eventually allowing for improved public health initiatives and quicker responses (Jolley et al., 2018). In the case of antibiotic resistance, it's even more complicated. Overall, the thoughtless use of antibiotics in clinics and farms, particularly in most developing countries—fuels the fire for resistant microbes. By monitoring both the use of antibiotics and resistance statistics, public health professionals identify hotspots and can do something about them. Occasionally, antibiotic remnants even find their way into animal foods, so tracking how they get transferred to us is quite critical. Effective surveillance bridges the gap between agriculture practices and human health, complementing a holistic approach that relies on surveillance to contain resistance (Manyi-Loh et al., 2018). International and local collaboration is also necessary Resistant pathogens do not acknowledge boundaries, so exchanging information, advice, and technology makes monitoring a lot smoother. Governments, health workers, and research centers sharing resources not only can identify outbreaks earlier but also lay the groundwork for informing citizens about wise antibiotic use. Such collaborative work—albeit not every time faultless—slows the chaotic development of antibiotic resistance and, in most instances, makes public health safer worldwide (Manyi-Loh et al., 2018).

8.2.3. Sentinel Surveillance

The use of sentinel surveillance systems has become a crucial element in public health, particularly when it is a matter of detecting disease trends and identifying outbreak patterns. The systems focus in on specific geographic locations or groups, accumulating information that is timely and relevant. For example, a glance at South Korea's HFMD sentinel surveillance revealed that although there were periods where it stumbled slightly with performance, it still did a good job remaining timely and having wide-ranging geography. That speaks to the effectiveness of well-designed surveillance structures to provide good leads for public health approaches, particularly during those volatile post-COVID years between 2020 and 2022 (Kim et al., 2024). Sentinel surveillance is not just a matter of marking epidemics; it also plays a central role in monitoring how germs evolve and sometimes resist, helping to fuel the use of antimicrobials more judiciously. Information directly from sentinel labs assists in monitoring conditions such as shigellosis, which, astonishingly, remains atop the list as a leading cause of diarrhea across much of the globe. A closer glimpse into trends—take the example of *Shigella sonnei* in Israel—showed that although there was a general decline in cases during the pandemic, an alarming spike in antimicrobial resistance (AMR) emerged later on. In general, such a glimpse emphasizes because ongoing surveillance must be conducted to inform astute public health actions and prevent antibiotic resistance (Cohen et al., 2024).

Ultimately, the actual power of these surveillance systems is in frequent reviews and adjustments to keep in line with changing public health requirements. Periodic re-examination prevents missed warning signs and improves overall performance; having the team well-equipped and on hand is also important, particularly once a crisis has taken hold. A retrospective on South Korea's HFMD surveillance experience highlighted the way that keeping personnel on their toes can be the difference between success and failure when disease volumes swing wildly. As diseases change due to social behaviors and the environment, sentinel surveillance needs to remain nimble and prepared, ensuring that agencies of public health never are without solid data for getting down into outbreaks and controlling diseases (Cohen et al., 2024; Kim et al., 2024).

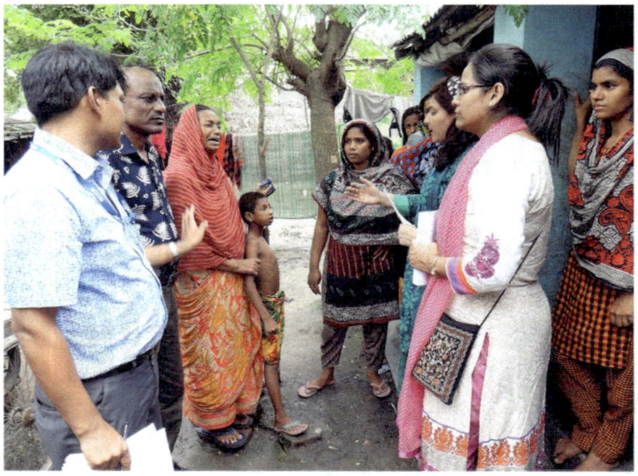

Source: By CDC Global - Contact Tracing During a Cholera Outbreak | Bangladesh, CC BY 2.0, https://commons.wikimedia.org/w/index.php?curid=64849467

8.3. Data Collection Methods

Gathering data is the foundation of how we monitor diseases and contain outbreaks. Health authorities rely on it to look for patterns and identify recurring trends, which subsequently allows one to intervene with solutions when necessary. You may discover methods such as cross-sectional surveys, cohort follow-up, or even case-control comparisons all used in an attempt to understand how an outbreak moves. In most instances, mixing traditional approaches with new technologies such as geographic information systems and mobile health apps—yes, those are still playing a significant role—shines the light on fast, near real-time information collection. Overall, having the right approach is basically what inspires us to have confidence in good public health responses.

When serious health challenges such as recent coronaviruses suddenly emerge, data collection cannot be overemphasized. Consider, say, quick-spreading respiratory disease; with current and reliable information assisting us in determining how these pathogens could be passed around and who gets sick. Too often, investigators rely on syndromic surveillance—gathering hints from symptoms reported in health-care settings—that sometimes rings a little like warning bells before an official outbreak is declared. Community-based surveillance, where information is collected directly from people on the ground, has a way of adding nuance to our knowledge. Quick deployment of established diagnostic testing at such times only serves to highlight how essential strong, adaptable data systems are to our response overall (Chan et al., 2020; Corman et al., 2020). Combining data from various corners certainly presents a more complete picture. When public health offices, schools, and hospitals are working together—sometimes in ways that are slightly messy—it makes things easier; for example, electronic health records can automatically pull in patient information, reducing the burden during emergencies. Incoming data from labs, field observations, and demographic databases tends to get shuffled together so you can drill a bit further into trends, even if the method is a little haphazard. Standardizing how information is gathered throughout an area typically makes comparisons more credible, which is an important aspect in developing strategies to reduce disease transmission and prevent future outbreaks.

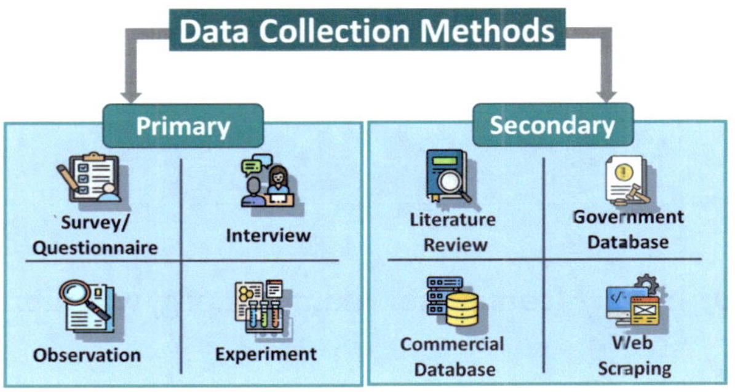

Source: EDUCBA. (2023). *Data Collection Methods*.

8.3.1. Use of Health Records and Reports

Medical records are increasingly incorporated into disease tracking in ways that seriously disrupt how outbreaks are explored. Large databases allow authorities to catch on to patterns of illness that tend to result in identifying likely outbreaks quickly. The figures drawn from these records sometimes indicate which populations are involved, suggest suspects in disease transmission, and inform responses made to varying communities. For example, examining health outcomes can indicate that diseases affect different ethnic groups differently—a nuance that aids in distributing resources more fairly. Such information, in general, becomes vital during crises such as the COVID-19 pandemic, where swift measures are required to curb transmission and shield the most at-risk (Kursumovic et al., 2020). Medical news reports from electronic medical records give a big publicity boost to public health messaging, too. Such regular updates allow public health agencies to share news of outbreaks with people in ways that enable them to make healthier decisions.

With the constant flow of information not only triggering alert messages to healthcare professionals within time, it also pushes communities as a whole toward awareness, and even to alter their behaviors during outbreaks occasionally. Most of these records pave the way for verifying whether public efforts, such as vaccination campaigns—are succeeding, by monitoring immunization rates in conjunction with declines in cases of disease (Spagnolo et al., 2020). This loop of data gathering, sharing, and verifying information illustrates just how closely health records and public health initiatives are interconnected. Simultaneously, it is difficult to deny the ethical aspect of utilizing personal health information for disease surveillance. There is always that chance, however minimal, that confidential information can get abused, therefore rigorous data governance is necessary. Establishing good frameworks that protect data while being open to a degree is essential in maintaining the trust of the public. Ethical care is also watching out so that these surveillance techniques do not, by the back door, expand healthcare access or quality gaps. As public health moves more and more into bed with tech for number-crunching, it's a genuine tightrope balancing act between the payoffs of tapping that data and the need to protect individual privacy (Kursumovic et al., 2020). Achieving that blend is critical to developing public health systems that are both effective and equitable in the long term.

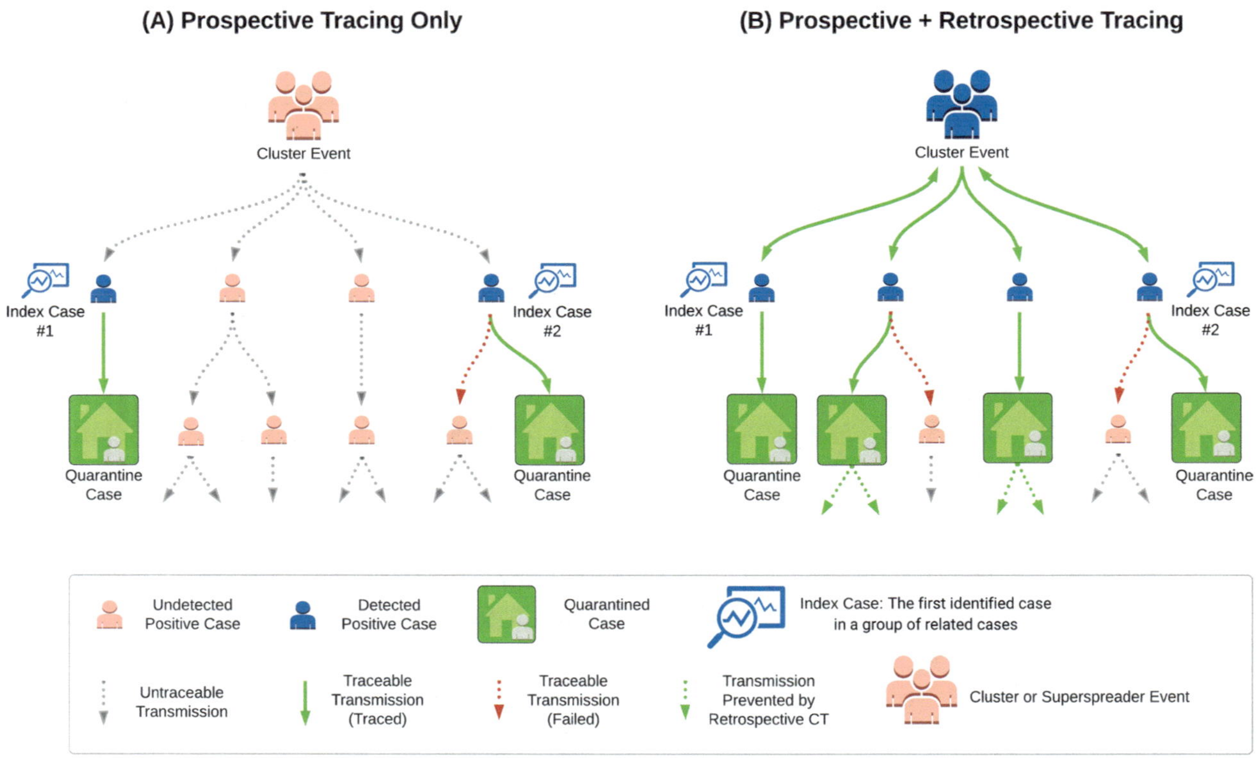

Source: By Adam Nagy - Own work, CC BY-SA 4.0, https://commons.wikimedia.org/w/index.php?curid=96784539

8.3.2. Surveys and Questionnaires

Data collection is central to monitoring disease and investigating outbreaks. Better questionnaires and surveys are not instruments—They are how we become aware of such things as how frequently a disease occurs, what dangers are present, and if our solutions are effective. Consider, for instance, a Vietnamese study of veterinary services; an online survey, revealingly, revealed gaps in the outbreak investigation capability among field vets. Such an evidence-based approach aids in determining where to direct resources and training, increasing overall disease surveillance and turning outbreak responses ever sharper (Auplish et al., 2024). What people think and do about health is important, too. In outbreak investigations, it helps to mix in both tales (qualitative information) and hard figures (quantitative data) for a better picture. During an outbreak of chikungunya in Pakistan, questionnaires were established to excavate risk spots such as where the mosquitoes breed and how the locals choose when to access care. When researchers overlaid these specifics with the actual occurrences of the disease, they were able to identify what triggered the spread—and then could calibrate their response accordingly. This combination of approaches deepens the portrait and informs decisions that seek to turn up the volume on prevention (Roghani et al., 2024). Strength in these surveys also lies in how nicely they adapt to various environments and groups. As diseases change and population demographics alter, it is ever more vital that such tools remain updated and culturally sensitive. Sure, a few problems here and there, such as low response rates or even a mistaken interpretation or two—can creep in, which is why a little trial and error, such as pre-testing with community feedback—is vital. Engaging local stakeholders makes the questions more on-point, which results in findings that truly support effective disease monitoring and outbreak strategies. More often than not, such a collaborative approach goes a great distance toward raising health outcomes on a larger scale (Auplish et al., 2024; Roghani et al., 2024).

8.3.3. Laboratory Testing and Diagnostics

Lab tests and diagnostics constitute an actual backbone when it comes to monitoring diseases—even more so in outbreak investigations. Their accuracy and speed reliability determine how quickly potential public health threats are identified and addressed. A study, for example, noted that Thailand's dengue surveillance system users require quicker, serotype-specific tests (Arkell et al., 2024). Folks there mentioned that meshing these new tests with what is already in place could seriously boost case reporting and create a friendlier environment for public health responses. It is not just about speeding up reports; these integrations also hand over timely, live info to health professionals, letting them read test results correctly and act quickly. Although laboratory diagnosis techniques have been leveling up their game, they tend to hit wither practical barriers that get in the way of efficient disease control. Consider the ACD outbreak in Brazil as an example. They employed a combination of techniques, such as peripheral blood smears and serological tests—yet the rate of success among these was quite disparate, revealing fundamental weaknesses in dependability. For the most part, these challenges demonstrate how important it is to adhere to established procedure; holding on to old habits can equate to poor monitoring and slow treatment, thus damaging patient care. Overcoming these speed bumps is essential for improved disease reaction and for reducing the overall effect of outbreaks. Increased lab test technology truly highlights the importance of innovation in public health measures. Usually, as with Thailand's emphasis on dengue diagnosis, real-world user input drives the development of technology that truly serves the surveillance system (Arkell et al., 2024). A large chunk of that advancement is about making tests not only extremely precise but also convenient enough for non-professionals to apply—bridging the divide for the average user. In addition, the rapid deployment and standardization of methods such as the polymerase chain reaction (PCR) have proven their value in managing outbreaks like ACD. By streamlining the testing process and accelerating how sensitive these tests are, public health teams can better track situations, move in quicker, and ultimately achieve better health outcomes.

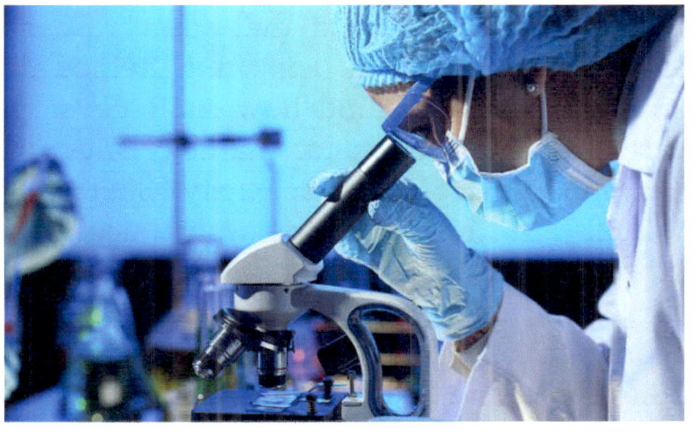

Source: Vincardiocenter. (2020). *Clinic Research.*

8.4. Role of Technology in Surveillance

Disease monitoring has taken a surprising turn over the years—technology now powers a shift that is impossible to ignore. Retrospective reporting used to involve handwritten logs and sluggish, hand-managed updates that frequently left gaps in vital information; then, obtaining accurate, real-time information was an ongoing struggle. Now, digital technology allows disease experts to assemble information as events happen, so patterns of disease transmission arise virtually instantaneously. Consider how electronic health records and mobile apps have assisted in ironing out reporting glitches. With these systems chomping up megabytes of data from everywhere, public health units can swiftly home in on emerging threats and act swiftly. By combining in these technological advances, officials enhance their preparedness and mitigate the impact of outbreaks, paving the way for a more agile and responsive means of monitoring public health. The jump to high-end sequencing and quick number-crunching has only served to heighten the excitement. Subtle analysis with genomic clues has basically overhauled the way we identify pathogens—even making the traditional techniques look bulky compared. In the majority of instances, integrating genomic data into surveillance networks has proven to be a game-changer, in that some research indicates that countries using this method can more clearly understand how AMR develops, nearly predicting resistance characteristics with an impressive degree of specificity (Bianconi et al., 2023). Not only does the system accelerate outbreak identification but it also charts the course for focused measures. By leveraging genomic insights, health officials can track how pathogens evolve over time, refining efforts to keep the spread at bay and treatments on target. COVID-19 put these advances into full spotlight. When SARS-CoV-2 first emerged, it soon became clear that rapid genomic insights were absolutely critical to creating effective measures. Overall, continuous sequencing of the virus has opened up our knowledge of its transmission, mutations, and even clues of its animal origin (Hu et al., 2020). Overlaying that genomic information with ground-level epidemiological data enabled officials to implement more rational containment efforts and vaccination efforts. This blend of technology not only strengthens our overall protection but also unites diverse nations and professionals in a truly cohesive way. Overall, combining contemporary technology and disease surveillance is not merely an improvement; it is becoming an integral pillar of today's public health initiatives—even if occasionally the journey to perfection happens to be a little rough.

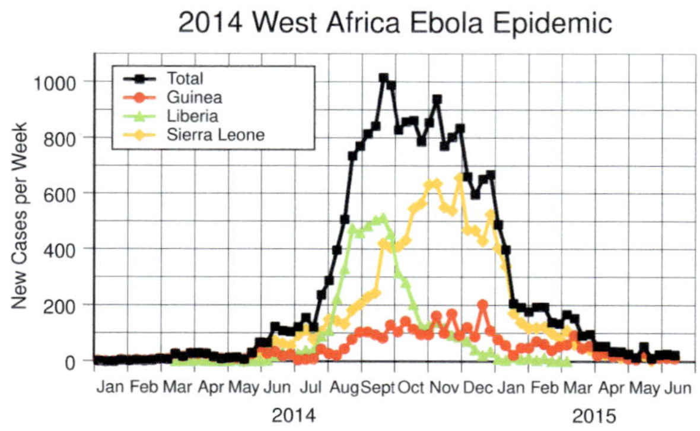

Source: By Delphi234 - Own work, CC0, https://commons.wikimedia.org/w/index.php?curid=37007270

8.4.1. Digital Health Records and Databases

Electronic health records and centralized databases have fundamentally altered the way we monitor diseases and investigate outbreaks. Rather than working with disorganized paper files, healthcare providers now bring together patient information in a single place, making it simpler to gather, verify, and exchange essential information about how frequently and where diseases emerge. They exchange information quickly—often even on an ad-hoc basis—so decision-makers can more intelligently allocate resources and deploy interventions with minimal delay. This shift also allows specialists to track patterns in diseases over extended periods of time, enabling them to determine whether public health measures are having an impact. In many instances, having such detailed information assists in identifying groups at increased risk and opens the door to more targeted prevention measures. In short, electronic health records enhance patient care directly and serve as a sort of spine for broad public health surveillance. The potential of electronic health records extends far beyond the clinic. Close examinations often uncover social, environmental, and even biological influences on our health, revealing a wider window into disease trends. Today, with smart technology such as AI in the equation, these massive heaps of data can be married to algorithms that pay attention to patterns and even predict outbreaks almost before they occur. For instance, one system may combine various health sets of data to correlate things like weather fluctuations or spikes in pollution with spikes in infections, essentially triggering early warning signs. Increasingly, there is also a perceived belief that such advances have the potential to take personalized medicine further, tailoring treatments to specific communities or groups based on age (Alowais et al., 2023). Overall, by reaching the full potential of digital records, our health systems will be able to shift from merely responding to issues to preventing them. Digital health records also create some special opportunities for at-risk populations. When those records are incorporated into our disease surveillance systems, access gets better – allowing more easily for people in rural or economically disadvantaged communities to reach care. It often entails individuals who might otherwise be confronted with geographic or budgetary barriers having access whenever needed, even remotely. This expanded, more integrated focus not only enables us to identify and deal with health disparities, but also pushes us toward achieving objectives such as those established by the United Nations for sustainable development (Mondéjar et al., 2021). In many cases, by strategically using digital records, public health officials boost immediate responses while also laying a foundation for long-term, sustainable practices that favor both equity and overall community well-being.

8.4.2. Geographic Information Systems (GIS)

GIS has revolutionized the way we manage disease surveillance and outbreak investigations, and that change is having a significant impact on public health responses. Rather than adhering to traditional data checks, spatial analysis allows us to observe how diseases spread about—sometimes catching concealed patterns you would otherwise miss. For instance, you can combine infection rates with demographic information to determine which populations may be more vulnerable, in effect joining seemingly unrelated dots. GIS software allows epidemiologists to examine all kinds of environmental variables as well, whether it is proximity to water or the clustering of cities; for the most part, these hints are involved in igniting outbreaks. This multi-layering proves to be essential while formulating focused interventions and increasing the health infrastructure, particularly keeping a view toward the possible epidemics. Essentially, GIS is more than merely elaborate mapping—it has become an absolute necessity as an ally to comprehending and combat emerging health diseases as well as in crafting overall strategy for epidemic responses. GIS also streamlines the manner results are disseminated between the authorities of health as well as among the general populace. By converting muddled data into graphics that are more intuitive, information disseminates more rapidly and individuals become better informed. In an epidemic, real-time mapping of cases can assist authorities in rapidly warning communities of surrounding risk areas and recommending required safety measures. Consider vaccine-preventable diseases for example: by superimposing vaccination rates over regions of high disease prevalence, GIS identifies locations that may require additional immunization drives. Platforms such as EPIWATCH sort of collect all these knowledge nuggets, triggering on-time action to prevent outbreaks from snowballing. This interactive feature also gets on board a combination of stakeholders—health officials, researchers, citizens—who all end up contributing in some form. On top of all that, combining AI and machine learning with GIS punches even more power. In general, these intelligent tools can sort through enormous volumes of spatial information quickly, it's easier to identify outbreak trends much earlier than ever. By combining historical data with real-time indicators, AI-powered GIS systems can even predict expected hotspots and upcoming patterns; such an advance notice encourages preventive measures instead of waiting for it to be too late. For instance, combining historical trends with present socio-environmental indicators allows these systems to predict where the next outbreaks will occur [extractedKnowledge1]. This integration of technology and GIS converts raw numbers into tactical actions that optimize health investments. Overall, as several initiatives have pointed out, integrating GIS into public health is not only a nifty added bonus—it is an important step toward the scaling up of surveillance and the construction of sound defenses in our increasingly interconnected world.

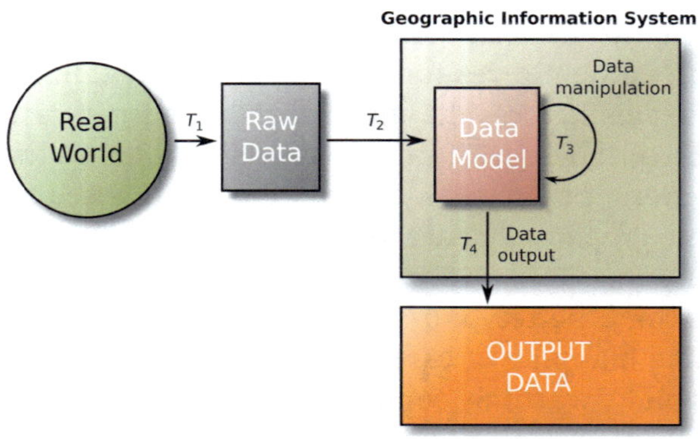

Source: By original image: Geo arbovectorization: Own work - Own work, CC BY-SA 3.0, https://commons.wikimedia.org/w/index.php?curid=18206891

8.4.3. Mobile Health Applications

Technology is disrupting the way we monitor health. Modern smartphone apps allow individuals to report rapidly during outbreaks and even enable self-testing for diseases like COVID-19. Users can easily submit their own test results through an app on their phone, and this method achieved an impressive 74.5% reporting rate. It also demonstrated how such systems can be used by everyone—even those who are not too at ease with high-tech devices. The professionals and community health workers contributed, too, which takes a lot of ways toward making the process accessible and equitable (Msuya et al., 2025).

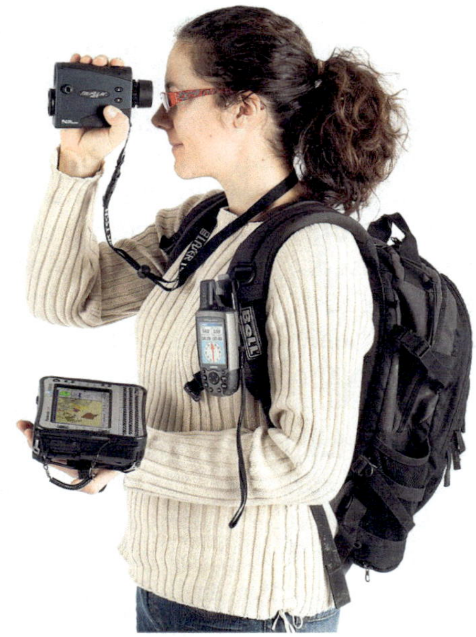

Source: By Claudiusmm - Own work, Public Domain, https://commons.wikimedia.org/w/index.php?curid=10787893

Mobile apps, in addition to that, are providing a boost to current health surveillance networks by collecting data in real-time. They combine in different diagnostic equipment from the get-go, making standardized screening and follow-up on patients much simpler. Many case studies have noted how these applications assist health organizations in maintaining a constant pulse on disease transmission and community health, and also enhance data quality with insights that inform public health actions. And how these apps interface with broader systems highlights just how strongly they can enable rapid reactions to emerging health dangers (Ambas et al., 2023). The rapidly evolving mobile health technology holds the promise for an actual revolution in public health policy, particularly duringpandemics around the world.

Not only do these technologies make reporting data easier, but they also accelerate our capacity to capture and analyze health information on an unprecedented scale. The combination of mobile technology and AI, for example, holds new potential to predict and suppress outbreaks before things get out of control. That being said, we still need to overcome issues such as privacy and data protection, which evidently impact the way such tools are developed. For the most part, as our reliance on technology for health monitoring increases, continuous innovation and collaboration will be essential for creating systems resilient enough to manage global health emergencies (Ambas et al., 2023).

8.5. Outbreak Investigation Process

When there is an outbreak, the initial response is to get to the bottom of what is happening—follow the source, learn how things are moving around, and identify who could be impacted. Disease surveillance is more than a phrase that gets thrown around; it refers to continuous gathering of information from all directions—from the lab to at-the-scene surveys—to pick up on any strange patterns that could be indicative of issues. Gathering pieces of data from hospitals, laboratories, and local health agencies can enhance the pace and accuracy of a response. In most instances, research has indicated that an integrated, comprehensive surveillance system ultimately informs intervention strategies that avoid outright public health emergencies (Das et al., 2024). The process itself usually plays out through several stages that do not necessarily occur in a particular sequence. At times, you begin by ensuring that indeed, there is an outbreak, followed by trying to nail down what constitutes a case, developing a working hypothesis of what is behind it, and lastly implementing control measures. Each component of the investigation requires rigorous scrutiny and meticulous data gathering—whether you rely on classical epidemiology or combine it with contemporary genomic shortcuts. For example, the recent emphasis on whole genome sequencing (WGS) has truly changed things by monitoring small genetic changes in pathogens to render responses more targeted. Resources such as the Pathogen Genomics in Public Health Surveillance Evaluation (PG-PHASE) Framework even allow officials to test how well they are doing as new data continues to arrive (Ferdinand et al., 2021). Ultimately, breaking the outbreak code depends on open, honest communication between all concerned. When the people of a community, the healthcare professionals, and the researchers share information promptly—even repeating a few facts—it accelerates decision-making. Being open also has a tendency to foster trust and gets individuals to stay with the recommended health practices, even if They are a little hesitant to begin with. Looking to the future, preparing for upcoming outbreaks is not merely ensuring a strong surveillance infrastructure but also continuously investing in public health systems that keep individuals on the same page, even when situations become complicated. Combining experience from previous occasions into plans for the future makes health systems usually much more resilient to infectious diseases (Das et al., 2024).

8.5.1. Identifying and Defining the Outbreak

Seeing that something is going on typically begins when you look around and see an uptick in illness that just does not ring true. Occasionally the numbers go way higher than usual for a particular period or location, suggesting something is afoot. You must go through all of it—epidemiological data, clinical documentation, and even snippets of environmental information—to cobble together what is happening. When you make clear guidelines, such as choosing some rise in cases as what defines an outbreak, then public health crews can easily mobilize resources and implement measures to contain it. Today, combining new tricks such as the use of pathogen genomics with the traditional surveillance techniques tightens up the identification of the cause in a short time, as stated in current research (Ong et al., 2024). Plotting where and how these events occur is a further insight. Consider the recent African swine fever (ASF) outbreak in Sweden—it hammered home the necessity of locally calibrated approaches. Scientists applied geo-localization to track where carcasses of animals were discovered, and tracing along those leads they mapped clusters in space and over time, although the process was a bit random. Local surveys, including those with hunting groups, can introduce additional information that can change our perspective about the dynamics of an outbreak. It is this combination of biological cues, environmental indicators, and human activities that demonstrates why determining an outbreak isn't merely a matter of lab results—it's also about where and whom (Chenais et al., 2024). Clearly defining what constitutes an outbreak is important for determining the appropriate intervention strategies. In most instances, determining whether an increase in cases is merely a typical seasonal surge or an actual emergency is everything to public health officials. It is useful to take into account underlying factors, such as changes in demographics, alterations in the local environment, and even human activity, which all combined may lead to a surge in illness. By monitoring these factors, experts can predict more effectively what can be expected next and adapt their plans for surveillance accordingly. And as pathogen genomics gradually insinuates itself into standard public health practice—albeit not yet in perfectly harmonized form—the potential for real-time monitoring and rapid signaling is beginning to redefine the characterization and control of outbreaks (Ong et al., 2024).

8.5.2. Case Finding and Contact Tracing

Rapid identification of who is ill and who may be at risk can truly make the difference in disease transmission. In the early days of COVID, individuals discovered that review of travel history – such as from a cruise vacation – sometimes provided an unexpected lead. For instance, scientists discovered that 149 travelers from Nile River cruises came back to the US with confirmed COVID, causing extensive community spread in many states because some areas enforced exhaustive contact screening. All this reveals that it is important to understand travel behavior and trends to make public health strategies effective (Guagliardo et al., 2022).

How a virus travels is almost everything when making plans for our next move. Consider the example of COVID-19 variants like Delta; studies tend to indicate that incubation periods can vary between groups. A study noted that variables such as age, gender, and how bad the disease becomes can adjust the mean incubation period – resulting in around 6.64 days for Delta. For the most part, these findings emphasize that being accurate in identifying cases and pursuing contacts is paramount, particularly when new variants begin to emerge (Wang et al., 2022). Combining rapid case identification with diligent follow-ups can truly get an outbreak into a manageable state. It's not only about seeing the ill; it is also about quickly reaching out to those who may have been exposed—albeit sometimes in a somewhat random manner. Referring back to that Nile River cruise scenario, focused tracing did more than merely isolate a handful of cases; it served to uncover the outline of how the disease moved around. Overall, assembling a system that combines rapid case finding with deep contact follow-ups proves to be a critical component of being prepared for public health problems (Guagliardo et al., 2022).

8.5.3. Implementing Control Measures

Outbreaks of disease require rapid, hands-on interventions. In Ajwan village, for instance, a case of mumps triggered an instant house-to-house survey – health workers went out, gathered information, and rapidly detected additional cases while distributing the appropriate medicine. This spontaneous action not only alleviated the immediate concern but also reminded everyone that spreading the message about mumps prevention is important, particularly when most individuals had not been vaccinated. In general, these measures reduce transmission and make public health emergencies more tractable (Debbarma et al., 2025). Chikungunya provides us with another perspective on how these controls operate. After an outbreak in Peshawar, authorities implemented a strategy that combined active case finding with rapid screening around areas where mosquitoes could breed. Surveys highlighted that standing water and insufficient mosquito shields were the main risk factors. Then, with targeting vector control and community discussions on prevention, the case numbers plummeted – a testament that loosely linked surveillance and swift action can make all the difference to community health (Roghani et al., 2024). Beyond quick solutions, long-term thinking counts too. Regular health education, vaccination campaigns, and increased community engagement are the pillars upon which avoiding future breakouts is built. For example, merely educating people about the reasons why vaccines , such as the one for mumps, are good, and establishing effective mosquito control systems can take far too long to prevent repeat breakouts. Additionally, developing local health expertise and encouraging people to come in earlier are significant steps. Both the mumps and chikungunya cases demonstrate that ongoing monitoring, combined with a consistent amount of control interventions, not only addresses existing issues but also bolsters the overall immune defense against what may come in the future (Debbarma et al., 2025; Roghani et al., 2024).

8.6. Challenges in Disease Surveillance

Monitoring disease is a complex undertaking that makes it necessary for public health systems to contend with all sorts of unforeseen issues. Investigations such as the one that transpired in an instance of a COVID-19 outbreak in a behavioral health facility illustrate how patient and healthcare worker interactions can abruptly trigger discrete groups of infection—even where units are shared. Researchers overall reported that interventions like point prevalence testing and molecular surveillance were instrumental in keeping the outbreak under control, while still attempting to provide basic care. Meanwhile, these findings remind us quite definitely that one tactic will not be effective everywhere (Rios-Guzman et al., 2024). Local limitations place another level on the dilemma. Usually, there are too old-fashioned public health frameworks that are overtaxed; lots of low-resource communities just can't react quickly enough when things get hot. Data gathering, for instance, usually gets disjointed because various agencies operate quite independently, with interventions fragmented and communication spotty. As a response, the Community-based Outbreak Investigation and Response (COIR) system recently emerged as an effective alternative that supports various groups to interoperate more harmoniously (Oza et al., 2023). Public health practitioners' and community members' trust indeed makes a big difference. Good surveillance is not merely about possessing sophisticated tools—it also greatly relies on the relationship between authorities and subjects. Even a bit of mistrust can undermine the reporting of cases and how well people comply with health measures. Therefore, it makes sense to increase open, honest communication and to engage locals seriously. When you consider it all together, technical competence as well as the local social-political climate are crucial to a successful response, so it is important to address these linked issues to improve outbreak investigation activities (Oza et al., 2023).

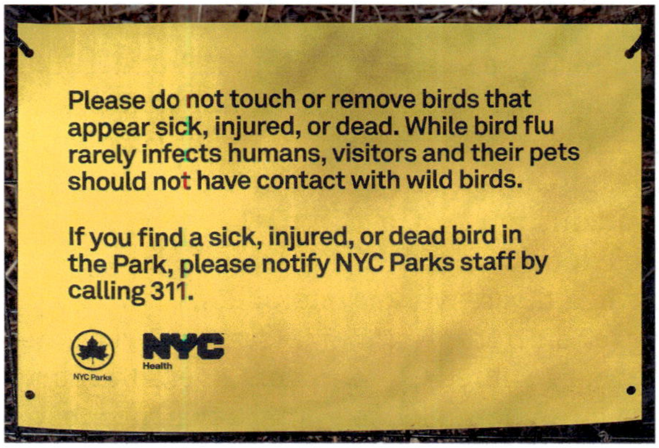
Please do not touch or remove birds that appear sick, injured, or dead. While bird flu rarely infects humans, visitors and their pets should not have contact with wild birds.
If you find a sick, injured, or dead bird in the Park, please notify NYC Parks staff by calling 311.
NYC Parks
NYC
Health

Source: https://en.wikipedia.org/wiki/Avian_influenza#/media/File:Bird_flu_sign_in_Central_Park_(83883).jpg

8.6.1. Data Privacy and Ethical Concerns

Disease surveillance has revolutionized public health—new monitoring technologies now form part of our daily battle against epidemics. Advances of this sort, however, bring their own set of privacy and ethics concerns. Consider Wastewater-Based Epidemiology (WBE) as an example; literally, it involves harvesting wastewater from the community to search for pathogens. This approach facilitates the monitoring of disease transmission in real-time but can also capture sensitive biological information such as individual genomic data. To most Indigenous peoples, this raises significant ethical issues, particularly since there has been a past history of research exploitation and since frequent informed consent is lacking. We genuinely need to develop individualized regulations that protect confidentiality but still achieve public health gains (Perreault et al., 2025). If these issues are not treated with caution, vulnerable populations may end up being left behind, which would be counterproductive to these efforts. The international landscape in health surveillance is not decelerating, and neither is the integration of AI with these technologies. AI is moving in to assist with outbreaks by processing information quickly and indicating patterns of disease, but its application isn't complication-free with privacy lapses and biases in algorithms. Obviously, there is an increasing effort to establish controls that prioritize transparency, accountability, and equitable data use. It is not merely a matter of adhering to regulations; positive measures must be taken to safeguard societies that could otherwise be damaged by abuse. Operational hand in hand, local health organizations and people—learning from other regions globally—can help shape more equitable AI solutions. Ultimately, keeping information confidential while realizing AI's ability is the answer to enhancing health outcomes across diverse populations (Tornimbene et al., 2025). Ethical concerns in disease surveillance resonate when you ponder how easily confidential information could get hijacked. Technologies such as WBE and AI-based surveillance are transparent about public health benefits but raise difficult issues of control over and benefit from data. The burden of historical exploitation in research particularly increases risks for Indigenous and other oppressed groups. This makes it important to establish ethical frameworks that value data ownership and obtain informed consent, fostering trust among health agencies and populations they serve. Communication, also, has to be clear enough so that affected communities know what is happening. Such an ethical strategy not only unites people but also creates a more equitable basis for contemporary disease surveillance. In short, proper tackling of these issues of privacy is necessary for promoting respect and cooperation in addressing public health emergencies (Perreault et al., 2025).

8.6.2. Resource Limitations and Funding Issues

Shortages of resources and funding challenges tend to disrupt our capacity to track disease and respond to outbreaks. Most health systems are just not able to mobilize sufficient finance, which in turn delays reactions to emerging threats and eats away at the wider public health system. Nations, for instance, tend to struggle to budget the money required for effective monitoring systems that are capable of detecting outbreaks early. This gap in funding consistently prevents in-depth studies that clarify how diseases work and inform effective interventions. COVID-19, as we learned, revealed how vulnerable health systems became excess technology and staffing problems accumulated, leading to sluggish responses and deepening the crises (Hale et al., 2021). The image becomes even cloudier when we examine funding disparities between wealthy and low-resource countries. In wealthy areas, strong health initiatives tend to receive funding, but much of the developing world is beset by debilitating budget issues that render it virtually impossible to spend money on sophisticated monitoring equipment and experienced personnel. This disparity, in general terms, becomes all the more apparent during large-scale health crises when outbreaks cross national borders. As diseases spread, the clamor for both national and international surveillance grows loud, yet underfunding remains a critical issue in less affluent regions. Such uneven distribution of resources can leave big gaps in our understanding of diseases, ultimately putting more people at risk (Amaral et al., 2020). Tackling these funding woes calls for creative, collaborative moves among governments, NGOs, and even private industries. A promising pathway is establishing global health funds that benefit disease surveillance in resource-scarce regions directly, enabling them to handle emergencies more effectively. Public-private partnerships, in all but a few instances, can also attract funds and brains, combining tech and research even during lean times. In addition to investing money in systems, developing local capacity through adequate training and education for public health workers is instrumental in keeping these initiatives around for the long term. Building up these foundational elements is necessary for building strong, enduring health systems that are capable of managing threats from disease, and in so doing, contribute to a safer global society (Hale et al., 2021).

8.6.3. Variability in Reporting Practices

Disease tracking relies heavily on how regularly cases are reported within various healthcare systems. Variations in how data is collected can completely scramble the picture and create gaps that impact public responses. Let's take COVID-19, for instance – Nigeria, Uganda, and many other nations didn't precisely stick to the same routine; their approaches to verifying cases and managing data tended to branch off in different ways. Every country struggled to develop its systems to track cases more effectively, yet staff shortages and issues in connecting data continued to arise. Overall, these different methods indicate the necessity of unified reporting standards that allow us to compare and take action quickly (Fawole et al., 2023). Mix-ups in surveillance and reporting can distort the epidemiological picture, and make it more difficult to track down outbreaks. Simple things like unclear case definitions or variations in writing down symptoms can lead us to underestimates the true effect of an illness. In most places, attention was on identifying people who had severe symptoms early, so mild or unusual symptom cases were missed. In general, this singular emphasis doesn't only delay immediate containment; it also distorts mortality estimates, as highlighted by initial inconsistencies in COVID-19 fatality rates (Klompas, 2020). Identification and investigation of these discrepancies are crucial to establishing firm risk models and allocating healthcare resources more equitably. Tech breakthroughs may be able to fill in these reporting gaps, even though the route is not a straight one to follow. Mobile reporting apps and real-time data-sharing platforms are proving promising in ironing out data collection in a variety of environments. Such new technologies have the potential to enhance how trends are monitored and enhance collaboration between public health authorities and providers. Yet in the majority of situations, implementing such technology must factor in disparate local infrastructure and resource availability. In addition, there is a need for training healthcare teams to become familiar with these tools in order that we might realize more timely and credible data—actions that end up making outbreak responses more effective (Fawole et al., 2023).

CLOSER LOOK

The Importance of Disease Surveillance in Public Health

In an interdependent world with ever more sophisticated global health challenges, recognizing and taking advantage of the power of disease surveillance has never been more important. What follows explores the value of disease surveillance in protecting our communities, its main challenges, and how groundbreaking technological innovation can transform public health organizations' capacities to detect, track, and respond to evolving health challenges.

What Is Disease Surveillance?

Disease surveillance refers to gathering, analyzing, and interpreting health information systematically to detect and respond to disease outbreaks. Traditionally, public health authorities have used manual data gathering and reporting, which confined its scope and efficiency. Today, advances in technology, digital tools, and other modern technologies have transformed disease surveillance, making it more actionable in terms of disease trends and public health threats.

Although methodologies and disease surveillance instruments have come far from John Snow's original efforts in the 1854 London cholera epidemic, the fundamental goal remains the same: delivering information that can be used to advance public health. It is a broad array of activities today that includes reporting notifiable diseases, laboratory diagnoses, and electronic health record analysis to give a complete picture of community health.

Why Disease Surveillance Matters

Disease surveillance is the foundation of public health. It offers a valuable system of monitoring that allows HCPs to detect, control, and manage infectious and chronic diseases. Through systematic data collection and analysis, a disease surveillance program can offer actionable information in guiding public health policies and informing long-term strategies for the protection of community welfare.

In the interconnected world with changing risks, this forward-thinking action is invaluable for safeguarding lives, minimizing healthcare inequalities, and enhancing resilience in the community.

SUMMARY

Disease surveillance and outbreak investigations demonstrate that combining methods is necessary when approaching public health hazards. Consider situations such as Group B Streptococcus outbreaks with chikungunya – they explain why combining new tools such as whole-genome sequencing (WGS) with good old-fashioned epidemiology can make all the difference. In a single episode of GBS, adherence to screening through regular screening plus adherence to infection prevention measures proved to be a key determinant in disease transmission, highlighting the importance of intensive site inspection and rule adherence in outbreak management (Lambert et al., 2025). These steps do not only allow us to respond quickly but also enhance how effectively public health campaigns operate, reminding us that constant reviews and adjustments in prevention procedures are crucial.

The chikungunya investigation illustrates, quite clearly, that to control outbreaks, it is important to seize timely and accurate information. By establishing strict standards for suspect cases and enlisting the help of local populations in reporting and prevention, public health squads can compile a more complete picture of disease outbreaks in infected regions. Identifying mosquito breeding grounds and conducting local information campaigns are reasonable steps that help reduce vector-borne diseases. For most instances, it highlights the demand for swift choices and instant responsiveness, placing health networks on notice for new threats (Mahadik et al., 2024). Ultimately, piecing together data from diverse sources and relying on new analysis provides the foundation for tomorrow's public health initiatives. Both GBS and chikungunya illnesses carry lessons that act as beacons for navigating future outbreaks. A culture of ongoing surveillance coupled with a proactive approach consolidates health systems to be stronger and better positioned to respond to unforeseen threats. Enhancing these foundations of disease investigation not only assists in managing crises in real time but also fosters a permanent foundation for public health security (Lambert et al., 2025; Mahadik et al., 2024).

Seeing how diseases are transmitted on farms illustrates why it is critical to monitor outbreaks. In farming, for instance, the severe economic blow from pathogens such as Foot-and-mouth disease (FMD) makes it obvious that governments need to support their biosecurity strategies with firm, effective actions. Australia and Denmark, both keen to remain FMD-free, went in different directions although they both emphasized making the best use of their resources and reducing costs. The island location of Denmark compelled them to concentrate intensely on preventing disease transmission within small areas through experiments in vaccination combinations, whereas Australia went in for a system that identifies cases early. When you take a closer look at local idiosyncrasies, it is evident that there is no one-size-fits-all solution to slashing the economic impact of such diseases (Wagner et al., 2025).

Technology now has an even larger part to play than ever before in monitoring public health. Recent initiatives, such as one by the NATO Centre of Excellence for Military Medicines, remind us how digital technology can deliver almost real-time information on what is going on out there. Even a pilot exercise in Kosovo used mobile devices to connect typical symptoms to emerging disease patterns. Although that trial did not detect any significant outbreaks, the early warning signs were a genuine boon for med teams on the frontline. Rapid alerts and a less frenetic flow of information enabled doctors to connect the dots, illustrating why combining modern technology with old-fashioned surveillance is so worth it (Lindfield et al., 2023). When you look at the cash side, there is no doubt that trade bans during disease scares hurt. Both Denmark and Australia have realized that accelerating exports after an outbreak can substantially ease the sting of trade bans. In most instances, reducing the time wasted means reducing significant financial losses, which makes swift, effective surveillance a victory for the economy as well. By placing smart investments in surveillance and quick response, nations can improve at catching outbreaks early. Ultimately, mixing new technology, local circumstances, and cost factors makes the best argument for a nimble, all-around strategy for handling health risks while buoying economies (Lindfield et al., 2023; Wagner et al., 2025).

KEY TERMS FROM THIS CHAPTER

- Passive surveillance
- Sentinel surveillance
- Primary case
- Cluster
- Attack rate
- Case-fatality rate
- Descriptive epidemiology
- Hypothesis generation
- Incubation period
- Public health response
- Laboratory confirmation
- Notifiable disease
- Active surveillance
- Syndromic surveillance
- Secondary case
- Epidemic curve (epi curve)
- Prevalence
- Contact tracing
- Analytic epidemiology
- Exposure
- Mode of transmission
- Field investigation
- Reporting system

REFERENCES

1. Alowais, S. A., Alghamdi, S. S., Alsuhebany, N., Alqahtani, T., Alshaya, A., Almohareb, S. N., Aldairem, A., et al. (2023). Revolutionizing healthcare: The role of artificial intelligence in clinical practice. *BMC Medical Education, 23*. https://doi.org/10.1186/s12909-023-04698-z.
2. Amaral, D. G., & de Vries, P. J. (2020). COVID-19 and autism research: Perspectives from around the globe. *Autism Research, 13*, 844–869. https://doi.org/10.1002/aur.2329.
3. Ambas, J., Dzikrullah, M., Prisusanti, R. D., Pangandaheng, T., & Sukmawaty, M. N. (2023). Innovations in global health: Leveraging technology for disease surveillance and pandemic preparedness. *Global International Journal of Innovative Research*. https://www.semanticscholar.org/paper/bb6c4a620d2c45d78863f092c335bff8cb650e0f (accessed on 6 May 2025).
4. Augustine, R., Das, S., Hasan, A., Pushpangadhan Abhilash, S. A., Salaam, S. A., Dalvi, Y. B., et al. (2020). Rapid antibody-based COVID-19 mass surveillance: Relevance, challenges, and prospects in a pandemic and post-pandemic world. *Journal of Clinical Medicine, 9*, 3372. https://doi.org/10.3390/jcm9103372.
5. Auplish A, Tra Vu TT, Pham Duc P, Green AC, Tiwari H, Housen T, Stevenson M and Dhand N (2024) Investigating the workforce capacity and needs for animal disease surveillance and outbreak investigation: a mixed-methods study of veterinary services in Vietnam. Front. Vet. Sci. 11:1410606. doi: 10.3389/fvets.2024.1410606 (accessed on 6 May 2025).
6. Besijn, E., Whelan, J., Bijkerk, P., Sips, G., Langeveld, J., Izquierdo-Lara, R. W., van Baarle, E., et al. (2024). Agile, on-demand wastewater surveillance of virus infections to support pandemic and outbreak response in Rotterdam-Rijn Mond, the Netherlands, 2020 to 2022. *Eurosurveillance, 29*. https://www.semanticscholar.org/paper/e2445b8b7b3004ab40c7803ab59be540c385e606 (accessed on 6 May 2025).
7. Bianconi, I., Aschbacher, R., & Pagani, E. (2023). Current uses and future perspectives of genomic technologies in clinical microbiology. *Antibiotics, 12*(11), 1580. https://doi.org/10.3390/antibiotics12111580.
8. Camará, M., da Costa, F. P., Chambe, G., Betunde, A., Cardoso, P., Johnson, K., Rullan-Oliver, P., & Lopez, A. (2023). Strengthening surveillance, disease detection, and outbreak response through Guinea-Bissau's Frontline Field Epidemiology Training Program: a cross-sectional descriptive study. *The Pan African medical journal, 45*, 133. https://doi.org/10.11604/pamj.2023.45.133.30807 (accessed on 6 May 2025).
9. Chan, J. F. W., Yuan, S., Kok, K. H., To, K. K. W., Chu, H., Jin, Y., Xing, F., et al. (2020). A familial cluster of pneumonia associated with the 2019 novel coronavirus indicating person-to-person transmission: A study of a family cluster. *The Lancet, 395*(10223), 514–523. https://doi.org/10.1016/s0140-6736(20)30154-9 (accessed on 6 May 2025).
10. Corman, V. M., Landt, O., Kaiser, M., Molenkamp, R., Meijer, A., Chu, D. K. W., Bleicker, T., et al. (2020). Detection of 2019 novel coronavirus (2019-nCoV) by real-time RT-PCR. *Eurosurveillance, 25*(3). https://doi.org/10.2807/1560-7917.es.2020.25.3.2000045.
11. Das, M., Albert, V., Das, S., Dolma, K., Majumdar, T., Baruah, P., Hazarika, S., et al. (2024). An integrated FoodNet in North East India: Fostering one health approach to fortify public health. *BMC Public Health, 24*. https://www.semanticscholar.org/paper/07979497179a19d8c589e3a0f3065af6ccd36b18 (accessed on 6 May 2025).

12. Ferdinand, M., Kelaher, C., Lane, C., Gonçalves da Silva, A., Sherry, N., Ballard, S., Andersson, P., et al. (2021). An implementation science approach to evaluating pathogen whole genome sequencing in public health. *Genome Medicine, 13*. https://www.semanticscholar.org/paper/753a96d4266ae0ec87805acb96a3da0cc7ca8e8a (accessed on 6 May 2025).

13. Florentino, P., Bertoldo Junior, J., Barbosa, G. C. G., Cerqueira-Silva, T., Oliveira, V. A., Garcia, M. H. d. O., Penna, G. O., et al. (2024). Impact of primary health care data quality on infectious disease surveillance in Brazil: Case study. *JMIR Public Health and Surveillance, 11*. https://www.semanticscholar.org/paper/1b80ead4b59baa72516d87b233a3f5d535fe06bc (accessed on 6 May 2025).

14. Hu, B., Guo, H., Zhou, P., & Shi, Z. L. (2020). Characteristics of SARS-CoV-2 and COVID-19. *Nature Reviews Microbiology, 19*, 141–154. https://doi.org/10.1038/s41579-020-00459-7.

15. Jolley, K. A., Bray, J. E., & Maiden, M. (2018). Open-access bacterial population genomics: BIGSdb software, the PubMLST.org website and their applications. *Welcome Open Research, 3*, 124. https://doi.org/10.12688/wellcomeopenres.14826.1.

16. Kursumovic, E., Lennane, S., & Cook, T. (2020). Deaths in healthcare workers due to COVID-19: The need for robust data and analysis. *Anesthesia, 75*, 989–992. https://doi.org/10.1111/anae.15116.

17. Lambert, M. C., Jones, S., Mueller, K., Maloney, M., Perera, N., Incekara, K., Petit, S., et al. (2025). Late onset invasive group B streptococcal disease outbreak in a neonatal intensive care unit identified through whole genome sequencing–Connecticut, 2020–2024. *Open Forum Infectious Diseases, 12*. https://www.semanticscholar.org/paper/34ba88a3e1b732362749d2eabb02ffd691bb8047 (accessed on 6 May 2025).

18. MacIntyre, C. R., Lim, S., & Quigley, A. (2022). Preventing the next pandemic: Use of artificial intelligence for epidemic monitoring and alerts. *Cell Reports Medicine, 3*, 100867. https://doi.org/10.1016/j.xcrm.2022.100867.

19. Mahadik, M. M., Jain, A., & Dzeyie, K. A. (2024). IJCM_292A: Chikungunya outbreak investigation at village Bolasa, Petlawat, Jhabua, Madhya Pradesh, India, September 2023. *Indian Journal of Community Medicine: Official Publication of Indian Association of Preventive & Social Medicine, 49*, S84, S85. https://www.semanticscholar.org/paper/11b76fbcc47fbb55b21999f829939a1e8400a0fd (accessed on 6 May 2025).

20. Manyi-Loh, C. E., Mamphweli, S., Meyer, E. L., & Okoh, A. I. (2018). Antibiotic use in agriculture and its consequential resistance in environmental sources: Potential public health implications. *Molecules, 23*, 795. https://doi.org/10.3390/molecules23040795.

21. Martin, R., & Fall, I. S. (2021). Field epidemiology training programs to accelerate public health workforce development and global health security. *International Journal of Infectious Diseases, 110*, S3–S5. https://doi.org/10.1016/j.ijid.2021.08.021.

22. Morton, V., Kandar, R., Kearney, A., Hamel, M., & Nadon, C. (2024). Transition to whole genome sequencing surveillance: The impact on national outbreak detection and response for *Listeria monocytogenes*, *Salmonella*, *Shiga Toxin-Producing Escherichia coli*, and *Shigella* clusters in Canada, 2015–2021. *Foodborne Pathogens and Disease*. https://www.semanticscholar.org/paper/46e7ed924a1a4464e06768b364beb2bd6ca1d567 (accessed on 6 May 2025).

23. Msuya, H. M., Ali, A. M., Mrisho, M., Lweno, O. N., Temu, S. G., Msuya, I., Kalabamu, F., et al. (2025). Feasibility of a mobile application for self and assisted reporting of Coronavirus

Disease 2019 self-testing results in Tanzania: A pilot study. *The American Journal of Tropical Medicine and Hygiene*. https://www.semanticscholar.org/paper/117e1a37277e0a3e65919ecfc812615c8d7e3d18 (accessed on 6 May 2025).

24. Ong, J. D. H., Zulfiqar, T., Glass, K., Kirk, M., Astbury, B., & Ferdinand, A. (2024). Identifying factors that influence the use of pathogen genomics in Australia and New Zealand: A protocol. *Frontiers in Public Health, 12*. https://www.semanticscholar.org/paper/8de760946a42e78358f5481b1c519217729c367f (accessed on 6 May 2025).

25. Palmeirim, M. S., Houngbedji, C. A., Barth-Jaeggi, T., Kouamé, J. P. Y., Krouman, A., Coulibaly, D., & Wyss, K. (2024). Key characteristics and perception of different outbreak surveillance systems in Côte d'Ivoire: Cross-sectional survey among users. *JMIR Public Health and Surveillance, 10*. https://www.semanticscholar.org/paper/3fcd1af7660929c5d3e578728fbb70afe8df0181 (accessed on 6 May 2025).

26. Perreault, M., & Goodridge, L. (2025). Indigenous data protection in wastewater surveillance: Balancing public health monitoring with privacy rights. *Genomic Psychiatry*. https://www.semanticscholar.org/paper/88a1dc026e7c9e553912268c42e97fe69a720135 (accessed on 6 May 2025).

27. Pulford, C. V., Perez-Sepulveda, B., Ingle, D., Bengtsson, R. J., Bennett, R., Rodwell, E. V., Pardos de la Gándara, M., et al. (2024). Global diversity and evolution of Salmonella Panama, an understudied serovar causing gastrointestinal and invasive disease worldwide: A genomic epidemiology study. *bioRxiv*. https://www.semanticscholar.org/paper/7c1f4b48489aa94142fb34dadbdaf547afab329f (accessed on 6 May 2025).

28. Salehinejad, S., Jangipour Afshar, P., & Borhaninejad, V. (2021). Rumor surveillance methods in outbreaks: A systematic literature review. *Health Promotion Perspectives, 11*(1), 12–19. https://doi.org/10.34172/hpp.2021.03.

29. Spagnolo, P. A., Manson, J. E., & Joffe, H. (2020). Sex and gender differences in health: What the COVID-19 pandemic can teach us. *Annals of Internal Medicine, 173*(5), 385, 386. https://doi.org/10.7326/m20-1941.

30. Tamayo Cuartero, C., Szilassy, E., Radford, A. D., Newton, J. R., & Sánchez-Vizcaíno, F. (2024). Setting clinically relevant thresholds for the notification of canine disease outbreaks to veterinary practitioners: An exploratory qualitative interview study. *Frontiers in Veterinary Science, 11*. https://www.semanticscholar.org/paper/e6318e6e29b1b197a56999b00efdc52b8a522649 (accessed on 6 May 2025).

31. Tesfaye, B., Makam, J. K., Sergon, K., Onuekwusi, I., Muitherero, C., & Sowe, A. (2020). The role of the Stop Transmission of Polio (STOP) program in developing countries: The experience of Kenya. *BMC Public Health, 20*. https://doi.org/10.1186/s12889-020-09196-1.

32. Tornimbene, B., Leiva Rioja, Z. B., Brownstein, J., Dunn, A., Faye, S., Kong, J., Malou, N., et al. (2025). Harnessing the power of artificial intelligence for disease-surveillance purposes. *BMC Proceedings, 19*. https://www.semanticscholar.org/paper/a09ec60dee41fabe75f63d19f85c6f3048dddcf3 (accessed on 6 May 2025).

33. Wang, K., Luan, Z., Guo, Z., Ran, J., Tian, M., & Zhao, S. (2022). The association between clinical severity and incubation period of SARS-CoV-2 Delta variants: Retrospective observational study. *JMIR Public Health and Surveillance, 8*. https://www.semanticscholar.org/paper/2f380a86b5a0a9f28d7ae2506e0f013a6ad210cc (accessed on 6 May 2025).

34. Wattamwar, A., Akwafuo, S. E., & Mistry, V. (2024). Data-driven real-time surveillance system for tracking disease outbreaks: A case study of Lassa fever outbreak. In *2024 IEEE 12th International Conference on Healthcare Informatics (ICHI)*. https://www.semanticscholar.org/paper/3108d3a29bc211f7e0c8b83c334c9ef0681049a3 (accessed on 6 May 2025).

35. Zhang, P., Moa, A., & Quigley, A. (2025). EPIWATCH®: A Rapid Epidemic Surveillance Tool for Detecting Early Signals of the First-ever Marburg Virus Outbreak in Equatorial Guinea. *Global Biosecurity*, *7*(1). https://doi.org/10.31646/gbio.279 (accessed on 6 May 2025).

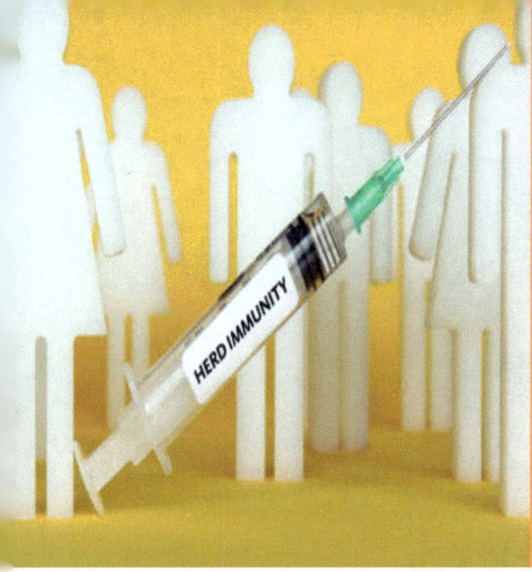

Chapter 9

VACCINATION AND HERD IMMUNITY

Contents

Introduction

Immunization is one of the pillars of public health today that not only establishes a preventive component in anticipation of the prevention of the majority of infectious diseases but also a fundamental practice of upholding the safety of community health. The history of discovery and utilization of vaccines has greatly minimized the occurrence of crippling diseases like polio, measles, and smallpox, thereby enhancing life expectancy and living standards for the global population. Vaccination has moved beyond scientific achievements to the development of new pathogens and adaptation with the evolving epidemiological realities. Vaccination is also associated with behemothic controversy that is accompanied by issues of safety, ethics, and policymaking. Understanding the complex nature of vaccination is important as societies deal with the endemic realities of vaccine hesitancy and access. In a bid to study history, changing trends, and the future trend of vaccination, this chapter tries to position its interest on its role in facilitating health and preventing disease in modern society (Figure 9.1).

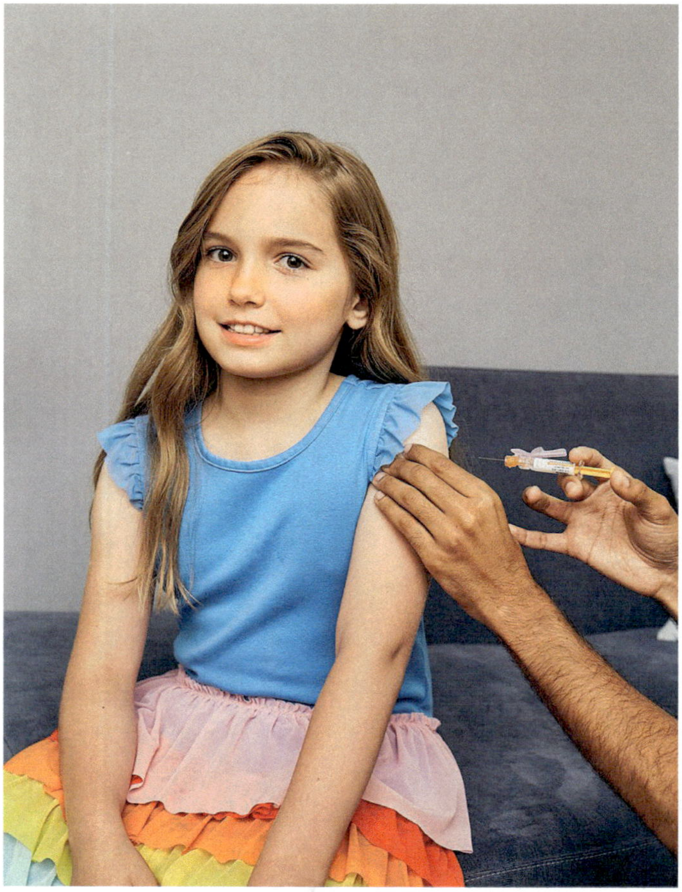

Figure 9.1. Vaccination.

Source: By SELF Magazine - Young girl about to receive a vaccine in her upper arm, CC BY 2.0, https://commons.wikimedia.org/w/index.php?curid=81631650

Definition of Vaccination

Vaccination is a protective measure of health that is designed to induce an immune response against specific infectious diseases to reduce the risk of getting ill and developing its complications. Basically, vaccination involves the introduction of a biological substance that is very much alike a disease-causing microorganism, which stimulates the immune system to detect and destroy the causative pathogen on future exposure. The value of vaccination is enhanced by its capacity to reduce morbidity and mortality from serious illnesses such as measles and pertussis. The case of measles vaccination, for instance, has led to a reduction in associated deaths through enhanced immunity, although there are issues arising from various case fatality rates in unvaccinated populations, especially for children below the age of five years (Aaby et al., 2009). Second, the dynamic changing epidemiological profiles of illnesses like pertussis show how, despite vaccine effects, ongoing requirements for booster immunization arise from the possible deterioration of immunity with time and consequently the demand for integrated approaches to vaccination in every age bracket (Bezzina et al., 2013) (Figure 9.2).

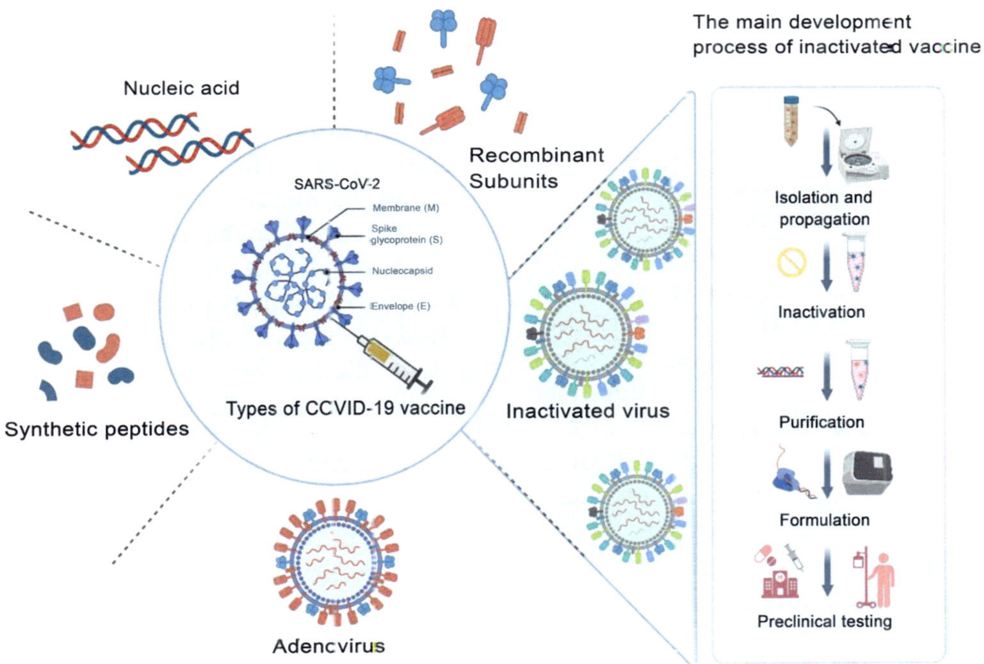

Figure 9.2. Vaccination.

Source: Hu L, Sun J, Wang Y, Tan D, Cao Z, Gao L, Guan Y, Jia X, Mao J. A Review of Inactivated COVID-19 Vaccine Development in China: Focusing on Safety and Efficacy in Special Populations. Vaccines. 2023; 11(6):1045. https://doi.org/10.3390/vaccines11061045

Historical Context of Vaccination

The historical background in vaccination defines its evolution as a critical public health intervention that has shaped future infectious disease control. Following the initial attempt by Edward Jenner in the late 18th century, the discovery of the smallpox vaccine opened up possibilities for the establishment of immunology and eventually the campaign against vaccination. This invention not only greatly reduced the frequency of smallpox, but also promoted the understanding of disease prevention via immunization. During the 20th century, polio vaccine advances, as well as improvements in vaccines against measles and other infectious illnesses, further highlighted the importance of vaccination in public health. However, growing antibiotic resistance and other challenges, as evidenced by the present world disease burden of such infections as enteric fever, once more also place emphasis on the need for ongoing vaccination and immunization strategy design to counter new pathogens and advance public health, again vindicating significant back-and-forth in development and contemporary challenges to vaccination (Hamdulay et al., 2024).

Importance of Vaccination in Public Health

Vaccination is a public health mainstay with outstanding advantages extending beyond personal protection to provide immunity to communities. Passages from the past through immunization demonstrate its capability for infectious disease prevention; smallpox eradication is the greatest triumph of immunization efforts, for example. In quantifying current challenges like the COVID-19 pandemic, we know that vaccine equity is of importance in upholding global health standards. The policymakers will have to grapple with the issues of cost-based vaccine systems, considering their impact on vaccine equity and public health policies (Wong et al., 2024). In addition, vaccines for children are especially pertinent as they cut morbidity and mortality due to preventable infections substantially, thus improving the productivity and schooling of society (Dobriyal et al., 2024). Finally, creating a culture of vaccination through education and availability programs of public health has to be done in an attempt to reverse misinformation and achieve long-term public health success (Figure 9.3).

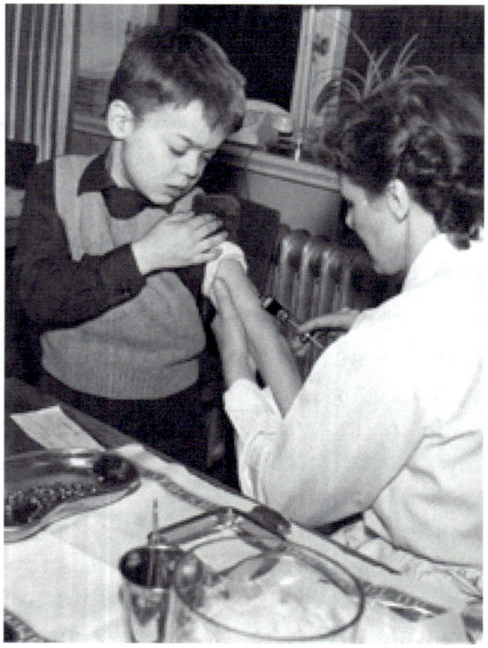

Figure 9.3. The importance of vaccinations protecting your health and community.

Source: By Ingemar Berling/Pressens Bild (Press photo) - http://pensionaren.pro.se/default.asp?a=2&lngItemID=3383, Public Domain, https://commons.wikimedia.org/w/index.php?curid=6040474

Overview of Vaccine Types

Vaccines are important in public health, and knowledge of the different types is key to understanding their advantages and uses. Generally, vaccines fall into live-attenuated, inactivated, subunit, and mRNA vaccines. Live-attenuated vaccines have weakened versions of the pathogen, which induce a robust immune response, like the measles, mumps, and rubella (MMR) vaccine. Conversely, inactivated vaccines utilize killed pathogens to elicit immunity, as in the case of the polio vaccine.

Subunit vaccines include particular fragments of the virus or bacterium, for example, proteins, that assist in the development of immunity without employing the live pathogen, whereas mRNA vaccines, such as the COVID-19 vaccines, employ genetic material to tell cells to make antigens that stimulate an immune response. Knowledge of these various types of vaccines is essential, particularly in light of current assessment of candidates under development, as emphasized in wider immunologic investigations (Cancellieri et al., 2020; Ricci et al., 2013) (Figure 9.4).

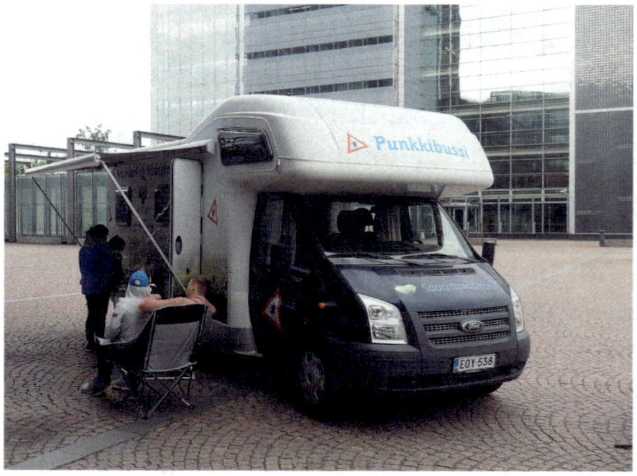

Figure 9.4. Types of vaccines.

Source: By JIP - Own work, CC BY-SA 4.0, https://commons.wikimedia.org/w/index.php?curid=92036727

Current Vaccination Rates Globally

The global rate of vaccination today offers a mixed picture, both in terms of success and shattering setbacks. While coverage has increased in the majority of regions, the COVID-19 pandemic, for example, has worked against immunization in much of the vulnerable world. Particularly, DTP (Diphtheria, Tetanus, Pertussis) vaccination coverage data has consistently risen by 1.2% between the years 2012 and 2021 in Africa; however, a fall of 3.5% between the years 2019 and 2021 was experienced in most Sub-Saharan countries, capturing an alarming trend of falling immunization during that period of the pandemic. On the other hand, countries such as Europe have registered increases in HPV vaccination that correlate with a dramatic drop in hospitalization due to cervical cancer, which indicates the effectiveness of visionary vaccination strategies (Amodio et al., 2023). Therefore, these diverse trends highlight the urgent need for a global concerted effort to provide repeated vaccine coverage, especially in low-income settings, to provide protection to public health.

Introduction to Vaccine Hesitancy

Vaccine hesitancy is a complex blend of individual and group determinants of attitudes and decisions regarding vaccination. Hesitancy tends to arise from lack of proper information regarding vaccines, complemented by uncredible sources of information and age-old myths regarding potential side effects. For instance, studies have identified how insufficient attention from healthcare providers (HCPs) is one of the leading reasons for misunderstanding vaccine efficacy and safety, leading to fear among individuals to be vaccinated (Adamo et al., 2017). Additionally, mass concern regarding the safety and efficacy of vaccines, especially that of COVID-19, further add fuel to hesitation. It has been shown through evidence that variables such as gender, level of education, and trust in the government play an important role in the willingness to be vaccinated. All these complicated issues should be resolved by open communication and education as an important means of decreasing vaccine hesitancy and facilitating public health (Figure 9.5).

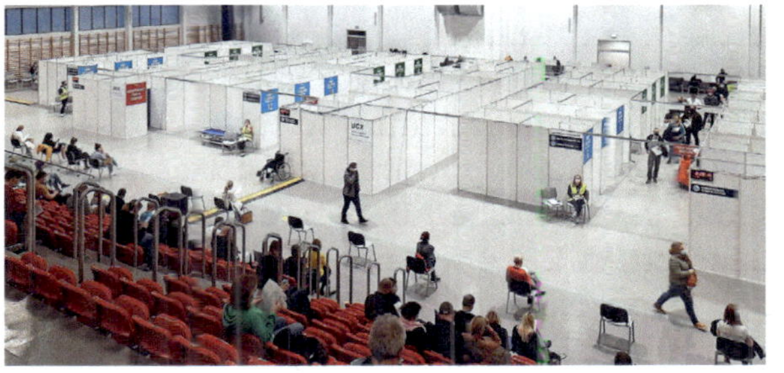

Figure 9.5. Vaccine hesitancy.

Source: By LukaszKatlewa - Own work, CC BY-SA 4.0, https://commons.wikimedia.org/w/index.php?curid=106052775

Brief Outline of Main Topics

The controversy over the vaccine includes a chain of events of utmost importance, all which correlate with public perception and health policy. Foremost among them is the evolution of vaccination over time, its inclination toward infectious disease prevention and increased public health benefit. Focus on processes used in vaccine production gives rise to scientific assessment that has to be implemented to determine safety and efficacy Secondly, the role of immunization activity in the public health policy agenda highlights the necessity of joint action by health workers, communities, and policymakers. Ethical considerations in vaccine practice such as equity of access and informed consent remain significant in contemporary health care. Finally, issues like vaccine hesitancy today have a direct implication for immunization coverage, and therefore myth-busting and trust in vaccination need to be increased. Recollection of the above broad topics provides a general impression of the diversified significance of vaccination to society as provided in most resource compendiums and academic literature (Hovi et al., 2001; Agarwal et al., 2015).

9.1. The Science Behind Vaccination

Understanding the vaccinology is crucial to addressing public resistance to immunization, and vaccines act by stimulating the immune system to recognize and counteract pathogens through an adaptive process but not causing the disease itself. This is based on the ability of the body to quickly recall antigens and mount a quicker and more efficient response to successive exposures. But persistent opposition to immunization, such as that for the HPV vaccine, points to challenges in effectively communicating scientific consensus and evidence. Evidence has identified that political orientation has a powerful impact on the reception of messages about vaccinations, most notably among self-identified Conservatives who may be more likely to be dubious of specialist lobbying (Gans et al., 2014). Also, understanding the nuances of health technology assessment and how this relates to health outcomes is essential since it informs decision-makers on the socio-economic determinants of vaccination policies (Briggs & Grieve, 2017). This is a complicated landscape that demands ongoing processes aimed at closing the science-to-people gap.

9.1.1. How Vaccines Work in the Immune System

The immune system operates through a complex network of cells and chemicals working together to defend the body against disease. Vaccines operate by mimicking exposure to a specific pathogen, prompting a response from the immune system without causing the disease.

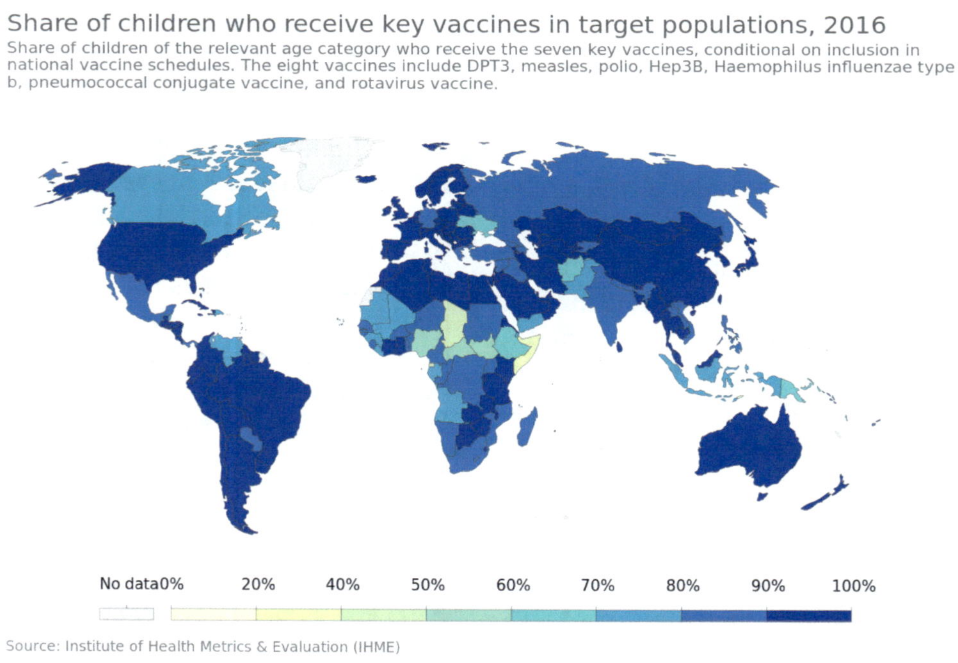

Figure 9.6. The immune system operates through a complex network of cells and substances that work together to defend the body against pathogens.

Source: By Our World In Data - https://ourworldindata.org/grapher/coverage-of-key-vaccines-sdgs, CC BY 3.0, https://commons.wikimedia.org/w/index.php?curid=86956836

This is commonly done through the use of weakened or killed versions of the pathogen, or parts of it, such as proteins. When they are vaccinated, the immune system recognizes these components as foreign and activates both the innate and adaptive immune responses. This cascade initiates the formation of memory cells that can recognize and destroy the actual pathogen when they become re-infected in the future. Furthermore, an appreciation of the role of vaccination against infection with infections like tuberculosis implies the need for more effective vaccines that utilize mucosal vaccine delivery approaches to deliver greater protection to vulnerable groups (Barclay et al., 2019). Immune senescence makes the response more problematic in older people, which underscores the need for ongoing vaccine innovation and age-related strategies (Nainu et al., 2025) (Figure 9.6).

9.1.2. Types of Vaccines: Live, Inactivated, and mRNA

The vaccination landscape has dramatically changed with the advent of different types of vaccines, i.e., live attenuated, inactivated, and mRNA vaccines. Weakened pathogens are used in live attenuated vaccines, which induce a strong immunity without leading to the disease and frequently result in long-term immunity through cellular and humoral means. On the other hand, inactivated vaccines employ killed pathogens, which are safer but less effective at times, as they do not induce strong cellular immunity relative to the live version. The latest breakthroughs introduced mRNA vaccines, which utilize genetic material to tell cells to make antigens, which lead to a specific immune response. As seen through the quick rollout of COVID-19 vaccines, which include those based on mRNA technology, these technologies show promise to generate immediate and potent protection against emergent infectious diseases, highlighting their importance in public health (Glezen et al., 2016; Masrar et al., 2021).

9.1.3. The Role of Adjuvants in Vaccines

The inclusion of adjuvants in vaccines is of major relevance in enhancing immune responses, particularly among the immunosenescent, i.e., the elderly. Since older bodies have challenges mounting an appropriate immune response, adjuvants can cause local inflammation, thereby enhancing the efficacy of vaccinations. Current research points out that those traditional methods of boosting immunogenicity, e.g., increased vaccine doses, are relatively ineffective compared to the methods that involve adjuvants. For instance, studies have revealed that different adjuvants can facilitate T follicular helper (Tfh) cell differentiation, which is an important factor in generating protective antibody responses. GLA-SE adjuvanted malaria vaccine increased Tfh cells substantially in clinical trials and again underscores the utility of tailored adjuvant formulations in immunization campaigns. Last but not least, as we continue to explore the complex interplay between vaccine-induced immunity and immune aging, adjuvants will be among the principal determinants of the best immunization outcomes in different populations (Hill et al., 2019; Pereira et al., 2020).

9.1.4. Vaccine Development Process

The vaccine development process is a multifaceted and crucial process involving much research and regulatory oversight to ensure safety and effectiveness. It usually begins with preclinical research, during which potential vaccine candidates are examined in laboratory and animal trials to assess their immune function. After successful preclinical results, candidates progress into clinical trials, which comprise three main phases increasingly involving human participants. Phase I deals with safety and dosing, then Phase II to evaluate immunogenicity and side effects, eventually leading to Phase III, where the vaccine is evaluated in a larger population for efficacy.

The process also involves co-ordination between scientists, healthcare providers, and regulatory agencies to manage the subtleties of varied public health needs. For instance, as during the COVID-19 pandemic, various nations, including Malaysia, initiated mass vaccination very early on to aid public health during the pandemic, emphasizing the urgency for effective vaccine development (Hamzah et al., 2021; Khindri, 2022) (Figure 9.7).

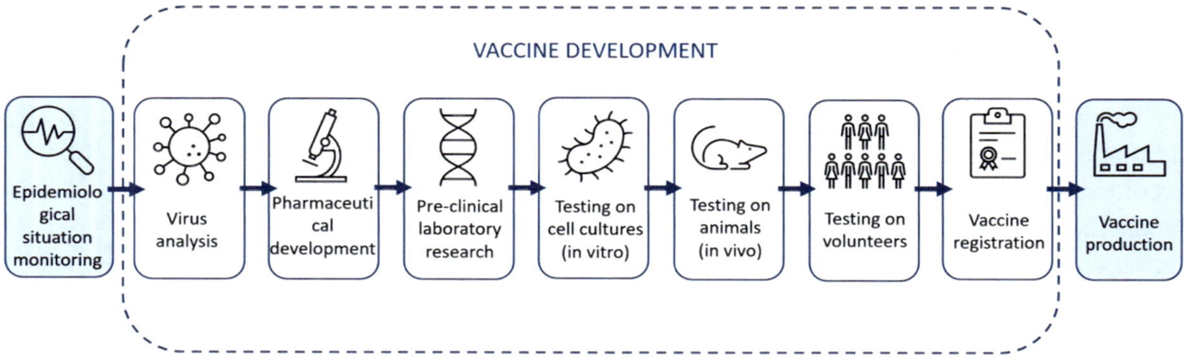

Figure 9.7. Vaccine development process.

Source: Ilin, I., Levina, A., & Kasyanov, I. (2022). Innovative ecosystem model of vaccine lifecycle management. *Journal of Open Innovation: Technology, Market, and Complexity. 85, Article 5.*

9.1.5. Clinical Trials and Safety Testing

Stringent clinical trials and safety testing are paramount in vaccine development, with guaranteed efficacy and public confidence. Any vaccine can only move through drawn-out phases of trials before being made available on the market, where its immunogenicity and safety profile are confirmed in various populations.

This systematic process is not only required for the identification of possible adverse effects but also for the establishment of the proper dosage and mode of administration. As indicated by the case of public health crisis like the outbreak of Zika virus, these trials have to straddle both regulatory and ethical environments that accommodate equilibrium between the right to health of an individual and the greater interests of society (Halabi et al., 2017). In addition, advancements in vaccine manufacturing as well as regulatory environments have also made the process easier while adhering to safety procedures. This cross-disciplinary analysis of vaccine manufacturing and regulation uncovered the quintessential place that clinical testing has in a responsively and effectively tackling diseases (Byrn et al., 2023).

9.1.6. Herd Immunity and Its Significance

Herd immunity is a pillar of public health, greatly reducing the incidence of vaccine-preventable diseases (VPDs) within a population. If a large majority of people are vaccinated, it indirectly affords protection to those who cannot be immunized for medical reasons, for example, allergies or poor immune function, thus acting as a buffer against disease transmission. This has been deeply exemplified by the success of laws such as California Assembly Bill 2109 (AB 2109) that sought to inform parents about vaccine safety and VPDs due to increasing personal belief exemptions (Goishi-Bessey et al., 2016).

The importance of having high vaccination levels goes beyond personal protection; it helps in overall societal health, lowering outbreaks and related healthcare expenditure. For example, the Centers for Disease Control and Prevention reports that the flu alone causes millions of illnesses each year, highlighting the importance of strong vaccination efforts to block widespread outbreaks and safeguard community health (Coburn et al., 2018) (Figure 9.8).

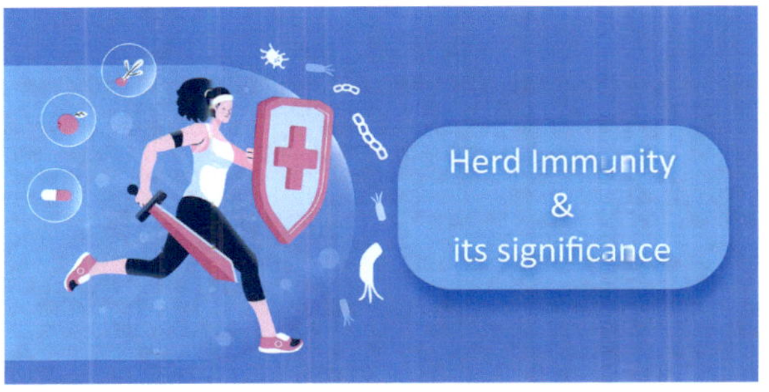

Figure 9.8. Herd immunity and its significance.

Source: Miracles Health. (2020). *Herd Immunity and Its Significance.*

9.1.7. The Impact of Vaccines on Disease Eradication

The development of vaccines has changed the course of public health history and, on the whole, is credited with the eradication of infectious diseases. One of the greatest success tales of such achievement is the worldwide eradication of smallpox, evidence of the success of mass vaccination campaigns to the World Health Organization (WHO) declaration of the disease eradicated in 1980. Such is an indication of the capability of vaccines to eradicate diseases that have afflicted man for centuries. But the disease discussion merely more vividly outlines an even more complicated world; as in recent quantitative models, optimum planning allows eradication by a planner, but monopolistic prices to treatment generally bar access and effectiveness (Coburn et al., 2018). Hence, where economics and vaccination policy overlap brings to the fore the significance of adopting a multi-pronged approach to eradicating diseases in that it stresses how success in public health is dependent upon effective vaccine development and equal methods of distribution.

9.1.8. The Role of the World Health Organization (WHO) in Vaccination

The WHO is of central importance in coordinating global vaccine efforts directed at preventing large-scale infectious disease outbreaks. Through worldwide surveillance networks and programmatic initiatives like the Global Polio Eradication Initiative, the WHO coordinates with nations to track polio cases, conduct vaccination campaigns, and leverage technological innovations like the AFRO GIS to quickly gather and analyze data (Kipterer et al., 2024). In addition, the WHOs recent classification of Noma as a neglected tropical disease reinforces its efforts toward bridging health inequalities and promoting vaccination in marginalized groups, specifically children in sub-Saharan Africa (Satapathy et al., 2024). By giving priority to fair access to vaccines and supporting strong immunization programs, the WHO not only fights current health emergencies but also enhances global health systems in the end with a view to protecting public health and averting future epidemics on a global level (Figure 9.9).

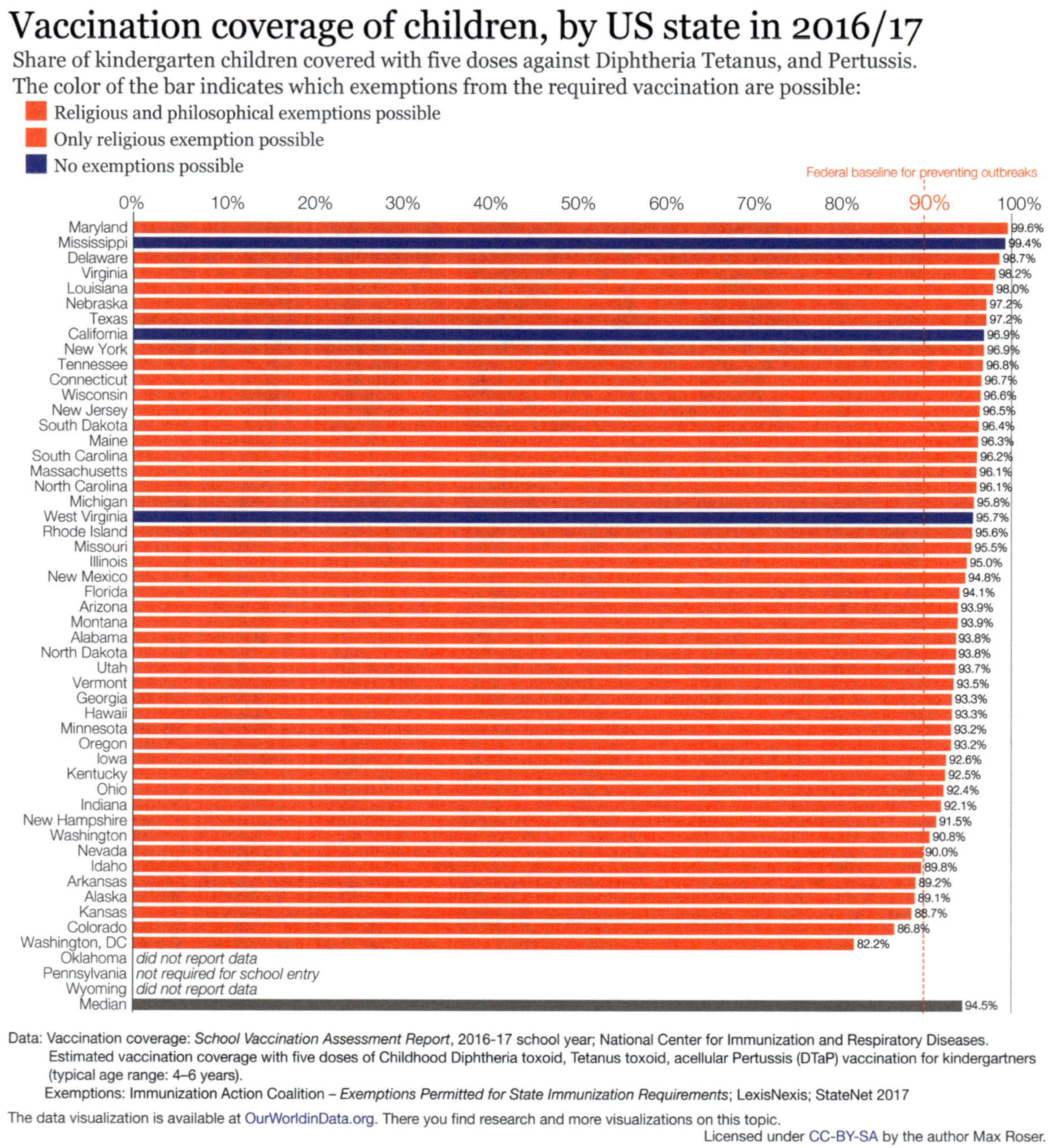

Figure 9.9. The role of the world health organization (WHO) in vaccination.

Source: By National Center for Immunization and Respiratory Diseases - https://ourworldindata.org/vaccination, CC BY 4.0, https://commons.wikimedia.org/w/index.php?curid=77613727

9.1.9. Future Advancements in Vaccine Technology

As vaccine technology continues to evolve, future developments will seek to improve the safety and effectiveness of vaccinations, ultimately solving future public health issues. Technologies like mRNA have already shown great potential, especially in fighting diseases like COVID-19, showing how quick development can address immediate health emergencies (Lain et al., 2020). In addition, the combination of synthetic biology methods would transform the design of vaccines, allowing for the development of more specific and powerful immunizations. The technologies also show promise against pathogens with multidrug resistance, as conventional antibiotics lose efficacy (Uddin et al., 2021). Highlighting the need for public acceptance and confidence, the effectiveness of these developments will hinge on transparent communication of how safe and effective they are. With each passing day, we use scientific advancements at a growing rate, and the future of vaccination can depend on not just technological advancement but also a collective effort to effectively involve the community in vaccination campaigns.

9.2. Benefits of Vaccination

The benefits of vaccination extend far beyond, contributing greatly to public health security and community immunity. Vaccines have critical roles to play in the prevention of infectious disease transmission, thereby safeguarding vulnerable groups of persons who are unable to receive vaccinations themselves due to existing health conditions. For instance, those suffering from chronic diseases, e.g., cancer or diabetes, exhibit higher susceptibility to severe outcomes of infections like COVID-19 and thus highlights the importance of widespread vaccination among such groups (Choi et al., 2023). In addition, historical data from pandemic influenza programs indicate the effectiveness of vaccination in eradicating hospitalization and reducing severity of illness in the overall population, for example, in Sweden during 2010/11 when monovalent vaccine significantly decreased deaths due to influenza (Widgren et al., 2013). In totality, these results highlight vaccination as a critical public health intervention in the sustenance of public health and prevention of disease outbreak (Figure 9.10).

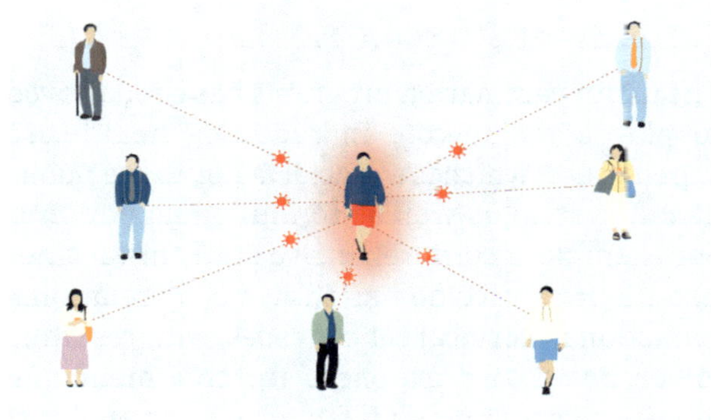

Figure 9.10. The benefits of vaccination extend far beyond individual health.

Source: European Vaccination Information Portal. (n.d.) *Mumps*.

9.2.1. Prevention of Infectious Diseases

Successful prevention of infectious diseases is greatly dependent on mass vaccination efforts that are specifically directed toward heterogeneous populations. Nations have come up with various mechanisms for providing immunization to vulnerable groups like migrants, who prove to experience health inequalities based on their status. For example, eight nations vaccinate all the vaccines in their national immunization program for migrant children, while others vaccinate some with emphasis on diseases like polio and measles (Declich et al.,

2017). Secondly, those with pre-existing medical conditions, like patients who have systemic sclerosis, are easily prone to infection and need specially formulated vaccines to be made immune from the prevalent pathogens (Benfaremo et al., 2021). Even after immunization improvement, there are still delivery gaps and access that need to be addressed by continuous research and cross-border coordination to ensure effective vaccination programs. These measures can be worth implementing to avert the transmission of infectious diseases and safeguard public health globally.

9.2.2. Reduction in Healthcare Costs

The use of vaccination programs has been proved to play a major role in reducing healthcare expenditure, which is a crucial factor to the public health system as well as to individual patients. For example, a comprehensive study of vaccines like the HPV vaccine has shown a correlational reduction in cervical cancer cases, with resulting lower healthcare expenses for treatment and long-term care among infected women (Babu et al., 2024). Similarly, the evidence for COVID-19 vaccinations also shows a significant decrease in hospitalizations and emergency department visits, resulting in diminished overall healthcare use and cost during the Omicron period (Pierre et al., 2023). These results highlight the cost savings associated with preventive care with vaccinations, where not only are improved health benefits seen but also where the financial cost to the healthcare system is diminished. In the end, investment in vaccination programs becomes an important measure toward fostering public health as well as decreasing the overall cost of healthcare.

9.2.3. Economic Benefits of Widespread Vaccination

Mass immunization not only decreases infectious disease transmission but also yields significant economic benefits to the individual and society. By lowering disease cases, immunizations lower healthcare costs by reducing hospitalization and medical interventions, which become extremely costly during epidemics. Further, a healthier population translates into higher productivity as individuals lose fewer workdays, thereby sustaining economic performance. The economic importance is most pertinent in low-income settings where the disease burden then ceases to be a problem of health but rather becomes a barrier to economic development. For instance, prevention of large diseases can avert large future healthcare expenses that the WHO asserts will amount to astonishing national health system savings. In general, the investment in immunization campaigns is not only justified for the improvement of health outcomes but also to facilitate robust economic growth and stability, which is in line with research that identifies the interconnectedness between health and economic policy (Howard et al., 2021; Bray et al., 2024).

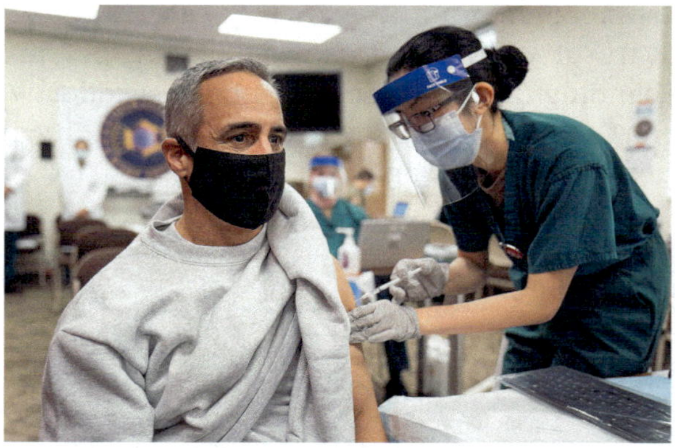

Source: By Chairman of the Joint Chiefs of Staff from Washington D.C, United States - 201221-D-WD757-1126, CC BY 2.0, https://commons.wikimedia.org/w/index.php?curid=97947808

9.2.4. Protection of Vulnerable Populations

Vaccination of vulnerable groups is an essential part of the vaccination process, especially to ensure equitable access to medical care.

Vulnerable groups like migrants and the poor do not have access to the vaccine in general, thereby increasing vulnerability to VPDs. These groups must be incorporated using strategies to gain utmost coverage of vaccinations to vaccinate a larger portion of the populations and gain herd immunity. For example, 2023 EUROGIN workshop findings highlighted the requirement for outreach programs in the most vulnerable populations and to extend catch-up immunization programs to enhance defense against human papillomavirus (HPV) and cervical cancer. Besides, lessons of hepatitis B immunization campaigns highlighted the applicability of the focal point approach to target marginal groups in an effort to achieve elimination goals. Thus, the consideration of these factors in immunization policy can maximize public health benefit and make sure that everybody, irrespective of their background, has access to immunization programs (Baussano et al., 2024; Pourbohloul et al., 2006).

9.2.5. Contribution to Global Health Security

The contribution that vaccination can make to global health security cannot be overemphasized with the current situation of the world facing the re-emergence of infectious diseases as well as the re-emergence of new pathogens. Vaccination programs have long been vital in restricting the spread of diseases, thereby not only creating individual immunity but also herd immunity that protects communities as a whole. This is especially crucial in low-resource settings where health infrastructure is expected to be lacking enough to contain outbreaks. Furthermore, the integration of improved epidemiological strategies, as highlighted in current research, allows improved surveillance and intervention responses to confront emerging health issues (Lewnard & Reingold, 2019). With the application of inter-disciplinary knowledge and advanced frameworks, such as those being pursued by agricultural research centers, the world can be more capable of reacting to public health crises. Vaccination, therefore, emerges as a cornerstone of global health security creating a safer and healthier world for future generations (Eijsackers et al., 2011).

9.2.6. Long-Term Health Benefits for Individuals

The long-term health consequence of vaccination is far beyond the instantaneous prevention of disease, and they have a significant influence on the health status of individuals in the long term.

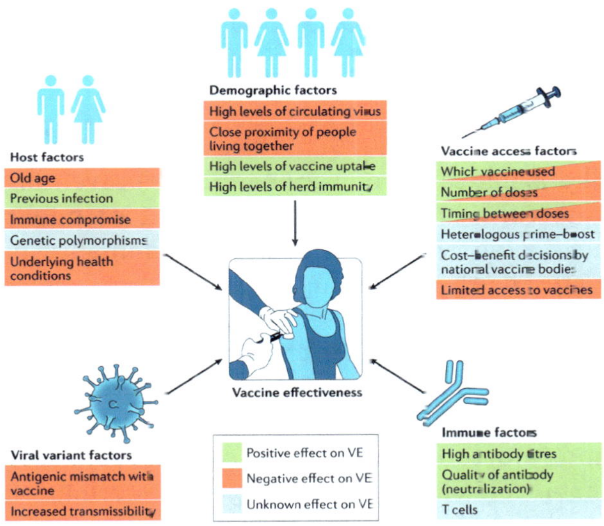

Figure 9.11. Long-term health benefits for individuals.

Source: Tregoning, J. S., Flight, K. E., Higham, S. L., Wang, Z., & Pierce, B. F. (2021). Progress of the COVID-19 vaccine effort: Viruses, vaccines and variants versus efficacy, effectiveness, and escape. *Nature Reviews Immunology, 21*, 626–636.

For instance, the widespread application of HPV vaccination is extremely important because it can reduce the occurrence of severe infections and their related cancers in both men and women. Studies indicate that the broadening of HPV immunization to men would reduce incidence by half, making its role in public health significant (Rongioletti et al., 2024). Secondly, the measles virus vaccination illustrates profound effects on overall health; research indicates that eliminating the virus not only enhances current health outcomes but also enhances educational and economic opportunities years later. In Mexico, for example, the measles vaccine has helped in generating employment and income, demonstrating its far-reaching effect on public health (Atwood et al., 2023). Vaccination is thus a keystone strategy in attaining long-term health benefits for individuals in various populations (Figure 9.11).

9.2.7. Role in Controlling Outbreaks

The significance of vaccination in preventing outbreaks cannot be overstated, as it is a public health intervention that has the influence of significantly curtailing the transmission of infectious diseases. Mathematical modeling has shown that strategic vaccination strategies, including pulse or constant vaccination, can have a significant impact on morbidities and mortalities during an outbreak. For instance, when the coverage of vaccination reaches 50%, pulse vaccination strategies can prevent approximately 45.61% of fatalities, demonstrating the impact of timely vaccination programs to prevent disease spread (Bolatova et al., 2024).

Additionally, in the case of emergent diseases such as human monkeypox, vaccination comes into play in preventing outbreaks, especially following the eradication of smallpox, leaving populations susceptible to associated viral threats (Maqbool et al., 2024). The use of vaccination strategies is therefore a preventive strategy as well as a proactive approach to combat emerging and re-emerging infectious diseases, ultimately protecting the health of the people and building community resilience.

9.2.8. Psychological Benefits of Vaccination

The psychological advantages of immunization reach far beyond the immunity it provides, having a significant effect on the mental health of individuals and communities. Immunization has the ability to reduce the widespread fear of contracting infectious diseases, allowing people to go about daily life with increased confidence. As parents observe the favorable consequences of immunization, e.g., low incidence of disease among children, they tend to feel empowered and more capable of controlling their family's health, which might improve parenting efficacy and satisfaction. Also, community vaccination activities promote a sense of shared responsibility and togetherness, which leads to social cohesion. As supported by research on parental education about flu vaccination, greater awareness of vaccines corresponds with greater immunization coverage, leading to the expectation that aware individuals are more likely to adopt immunization as a preventive measure for their own and their relatives' well-being (Chughtai & Chughtai, 2022). These programs eventually translate to a strong public health view, supporting the psychological benefits of taking part in vaccination programs (Alogaily et al., 2022).

9.2.9. Case Studies of Successful Vaccination Programs

The analysis of effective vaccination programs in different settings shows a common thread: the paramount role of strategic planning and community outreach. For example, programs in nations like Rwanda have shown how focused vaccination campaigns can significantly lower infectious diseases, thus enhancing public health outcomes. These programs highlight not just the necessity of mass vaccine distribution but also the importance of education in addressing vaccine hesitancy. Furthermore, results of a systematic review of COVID-19 vaccination suggest that indirect protection is just as important as direct immunity, showing the success of the program in lowering the rates of transmission among both vaccinated and non-vaccinated populations (Oordt-Speets et al., 2023). High-quality metrics in tracking progress, as observed in many case studies, support the importance of reflective practice in public health interventions, implying that responsive and locally relevant approaches may improve general effectiveness (Naz et al., 2024).

9.3. Vaccine Hesitancy and Misinformation

Vaccine hesitancy is a multifaceted public health issue, mostly fueled by the widespread dissemination of misinformation, especially on social media. Hesitancy is not homogeneous; it may take on highly diverse forms across various demographic sections, based on cultural beliefs and access to credible information.

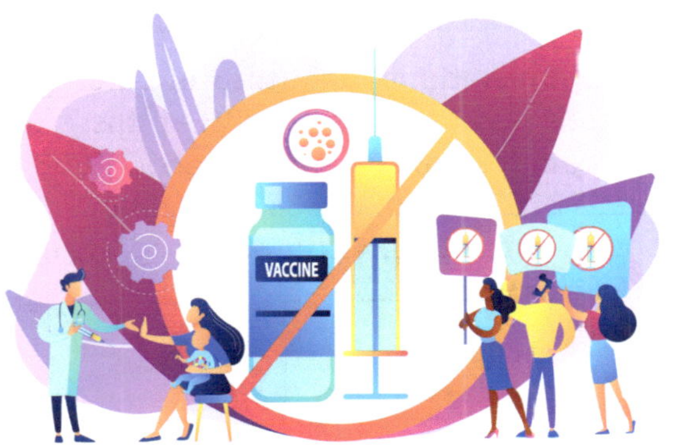

Figure 9.12. Vaccine hesitancy and misinformation.

Source: Net Vector. (n.d.). Antivaccination protest, people rejecting preventive medicine. *Shutterstock.*

Research shows that those who feel that they are healthy tend to be influenced by overstated information about vaccine side effects, and thus think that vaccination risks are greater than the risks of the diseases themselves. As an example, misinformation about fertility has significantly influenced women's choices about COVID-19 vaccinations, highlighting the importance of certain targeted public health communication to reduce these fears (Kostkova et al., 2022). In addition, the mistrust in health systems and information sources remains a major correlate of vaccine hesitancy and indicates that such interventions need to account for context-specific subtleties and efforts toward restoring communities' trust (Bliuc et al., 2021) (Figure 9.12).

9.3.1. Definition and Causes of Vaccine Hesitancy

Vaccine hesitancy is now increasingly identified as a major public health issue that undermines efforts to attain mass immunization. As reluctance or refusal to be vaccinated despite the existence of vaccines, this occurs due to many reasons such as fear of vaccine safety, effectiveness, and misinformation.

Studies have shown that expectant mothers, for example, will recognize the value of vaccinations for their offspring but also have misconceptions that contribute to lower confidence in the immunization procedure (Baccolini et al., 2020). Moreover, social pressures and digital media intensify this reluctance, whereby misinformation against vaccines is more emotionally attractive than pro-vaccine messages, which are thus more likely to be shared (McGee et al., 2020). It is essential to address these fears through appropriate communication tactics in turning reluctance into acceptance, highlighting the importance of healthcare professionals communicating with reluctant individuals compassionately to guide them into making well-informed vaccination decisions.

9.3.2. The Role of Social Media in Spreading Misinformation

The advent of social media has revolutionized the public health communications landscape, with special reference to immunization campaigns. While Facebook and Twitter have emerged as primary sources of information, they also act as channels of misinformation. There are countless examples where false information about vaccines has spread on the web, and the public health consequences have been staggering. For instance, during the Pakistan polio immunization campaigns, unsubstantiated rumors about side effects of the vaccine spread quickly across social media channels, eroding confidence in public health institutions and fueling refusals of vaccines (Ittefaq et al., 2024). Likewise, the pandemic situation during the COVID-19 outbreak demonstrated how social media amplified both correct health information and misinformation, making it difficult to have a public response to vaccination drives (Ngoma et al., 2024). This twofold responsibility highlights the need for public health agencies to act on social media in a calculated manner, ensuring digital literacy and disseminating accurate information to neutralize the wide-ranging spread of misinformation.

9.3.3. Historical Examples of Vaccine Hesitancy

Vaccine skepticism has existed in many forms throughout history, indicative of entrenched societal anxiety and opposition to immunization routines. The Victorian period is a deep reflection, the resistance to compulsory smallpox vaccination after the 1853 Vaccination Act being a great example, which shows mass anger against forced medical procedures. This time witnessed the growth of a large corpus of anti-vaccination texts, summarized in the Victorian Anti-Vaccination Discourse Corpus (VicVaDis), consisting of 133 pamphlets between 1854 and 1906. The language used in these works not only raised concerns regarding vaccinations safety and effectiveness but also provoked discussions regarding individual freedom and state control (Coltman-Patel et al., 2023). Additionally, recent research finds that such feelings continue to exist, as experienced during the COVID-19 pandemic, where vaccine talks became controversial, especially in ethnic minority groups, echoing past distrust toward health organizations and communication processes (Martin et al., 2024). Such historical instances prove the long-standing nature of vaccine reluctance and its intricate interaction with socio-cultural factors.

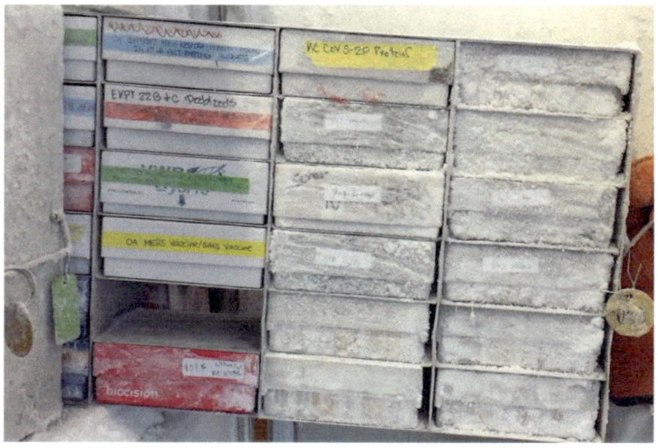

Source: By National Institute of Allergy and Infectious Diseases (NIAID), NIH - https://www.flickr.com/photos/niaid/49465177603/in/album-72157629102873393/, Public Domain, https://commons.wikimedia.org/w/index.php?curid=98227212

9.3.4. Psychological Factors Influencing Vaccine Acceptance

It is important to understand the psychological drivers of vaccine uptake in establishing effective public health interventions. Beliefs and emotions of individuals tend to play a great role in their acceptance of vaccines. According to literature, lack of knowledge and negative emotions have been found to play a great barrier against uptake, showing that individuals with low awareness or misinformation regarding vaccine safety and effectiveness tend to be more resistant to vaccination campaigns (Songthap et al., 2012). Besides, social factors, including peer attitudes and cultural beliefs, may provide a setting in which vaccine hesitancy can thrive. More so, research on Italian adults indicates the role of psychological factors in that people with a conspiracy mindset and those who experienced a violation of fundamental beliefs amid the pandemic showed heightened vaccine hesitancy (Barazzetti et al., 2024). This calls attention to the need for psychological and social considerations in vaccine communication campaigns to promote acceptance and eventually improve public health results.

9.3.5. Strategies to Combat Misinformation

To combat misinformation on vaccination, winning strategies have to be strong, holistic, and community-based to increase public trust and participation. Initiatives like the CDCs Partnering for Vaccine Equity (P4VE) have shown success in channeling funds toward national and local entities that foster vaccine confidence and respond to access barriers, especially among vulnerable populations (Taylor et al., 2023). In parallel, studies emphasizing the need-to-know community-level misinformation patterns ascertaining the value of context-specific interventions following comprehensive needs assessments underscores the value of adapting messaging according to cultural and social contexts of their recipients with the help of data from expansive social media monitoring projects and feedback from communities to enable better communication (Cohen et al., 2023). Such an approach not only enlightens people with authentic information but also prepares a socially responsible climate in which public health campaigns can thrive, ultimately improving vaccine uptake and community health outcomes.

9.3.6. Importance of Community Engagement

Community involvement plays a central part in boosting vaccine coverage, especially amid vaccine hesitancy and access problems. Through participation of citizens in vaccination programs, local health agencies can more easily grasp and resolve individual concerns and cultural factors behind influencing public perceptions toward vaccines. Quality community involvement helps to build confidence and openness, which are imperative in mitigating concerns about vaccine safety and performance. For example, in Nepal, Senegal, and Zambia, effective governance and community-based programs markedly raised immunization levels by aligning vaccination programs with local demands and insights (Sakas et al., 2022). Moreover, context-specific communication strategies that include community leaders help to reach vaccine-hesitant populations, thereby ultimately increasing vaccine acceptance and eliminating misinformation (Tuckerman et al., 2022). Therefore, the prioritization of community participation in vaccination activities not only is an effective mobilization of resources but also creates a well-informed population, translating into better health outcomes for populations

9.3.7. Role of Healthcare Professionals (HCPs) in Addressing Concerns

HCPs are important to handle concerns about vaccinations, especially with increased vaccine hesitancy among parents and communities. With their competence, they can give correct information regarding the advantages and disadvantages of vaccines, as shown in research suggesting that parental decisions to give childhood vaccinations are highly influenced by perceptions of vaccine risk (Leder et al., 2015). By clearly conveying the significance of immunization, healthcare professionals can dispel misconceptions and myths about vaccines. Studies indicate that trust in HCPs and information obtained from them, e.g., general practitioners, has a positive relationship with the decrease in vaccine-related misconceptions (Bert et al., 2020). Thus, improving healthcare professionals' communication skills and building trust among communities are critical measures to boost vaccination rates and enhance public health outcomes. Finally, the role of HCPs is not limited to the simple administration of vaccines but also includes informing and reassuring concerned population groups to facilitate well-informed decision-making regarding immunization.

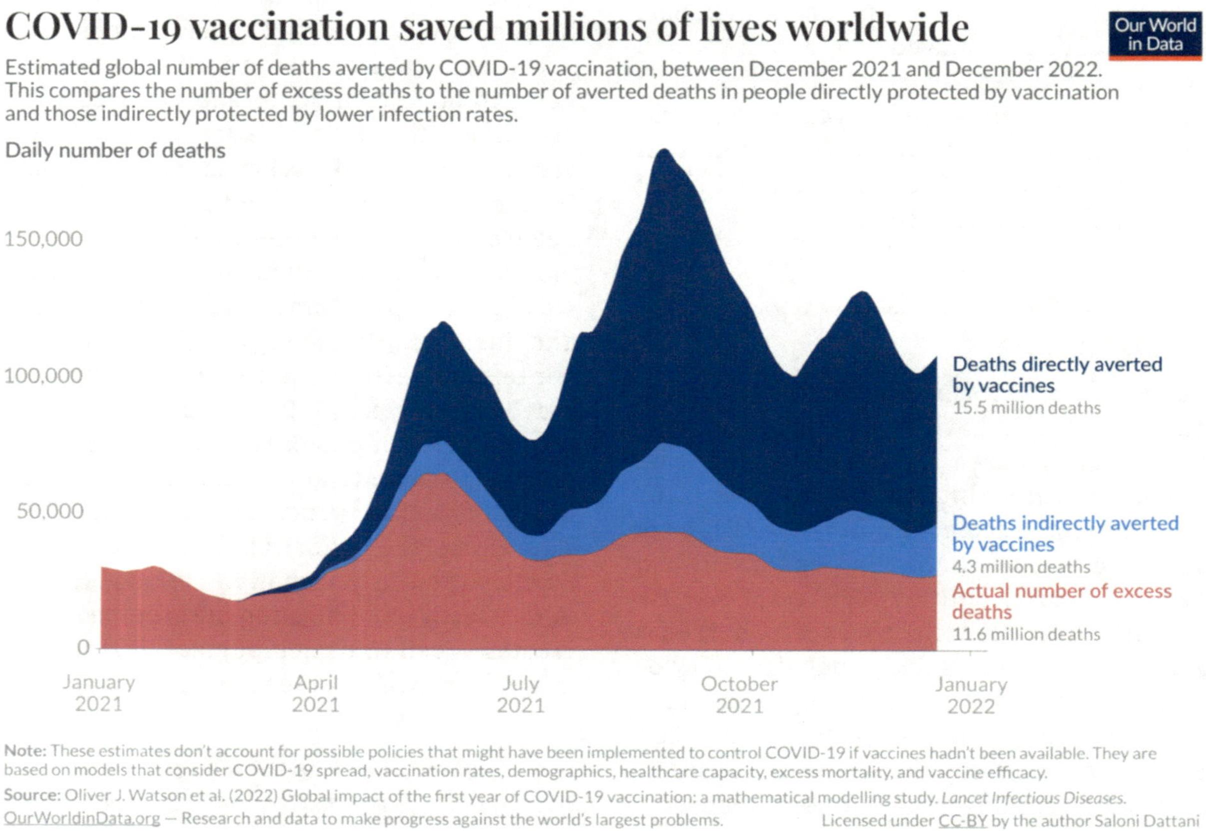

Source: By Saloni Dattani and Lucas Rodés-Guirao - https://ourworldindata.org/key-charts-understand-covid-pandemic, CC BY 4.0, https://commons.wikimedia.org/w/index.php?curid=155869825

9.3.8. Government Policies to Promote Vaccination

To successfully promote vaccination, governments have put in place various policies that seek to raise public awareness and accessibility. Such efforts usually include public health campaigns that inform citizens of the advantages of vaccination, thus combating vaccine hesitancy and misinformation. For example, the creation of specialized units within health authorities, like the new Coronavirus and other Respiratory Viruses Division, represents a strategic move to boost vaccination in times of public health emergencies. In addition, certain policies take on social measures designed to encourage community participation, using strategies that take advantage of feelings of social obligation among parents to promote child immunization (Wiley et al., 2017). By integrating education outreach with community-based projects, these government policies promote not only increased vaccination rates but also help to establish a sustained public confidence in health systems that is absolutely essential for efficient disease prevention.

9.3.9. Case Studies of Successful Interventions

Reviewing case studies on successful interventions indicates the strong influence of vaccination strategies on public health outcomes. One notable example is the international effort against pandemic influenza, whereby nations with strong preparedness plans managed to successfully contain outbreaks. The research suggests that successful containment of moderately infectious viral strains is possible through proper planning and resource input, and that a mix of policies can ward off the spread of more infectious types. In particular, the probability of success of containment in first-line risk nations is increased by propitious conditions, emphasizing the need for interventions customized according to context. In addition, the eradication of Rinderpest by vaccination not only improved livestock health but also served to enhance food security among millions, demonstrating the wider implications of immunization campaigns in human and animal populations (Dutta, 2008). Such cases reinforce the crucial function vaccinations serve in disease control, hence emphasizing the necessity for continued investment in vaccine development and dissemination.

9.4. Ethical and Legal Considerations

Ethical and legal concerns about vaccination are key to the formulation of effective public health policy. At the center of this discussion is the balancing of individual freedom versus the societal obligation to safeguard public health. With declining rates of vaccination, policies tend to incorporate mandates that require vaccination, presenting ethical issues related to informed consent and individual liberty. This emphasizes the importance of transparency in communication policy, as citizens need to have faith that information communicated is true and understandable, enabling informed choice. In addition, the equitable allocation of vaccines among various groups brings with it considerable moral challenges, especially in responding to disparities between developed and developing countries (Ogugua et al., 2024). Legal frameworks, in turn, need to evolve to accommodate these nuances so that strict compliance with public health policies does not impinge on individual rights. It is with this understanding that policymakers must walk in the complex world of vaccination strategies (Figure 9.13).

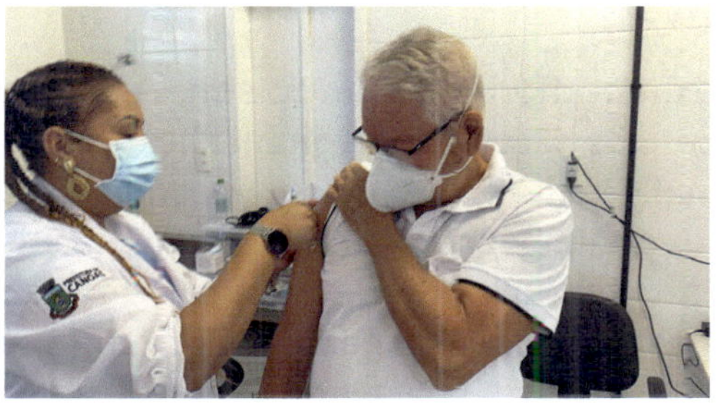

Figure 9.13. The ethical and legal considerations.

Source: By Eduardo Gerhardt Martins - Own work, CC BY-SA 4.0, https://commons.wikimedia.org/w/index php?curid=105119887

9.4.1. Informed Consent in Vaccination

The phenomenon of informed consent is central to the discussion regarding vaccination so that individuals are well informed prior to receiving any vaccine. The process needs proper communication regarding the advantages and disadvantages of vaccinations for fostering autonomy and trust between patients and healthcare providers. For example, in research assessing the safety and effectiveness of new interventions, including newborn administration of azithromycin, ethical concerns related to informed consent are critical to safeguard vulnerable groups (Bagagnan et al., 2019). In addition, knowledge of the wider social contexts affecting vaccination uptake, for example, religion, political ideology, and education policy, can improve informed consent procedures. HPV vaccine research suggests that identification of individual and macro-level variables can empower patients in making health-related decisions (Brownson et al., 2019). Therefore, informed consent not only honors individual rights but is also an essential tool in public health promotion through the delivery of efficient vaccination strategies.

9.4.2. Mandatory Vaccination Policies

Implementation of compulsory vaccination policies has become a key public health strategy, especially in the prevention of infectious diseases such as meningococcal disease and mitigation of risks posed by high-density settings, for example, mass gatherings. The policies not only seek to drive up vaccination coverage but also to create herd immunity, thus safeguarding susceptible persons. For example, in environments such as the Hajj pilgrimage, where large numbers of people gather, enforced vaccinations are essential to averting outbreaks that may pose widespread health consequences. Additionally, research indicates that such measures go a long way in curbing rates of transmission in communities, demonstrating their effectiveness in protecting public health. Nonetheless, as much as mandatory vaccination can have beneficial effects, issues like vaccine hesitancy and access inequities need to be addressed to provide equal health benefits to all groups. Hence, continued efforts to address the balance between public safety and individual rights are critical to the debate on mandatory vaccination.

9.4.3. Ethical Implications of Vaccine Distribution

The ethical considerations of vaccine distribution are complex, often overlapping public health interests with social justice principles. Central to the controversy is fair access to vaccines, especially for vulnerable groups who might face systemic barriers to care.

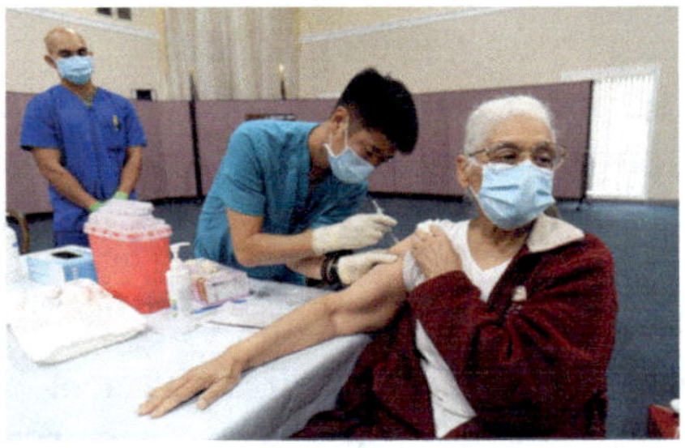

Figure 9.14. Ethical implications of vaccine distribution.

Source: The Nation's Health. (n.d.). *Image Depicting Health-Related Content*. https://www.thenationshealth.org/content/nathealth/51/2/1.1/F1.medium.gif

The integration of vaccines into mandatory school attendance, like the national Advisory Committee on Immunization Practices (ACIP) recommendation of meningitis vaccination, highlights the importance of public health interventions in safeguarding high-risk adolescents from severe illness. But in states like Alaska, where these kinds of policies do not yet exist, the projects require advocacy shows that legislative backing and community education are necessary (Hulstine et al., 2017). In addition, successful vaccination efforts, such as those assessed in rural Kenya, show the significance of coverage among populations that would otherwise be neglected; not only do these efforts decrease disease susceptibility, but they also work to redress public health disparities more generally (Figure 9.14).

9.4.4. Equity in Access to Vaccines

The doctrine of equity in access to vaccines has become a core pillar in public health thinking, particularly brought into sharp focus by the COVID-19 pandemic. While vaccines have been identified as essential for disease prevention, inconsistencies in distribution and administration continued to be a feature, albeit further worsened by vaccine nationalism, which derailed efforts toward global health equity (Harmon et al., 2024). Mitigating this disparity requires a multi-dimensional process involving the active engagement of impacted populations and countries within international discourse, so that local needs within health systems are addressed, as well as building confidence and vaccine acceptance among varied populations (Privor-Dumm et al., 2023). There is a need not only to expand vaccine availability but also to align local health priorities into global vaccination efforts, thereby fostering an inclusive, equitable public health environment. Therefore, political will and investment over the long term are crucial in ensuring an environment where vaccine is achieved, especially in low- and middle-income countries (LMICs).

9.4.5. The Role of Pharmaceutical Companies

The contribution of pharmaceutical firms toward vaccination has been pivotal, especially in the wake of international health crises like the COVID-19 pandemic. In the wake of sudden appearance of the severe acute respiratory syndrome coronavirus 2 (SARS-CoV-2), pharmaceutical companies marshaled unprecedented resources to create vaccines. This was made possible by strong international cooperation and large-scale funding, which allowed researchers to accelerate vaccine trials and monitored mass production. By December 8, 2020, the first vaccine outside of a clinical trial was given, prompting global vaccination rollouts that eventually saved an estimated 19.8 million lives in the first year alone (Watson et al., 2022). Disparities in vaccine availability, though, reinforced the call for fair distribution, particularly in low-income nations where the shortage prevented potential gains (Chavda et al., 2022). Therefore, although the pharmaceutical industry was instrumental in responding to the pandemic, global vaccine equity is still a relevant issue.

9.4.6. Vaccine Patents and Global Access

The crossroads of vaccine patents and universal access is now more essential in confronting health inequities, especially in LMICs. Although patents aim to encourage innovation, they mostly create inflated prices for vaccines that limit access among vulnerable groups.

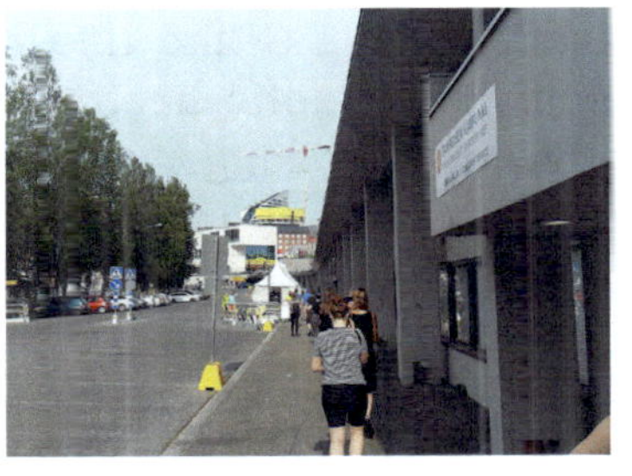

Source: By OP995 - Own work, CC BY-SA 4.0, https://commons.wikimedia.org/w/index.php?curid=106845348

For instance, uptake of the HPV vaccine, with potential to avert cervical cancer mortality, is strongly hampered in these areas by high costs and resistance on cultural grounds, as discussed in Ewongwo et al. (2024). In addition, throughout the COVID-19 pandemic, vaccine inequities were further fueled by the prioritization of patent rights over equitable distribution, leading to few vaccination centers in highly populated regions such as Los Angeles County, as documented in Aljohani et al. (2024). This reveals the pressing need for global cooperation to relax patent limitations so that life-saving vaccines become accessible to all, irrespective of socioeconomic position. Resolving these issues is crucial to meet global vaccination objectives and advance public health results.

9.4.7. Balancing Individual Rights and Public Health

The convergence of individual rights and public health has, however, become a highly complicated issue due to recent health emergencies, especially amid the Covid-19 pandemic. Governments, as a move to protect the public health, have implemented policies that tend to invade individual freedoms, thus raising questions regarding their validity. For example, Italy had enforced strict mobility controls and launched the Green Covid-19 Certificate, which not only controlled the entry to places but also impacted basic rights such as education and work. This situation is the best example of the fine line needed to be drawn between public health needs and liberties, and how the danger exists of short-term measures becoming an enduring part of governing (Pignataro et al., 2022). In addition, the theoretical approaches to healthcare justice, especially those by Ronald Dworkin, tend to fail in informing such pivotal choices during pandemics since they presuppose a falsity of harmony between general rights and common needs for healthcare (Biondo, 2023). This highlights the importance of solid deliberation processes that provide accountability and transparency during policy-making.

9.4.8. Legal Challenges Related to Vaccination Mandates

The constitutional challenges related to vaccination mandates have come up as a controversial issue, marked by a precarious equation between public health needs and individual rights. As policymakers face the challenge of imposing vaccine mandates, especially in the case of COVID-19, they need to traverse legal and ethical minefields which may trigger massive outrage. Most importantly, mandates are also seen to intrude on individual autonomy and decision-making, highlighting the problem of overreach by the state (Angus et al., 2022). Additionally, the idea of `vaccine apartheid` highlights the threat of social polarization and discrimination against non-vaccinators, muddying the waters of public health policy (Angus et al., 2022). Moreover, particular vaccine mandates, for instance, the meningitis vaccine within school attendance policies, underscore the difficulties of legislative lobbying across various jurisdictions, as indicated by lackluster responses in a few cases. These intricacies underscore the need for careful deliberation and public consultation within the creation of vaccination policy.

9.4.9. International Laws Governing Vaccination

The system of global laws that regulate vaccination is central to reconciling public health issues across borders. These laws, which are derived from both international health bodies and treaties, seek to enhance worldwide access to vaccines while guaranteeing that vaccination procedures are safe, efficient, and ethically provided. For example, the WHO has set guidelines highlighting the significance of vaccinations as a key aspect of disease prevention and public health policy. Further, changing challenges like vaccine hesitancy and the spread of misinformation require robust legal frameworks that evolve with these trends. Nations have to bring their national legislation into line with international norms, as captured in agreements that foster cooperation in the development and distribution of vaccines. Such regulation harmonization is necessary not just to fight infectious diseases but also to ensure global cooperation in a sustainable health response (Nidhi & Bala, 2024; Phuong, 2024).

CLOSER LOOK

Vaccine Hesitancy

Vaccine hesitancy is a reluctance to accept or delay the uptake of vaccines in the presence of available vaccination services. It's an intricate and context-dependent phenomenon driven by confidence, complacency, and convenience—commonly referred to as the "3 Cs."

- Confidence is about trust in the safety and efficacy of vaccines, the healthcare system, and policymakers.
- Complacency arises due to a low perceived risk of the disease and results in individuals feeling that they do not need vaccination.
- Convenience refers to access problems such as proximity, affordability, and ease of receiving vaccination.

Vaccine reluctance is not confined to a single population or region and can occur in high- as well as low-income nations. It is motivated by numerous different factors, such as misinformation, religious or philosophical conviction, past mistrust, and individual experience with healthcare.

The impact of vaccine hesitancy can be severe. It has resulted in the re-emergence of once-contained infections such as measles and can disrupt the efforts to develop herd immunity during pandemics like COVID-19. Clear communication, community mobilization, and well-respected healthcare providers are necessary to resolve vaccine hesitancy. The strategy needs to be adjusted based on population and concerns to promote informed and assertive vaccine uptake effectively.

SUMMARY

The cost-effectiveness analysis of vaccination programs offers valuable lessons for policymakers who seek to improve public health outcomes. In situations such as Bangladesh, where rotavirus infection is a major cause of childhood mortality, the introduction of a rotavirus vaccination program may help curb healthcare expenditures as well as disease burden, guiding decision-makers about the best vaccinations to use and how this affects public health expenditures (Pinky, 2023). Equally, the systematic review of hepatitis B virus (HBV) vaccination emphasized its economic viability in diverse settings, reinforcing calls for universal vaccination and programs targeted at-risk groups (Colamesta et al., 2016). By incorporating these analyses into public health policy, nations can more appropriately allocate finite resources and target interventions that maximize health benefits, ultimately leading to healthier populations and better economic stability. The overall message is that successful vaccination measures are not just health policy but also economically sound options.

In summarizing the salient points about vaccination, it is important to note both the effectiveness and pitfalls related to different vaccination schemes. For example, research emphasized the consistent ability of point-of-care (PoC) test kits such as Witness and Anigen Rapid to discriminate between vaccinated and infected cats, emphasizing the significance of knowing antibody production after vaccination (Hall et al., 2016). This realization is crucial in guaranteeing proper diagnosis and veterinary healthcare management. In contrast, problems still exist as can be seen through the slow expansion of civilian vaccination during increased security issues surrounding bioterrorism, where operational factors delayed the smallpox vaccination program despite sufficient vaccine availability (Bloem & Bicknell, 2003). Together, these conversations shed light on the intricacies of vaccine strategies, highlighting the necessity for ongoing review and realignment in line with upcoming health challenges as well as maintaining public and animal health security.

KEY TERMS FROM THIS CHAPTER

- Vaccine
- Herd immunity
- Antibody
- Vaccine effectiveness
- Vaccine hesitancy
- Breakthrough infection
- Inactivated vaccine
- mRNA vaccine
- Cold chain
- Immunization
- Antigen
- Vaccine efficacy
- Vaccine coverage
- Booster dose
- Live attenuated vaccine
- Subunit vaccine
- Adjuvant
- Contraindication

REFERENCES

1. Aaby, A., Bhatia, R., Bhuiya, A., Bosu, W., et al. (2009). Estimates of measles case fatality ratios: A comprehensive review of community-based studies. *International Journal of Epidemiology, 38*(1), 192–205. https://core.ac.uk/download/pdf/9417568.pdf (accessed on 6 May 2025).
2. Adamo, G., De Soccio, P., De Vito, C., Marzuillo, C., et al. (2017). Childhood vaccinations: A pilot study on knowledge, attitudes, and vaccine hesitancy in pregnant women. *Epidemiology Biostatistics and Public Health, 14*(4), e12625-1–e12625-5. https://core.ac.uk/download/154948381.pdf (accessed on 6 May 2025).
3. Ajeigbe, O. F., Arage, G., Besong, M., Chacha, W., Desai, R., Doegah, P. T., Hamoonga, T. E., et al. (2022). Culturally relevant COVID-19 vaccine acceptance strategies in sub-Saharan Africa. *The Lancet Global Health, 10*, e1090–e1091. https://doi.org/10.1016/s2214-109x(22)00251-0.
4. Alogaily, R. S. (2022). *Essays in behavioral economics and neuroeconomics* (CGU Theses & Dissertations, 398). https://core.ac.uk/download/534379341.pdf (accessed on 6 May 2025).
5. Amodio, E., Casuccio, A., Maiorana, A., Maranto, M., et al. (2023). Impact of preventive strategies on HPV-related diseases: Ten-year data from the Italian hospital admission registry. *Cancers, 15*(5), 1452. https://core.ac.uk/download/576924411.pdf (accessed on 6 May 2025).
6. Atwood, A., & Pearlman, S. (2023). The long-term benefits of vaccination campaigns: Evidence from measles. *Journal of Health Economics, 101*, 102974. https://www.semanticscholar.org/paper/7e1b9850f48ec5a79a72d08d2404290f049d1afc (accessed on 6 May 2025).
7. Baccolini, V., De Vito, C., Marzuillo, C., Massimi, et al. (2020). Factors affecting the vaccination choices of pregnant women for their children: A systematic review of the literature. https://core.ac.uk/download/323192079.pdf (accessed on 6 May 2025).
8. Barazzetti, A., Milesi, S., & Negri, A. (2024). Exploring factors influencing COVID-19 vaccine hesitancy and refusal: A study in Italy during the vaccine rollout. *International Journal of Environmental Research and Public Health, 21*, 331. https://core.ac.uk/download/630962039.pdf (accessed on 6 May 2025).
9. Barclay, W. R., Stylianou, E., McShane, H., Paul, M. J., Reljic, R., Co, T. R., Rodríguez, A., et al. (2019). Mucosal delivery of tuberculosis vaccines: A review of current approaches and challenges. *Expert Review of Vaccines, 18*(12), 1271–1284. https://core.ac.uk/download/286270868.pdf (accessed on 6 May 2025).
10. Baussano, I., Bruni, L., Dillner, J., & Elfström, K. (2024). Scientific approaches toward improving cervical cancer elimination strategies. *International Journal of Cancer, 154*(9), 1537–1548. https://doi.org/10.1002/ijc.34839.
11. Benfaremo, D., Cardamone, C., Delfino, L., Gangemi, S., Icardi, G., Lunardi, C., Maule, M., et al. (2021). Current take on systemic sclerosis patients' vaccination recommendations. *Vaccines, 9*, 1426. https://core.ac.uk/download/541259743.pdf (accessed on 6 May 2025).
12. Gostin, Lawrence O. and Berkman, Benjamin E., "Pandemic Influenza: Ethics, Law, and the Public's Health" (2007). Georgetown Law Faculty Publications and Other Works. 449. https://scholarship.law.georgetown.edu/facpub/449 (accessed on 6 May 2025).
13. Bert, F., Olivero, E., Rossello, P., Gualano, M. R., Castaldi, S., Damiani, G., D'Errico, M. M., Di Giovanni, P., Fantini, M. P., Fabiani, L., Gabutti, G., Loperto, I., Marranzano, M., Masanotti, G., Nante, N., Rosso, A., Squeri, R., Signorelli, C., Siliquini, R., & Collaborating Group (2020).

Knowledge and beliefs on vaccines among a sample of Italian pregnant women: results from the NAVIDAD study. *European journal of public health, 30*(2), 286–292. https://doi.org/10.1093/eurpub/ckz209 (accessed on 6 May 2025).

14. Biondo, F. (2023). Ai ricci importa la salute pubblica? La teoria dei diritti di Dworkin, i beni pubblici e le sfide della pandemia. https://core.ac.uk/download/576922720.pdf (accessed on 6 May 2025).
15. Bliuc, A. M., & Courtney, D. S. (2021). Antecedents of vaccine hesitancy in WEIRD and East Asian contexts. *Frontiers in Psychology, 12*, 747721. https://core.ac.uk/download/492525414.pdf (accessed on 6 May 2025).
16. Bloem, K. D., & Bicknell, W. J. (2003). Smallpox and bioterrorism: Why the plan to protect the nation is stalled and what to do. https://core.ac.uk/download/71341573.pdf (accessed on 6 May 2025).
17. Branca Pereira, A., Xu, X. N., & Akbar, A. N. (2020). Targeting inflammation and immunosenescence to improve vaccine responses in the elderly. *Frontiers in Immunology, 11*, 583019. https://doi.org/10.3389/fimmu.2020.583019.
18. Bray, F., Laversanne, M., Sung, H., Ferlay, J., Siegel, R. L., Soerjomataram, I., Jemal, A., et al. (2024). Global cancer statistics 2022: GLOBOCAN estimates of incidence and mortality worldwide for 36 cancers in 185 countries. *CA: A Cancer Journal for Clinicians, 74*, 229–263. https://doi.org/10.3322/caac.21834.
19. Briggs, A., & Grieve, E. (2017). A methodological approach for measuring the impact of HTA. https://core.ac.uk/download/80697121.pdf (accessed on 6 May 2025).
20. Brownson, R. C., Franco, M., Mazzucca, S., Padek, M., et al. (2019). Going beyond the individual: How state-level characteristics relate to HPV vaccine rates in the United States. *BMC Public Health, 19*, 246. https://core.ac.uk/download/223009500.pdf (accessed on 6 May 2025).
21. Brujić, M. (2024). Personal responsibility for the common good: The MMR vaccination discourse in contemporary Serbian daily newspapers. *Journal of Applied Journalism & Media Studies*. https://www.semanticscholar.org/paper/b6cdcdf31c0b88fab55a8904e285075b1dfcced2 (accessed on 6 May 2025).
22. Byrn, S. R., Clase, K. L., & Milton, N. (2023). BIRS course: RNA vaccine manufacture and assessment of regulatory documents for RNA vaccines. *BIRS Technical Report Papers*, Paper *2*. https://core.ac.uk/download/586533213.pdf (accessed on 6 May 2025).
23. Cancellieri, A., Capuano, A., de Waure, C., Ferlazzo, M., et al. (2020). Potential effects of vaccinations on the prevention of COVID-19: Rationale, clinical evidence, risks, and public health considerations. *Expert Review of Vaccines, 19*(10), 919–936. https://core.ac.uk/download/401894062.pdf (accessed on 6 May 2025).
24. Chavda, V. P., Yao, Q., Vora, L. K., Apostolopoulos, V., Patel, C., Bezbaruah, R., Patel, A., et al. (2022). Fast-track development of vaccines for SARS-CoV-2: The shots that saved the world. *Frontiers in Immunology, 13*. https://doi.org/10.3389/fimmu.2022.961198.
25. Chughtai, N., & Chughtai, N. (2022). Parental education to increase the rate of flu vaccination in children ages six months to 17 years: A quality improvement project. *Nicole Wertheim College of Nursing Student Projects, 91*. https://core.ac.uk/download/515576506.pdf (accessed on 6 May 2025).

26. Coburn, H. (2018). Vaccine epidemiology and decision-making: A Bryant student focus. https://core.ac.uk/download/158246439.pdf (accessed on 6 May 2025)

27. Cohen, T., Cuccaro, P., Dominguez, O., Fernandez, A., et al. (2023). Lessons learned from interdisciplinary efforts to combat COVID-19 misinformation: Development of agile integrative methods from behavioral science, data science, and implementation science. *JMIR Infodemiology, 3*, e40156. https://core.ac.uk/download/604668993.pdf (accessed on 6 May 2025).

28. Coltman-Patel, T., Dance, W., Deignan, A., Demjen, Z., & et al. (2023). The Victorian anti-vaccination discourse corpus (VicVaDis): Construction and exploration. *Digital Scholarship in the Humanities, 2023*(00), 1–13. https://core.ac.uk/download/590344668.pdf (accessed on 6 May 2025).

29. Declich, S., Del Manso, M., Dente, M. G., Giambi, et al. (2017). Immunization strategies targeting newly arrived migrants in non-EU countries of the Mediterranean basin and Black Sea. *International Journal of Environmental Research and Public Health, 14*, 459. https://core.ac.uk/download/98348059.pdf (accessed on 6 May 2025).

30. Dobriyal, A., Dobriyal, S., & Kumar, K. (2024). Safeguarding the future: The critical role of child vaccination in cultivating a healthy generation. *Himalayan Journal of Social Sciences and Humanities, 18*(1), 25–30. https://doi.org/10.51220/hjssh.v18i1.4.

31. Dudley, M., Goldney, R., Jureidini, J., Mansfield, R., & et al. (2005). Depressed youth, suicidality, and antidepressants. *Medical Journal of Australia, 183*(5), 275–276. Dutta, Arin, The Effectiveness of Policies to Control a Human Influenza Pandemic: A Literature Review (February 1, 2008). World Bank Policy Research Working Paper No. 4524, Available at SSRN: https://ssrn.com/abstract=1096847 (accessed on 6 May 2025).

32. Eijsackers, H. J. P., & Scholten, M. C. T. (2011). Livestock farming with care: Summaries of essays. https://core.ac.uk/download/pdf/29230069.pdf (accessed on 6 May 2025).

33. Gans, R. (2014). The politics of HPV vaccination advocacy: Effects of source expertise on the effectiveness of a pro-vaccine message. *Proceedings of the New York State Communication Association, 2013*, Article 3. https://core.ac.uk/download/56705918.pdf (accessed on 6 May 2025).

34. Grace, D., Knight-Jones, T. J. D., Melaku, A., Alders, R., & Jemberu, W. (2024). The public health importance and management of infectious poultry diseases in smallholder systems in Africa. *Foods, 13*. https://www.semanticscholar.org/paper/c3deddc7ba59ad563d6ff215ea783ddf143b921e (accessed on 6 May 2025).

35. Hamdulay, K. F., Rawekar, R., Tayade, A., Kumar, S., & Acharya, S. (2024). Evolving epidemiology and antibiotic resistance in enteric fever: A comprehensive review. *Cures, 16*. https://www.semanticscholar.org/paper/c474246486619a0b32c27b851b6fdc9122242716 (accessed on 6 May 2025).

36. Hill, D. L., Pierson, W., Bolland, D. J., Mkindi, C., Carr, E. J., Wang, J., Houard, S., et al. (2019). The adjuvant GLA-SE promotes human Tfh cell expansion and emergence of public TCRβ clonotypes. *The Journal of Experimental Medicine, 216*, 1857–1873. https://doi.org/10.1084/jem.20190301.

37. Howard, J., Huang, A., Li, Z., Tüfekçi, Z., Ždímal, V., van der Westhuizen, H., von Delft, A., et al. (2021). An evidence review of face masks against COVID-19. *Proceedings of the National Academy of Sciences, 118*. https://doi.org/10.1073/pnas.2014564118.

38. Khindri, N. (2022). Our fundamental knowledge of ozone atmospheric chemistry over metropolitan Detroit, Michigan. https://www.semanticscholar.org/paper/76bb19d1d263bb80a73f414394cd475154ffa09c (accessed on 6 May 2025).

39. Lainé, C., Cotton, D., & Moyer, D. V. (2020). COVID-19 vaccine: Promoting vaccine acceptance. *Annals of Internal Medicine, 174*, 252–253. https://doi.org/10.7326/m20-8008.

40. Leder, L. (2015). Vaccination hesitation: Investigation why parents decline pediatric influenza vaccines in Juneau, Alaska. https://core.ac.uk/download/162577318.pdf (accessed on 6 May 2025).

41. Lewnard, J. A., & Reingold, A. L. (2019). Emerging challenges and opportunities in infectious disease epidemiology. *American Journal of Epidemiology, 188*(5), 873–882. https://doi.org/10.1093/aje/kwy264.

42. Lydeamore, M., Zachreson, C., Conway, E., Shearer, F., Baker, C., Ross, J., Miller, J. C., et al. (2024). Border quarantine, vaccination, and public health measures to mitigate the impact of COVID-19 importations: A modelling study. https://www.semanticscholar.org/paper/1f21ec22b490b461065aba59954cf78faf7e601e (accessed on 6 May 2025).

43. McGee, L. U., & Suh, J. (2020). Communication strategies to address vaccine hesitancy in healthcare settings and on social media. *Journal of Applied Research on Children: Informing Policy for Children at Risk, 10*(2), Article 7. https://core.ac.uk/download/323216373.pdf (accessed on 6 May 2025).

44. Mechoulan, S. (2025). Market structure and communicable diseases. https://core.ac.uk/download/pdf/9305730.pdf (accessed on 6 May 2025).

45. Meghani, M., Pike, J., Tippins, A., & Leidner, A. (2024). Cost-effectiveness analysis of routine outreach and catch-up campaign strategies for measles, mumps, and rubella vaccination in Chuuk, Federated States of Micronesia. *Public Health Reports*. https://www.semanticscholar.org/paper/6f50cc31a0041b7da2b27432b8abdffffcd605ba (accessed on 6 May 2025).

46. Mutsigiri-Murewanhema, F., & Murewanhema, G. (2021). Drivers of the third wave of COVID-19 in Zimbabwe and challenges for control: Perspectives and recommendations. *Pan African Medical Journal, 40*(46). https://core.ac.uk/download/544239798.pdf (accessed on 6 May 2025).

47. Nainu, F. (2025). The impact of immunosenescence on immune responses: A challenge on influenza vaccination in the elderly. *The Impact of Immunosenescence on the Immune Responses, 16*(1), 7–12. https://core.ac.uk/download/pdf/25493748.pdf (accessed on 6 May 2025).

48. Ngoma, C., Matatiyo, A., Oke, G., Adebisi, Y., & Shomuyiwa, D. (2024). Navigating the digital frontier during the COVID-19 pandemic and EVALI epidemic: The impact of social media on public health. *Public Health Challenges*. https://www.semanticscholar.org/paper/787f37d2ebcd0be0a49ec2498fd1ec72b1727ce8 (accessed on 6 May 2025).

49. Nidhi, R., & Bala, M. (2024). Bio-medical waste and environmental protection laws and policies in India: Management and solutions to tackle its effects in India. *International Journal for Multidisciplinary Research*. https://www.semanticscholar.org/paper/766274628fd05499b8700624b18bf6a33910488e (accessed on 6 May 2025).

50. Pierre, V., Draica, F., di Fusco, M., Yang, J., Nunez-Gonzalez, S., Kamar, J., Lopez, S. M. C., et al. (2023). The impact of vaccination and outpatient treatment on the economic burden of

COVID-19 in the United States Omicron era: A systematic literature review. *Journal of Medical Economics, 26*, 1519–1531. https://www.semanticscholar.org/paper/7ced7920e73a8b65fde19c4a7a9bf954d60660b3 (accessed on 6 May 2025).

51. Pinky, A. (2023). *Cost-Effective Analysis of Rotavirus Vaccination in Dhaka, Bangladesh Using a Dynamic Model of Rotavirus Transmission* (Public Health Theses No. 2324). https://core.ac.uk/download/571280654.pdf (accessed on 6 May 2025).
52. Pourbohloul, B., Brandriss, M., Grenfell, B., Cauchemez, S., Dauer, M., Dezso, Z., et al. (2006). A comparative analysis of influenza vaccination programs. *PLoS Medicine, 3*(10), e387. https://doi.org/10.1371/journal.pmed.0030387.
53. Rongioletti, M., Vaccarella, C., Mariani, S., Bucossi, S., D'Andrea, B., Pietricola, S., & Squitti, R. (2024). Long-term outcomes of high-risk human papillomavirus in anal infection support HPV men vaccination. *American Journal of Clinical Pathology*. https://www.semanticscholar.org/paper/1f7bc07ff2f1af4de5664e211ed6fb28ea432055 (accessed on 6 May 2025)
54. Taylor, A., Heinrichs, A., Azizi, A., Megibow, E., Allen, E. H., & Emmet, S. (2023). Advancing vaccine equity through community-based organizations: Partnering for vaccine equity program annual evaluation report, Year One. https://core.ac.uk/download/591044576.pdf (accessed on 6 May 2025).
55. Tuckerman, J., Kaufman, J., & Danchin, M. (2022). Effective approaches to combat vaccine hesitancy. *The Pediatric Infectious Disease Journal, 41*, e243–e245. https://doi.org/10.1097/inf.0000000000003499.
56. Uddin, T. M., Chakraborty, A., Khusro, A., Matin Zidan, B. R., Mitra, S., Emran, T. B., Dhama, K., et al. (2021). Antibiotic resistance in microbes: History, mechanisms, therapeutic strategies, and future prospects. *Journal of Infection and Public Health, 14*, 1750–1766. https://doi.org/10.1016/j.jiph.2021.10.020.
57. Visseren, F. L. J., Mach, F., Smulders, Y. M., Carballo, D., Koskinas, K. C., Bäck, M., Bénétos, A., et al. (2021). 2021 ESC guidelines on cardiovascular disease prevention in clinical practice. *European Heart Journal, 42*, 3227–3337. https://doi.org/10.1093/eurheartj/ehab484.
58. Wong, L. P., Lee, H. Y., Alias, H., Zimet, G., Liu, T., Lin, Y., & Hu, Z. (2024). Cost-based COVID-19 vaccination and willingness to pay: A post-pandemic review. *Human vaccines & immunotherapeutics*, *20*(1), 2313860. https://doi.org/10.1080/21645515.2024.2313860 (accessed on 6 May 2025).

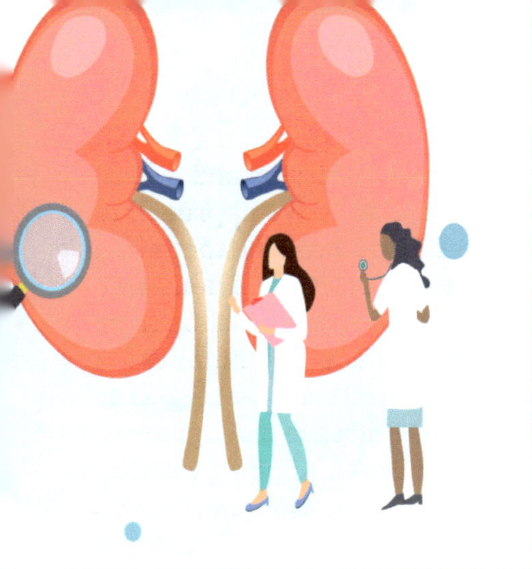

Chapter 10

INTERVENTION STRATEGIES AND DISEASE CONTROL

Contents

Introduction

These recent years have taught us just how desperately we require more intelligent means of managing disease outbreaks. Consider what occurred all those years ago in 2021 when Thailand was confronted by lumpy skin disease; that experience highlighted the importance of having a wide, diversified approach. With cases starting to peak, authorities not only initiated a nationwide immunization campaign but also established regulations to restrict travels and augmented surveillance. Individuals began to dig into how these combined strategies interacted with each other, and informal impact analysis—yes, that statistical software—assisted in painting a better picture of how these interventions correlate with new cases (Punyapornwithaya et al., 2024). Changing gears to chronic diseases, individualized treatment is becoming a game changer. Consider children with Crohn's disease, for instance. Rather than holding fast to generic dosing, some medical teams are now experimenting with precision dosing designed specifically for each patient. Typical protocols fall short because not everyone responds identically to medications. With methods such as active drug monitoring and personalized infliximab doses, physicians are now achieving superior, longer-term outcomes—sustained remission and overall enhanced health results, in fact. Clinical trials suggest a move toward a more adaptive approach to treatment, and although more needs to be done to support these findings more broadly, the initial data looks promising (Minar et al., 2024). When you take a step back, however, it is obvious that our intervention strategy needs to continue to evolve. The efficacy of mass vaccination campaigns and more targeted treatments indicates that fine-tuning our approaches can reduce case numbers of disease and improve how patients do generally. Throw in intelligent early surveillance strategies to refine treatments in progress, and you've got a blueprint for improved chronic disease management. These lessons provide valuable lessons for both healthcare professionals (HCPs) and policymakers, emphasizing in most instances that relying on robust, evidence-driven research is most important. As new infectious challenges and intransigent chronic diseases arise with increasing frequency, constructing a flexible and adaptable intervention system just may be our best option moving forward (Minar et al., 2024; Punyapornwithaya et al., 2024).

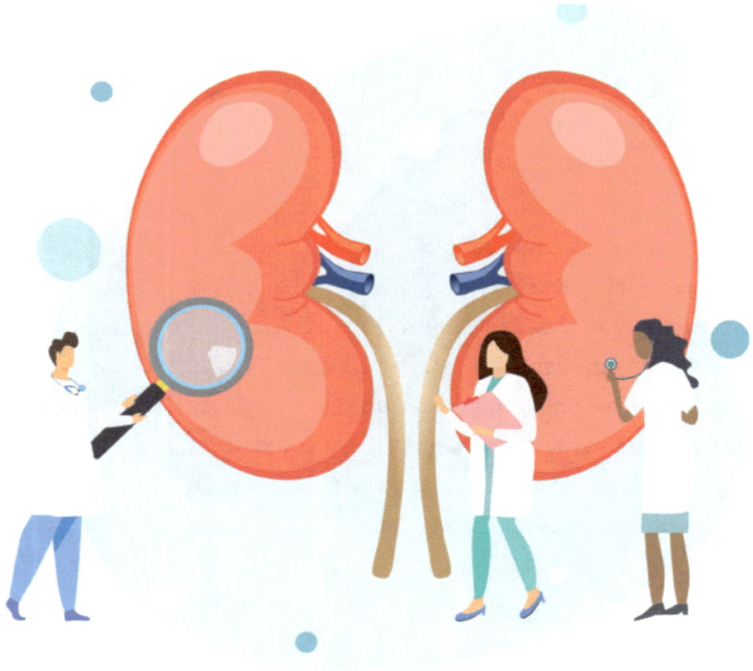

Source: https://d8tzmbmuvomgp.cloudfront.net/medialibrary/00011/93D9D070-0B60-4AB4-B7A4-88D23EF409FC.png

Definition of Intervention Strategies

Public health relies on having a clear, solid strategy to reduce the spread and damage of diseases. Rather than adhering to any single formula, people typically combine a few approaches to preventing illness—sometimes addressing risk factors directly (what we would term primary prevention) and other times identifying early warning signs or treating conditions that have already appeared (that's secondary and tertiary prevention at work). The success of such actions is very much dependent on sound epidemiological information and the way communities act, so there is always an impetus for focused campaigns specifically addressing various groups. Essentially, these types of blueprints guide both policy planners and health workers through the sometimes-sloppy disease control maze. Going a bit deeper, a central aspect of sorting out intervention strategies is determining what method is applicable to a specific situation. At times the solution is at the individual level, such as receiving a vaccination or rudimentary health education, and sometimes authorities implement larger-scale measures—think quarantine or travel bans when outbreaks are happening. The WHO tends to emphasize that plans must be versatile enough to adapt to changing patterns of disease. For new diseases, for instance, rapid initial containment has become a key; just consider how states hustled during the COVID-19 outbreak to enact firm controls, even new details still coming out. And combining new tech with data analysis can enhance the overall performance of these strategies. And yet, one cannot help noticing how social, economic, and even environmental considerations come into play in these strategies. Identifying these factors provides a more nuanced perspective on disease control that can help get communities on board—even if, sometimes, it makes things slightly more complicated. Research indicates that cultural beliefs, healthcare access, and educational resources available all contribute significantly to effective public health initiatives. And in addition, when governmental and non-governmental institutions collaborate (sometimes in a rather ad hoc manner), it is easier for them to share information and resources. As the science of disease control continues to develop, having multi-faced and well-rounded strategies is essential to maintaining both health outcomes and overall well-being in our communities.

Importance of Disease Control

Public health relies on good disease control, particularly where there are areas of the world that are still finding their footing—because epidemics can literally set societies off course. Central Vietnam has seen a spike in fascioliasis, which does mean that our standard procedures aren't working. Cases leapt unexpectedly from about 1,500 in 2004–2005 to nearly 9,985 in 2011; this spike indicates that relying only on triclabendazole chemotherapy is limited since resistance begins to emerge. We truly need to shake things up by rethinking old designs and incorporating local risk and learning-about-health data—measures that, in most instances, are needed for keeping things together (Quy et al., 2016). Disease control isn't merely about keeping people healthy immediately; it also fits into the overall scheme of keeping society stable and even helping the economy. Consider multidrug-resistant tuberculosis (MDR-TB) in India, for instance. Approximately 630,000 new patients emerge annually, and poor treatment programs merely exacerbate the issue. When the health systems fail to remain linked or maintain a good surveillance and treatment regimen, the entire exercise collapses. In general terms, rapid drug susceptibility testing and improved community health literacy (HL) may be the game changer in such situations. If India could transform its public health system based on the examples that are to be found in countries with fewer cases of MDR-TB, then it might not only stop the disease from spreading but also set the stage for a healthier, more prosperous society (Gamon et al., 2013). Ultimately, gaining control over diseases is a foundation for enduring progress. Prioritizing intervention measures allows health systems to mitigate the impact of infectious diseases and accrue resilience in populations affected. A combination that includes education, community participation, and enhanced access to healthcare is crucial. For example, establishing a widely based model of control for fascioliasis could prevent further deterioration among vulnerable populations. Similarly, addressing the MDR-TB crisis involves providing wise investments into healthcare to enable quick recovery. These frameworks do not simply extinguish a fire—they provide the foundation for healthier societies that foster overall public health, economic development, and social justice. In the absence of these efforts, the disease cycle continues to strangle development across the board (Gamon et al., 2013; Quy et al., 2016) (Figure 10.1).

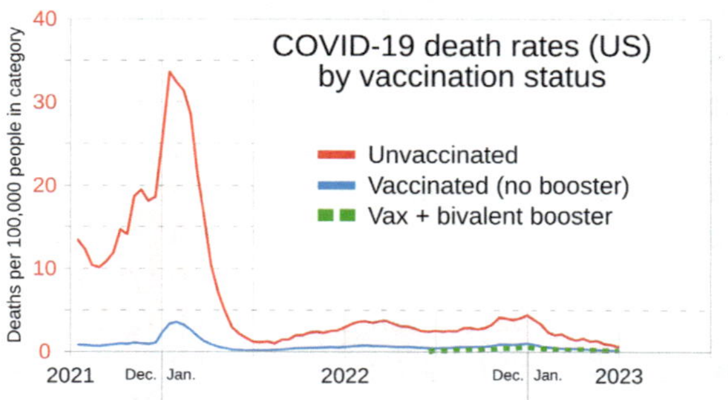

Figure 10.1. Importance of disease control.

Source: By RCraig09 - Own work, CC BY-SA 4.0, https://commons.wikimedia.org/w/index.php?curid=139711160

10.1. Historical Context of Disease Control

History and discovery have always been an important factor in how we treat diseases. People way back when relied primarily on quarantine and isolation—practices that were effective, although rather rudimentary. Consider the 14th-century bubonic plague; the early strategies, however simplistic they appeared to be, laid the groundwork for subsequent, more systematic public health actions. Then, in the 1800s, came germ theory and flipped our understanding on its head. In general, it was not long after that people began taking proactive measures, such as increasing sanitation measures and implementing vaccinations. That advance also pushed governments to realize the importance of concerted effort and prudent policymaking when managing health emergencies. Epidemiology entered the scene next, altering our perception of disease transmission in ways that frequently caught everyone off guard. By monitoring trends in prevalence and incidence, authorities could identify risk factors and target the proper areas for intervention—now and then in the most surprising ways. For the majority, combined statistical techniques are used to provide some dash of credibility for public health programs. Systematic reviews, as described by Page et al. (2021), created a turning point, establishing typical frameworks even if things were not clear. Consequently, policymakers were left with evidence-based data that it became simpler to determine the best practices and organize resources better in times of crisis. Our present strategies have roots that run deep in history and society's response to challenges. Large outbreaks—consider the 1918 influenza pandemic, for instance—rattled things up and led to a move toward more integrated, cross-sector responses. At such a difficult time, health officials fought not only the disease but also a tidal wave of misinformation and fear, making open and clear communication imperative. The lessons of the time continue to resurface in today's guidelines, such as those by AASLD (Northup et al., 2020). When you put it all together, the mix of historical events, scientific insights, and evolving public reactions reveals a dynamic, sometimes messy, but always determined effort to curb disease and protect us all.

10.1.1. Major Pandemics and Their Impact

Pandemics have long disrupted our ordinary lives out of kilter, disrupting not only our health strategies but also how we live among ourselves. You can observe that with COVID-19 , it wasn't simply a fight against a virus; it activated a lot of mental tension as well. Stress, anxiety, and emotional storms intensified in ways that demonstrated the extent to which our minds could be shaken about when crises come. Young people were especially hard hit – having more episodes of low mood, disturbed sleep, and difficulty relating to others, partly due to lockdowns and school closures. It then becomes quite clear that addressing these mental health challenges needs to be a priority. A few art-based interventions and clinician-led support services have been promising, albeit we still badly need approaches to suit various needs, particularly when imminent outbreaks may just add to the pressure (Meherali et al., 2021). It is not just our mental wellbeing that is affected; our body can also suffer. Following a large-scale outbreak, daily routines can change dramatically – and one definite casualty appears to be our cardiovascular health. With people being less active and schedules interrupted, markers such as obesity, hypertension, and diabetes seem to inch up. The Global Burden of Disease (GBD) Study, to illustrate, reports an alarming tale: between 1990 and 2019, problems related to cardiovascular health and the accompanying rates of death have risen consistently.

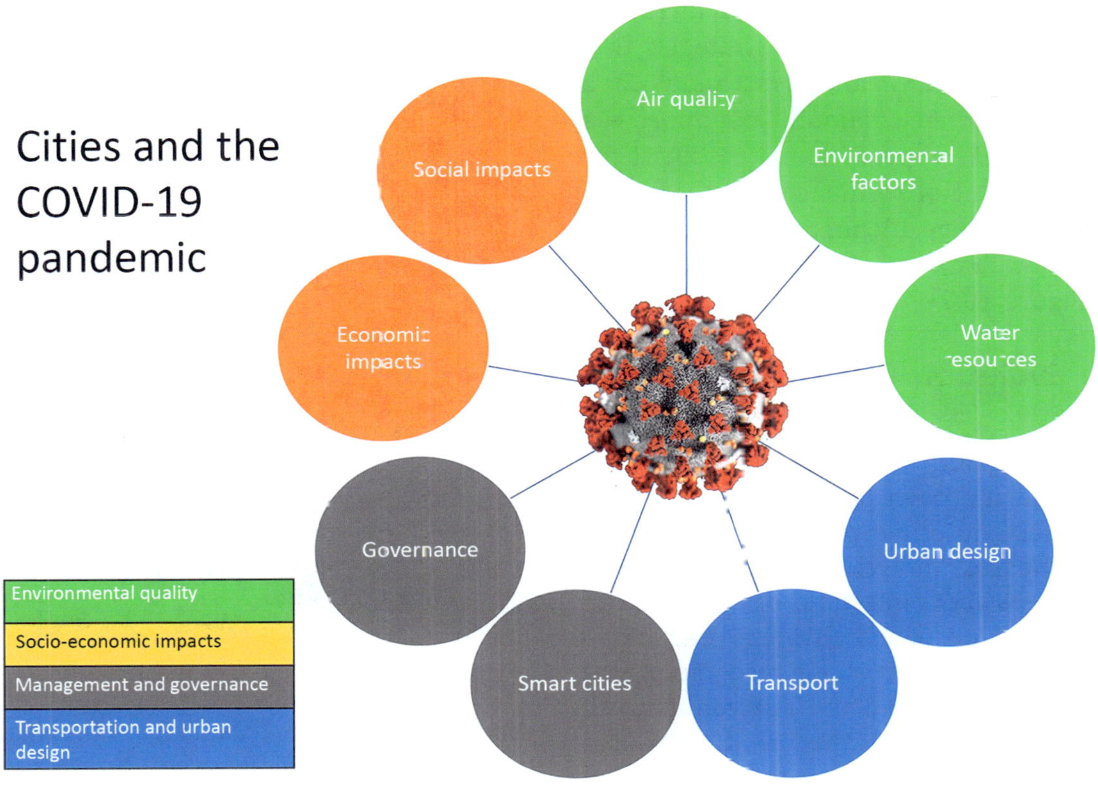

Figure 10.2. Major pandemics and their impact.

Source: Sharifi, A., & Khavarian-Garmsir, A. R. (2020). *The COVID-19 pandemic: Impacts on cities and major lessons for urban planning, design, and management. Science of The Total Environment, 749*, 142391.

While our life patterns turn in unforeseen directions following pandemics, it is reasonable, in a broad sense, to rely on health conversations facilitated by communities and public announcements that encourage us toward improved practices. More often than not, the solution lies in recognizing our mental and physical health as pieces of the same jigsaw puzzle (Roth et al., 2020). On top of all that, there is a significant economic cost to bear. Sizable outbreaks can run shockwaves through our healthcare systems, causing a reallocation in budgets that all too often leaves long-term health concerns in the shadows. That uneven distribution can lead to delays in addressing chronic issues – delays that could escalate once the immediate crisis has passed. Interventions, studies say, can ease both the short-term budget blow and the longer-term burden on our healthcare systems. Spending a little extra on mental health services and providing preventive care more widely, for example, could pay dividends in the long run. Looking back at previous pandemics, increased support overall is observed for strategies that combine integrated health systems with a generous helping of community support – a combination that appears to be essential for the establishment of resilience and the better addressing of future dilemmas, both physically and mentally (Roth et al., 2020; Meherali et al., 2021) (Figure 10.2).

10.1.2. Evolution of Public Health Policies

Public health policy has been changing a lot recently, and it's been powered by emerging health issues and our evolving understanding of how illnesses function. In the old days, everything was about infectious diseases—strict quarantine and lots of strict hygiene practices—but today there is an increasing recognition that things such as diet and the environment all blend together in complicated ways. Consider, for instance, the way malaria and anemia can strike populations simultaneously; it illustrates that we cannot simply address one disease without considering the larger picture. Such a knotty scenario forces policymakers to design interventions that break free from addressing only a single disease, instead untangling the social causes underlying them, all while loosely aligning with frameworks such as the Sustainable Development Goals (Achieng, 2025). Data science and predictive analytics have also leaped into the battle, disrupting things even further. These emerging technology tools now probe deeply into patterns of disease and aid in getting resources out more resourcefully, a development that has been fairly dramatic. In the US, for example, data indicators allow health administrators to identify populations vulnerable to chronic diseases and assemble interventions that perfectly fit. Over in Africa, other data-driven initiatives are making significant progress in managing infectious diseases. Public health systems are running against technology in a never-ending race, they want to be nimble so that every tactic remains both equitable and effective (Odilibe et al., 2024). On top of all this, ethical considerations are ever more part of the debate as these policies change. Data-driven approaches tend to raise eyebrows over privacy, equity, and even biases creeping into health information.

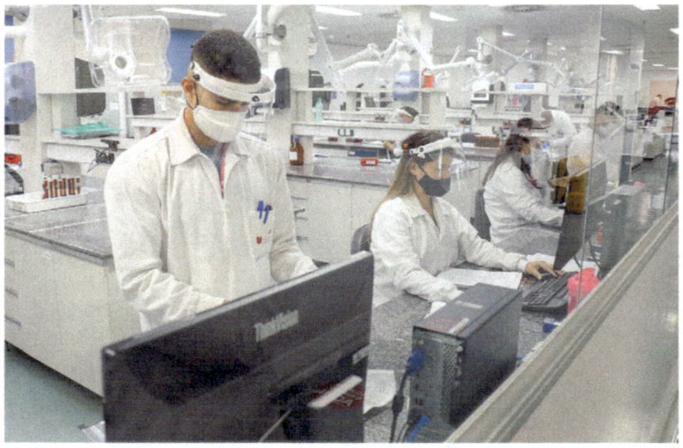

Figure 10.3. Evolution of public health policies.

Source: By Agência Brasília from Brasília, Brasil - Fábrica do DF produz vacina Sputnik V, CC BY 2.0, https://commons.wikimedia.org/w/index.php?curid=99262062

Health officials, balancing these slippery concerns, must work twice as hard to gain public confidence and seek community input when they influence policy. It is a fine balancing act—leveraging the cool insights data provides while ensuring everyone is treated equally. As policies continue to evolve to address fresh challenges, integrating ethical considerations becomes central to constructing a healthcare system as equitable as it is effective, ultimately enhancing the impact of intervention strategies and disease control measures (Odilibe et al., 2024) (Figure 10.3).

10.1.3. Lessons Learned from Past Interventions

Intervention programs have evolved a lot due to what we gained from previous public health experiments. Let's take the COVID-19 pandemic for instance—in hindsight, it's quite clear that having warning systems in place early and healthcare solutions rapidly is a requirement. We realized those interventions such as isolating people and accelerating vaccinations work, but so is establishing consistent, transparent channels of communication so that updates reach everyone on time. This cluttered history informs us that to keep pace with new diseases, we must continue to modify our playbook. More often than not, applying these lessons contributes toward constructing a health system that is capable of managing surprise challenges (Adams et al., 2025). There is also community engagement. Previous initiatives, as it were, quite literally demonstrate how remaining in touch with the people at the local level pays dividends. Studies on initiatives such as community-based cancer prevention (CBPR)—in which locals impart their own expertise—continuously remind us that individuals most know their own conditions. Strengthening and maintaining those relationships, even if it means some occasional backpedaling, has smoothed the implementation of programs and even reduced health disparities for under-served populations. As it happens, when we appreciate the daily life as much as the specialist plans, our interventions become a little more adaptive, a bit more culturally resonant, and, Overall, more resilient (Adams et al., 2025). Then, recalling the more challenging moments such as the Ebola and H1N1 scenarios, sure enough the system was not quite equitable for all. Witnessing those holes in access to healthcare prompted a shift of focus toward equity as a central concept. We discovered—sometimes at great pain—that strong, comprehensive systems for health matter in cushioning the impact when new dangers emerge. Getting more noise and collaboration among worldwide health agencies appears to be fairly vital if we are going to level out the patchy assistance to marginalized communities. Overall, combining these past experiences with fresh strategies would lay the groundwork for greater equal access to health care, making our overall response to disease crises that much more robust (Aati et al., 2024).

10.2. Types of Intervention Strategies

Modern health interventions have evolved into a motley collection of concepts intended to address the prevention as well as the treatment of disease. Physiotherapy, for example, is widely regarded – particularly with conditions such as Parkinson's disease – where constant motor exercises and rehabilitation methods have proven effective. Researchers tend to classify these approaches as either resistance training, aerobic exercise, or even unorthodox alternatives like exergaming or hydrotherapy. A meta-analysis, for instance, reported that such standard methods promote motor skills, balance, gait patterns, and overall quality of life, which is a strong argument to incorporate them into daily care (Radder et al., 2020). Emerging strategies are also emerging as health demands change. Older practices are being more and more supplemented with new concepts such as telehealth services and community health programs, and in most instances, that makes it more accessible to deliver care while also generating more patients' interest. Those new methods entice individuals by providing them with personalized health advice and self-help instruments – occasionally in the form of mobile apps that allow patients to contact their physicians in real-time. Doing so, they promote individuals to play an active part in controlling their health, combining traditional with innovative methods to establish a comprehensive system that effectively empowers individuals during the course of their care (Burnett et al., 2018). It is equally difficult not to consider the influence of shared decision-making when selecting the most appropriate treatment route. When patients and doctors talk and decide together, it typically leads to care plans that better accommodate individual needs and preferences. Health workers who present clear information about a variety of treatment options - rather than only the standard options - enable patients to make well-informed decisions that lead to longer compliance with their plans. In short, combining the use of different treatment concepts with engaged patient participation sets the stage for successful disease management. The more healthcare continues to evolve, more turning toward a combination of approaches and a more participatory decision-making style will likely be the key to achieving the most desirable outcomes (Radder et al., 2020) (Figure 10.4).

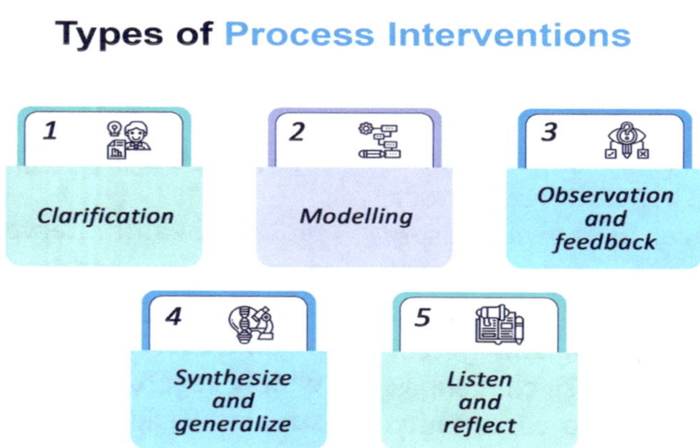

Figure 10.4. Types of intervention strategies.

Source: AIHR. (n.d.). Types of Process Interventions.

10.2.1. Preventive Measures

Preventative measures are more or less the first line of defense against outbreaks - it is not so much a matter of having a plan as implementing smart, day-to-day precautions. If you examine the mechanisms of disease transmission, it becomes apparent that drawing on community sentiment and even altering our environment is a must. New studies frequently indicate that models—yes, even simple room-based ones—cause us to understand how humans engage with one another, which in turn reveals that measures like quarantine and immunization can indeed stop a disease's progression. In the majority of instances, such flexible strategies provide health systems with the advantage required to respond quickly to new threats; they sort of chart the complicated connection between our everyday routines and the path that diseases travel along, highlighting how important prevention is Chatterjee et al. (2023). In another arena, the financial aspect of it all is connected to these prevention measures, particularly when considering disease management in farms. Consider Porcine Reproductive and Respiratory Syndrome (PRRS) for example—several plans have been bandied about to test what is best coastwise where disease severity shifts between mild and severe. Simulations that replicate strategies like mass vaccinations and intensified biosecurity protocols offer a glimpse into the ways these measures not only maintain animals healthier but also improve overall productivity. In most moderately impacted herds, measures such as close & roll-over (C&R) combined with mass vaccination of sows and piglets appear as viable, cost-saving interventions, suggesting that prevention can narrow the economic blow while cementing farm resilience (Alarcon et al., 2018). When a broader public health perspective is zoomed out, prevention's tale extends far beyond the farm. Urban populations today confront the double threat of new infectious diseases and persistent health gaps, so combining endeavors such as educational campaigns, enhanced sanitation, and greater access to vaccines becomes central. In general, when a population invests in a culture of prevention, individuals not only equip themselves with essential know-how but also create a collective safety net. This combination of evidence-based prevention and routine action builds both individual responsibility and more robust group health outcomes, setting the stage for a more adaptable response to the next outbreak. Prevention is, in a sense, not merely an option – it is the cornerstone of how we hold off epidemics (Chatterjee et al., 2023).

10.2.2. Therapeutic Interventions

Treatment measures that address chronic diseases and micronutrient deficiencies truly make a difference—for most communities, these measures do double the work by addressing existing issues and preventing future ones. A closer look at economic research in low- and middle-income countries reveals that interventions such as preventive interventions and food fortification receive much focus, as they are important in reducing undernutrition and its cascading effects. Nevertheless, one cannot help but observe that most of these studies overlook solid modeling techniques, which—honestly—reduces their value in informing healthcare plans (Ramponi et al., 2020). This trend, in general, makes it apparent that we require a more systematic approach to ranking interventions that improve health outcomes while monitoring costs. In managing complex illnesses, the scenario becomes even more intriguing. These instances depend on fairly novel models that reveal how biologic systems interact. With techniques such as network control, practitioners can get down to the nitty-gritty of how disease operates by highlighting critical elements of a network; messing around with these critical nodes is able to initiate ripple effects that spread through a course of treatment.

For instance, precisely fine-tuning certain genes or proteins can guide cells toward programmed suicide—consider apoptosis in cancer treatment contexts (Yang et al., 2018). This selective approach not only increases treatment efficiency but also facilitates easier resource management, combining technical acumen and practical requirements in creative ways. In addition to managing individual health, these interventions act as bridges that connect a cluster of sectors that aim at disease control. Combining health outcomes with non-health outcomes broadens discussions of nutrition and its broader social implications. Recently, greater economic assessments began to extend beyond mainstream healthcare, suggesting that successful strategies can also promote economic sustainability by increasing productivity and overall well-being (Ramponi et al., 2020). Policymakers are generally urged to consider more deeply—trading off short-term care against long-term socioeconomic benefits. Overall, such an integrated perspective fuels a multidisciplinary debate that is necessary for refining intervention approaches and finally producing improved outcomes in disease management.

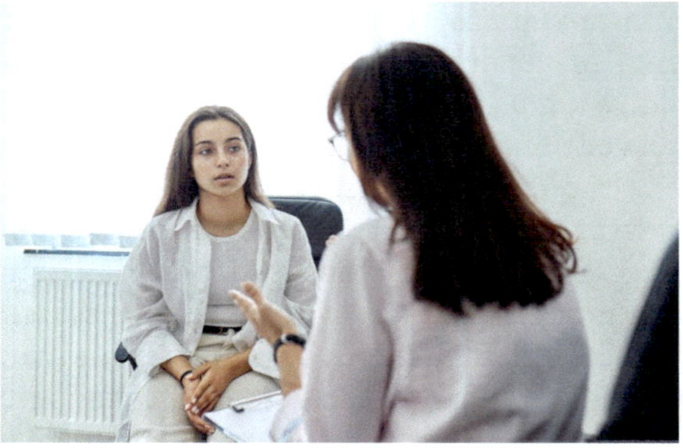

Source: Keele University. (2025). *Therapeutic Interventions Lead to Fewer Suicide Attempts in Adolescents, Research Finds.*

10.2.3. Educational Campaigns

Education is now a key weapon against disease, particularly diseases transmitted by insects. When groups get together, they appear to enhance prevention in ways you may not anticipate—consider how the Aedes mosquito transmits illness in communities affected with arboviral disease outbreaks. I remember one overview that indicated, in fairly straightforward language, that local initiatives tend to persist and perform more effectively in the long run. In many instances, when ordinary citizens get involved, a sense of cooperativeness is created that supports changing behaviors and eventually public health results (Heyrani et al., 2024). It is fascinating to see how educational campaigns may modify themselves according to local tastes so that the entire effort becomes more sincere. These types of programs could add a surprise combination of workshops, small-group classes, and even hands-on training that shares the sort of essential information required to avoid infections. This combination not only reinforces what people know but also establishes a collective understanding of the way diseases are transmitted, providing communities with that added incentive to protect themselves. For example, recent research on the Zika virus indicates that when education is combined with other control strategies, the advance is quite significant; in most instances, theory supports the premise that integrating health learning into larger plans produces a form of layered protection that builds resilience in communities. As countries grapple with the messy realities of disease control, the role of educational initiatives is difficult to overestimate. Overall, long-term success depends upon keeping individuals engaged and prepared to overcome new public health challenges as they arise. Maintaining these programs quite often involves steady effort, periodic review, and – yes – a wide-ranging teamwork strategy that spans multiple disciplines. Combining education with control measures for these pathogens does not merely sum; it ensures that individuals remain educated and willing to take action. Ultimately, smarter, more active communities constitute one of the strongest defenses against coming, and even resurgent, health dangers, underscoring the fact that education truly is a line of defense (Heyrani et al., 2024).

10.3. Role of Government in Disease Control

Governments dictate how health problems are addressed. They establish policies and construct structures to address issues such as malnutrition and chronic illnesses—a step that occasionally appears somewhat scatterbrained. For instance, the World Health Organization (WHO) has assisted countries such as Tanzania in combating malnutrition, which indicates that leaders should have strong, comprehensive plans for providing services and establishing regulations. Recent research even indicates that some of the policies today fall short, particularly for childhood obesity. More often than not, what is needed is an amalgamation of sectors to collaborate—bringing in varied voices—to intervene meaningfully (Mahiti et al., 2025). Keeping regulations up to date and disseminating public awareness, in fact, can significantly contribute to community health. Another large aspect of what governments do is collecting and examining data that in turn informs policy decisions. Urbanization, for example, accelerates problems such as vector-borne illnesses (VBDs) like dengue fever. In Malaysia, people have been keeping their hands full tracking and controlling dengue, which highlights the challenge of coping with limited resources in the face of increasing health demands.

The general success of these plans also depends on many agencies acting, at times chaotically, together—developing a synchronized response to crises. By drawing on evidence to inform decisions about where to target effort and resources, governments can identify high-risk areas more sharply and manage prevention of disease more effectively, with results that improve overall public health incrementally. Governments can also affect normal health behaviors by regulation and by plain education. Offering nutrition classes in schools, for example, is not merely a matter of feeding children facts but also guides families toward the option of healthier living. Efforts like these often double as community programs, making it easier to get everyone on board with better ways of living, even if this means repeating important points in varied formats. Additionally, placing some restrictions on marketing unhealthy food to children can gradually push eating habits in the correct direction, helping lower obesity rates. Evidence indicates that pairing policy adjustments, community action and hands-on education outreach is typically crucial to keeping disease at bay (Mahiti et al., 2025). Whenever governments intervene as true champions of public health, they can initiate reforms that reduce disease incidence and improve health more generally (Figure 10.5).

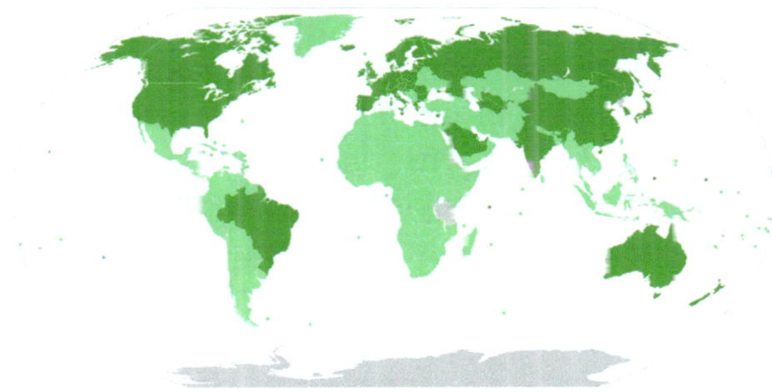

Figure 10.5. Role of government in disease control.

Source: By BlankMap-World6.svg: Canuckguy (talk) and many others (see File history)MSG17 - Own work based on: COVID-19 vaccine#Vaccine candidates, CC BY-SA 4.0, https://commons.wikimedia.org/w/index.php?curid=97386856

10.3.1. Policy Formulation and Implementation

Creating and implementing policies is a significant thing when it comes to fighting diseases. You need to understand what's happening—what health problems are striking hardest, what various populations require, and what you can draw on as resources. Consider dental caries in regions of Latin America and the Caribbean—individuals have discovered that applying fluoride with reduced sugar can be rather effective. It's usually a good idea to put health experts, policymakers, and voices from the community in a room together so that the strategies ultimately align with what people go through. Only by involving everyone can we ensure no vulnerable group gets inadvertently left behind, and the allocation of health resources becomes a little more equitable. In fact, making policy concepts into actual action is all about coordinating at all levels of government and across sectors. In most instances, when working with conditions such as dental caries, a regular check on how policies are performing is essential. For instance, those that provide fluoride—be it in water or salt—require frequent checks to enhance their impacts while averting challenges such as dental fluorosis. And, you know, obstacles like there just not being enough money or a lack of public awareness can drag things out; dealing with these through targeted education and strategic resource shifts is the way to go. Engaging the community in planning and action can also help generate additional support and make the entire effort feel lived-in. Circumstances do change, so policies must be poised to shift mid-steam. Generally speaking, even strategies such as limiting sugar intake should be reviewed and tweaked now and then, to keep up with shifting diets and new research. Taxes on sugary drinks and tighter rules on ads can work pretty well as tools to cut down on sugar—truly important for protecting kids, for example. Collaborating with people from education and food industry professionals in conjunction with public health organizations usually yields more success. These sort of mix-and-match strategies not only improve health but also create good blueprints for the future; it is, after all, a constant process of working out the entire plan. Finally. By constantly monitoring and revising these policies, we guarantee that our strategies remain afloat in an evolving public health environment (Williams et al., 2018; Ricomini-Filho et al., 2021).

10.3.2. Funding and Resource Allocation

Funding options determine how effectively we combat diseases. In much of rural Uganda, say, in combating malaria, not having sufficient money makes the health conditions even more acute. When there is little money, hospitals and clinics fall short on proper infrastructure and sufficient trained personnel—thus retarding any well-conceived intervention strategies. Unbalanced allocation of resources occasionally results in failing to provide for the distinct requirements of such rural communities, effectively perpetuating the cycle of ill health. Generally, investing in the proper locations on firm evidence can increase the entire system's capacity for fair and efficient provision of care (Ali, 2025). Models relying on innovative finance and engaging the voice of place have proven to be a game-changer. In disease-stricken populations such as those struck by malaria, employing technologies in addition to taking local feedback makes each dollar go a long way.

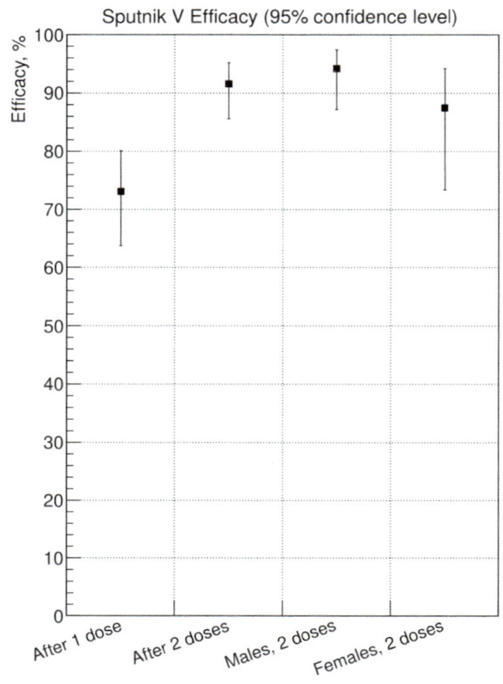

Figure 10.6. Funding and resource allocation.

Source: By V1adis1av - Own work, CC BY-SA 4.0, https://commons.wikimedia.org/w/index.php?curid=101868251

Overall, these strategies do more than merely make funding more evenly distributed—they involve empowering individuals with a voice in creating their own destiny regarding health. A few inspiring case studies point out that when governments, NGOs, and private sector partners collaborate, there is a higher likelihood of igniting new, creative financing solutions that respond to local priorities (Ali, 2025). As for treating life-threatening conditions, like major burn injuries, how funds are allocated between emergency care and long-term treatment significantly affects patient healing. Recent studies suggest that the use of vasopressors early in treatment may be a marker for a more challenging case; these patients tend to have longer hospital stays and ultimately require additional surgeries. This trend indicates a greater clinical load that requires judicious budgeting. In general, relying on such clinical markers can help direct which areas receive increased attention, making sure each dollar goes toward improving patient care and ultimately translating to improved outcomes for those who are in need the most (Figure 10.6).

10.3.3. Collaboration with International Organizations

Tackling global health issues requires a combination of approaches, and a large component of that is collaborating with communities from around the world. Consider organizations such as the WHO or other non-governmental organizations—truly they bring things into action in other places. When these organizations collaborate, they merge resources, expertise, and experience, which is what drives the effort toward equity in health. For instance, when they collaborate, they not only provide funds but also provide straight, pragmatic advice that is responsive to local tradition and necessity. Such cooperative steps bring to mind communities that can overcome adversity, demonstrating the power of collective strength to catalyze innovative, sustainable remedies for health. Collaboration with these international organizations also helps disseminate vital, tested methods for disease management. In general, through systematic reviewing and consultation with stakeholders, they learn the key pieces that make interventions more effective. Research from projects such as the DEterminants of DIet and Physical Activity (DEDIPAC) Knowledge Hub even highlights that a deliberate approach can mobilize robust backing for these measures (Brug et al., 2015). By resting on instruments like the RE-AIM framework, groups can deconstruct effectiveness into components such as reach, adoption, and sticking power over the long haul. This type of evidence is crucial for refining plans for coping with challenging circumstances, which tends to enhance the chances for favorable health results within various groups. Collaborating across borders also creates the platform for a responsive reaction to evolving public health emergencies—pandemics or chronic disease, for example. With our increasingly globalized world, getting health policies in sync across nations is a big deal now. Collaborations allow nations to share best practices, monitor trends, and mobilize resources rapidly. International cooperation comes in when it is about unraveling the complicated aspect of health policies and legal regulations. International organizations intervene to smoothen the experience. Such mutual coordination optimizes the influence of health actions, as viewed in models delineating the foremost conditions for the success of policy (Brug et al., 2015). In such a perspective, cooperation is not merely an added measure; it is the stimulant that gives impetus to wide-ranging successful disease control action.

10.4. Community-Based Interventions

Community-based care initiatives are receiving much focus, particularly now that issues such as heart disease continue to increase. Neighborhood arrangements have become a sort of homegrown answer—making use of what's already available in communities so services reach the areas which truly require them. Consider, for instance, how Clinical Pharmacists (CPs) have filled the gap in community pharmacies. One study of around 900 individuals in 55 various pharmacies revealed that when CPs emphasize patient education and closely monitor medication, the risk of heart problems declines in a significant manner. This type of hands-on, local intervention not only raises individual health scores but also generates community engagement, creating a wider barrier against disease (Obeagu, 2024). New technology is providing these community shifts with an added boost, particularly for seniors. Virtual reality isn't merely for games anymore—it's being utilized to assist in keeping the mind active. In one example, community-residing seniors participated in some guided VR sessions, and what were the results? An improvement in executive functions many found quite impressive.

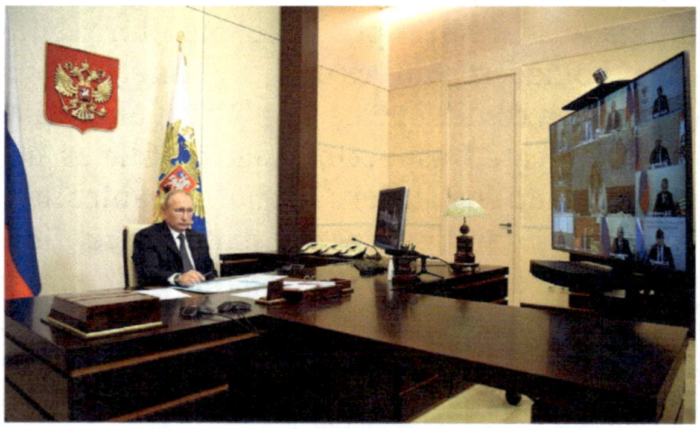

Source: By Kremlin.ru, CC BY 4.0, https://commons.wikimedia.org/w/index.php?curid=93048476

All in all, such customized, tech-based programs not only engage or entertain but also do a great job warding off age-related cognitive decline. By incorporating these brain-stimulation methods into daily community environments, public health initiatives can address challenging problems while providing a little added help to those who need it (Makmee et al., 2022). Aside from the individual benefits, these grassroots interventions are central to ensuring our healthcare system remains viable. By taking care out of large hospitals and into the immediate community, the pressure on emergency services is relieved and more energy is devoted to preventing people from getting ill in the first place. For example, when community members take a positive role in caring for conditions such as CVD, health literacy (HL) increases and people begin to take responsibility for their own behaviors. Research, in most instances, demonstrates that the collaboration of healthcare professionals (HCPs) and community groups yields a networked community dedicated to disease prevention. This comprehensive strategy does not merely enhance figures on paper—it also aligns with broader public health objectives aimed at reducing the long-term effects of chronic diseases (Makmee et al., 2022).

10.4.1. Grassroots Health Initiatives

Public health today relies on the initiative of local communities. Those people on the ground bring their own expertise and cultural flair to the battle against disease, so solutions are developed from real-world problems. Consider those community-organized HIV prevention initiatives—they've established trust and ignited meaningful participation through neighbor-to-neighbor sharing. Messages that originate directly from the community are more likely to resonate with vulnerable individuals, pushing them toward healthier behaviors. It has been proven that such in-your-backyard initiatives commonly increase testing and maintain individuals on their treatment regimens, showing that locally sourced concepts typically have greater success than distant, top-down mandates (Obeagu, 2024). With local resources combined with a sense of ownership, disease rates fall and overall well-being increases. How we turn over health provision has also been an assist to such community schemes. Changes in financing—funding coming from various sectors as opposed to one prime source—means local communities fill the breach, frequently taking the lead with respect to plans to improve health. With backing from national organizations and even the Center for Medicare and Medicaid Innovation (CMMI), these neighborhood teams can obtain the support they require to experiment with layered health interventions. They even create accountable health communities (AHCs) that bring together professionals from various disciplines, not only clinical care but also social factors such as poverty and education (Corrigan et al., 2015). By sharing resources and making unlikely alliances, they build enduring solutions to health inequities. Sustainability is a finicky animal, overall. It all depends on consistent cash flow, engaged community voice, and savvy means of measuring impact. Too often, inconstant government backing and money that appears and then vanishes can impede advance. Generally, grassroots groups must establish mutual accountability with health providers and local people—even though sometimes it is necessary to introduce a little chaos for creativity. One suggestion is to direct a portion of hospitals' community benefits back into local activities, weaving together a more cohesive health system. Through collaboration and a shared, if occasionally confused, vision for health equity, these efforts can continually adapt, evolve to address the changing challenges of disease control (Corrigan et al., 2015).

10.4.2. Role of Local Health Workers

Local health workers truly make an impact on disease control. They are not mere pieces in the medical apparatus but are the connecting bridge that interfaces clinical services with the day-to-day neighborhoods. They understand the habits, language habits, and traditions of their community very well, and this intimate understanding allows them to mold health interventions that resonate with people. Most of the time, solutions developed for specific needs conquer challenges that more general techniques overlook. Consider type 2 diabetes, for instance—DIABETHIC demonstrated that when these workers and patients' collaborate to identify issues and come to mutual agreements, trust develops organically, and patients adhere more to treatment. By banding together to address such concerns as culturally attuned dietary guidance and greater social support access, they inadvertently increase treatment compliance as well as general well-being (Bonvicini et al., 2025).

Community health workers also lead the way in preventing issues from arising in the first place, particularly for the most at-risk individuals. For instance, the DREAMS Initiative in Sub-Saharan Africa, which focuses on adolescent girls and young women, shows how these workers do more than just provide medical care—they spark community conversations and help clear up long-held myths about things like HIV Pre-Exposure Prophylaxis (PrEP). They are not merely service providers; They are advocates whose voices ensure that even the sidelined are heard. An idea like the safe space model highlights very nicely how the addition of a community-centric twist to health concepts can dismantle stigma and misconceptions, leading the way for improved measures and results for vulnerable groups (Jackson-Gibson et al., 2021).

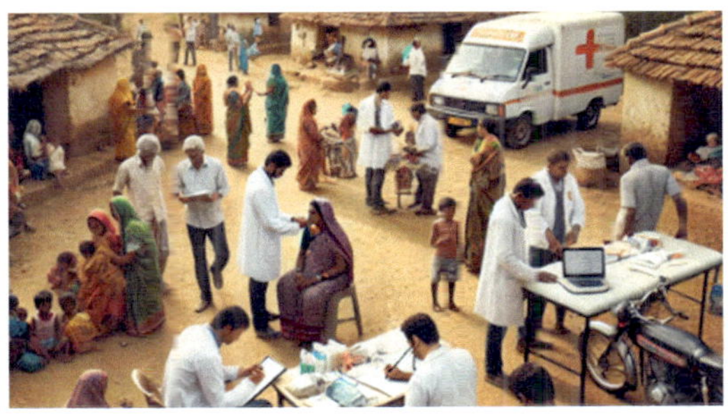

Figure 10.7. Role of local health workers.

Source: Indian Association of Preventive and Social Medicine. (2025). *Strengthening Healthcare Through Collaboration.*

In the long run, local health workers' participation sets the stage for long-term health gains. Being regarded as part of the communities and not outsiders, they foster long-term relationships that keep health messages alive and resilient. Overall, such close relationships facilitate ease in identifying new challenges as they arise, and adjusting strategies in the moment. Their constant communication with residents regularly leads to seeing issues before they spiral, allowing interventions to arrive at precisely the right time. Overall, this consistent, grassroots mobilization not only addresses current issues but also creates more robust health systems capable of addressing future problems (Bonvicini et al., 2025) (Figure 10.7).

10.4.3. Community Engagement and Participation

Local knowledge is what gets results when combating diseases – outcomes in public health rely heavily on individuals familiar with their own communities. Successful interventions now rely on regular citizens to contribute wisdom on their own social networks and cultural idiosyncrasies, so initiatives such as mosquito control or health education can be adapted to resonate more with locals. Aedes mosquito control projects, for example, demonstrate that the participation of specialists across various disciplines with the voices of local people generally leads to outcomes that last. It is evident that sustaining efforts is not only a matter of policy but also the ability of the community to take action based on its own knowledge, the active engagement of the people being at the center. In diverse cultural contexts, trust in the community can also increase access to care and knowledge about health. Consider the Health and Faith Initiative in Koreatown: this initiative leverages established social networks such as churches to disseminate health education and establish disease screening for immigrant communities. Bilingual church leaders were equipped to facilitate cancer education workshops, which alleviated challenges such as language barriers and economic barriers in a very practical manner. This model, in numerous instances, highlights how community institutions bridge gaps in health services, particularly for individuals facing additional barriers. By relying on these trusted community leaders, the project not only funneled resources efficiently but also facilitated an environment in which disease control plans could be discussed freely. Also, when community members are engaged in disease control designs, they are more likely to take ownership of the process and enhance the overall effectiveness of health programs. A recent assessment of Aedes mosquito control operations overall demonstrated that methods constructed around local participation emphatically outperform ones imposed top-down. Where individuals engaged in this activity, mosquito-borne diseases fell significantly – an indicator that collaborative efforts compound the effects. Overall, maintaining these efforts relies on maintaining open dialogue and adapting as local conditions evolve, even if the process isn't flawless every time. Overall, a continuous, occasionally flawed, conversation between authorities responsible for public health and local communities lays the groundwork for solutions that are both successful and organically part of their own cultural fabric.

10.5. Technological Innovations in Disease Control

Technology and public health cooperate in some quite surprising ways. New methods of disease combat now also pay attention to our environment. Integrated vector management (IVM), for instance—is a practice that combines knowledge about disease research and plain green concepts. IVM combats insect-borne diseases while reducing the likelihood that insects turn cunning against pesticides; it's truly a two-pronged approach that alters how we address health concerns. Gwadabe et al., (2025) note that coupling health movements with nature issues is a potent way to augment their influence as well as residual presence. Ultimately, such fusion enables us to treat ailments at present and regulate our environment concurrently. Predictive modeling through AI and machine learning has also upset hospitals and medical clinics. Large caches of data enable early detection of risky areas so that outbreaks can be caught in the early stages. These intelligent models not only alert us to potential issues—they assist in getting the resources to where they are necessary, occasionally reducing waste. A study indicates that when these models team up with IoT-based tracking, they drive improved cleanup methods and reduce contamination risks significantly (Palla & Iwunwa, 2025). This proactive approach empowers most of the health workers to make evidence-based decisions to make the overall system more robust, even though the details at times appear to be somewhat exaggerated. Mobile health (mHealth) is yet another fragment of this changing picture. These technologies provide healthcare providers with immediate access to the patient's information and enable patients to stay connected, particularly where resources are limited. mHealth not only enables it to be easier to collect vital health information, but it also assists the patients in making sense of and adhering to treatment plans—something that's been the case in many instances (Gwadabe et al., 2025). As our battle against illnesses becomes increasingly about real-time information and community connection, mHealth is pushing us toward a more personal and responsive approach to caregiving. Overall, combining common-or-garden technology with traditional public health tactics is a giant leap forward in being one step ahead of infectious disease, even if the strategy occasionally is a bit rough around the edges (Figure 10.8).

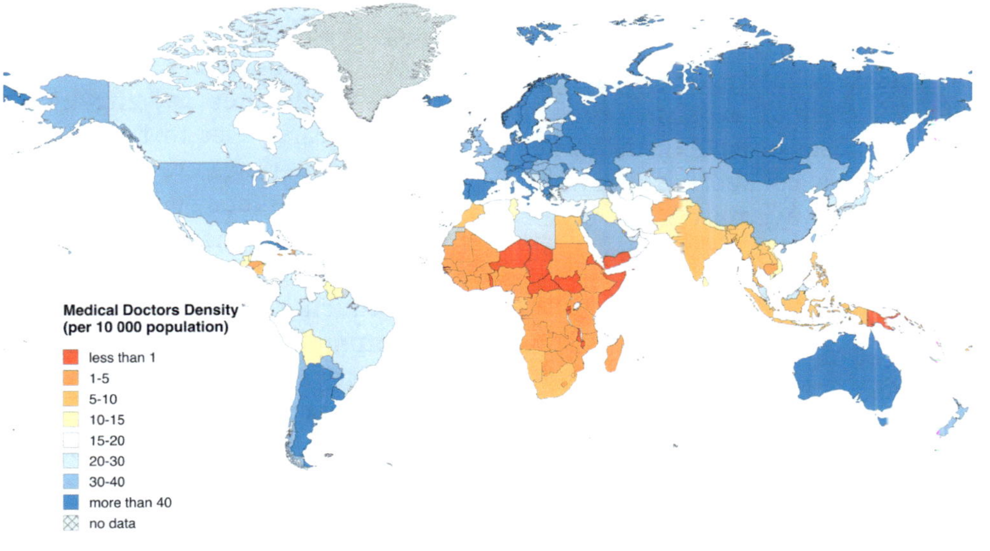

Figure 10.8. Technological innovations in disease control.

Source: By ThatNerdyHylian - Own work, CC0, https://commons.wikimedia.org/w/index.php?curid=165512568 https://www.statnews.com/wp-content/uploads/2018/03/1500pixels.jpg

10.5.1. Use of Data Analytics and Surveillance

Data analytics is disrupting how we monitor diseases nowadays Real-time data allows healthcare professionals to identify warning signs and, quite honestly, enhance patient outcomes significantly. It is not about getting ahead of issues; it is also about utilizing resources more intelligently and managing chronic conditions. Individuals tend to note that predictive analytics—basically that ability to crunch real-time data—assists administrators in making difficult decisions, even though the discussion occasionally goes into thick technicalities. The entire arrangement ends up enhancing efficiency in health facilities, paving the way for improved care and more effective disease control practices (Kosaraju, 2024). Then there is the One Health concept, which has emerged as a means of viewing how all people, animals, and the environment interconnect. When considering monitoring antibiotic consumption—from the international arena down to neighborhood farms—the necessity of multi-strata attempts at data gathering becomes extremely evident. Current research continues to point out that the spotty monitoring of antimicrobials in the animal population can be a monkey wrench in the works of public health outcomes. By drawing on tools such as the United States Center for Disease Control and Prevention Policy Analytical Framework, people can begin to calculate what type of strategies will prove effective. Such an expansive type of surveillance not only feeds into public policy but also pushes international collaboration forward, all while improving the overall quality of the data utilized to combat diseases (Ching et al., 2024). Meanwhile, it is difficult to avoid all the hype surrounding ethics with regard to data privacy and regulation in these technology-influenced strategies. Organizations are relying more and more on these systems for disease tracking and intervention, and that usually means walking the fine line between patient trust and protecting personal information. In most instances, establishing robust—but not rigid—data governance structures is the way to go, as they both safeguard individual privacy and establish how data is used. Tackling these ethical puzzles head-on turns out to be vital for the trustworthiness of any data-heavy health strategy. As predictive analytics continues to steer healthcare interventions, being careful and responsible with data is not just a nice-to-have—it is essential for winning and keeping public confidence (Kosaraju, 2024).

10.5.2. Advancements in Medical Technology

Healthcare is evolving rapidly, and there are emerging technologies beginning to transform the way we prevent and cure diseases. Nanorobots, for instance, provide a clear spin by getting medications directly to target cells. This mini technology usually reduces side effects and increases the effectiveness of treatments. In some cases, the robots even enable doctors to use less invasive procedures, allowing patients to heal faster. Most often, this is going to turn the field of oncology on its head, although it also comes with some ethic and practical issues that remain to be resolved. In general, such breakthroughs promise a new way of designing and delivering treatments in the clinic—one which requires continued research and collaboration across disciplines (Zoheb et al., 2025). One of the fascinating aspects is how these advances are addressing chronic diseases—diabetes specifically. Conventional therapies rarely get to the root of the causes and can sometimes create additional miseries. Innovative methods such as gene therapy, stem cell methods, and nanotechnology are unveiling unforeseen avenues for managing blood sugar and reducing complications. A combination of contemporary nutrition recommendations and lifestyle adjustments further emphasizes the importance of a balanced treatment plan. Nevertheless, implementing these innovations is not without their bumps along the road, from patients' ability to adhere to their plans to refining how treatments are administered. Overall, combining these new ideas with proven approaches appears essential to creating management frameworks that remain resilient (Landge, 2025). New technology is also providing innovative means to contain disease and improve patient care. Wearable sensors and mobile medical apps now enable individuals to monitor vital signs and other health indicators in real time—providing both patients and physicians helpful hints for making informed decisions. These technologies enable more patient control while providing clinicians with information that they can use. Telemedicine, which gained momentum following disruptions such as the COVID-19 pandemic, has become an efficient means of consultation. This change in receiving care, particularly for vulnerable populations, serves to bridge some gaps in public health. In short, when healthcare and technology converge, we not only witness developments in treatment techniques but also experience a shift toward more collaborative and open care (Landge, 2025; Zoheb et al., 2025) (Figure 10.9).

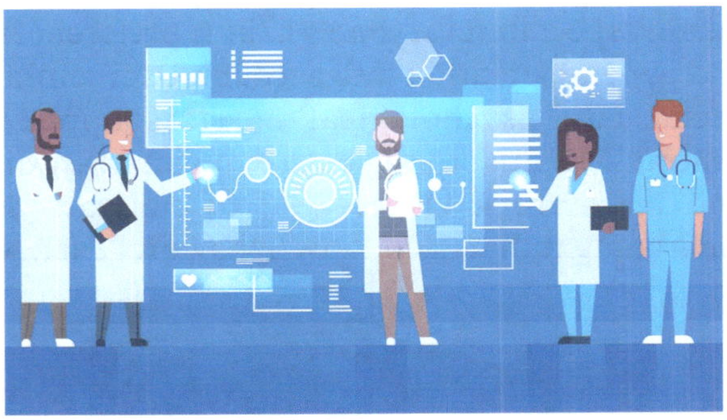

Figure 10.9. Advancements in medical technology.

Source: https://media.licdn.com/dms/image/v2/D5612AQGqveA9-Qwh0g/article-cover_image-shrink_720_1280/article-cover_image-shrink_720_1280/0/1687454511447?e=2147483647&v=beta&t=q0exchy-xrL9ptXGo3geBTiPSAHFNcx3IHL8bT6GMoI

10.5.3. Telehealth and Remote Monitoring

Technology is transforming healthcare in ways you can't ignore. Remote monitoring and telehealth have exploded onto the scene as go-to means of getting interventions accomplished right. Healthcare systems, attempting to deduce a combination of needs, particularly for individuals who are older or who have chronic conditions—are currently employing these digital technologies to engage patients more in their own health care. The Advancing Care Coordination & Telehealth Deployment (ACT) Program, for example, shows that physicians and patients don't always view care in exactly the same way. As a general rule, this disparity demonstrates why establishing coordinated telehealth services—with emphasis on understandable speech and patient comprehension—is so critical. By doing this, telehealth not only encourages patients to become active participants, it can also result in improved outcomes and more stable treatment plans. Primary care is at the forefront of having telehealth work effectively. With good technology, primary care physicians are not merely throwing in additional bells and whistles; They are streamlining care coordination, particularly for individuals facing several health complexities. Remote monitoring translates to being able to monitor health information in real-time and intervening before a condition rapidly declines. Studies all in all indicate that good handling of these problems is important—it not only provides patients with the care they require but also reduces the burden on hospitals. And having telehealth become standard in primary care clinics creates a sort of teamwork whereby patients and caregivers both contribute toward making healthcare more accessible and efficient. Nevertheless, all is not sailing smoothly. Teething issues persist when attempting to implement and optimize telehealth initiatives within primary care. Challenges such as patchy data availability and extremely homogenous resources make it difficult to assess how effective such programs are. As per the ACT Program, organizational structure can influence what patients anticipate and feel. More often than not, primary care providers must modify their day-to-day practices so that these new instruments fit seamlessly into place—so that the transition doesn't simply appear good on paper but puts the patient at the forefront. As the medical field continues to develop, close-fisted observation, and constant adjustments will be essential to finding a balance between controlling disease and better outcomes in a highly varied patient population.

10.6. Challenges in Implementing Intervention Strategies

Health systems today frequently encounter a great many unforeseen challenges when experimenting with innovative intervention approaches. One of the big problems is that there simply are not enough resources available—due to this shortage, frequently healthcare providers are not receiving the type of training they require. Family physicians, for instance, who are meant to provide dietary recommendations for long-term ailments such as diabetes, find themselves pushed by timed schedules and a shortage of specialized expertise. In the majority of instances, Abdullah et al. (2024) demonstrate that these limitations prevent the effective promotion of healthy eating habits, hence disrupting patient outcomes and long-term care. In short, filling these knowledge gaps with well-targeted training and improved systems of support is crucial. Still, another snag exists in attempting to partner with all the right parties; things are particularly ugly when different stakeholders have to collaborate together. The One Health initiative is a prime example—it requires collaborations among individuals in human health, animal health, and environmental authorities, and getting all those parties aligned with each other is no easy task. In general terms, effective coordination and communication are the core of integrated surveillance systems that assist in warding off public health threats, particularly those associated with zoonotic diseases. As Ojeyinka & Omaghomi (2024) discuss, assembling coordinated surveillance activities implies facing regulatory hurdles and chop-chop data systems that can urgently put the brakes on. Constructing robust, cross-sectoral frameworks that facilitate open data sharing and concerted action is necessary to keep disease in check. Individuals' mindsets and day-to-day behaviors introduce another level of complexity. Frequently, people resist lifestyle changes aimed at preventing disease, in part due to cultural beliefs, occasionally due to misinformation, or simply due to lack of motivation. For example, when nutritional interventions are applied to treat chronic diseases, patients may find the recommendations too stringent or limiting to maintain. Abdullah et al. (2024) point out that the real worth of nutritional counseling depends on a patient-centered approach that takes respect for everyone's habits, preferences, and general situation into account. Overcoming social and psychological barriers appears central if health strategies are to gain traction, and therefore it is essential to cultivate an environment that facilitates behavioral change.

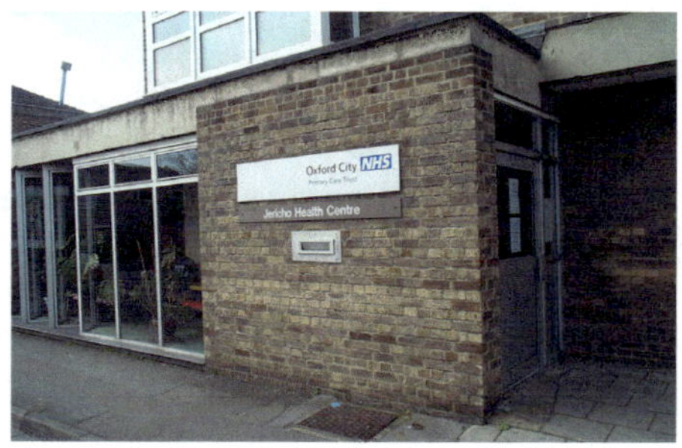

Source: By Kaihsu - Own work, CC BY-SA 3.0, https://commons.wikimedia.org/w/index.php?curid=90005

10.6.1. Socioeconomic Barriers

Financial issues and societal hurdles go far when it comes to our well-being, particularly with long-term disease. Individuals with lower incomes tend to have so many hurdles that it becomes quite difficult to obtain quality healthcare or simply lead a healthier lifestyle. Not being able to afford it leads to missing out on quality physician visits, required medications, and simple check-ups. And it is not only about cash; where people live matters too – many neighborhoods lack fresh food stores or safe areas for exercise, which only makes things worse. All of these issues tend to feed off one another, creating a loop of ongoing illness and poverty that generally calls for intervention strategies crafted specifically for those hit hardest. Local, grassroots-based initiatives can at times be the solution to these hard obstacles. Studies indicate, in many instances, that educational initiatives that engage people, particularly those in underserved populations—can have significant impact. For instance, churches in rural Alabama joined forces with community organizations to offer focused health education to better cope with hypertension among Black adults. By relying on already established community institutions, these programs not only enable individuals to receive the care they require but also create a feeling of belonging and responsibility—closing the socioeconomic divides that too often block the path to improved health. New, innovative solutions that combine various aspects of health services provide a balanced path forward for the care of chronic disease. See how combining sports activities with healthcare at the community level can create strength in the community and reduce the risk of chronic illnesses. When you combine simple health education, convenient access to medical services, and firsthand training for residents, you are producing a type of culture that is all about awareness and activity. This concerted effort, in most instances, can narrow the economic disparities that usually result in poorer results. Finally, creating a health system that addresses the needs of high-risk individuals continues to be central in our continuous battle against chronic disease.

10.6.2. Cultural Resistance to Interventions

If you consider halting diseases, you simply can't neglect the cultural aspect of things—even when the science underpinning an intervention is sound. History teaches us that good designs frequently encounter resistance since individuals' beliefs and traditions play a great deal of importance. Consider initiatives that distribute insecticide-treated beds for malaria; if people don't believe the nets will work or are safe to use, the entire concept starts to collapse. Misinformation, deep-seated religious beliefs or plain old traditions can cause individuals to avoid using these initiatives, and that undermines our battle against disease. It turns out that getting what a community thinks and involving them right from the start is key to building trust and making these health measures stick. After noticing this cultural resistance, it becomes clear that getting the community involved is not just a nice add-on—it is essential. Programs must employ hands-on approaches that invite local feedback so that interventions are compatible with the values and lifestyles of the people. For instance, combining public health strategies with known cultural traditions can enhance how well the people accept the concept when addressing schistosomiasis. Forcing local leaders to support the interventions can increase trust in the message so that everyone feels They are on the same team. And when new measures are anchored in things that are already a part of daily life, such as traditional methods for managing water—they are more likely to be adopted naturally. This type of approach not only gains more buy-in but also leverages what locals already know, creating ideas that feel both new and culturally on-target. Ultimately, whatever strategy succeeds must pay attention to how cultural landscapes evolve and how external influences may reorder those opinions. Globalization and climate change, for example, shake things up so that well-established beliefs and practices can shift, which could disrupt health interventions. Ongoing research and open discussions with community members help catch these changes, ensuring plans remain relevant and effective. One such good example is modifying housing to become more climate-resilient—as some recent research has pointed out—while not only assisting in the mitigation of malaria transmission but also aligning with how the locals handle climate issues (Mukamurera, 2025). In the same way, exploring the social and economic origins of schistosomiasis, such as environmental effects and general health within communities, remains important to bypassing resistance (Mwinzi et al., 2025). In general, the combination of cultural knowledge with flexible methods enhances overall success in disease control and maintains efforts sustainable in the long run.

10.6.3. Global Disparities in Healthcare Access

Health results vary greatly when healthcare is not accessible evenly. Most low and middle-income countries have individuals who are devastated because services simply are not there when needed. There is a combination of things that cause this – such as having sufficient funds, being able to get an education, and even the design of neighborhoods.

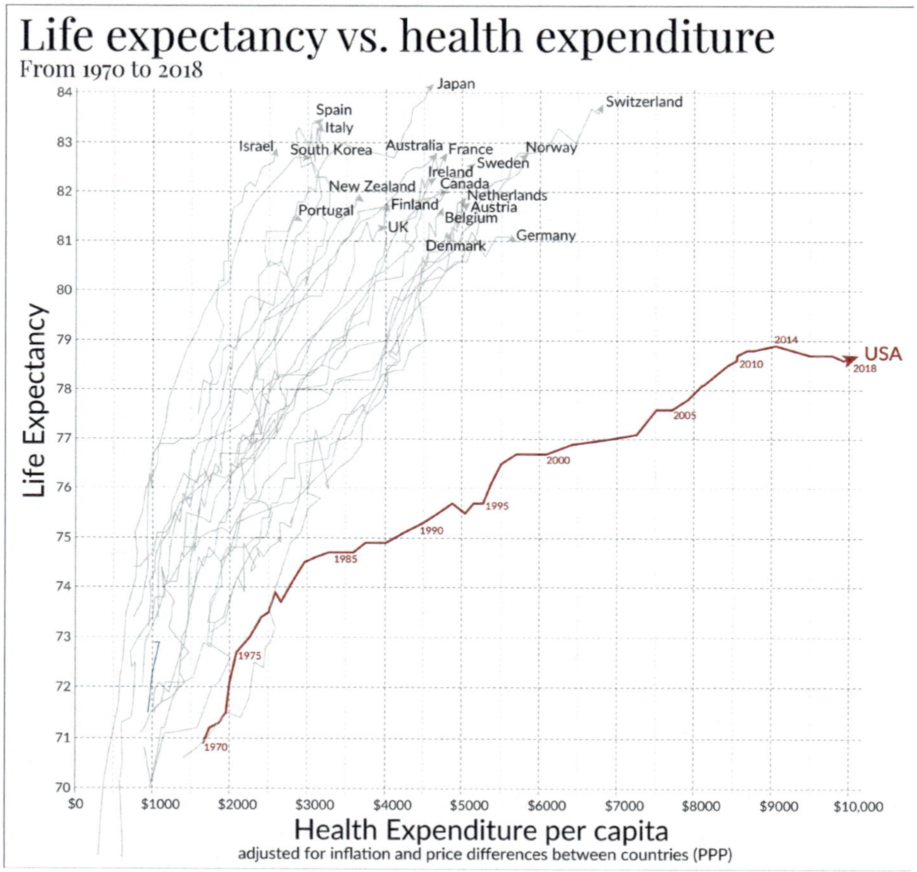

Figure 10.10. Global disparities in healthcare access.

Source: By Max Roser - Link between health spending and life expectancy: US is an outlier (archive link). May 26, 2017. By Max Roser at Our World in Data. Click the sources tab under the chart for info on the countries, healthcare expenditures, and data sources. See the later version of the chart in the Oct 29, 2020 article by Max Roser: Why is life expectancy in the US lower than in other rich countries?., CC BY-SA 4.0, https://commons.wikimedia.org/w/index.php?curid=21270608

The CDC indicates that these things determine how far the health system. Without wise, effective steps to address the gaps, healthcare costs could balloon out of control—some projections even suggest more than a trillion dollars annually by 2040 (Srinivasaiah, 2024). When you consider it, the suffering of entire communities, rather than individual people, illustrates quite how far-reaching these problems are. Take the example of illnesses such as malaria. More than 90% of malaria infections strike Africa, particularly children and expectant mothers. In most of those places, poor infrastructure means life-saving treatments and preventive measures just do not make it to the patients who need them the most (Kamanzi, 2024). Even when there are established tools, such as Insecticide-Treated Bed Nets and high-quality antimalarial medicines—their impact gets diluted because the systems for delivering them are too weak or patched up unevenly. This scenario brings home the importance of targeted actions that not only address disease immediately, but also create a more robust healthcare system as a whole. A combination of grassroots efforts and technology is the key to closing these gaps. It's reasonable to have local people play a hands-on part in implementing these health initiatives so that they function in the long term—even if the strategy is rehashed multiple times. Furthermore, leveraging data analytics can provide some seriously useful information about how to allocate resources and provide services more efficiently to various regions. In most instances, getting together on a global front is the sole path to enhancing aggregate access that in return will reduce costs and enhance results. Overall, addressing such disparities is not merely the appropriate thing to do; it is also an intelligent decision for disease control and driving public health (Srinivasaiah, 2024) (Figure 10.10).

CLOSER LOOK

COVID-19

COVID-19 is an extremely contagious respiratory illness brought on by the SARS-CoV-2 virus. Initially discovered in late 2019 in Wuhan, China, it immediately spread into a worldwide pandemic, impacting countless lives and economies globally. The virus is mostly transmitted through respiratory droplets after coughing, sneezing, or speaking, but also through aerosols and contaminated surfaces. Symptoms are mild (cough, fever, tiredness) to severe (pneumonia, acute respiratory distress syndrome, organ failure), and some carry no symptoms but remain infectious.

COVID-19 has a disproportionate impact on older people and those with comorbidities like diabetes, heart disease, and obesity. It has uncovered and made more entrenched existing disparities in healthcare access among populations.

Public health measures have ranged from mask requirements, lockdowns, and travel bans to most crucially, large-scale vaccination campaigns. mRNA vaccines such as Moderna and Pfizer-BioNTech have been most important in slowing severe disease and death, although new variants have continued to pose challenges.

COVID-19 has also spurred innovation in telemedicine, vaccine production, and public health monitoring. Though significant advances have been achieved, the virus continues to mutate, and hence global collaboration, vaccine equity, and readiness for future pandemics are essential.

SUMMARY

There are numerous attempts being made to control diseases, and when you combine various intervention strategies, it then becomes apparent that one size fits all doesn't work since demographic and socioeconomic variations do count. It is somewhat like experimenting with a new recipe: you must tailor it to what you have. New technologies such as remote blood pressure monitoring (RBPM) are creating new pathways for the management of chronic disorders like stroke and cardiovascular disease. In the majority of cases, research demonstrates that compliance with RBPM is directly linked to improved health outcomes among at-risk individuals; this supports the necessity of prevention practice based on evidence. And by focusing on minority populations, which tend to have a greater burden of vascular issues, these plans can be adjusted to reduce health disparities and ultimately improve public health levels in these at-risk populations (Kurzman et al., 2025). Community engagement proves to be a giant component in programs combatting non-communicable diseases. Occasionally, getting people together has the effect of stirring up resources and creating support systems that function near magic—keeping healthcare initiatives alive. Recent research indicates that community-driven solutions, such as peer support networks and even specific health classes, can get people to stick with healthy habits over the long term. As you blend in culturally appropriate concepts with technology today, even poor regions can catch up, developing not only resilience among residents but also a sort of blueprint for sustainable, scalable NCD prevention (Banerjee et al., 2024). All these various strategies, taken together, provide us with a comprehensive framework that addresses the numerous tiers of disease control. As studies continually uncover what's stopping us and what's driving us forward, stakeholders absolutely need to have flexibility and inclusiveness at the forefront. Delving deeper into more tech innovations along with community engagement appears to create a synergy that increases our overall prevention power. Getting together public health professionals, policymakers, and community members—sometimes in innovative ways—will be instrumental to refining these strategies and ensuring that they hold up over time. Ultimately, as chronic diseases continue to escalate, that combination of hands-on community activity and high-tech innovation seems like our best option for achieving our public health objectives (Banerjee et al., 2024; Kurzman et al., 2025).

Good disease management requires combining various means of observing and acting early. The recent review of SARS-CoV-2 testing, for example, indicates that catching cases before symptoms even appear can make a big difference; waiting to see who feels ill captures much of the picture. In Germany, a hands-on approach proved to identify many silent carriers—individuals who unknowingly allow the virus to quietly make its way into communities. For the most part, these initial actions, such as those piloted in the CoV-Surv Study, ultimately provide local health crews more indications of how prevalent the issue may become, and can then guide practical responses prior to outbreaks raging out of control (Deckert et al., 2021). Customizing support to meet one's own requirements can also raise outcomes across groups. When researchers examined disability support systems, they discovered that initiating assistance early not only improves individuals' health but also is cost-saving in the long term. Consider Australia's National Disability Insurance Scheme (NDIS)—it demonstrates that allowing people to direct their own care makes support both accessible and appropriate to individual situations. This type of flexible thinking can be used elsewhere as well, indicating that some personalized care could potentially redesign how we manage chronic health problems and other complications in communities (Gilchrist et al., 2021). Finally, consideration of cost-effectiveness is essential to maintaining these strategies. Verifying how much each approach costs, such as in the CoV-Surv Study, where numbers like cost per correctly screened individual and detection rate are involved—assists authorities in selecting choices that pay. Examining how increasing employment opportunities for individuals with disabilities can advantage all parties also underscores why intelligent investments in health are significant. Overall, while our health systems continue to change, frequent re-evaluation of intervention plans becomes a necessity for keeping up with disease control and creating communities that can recover (Deckert et al., 2021; Gilchrist et al., 2021).

KEY TERMS FROM THIS CHAPTER

- Intervention
- Eradication
- Prevention
- Isolation
- Health education
- Chemoprophylaxis
- Social distancing
- Hygiene promotion
- Travel restrictions
- Risk communication
- Disease control
- Elimination
- Quarantine
- Contact tracing
- Personal protective equipment (PPE)
- Mass drug administration (MDA)
- Lockdown
- Disinfection
- Behavioral change communication (BCC)
- Outbreak response

REFERENCES

1. Adams, S. A., Workman, L., Sakhuja, M., Yelton, B., Wickersham, K. E., Fairman, C., Eberth, J., Heiney, S., Hebert, J. R., King, J. H., Hucek, F. A., Schaurer, L., & Friedman, D. B. (2025). Reflecting on partnerships established and sustained over four cycles of a federally funded cancer prevention and control research program: lessons learned for community-academic networks. *Frontiers in public health, 12,* 1384588. https://doi.org/10.3389/fpubh.2024.1384588 (accessed on 6 May 2025).
2. Alarcon, P., Alexopoulos, C., Amirpour Haredasht, D., Arruda, A. G., Nathues, H., Cano, J. P., Corzo, C., et al. (2018). Modelling the economic efficiency of using different strategies to control Porcine Reproductive & Respiratory Syndrome at herd level. *Preventive Veterinary Medicine, 152,* 89–102. https://core.ac.uk/download/153498728.pdf (accessed on 6 May 2025).
3. Baroni, I., Barrett, D., Bescos, C., Buskens, E., et al. (2015). *What Does it Take to Make Integrated Care Work? A 'Cookbook' for Large-Scale Deployment of Coordinated Care and Telehealth.* https://core.ac.uk/download/155776181.pdf (accessed on 6 May 2025).
4. Bonvicini, L., Venturelli, F., Bononi, F., Balestra, G. L., Iorio, G., Ghirotto, L., Petrelli, A., et al. (2025). A randomized trial to evaluate a complex, co-created, culture-sensitive intervention to promote healthy lifestyles and compliance to therapy in immigrants with type 2 diabetes: A protocol of a multicenter Italian study. *PLOS One, 20.* https://www.semanticscholar.org/paper/fa265aa918b3e0258471d5d9494dd5fcc8b8adfc (accessed on 6 May 2025).
5. Brug, J., De Bourdeaudhuij, I., Hayes, C. B., Hendriksen, M., et al. (2015). Implementation conditions for diet and physical activity interventions and policies: An umbrella review. *BMC Public Health, 15,* 1250. https://core.ac.uk/download/55847893.pdf (accessed on 6 May 2025).
6. Burnett, A. L., Nehra, A., Breau, R. H., Culkin, D. J., Faraday, M. M., Hakim, L., Heidelbaugh, J. J., et al. (2018). Erectile dysfunction: AUA guideline. *The Journal of Urology, 200,* 633–641. https://doi.org/10.1016/j.juro.2018.05.004.
7. Chatterjee, S., Rastogi, S., & Zehmakan, A. N. (2023). A novel room-based epidemic model: Quarantine, testing, and vaccination strategies. *arXiv.* http://arxiv.org/abs/2310.12171 (accessed on 6 May 2025).
8. Gamon, M. (2013). *Multidrug-Resistant Tuberculosis in India: Solving A Problem by Reconstructing the Public Health Infrastructure.* Ronald E. McNair Scholars Program, 2013 (Book 12). https://core.ac.uk/download/67755957.pdf (accessed on 6 May 2025).
9. Gilchrist, T. E., & Perks, B. (2021). *NDIS Green Paper 5: NDIS Industry Literature Summary—A Review of The Collection of Industry, Government, And Academic Reports. SSRN Electronic Journal.* https://www.semanticscholar.org/paper/706adff36594bc72217c8707634bf23f0ffe0a92 (accessed on 6 May 2025).
10. Heymann, D., & Shindo, N. (2020). COVID-19: What is next for public health? *The Lancet, 395,* 542–545. https://doi.org/10.1016/S0140-6736(20)30374-3.
11. Kosaraju, D. (2024). Predictive analytics in healthcare: Leveraging AI to anticipate disease outbreaks and enhance patient outcomes. *Galore International Journal of Health Sciences and Research.* https://www.semanticscholar.org/paper/3de05adec9be85f1526f2b1c1233927626aac832 (accessed on 6 May 2025).

12. Meherali, S., Punjani, N. S., Louie-Poon, S., Abdul Rahim, K., Das, J. K., Salam, R. A., & Lassi, Z. S. (2021). Mental health of children and adolescents among COVID-19 and past pandemics: A rapid systematic review. *International Journal of Environmental Research and Public Health, 18*(7), 3432. https://doi.org/10.3390/ijerph18073432.

13. Menzies-Gow, A., Bafadhel, M., Busse, W. W., Casale, T. B., Kocks, J., Pavord, I., Szefler, S. J., et al. (2019). An expert consensus framework for asthma remission as a treatment goal. *Journal of Allergy and Clinical Immunology, 145*, 757–765. https://doi.org/10.1016/j.jaci.2019.12.006.

14. Nesbitt, T. S., & Young, H. M. (2017). Increasing the capacity of primary care through enabling technology. *Journal of General Internal Medicine, 32*(4), 398–403. https://doi.org/10.1007/s11606-016-3952-3.

15. Northup, P. G., García-Pagán, J. C., García-Tsao, G., Intagliata, N. M., Superina, R., Roberts, L. N., Lisman, T., et al. (2020). Vascular liver disorders, portal vein thrombosis, and procedural bleeding in patients with liver disease: 2020 practice guidance by the American Association for the Study of Liver Diseases. *Hepatology, 73*, 366–413. https://doi.org/10.1002/hep.31646.

16. Ojeyinka, O. T., & Omaghomi, T. T. (2024). Integrative strategies for zoonotic disease surveillance: A review of one health implementation in the United States. *World Journal of Biology Pharmacy and Health Sciences*. https://doi.org/10.30574/wjbphs.2024.17.3.0124: https://www.semanticscholar.org/paper/14a36c29aff45152e6e0acf02aa87c449c24c683 (accessed on 6 May 2025).

17. Page, M. J., Moher, D., Bossuyt, P. M., Boutron, I., Hoffmann, T., Mulrow, C. D., Shamseer, L., et al. (2021). PRISMA 2020 explanation and elaboration: Updated guidance and exemplars for reporting systematic reviews. *BMJ, 372*, n160. https://doi.org/10.1136/bmj.n160.

18. Palla, U., & Iwunwa, M. G. (2025). Leveraging predictive models to enhance infection control and reduce cross-contamination in public health settings. *International Journal of Research Publication and Reviews*. https://www.semanticscholar.org/paper/471be7429ec568067fea0cc7a399c7db7d75d031 (accessed on 6 May 2025).

19. Ricomini-Filho, A. P., Chávez, B. A., Giacaman, R. A., Frazão, P., & Cury, J. A. (2021). Community interventions and strategies for caries control in Latin American and Caribbean countries. *Brazilian Oral Research, 35*, e0054. https://doi.org/10.1590/1807-3107bor-2021.vol35.0054.

20. Roth, G. A., Mensah, G. A., Johnson, C. O., Addolorato, G., Ammirati, E., Baddour, L. M., Barengo, N. C., et al. (2020). Global burden of cardiovascular diseases and risk factors, 1990–2019. *Journal of the American College of Cardiology, 76*, 2982–3021. https://doi.org/10.1016/j.jacc.2020.11.010.

21. Williams, B., Mancia, G., Spiering, W., Rosei, E. A., Azizi, M., Burnier, M., Clement, D. L., et al. (2018). 2018 ESC/ESH Guidelines for the management of arterial hypertension. *European Heart Journal, 39*, 3021–3104. https://doi.org/10.1093/eurheartj/ehy339.

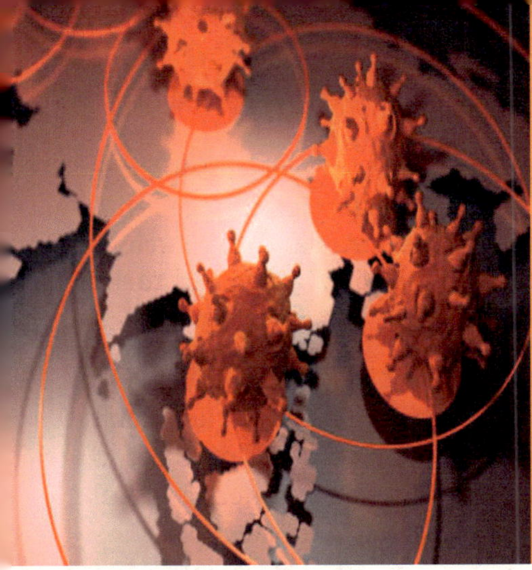

Chapter 11

MODELING EPIDEMICS AND PREDICTING OUTBREAKS

Contents

Introduction

Infectious diseases, with their maddening turns, continue to challenge our health systems worldwide. Urbanization and greater interconnectivity between people only aggravate the potential for outbreaks, pushing us toward new, sometimes unpolished, modes of thinking about what's around the corner. Scientists are delving into math models and computer simulations to test hundreds of "what if" scenarios—adjusting the rate at which infection spreads and how treatments can be effective. It's not just about reliving old epidemics; it's also about outlining plans to avoid future threats. AI now becomes part of the equation, offering cutting predictions and healthier decisions (Mustafa et al., 2025). In some respects, combining old-fashioned math-y epidemiology with new-fangled technology is directing us toward new, unorthodox means of combating infection—and it puts into context just why more investment in technology and research is so desperately required. Machine learning is truly disrupting how we predict outbreaks. Rather than hanging on to age-old surveillance techniques that are slowed down by delays and spotty data, modern ML algorithms dig through mountains of information—from medical trials to social media buzz—to provide quicker, more precise predictions (Ehsan, 2024). These methods, while sometimes a tad adaptive in tendency, can pick up cues that older models may readily overlook, even considering varying strains of the virus and the unclear nature of disease transmission. As we unravel the layers of viral spread, how ML zigzags and turns to make its best bets is pure gold.

This development sort of nails technology's ongoing position as a front-runner in staying ahead of new threats to public health. Naturally, inserting AI and ML into epidemic models isn't without its bumps. Large problems such as unbalanced data quality, models that are difficult to read, and excessively stringent validation procedures still hang in the air. There is a heavy moral implication to contend with as well—fired-up predictions trigger intervention mistakes with far-reaching consequences. Specialists across diverse fields must collaborate, revising data gathering and ensuring models are as solid as possible. In our effort to leverage technology in improving outbreak management, constructing systems that marry these new tricks with old public health tricks is still essential (Ehsan, 2024; Mustafa et al., 2025). The future of epidemic modeling ultimately relies on clever, if occasionally flawed, cooperation between state-of-the-art tools and timeless health lessons.

Definition of Epidemics and Outbreaks

If you consider how diseases develop over time, it is obvious that the language that we use determines what the public perceives as well as how scientists discuss them. There isn't a hard line, you understand—a flare-up is usually considered a spike in cases limited to one population, something that, for the most part, can be corralled with targeted control measures. Epidemics, on the other hand, tend to spread more broadly across large groups of communities or even districts and sometimes overwhelm healthcare services. Often, pinning down these distinctions is crucial for developing models that predict how rapidly an illness could spread and inform public health interventions. Consider COVID-19—a very real-world example that illustrates how problematic these terms can be. The Coronaviridae Study Group pointed out that infections can spread very quickly from a small local problem to a global one, emphasizing how speedily it is possible to transmit the disease in today's globalized world.

Considering SARS-CoV-2 and its status as a prominent human pathogen, epidemics could even begin with animal-to-human transmissions, which in most instances reminds us to reset our healthcare preparedness. Decomposing these words allows researchers to monitor upcoming threats and refine health systems as well as global collaboration in dealing with crises (Gorbalenya et al., 2020). Social media has genuinely shaken things up in the matter of disseminating epidemic news. Sites now disseminate not only solid, factual information but also a decent amount of false talk, sort of reflecting how an illness can spread. Observing how health-related messages circulate on the web even provides hints regarding true disease dynamics—for example, how rumors propagate on such networks is sometimes similar to the simple reproduction numbers (R_0) employed in viral dynamics. This demonstrates that how we transmit information and how diseases are transmitted are closely intertwined, and so it is crucial to understand these communication patterns when attempting to anticipate and react to outbreaks (Cinelli et al., 2020) (Figure 11.1).

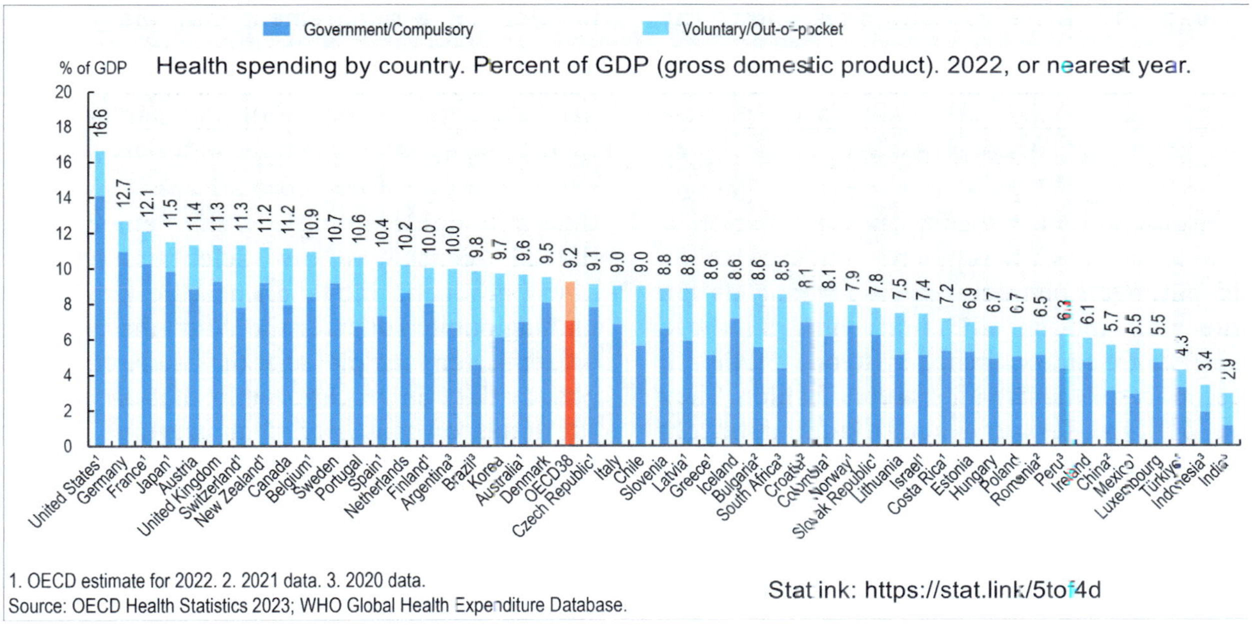

Figure 11.1. The epidemics and outbreaks.

Source: By OECD. Also, text was added via an image editor such as freeware IrfanView. - To get the bar chart click the PDF link under the section titled "Health expenditure in relation to GDP" in the pages below.https://www.oecd-ilibrary.org/docserver/d5dbe32a-en.pdf?expires=1733790258&id=id&accname=guest&checksum=0FC70491793AE05DB0949075484BEF1Dhttps://www.oecd-ilibrary.org/docserver/d5dbe32a-en.pdf?expires= 1733760516&id=i d&accname= guest&checksum= B1F710F0E233C802D094F1CE7E10ADEAStatlink: https://stat.link/5tof4d, Public Domain, https:// commons.wikimedia.org/w/index.php?curid=130444985

Importance of Modeling in Public Health

Disease transmission isn't a neat process—neither is it predictable or clean, particularly today when new cases are popping up all the time. Scientists aren't being wedded to any one approach; they switch from one method of modeling to the next to both visualize and predict outbreaks. Consider Rift Valley fever (RVF) as an example—certainly for most cases, applying a kind of maximum entropy method produces a rough outline of where the mosquito-borne carriers would likely be lurking. This technique points a spotlight at probable environmental hotspots, suggesting possible outbreak areas. It is not hypothetical; these models directly contribute to actual public health responses by assisting with the establishment of targeted surveillance and timely intervention in between epidemic waves, ensuring more effective use of resources (Abdo-Salem et al., 2013). Obtaining realistic demographic information is crucial as well, particularly for diseases in livestock such as foot and mouth disease (FMD). Older approaches tend to have a wide, aggregated perspective that misses local details. With software such as the Farm Location and Agricultural Production Simulator (FLAPS)—essentially plotting where farms are—scientists can observe how farms are grouped in the real world. In general, this results in simulations with a greater basic reproductive number (R_0) for FMD outbreaks than if you simply assumed that farms were randomly distributed. Subdividing the data into these realistic bites allows the predictions more accurately represent what could occur, opening the doors to wiser public health interventions and control efforts (Burdett et al., 2020). Public health modeling is not simply for predicting things; it is a means of gaining an intuition about the complex combination of variables such as environment, human behavior, and pathogen characteristics. As long as it's done well, models illuminate how all these elements are sort of hitched up to one another in a complicated, nearly unexpected fashion. They give policymakers and health administrators a loose blueprint against which to try various types of intervention and derive insights that inform the decision-making process. By marking high-risk areas, mapping out resource allocation, and charting potential disease routes, modeling transforms otherwise raw information into an active game plan for epidemic management. It is more than mere number-crunching in most instances—it is a hands-on means of guarding public health in our increasingly interdependent world.

11.1. Historical Context of Epidemic Modeling

Epidemic modeling has truly transformed how public health responds to outbreaks. At first, models were quite basic-even nearly primitive-and they assisted individuals in getting their heads around the way that diseases transmit. In the 20th century, however, things started to transform when individuals began incorporating statistical approaches, and this caused models to function slightly better. The turning point came with the SIR model—breaking people down into the susceptible, the sick, and the recovered—and provided scientists with a new framework to conceptualize disease transmission. Early concepts provided simulation of various outbreak situations and eventually led to models incorporating social and demographic information, a requirement that finally struck a chord in times of crisis such as the COVID-19 pandemic. Technology has taken these models to new levels, as well. Today, the demand for rapid, real-time analysis combines with technological advances to produce more advanced methods. Genomic epidemiology, which emerged in the 21st century, allows scientists to track how pathogens move on a scale previously unimaginable. Consider the West African Ebola epidemic, for example; scientists there employed genetic data and location information to catch subtleties of contagion that previous models would have overlooked.

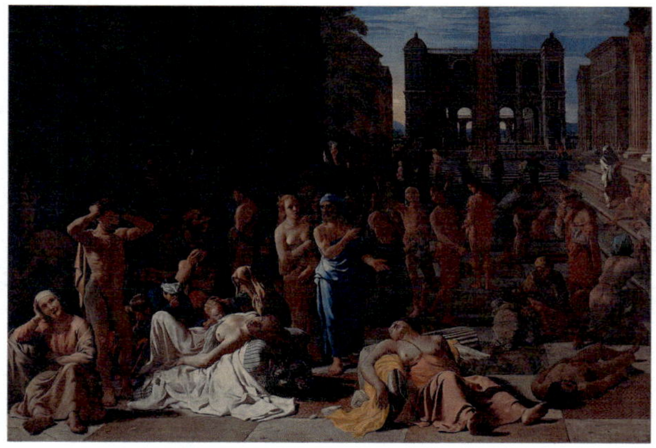

Figure 11.2. Historical context of epidemic modeling.

Source: By Michiel Sweerts - Image: http://collections.lacma.org/sites/default/files/remote_images/piction/ma-31770455-O3.jpgGallery: http://collections.lacma.org/node/183358 archive copy at the Wayback Machine, Public Domain, https://commons.wikimedia.org/w/index.php?curid=27201183

By connecting simple genetic information to other facts such as where individuals lived and how they interacted, scientists came to perceive the bigger picture in a manner that resulted in more targeted interventions—things previously almost impossible a few decades before. Health modeling is more than mere cold calculation—it also prods individuals to change their behavior and shapes policy. As discussion of airborne transmission increased, particularly during the COVID pandemic, public health guidance needed to catch up in short order, and mask-wearing moved from being optional to effectively mandatory. Mask-wearing became a sign of how these models could influence everyday behavior as much as they influenced scientific tactics. Yes, the combination of data science and regular life can become a bit complex here and there, but it also illuminates how bringing strands together, numbers, human conduct, and public policy, can make a meaningful impact in managing health crises (Figure 11.2).

11.1.1. Early Mand Their Limitations

Initially, prediction models for outbreaks were quite rudimentary and failed to truly reflect the chaotic nature of how viruses spread. In those days, most models were so simplistic that they neglected the constantly shifting patterns of human behavior and demographics. Consider the SIR model—it was soon a top epidemiology tool, but its concept of a fixed doubling time ignores how rapidly social distancing behavior and policies can change (Weissman et al., 2020). Criticisms have noted that this type of neglect creates a huge disconnect between what the model predicts and reality, so there is certainly a need for frequent, iterative updates. If you look at actual pandemic situations, you find even more errors in those original models. Granted, the SIR model has been subjected to quite a lot of modification over the years, but it still tends to gloss over important points such as asymptomatic transmission or distinguishing between severe and mild cases. More recent models such as the SEMCR take a cue from their SEIR predecessors by incorporating slight refinement in the way they measure population processes and intervention measures. This method reflects what has been seen in recent epidemics, with linking exposed patients more specifically to recoveries being central (Yang et al., 2020). In most instances, making this transition to these more precise models is not only beneficial—it is necessary to understand the complete situation of infectious disease transmission. Due to these difficulties, it is difficult to emphasize too much the need to continue testing and refining our models. Early approaches provided us with a crude beginning, but as new data keeps coming in, our instruments must be periodically adjusted to keep us on course. Most recent studies indicate that validating models such as CHIME against actual data has improved our capacity for anticipating healthcare demand and keeping strategies in line (Weissman et al., 2020). And beyond that, burgeoning evidence of a large number of mild or undetected cases only contributes to the challenge of providing easy predictions (Yang et al., 2020). Ultimately, by understanding the limitations of our early models, we stand a better chance of predicting and addressing future outbreaks—no matter if that means our own work is always a little of a moving target.

11.1.2. Key Historical Epidemics and Their Impact

Historical epidemics shake up more than medicine—they turn entire societies upside down. Consider the 14th century plague, for instance; it killed enormous segments of Europe's population and disrupted the organization of labor. With so many dead, the living could demand higher wages, which slowly undermined the previous feudal system. This shift, in many cases, set the stage for today's modern workforce and rewrote European economic narratives. And let us not forget the persisting mental toll: people were left with a deep, lasting fear and mistrust that seeped into everyday cultural and social life. More recently, the HIV/AIDS crisis in the late 20th century exposed some pretty glaring gaps in both healthcare systems and societal attitudes toward illness. The stigma attached to HIV/AIDS tended to hinder effective public health measures, making it difficult for the infected to access assistance. Fearless activism and continuous advocacy finally prompted significant advances in treatment and prevention – turning the narrative from despair to a stronger one. This long-fought struggle demonstrates how important community action can be when dealing with medical emergencies, and it reminds us still today of the importance of equitable access to healthcare and proper, accurate information, particularly when false news is so prevalent.

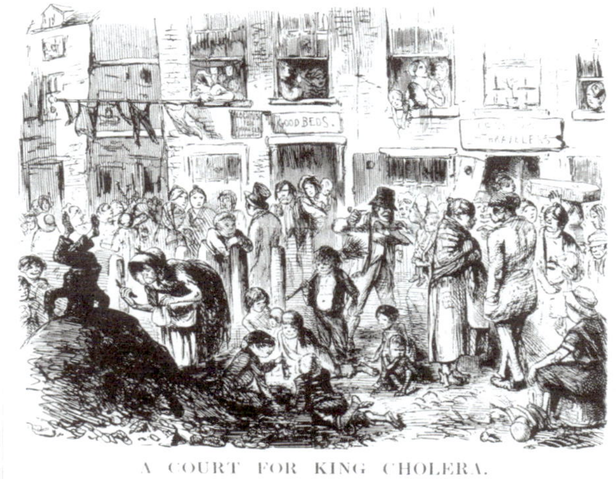

Figure 11.3. Key historical epidemics and their impact.

Source: Public Domain, https://commons.wikimedia.org/w/index.php?curid=680455

Then came along COVID-19, and it made one thing abundantly clear: modeling epidemics isn't an easy job. As numbers skyrocketed, health systems across the globe had to scramble, with each region reacting differently according to resources and political climates at hand. Scientists even consulted earlier outbreak data – employing methods such as ARIMA models – in an attempt to predict what would come next, mixing history with real-time numbers. However, such a predict is fraught with uncertainty; much relies on how well guidelines are obeyed and the emergent behavior of new variants. Overall, reflecting on previous epidemics provides us with significant clues for present and future prevention and control, ranging from public health and the economy to day-to-day life (Katoch et al., 2021). The COVID-19 pandemic has particularly put the spotlight on the necessity of flexible, resilient healthcare systems as societies move through the complex of health issues, anxieties, and shifting social norms (Clauw et al., 2020) (Figure 11.3).

11.1.3. Evolution of Modeling Techniques Over Time

Modeling techniques in epidemiology have come a long way, revealing just how much our understanding of disease spread has deepened over time. Early on, models were built on fixed, deterministic ideas that gave us a basic picture yet often missed the random, unpredictable twists found in real outbreaks. With increased processing power and improved methodologies for collecting data, researchers have begun incorporating more challenging factors into their research, which—overall—improves prediction accuracy. For instance, certain new studies mix nonlinear and random components to create simpler models that still maintain a firm connection with the larger-scale, complex versions. This revolution is necessary to capture the insidious, subtle movement of outbreaks, particularly when novel infectious agents appear and spread within communities, requiring models that must be flexible but also accurate (Forgoston & Schwartz, 2013). Stochastic modeling has opened our eyes to how disease jumps across species, something that is particularly significant in the case of zoonotic disease. Studying avian influenza, for example, indicates that wild bird-domestic poultry mixing contributes significantly to epidemic prediction. Scientists have modeled potential outbreaks that begin with such contact using continuous-time mathematics models and conclude that interventions such as decreasing the frequency of contact or ramping up culling can considerably reduce the risk. These results further support the notion that combining ecological information with epidemiological data makes our entire strategy for predicting and controlling outbreaks significantly stronger (Gralinski & Menachery, 2020). Real-time data analysis is also now at the heart of contemporary modeling. Contemporary epidemiological practice depends on real-time inputs, permitting continuous fine-tuning as infection dynamics evolve—a capability that becomes crucial in times of public health crisis. For the most part, coupling traditional disease models with technologies such as geographic information systems (GIS) constructs a spatially intelligent paradigm, one that is informative regarding how parameters like mobility and population density influence spread. Overall, this paradigm shift in modeling not only clarifies the complex dynamics of infectious diseases but also serves to support the development of practical interventions for the prevention and control of outbreaks.

11.2. Mathematical Models in Epidemiology

Biological complexities and environmental interactions often throw us off balance, making it necessary to use creative frameworks when trying to grasp how epidemics work. Math models come in handy for picturing these connections—and sometimes they even hint at where outbreaks might flare up. In one Rift Valley fever (RVF) study conducted in East Africa, a maximum entropy method was applied to highlight potentially viable regions for chief mosquito species; statistically significant according to most metrics, the findings revealed that mosquito populations concentrate within proximity to past epidemic areas (Abdo-Salem et al., 2013). In the end, these findings typically confirm that these models assist us in unraveling transmission dynamics and inform public health interventions. Another significant aspect is the way modeling can elucidate vaccination strategies for various groups. Scientists tend to look to contact network epidemiology to test whether a focused vaccine strategy can reduce both illness and mortality from illnesses such as influenza. The analysis generally indicates that the optimal plan significantly hinges on the reproductive rate of the virus; for moderately spreading strains, measures intended to curb morbidity tend to beat ones aimed at merely reducing mortality, while highly infectious strains require high-risk group priority (Pourbohloul et al., 2006). This type of dynamic insight, in the majority of instances, provides public health authorities with a more detailed snapshot to design interventions and allocate resources better, ultimately contributing to more effectively containing vaccine supplies and distribution. Incorporating environmental and social elements with mathematical models further enhances their predictive strength. When factors like travel habits, population levels and day-to-day social habits come into play, the models begin to unveil more of the complicated nuances behind disease transmission. In the case of an epidemic, for instance, such models can sometimes predict possible routes of transmission and even identify hotspots for intervention, especially in the case of diseases that have alternate means of transmission, such as influenza and other airborne viruses. Employing a strong model in time of crisis allows officials to project pressing needs ahead of time and allocate resources—though not always ideally—which goes a great distance toward minimizing the disease's overall burden. Ongoing improvement and field verification, as a general rule, are important to maintaining these models' utility in the constantly evolving environment of epidemic response (Figure 11.4).

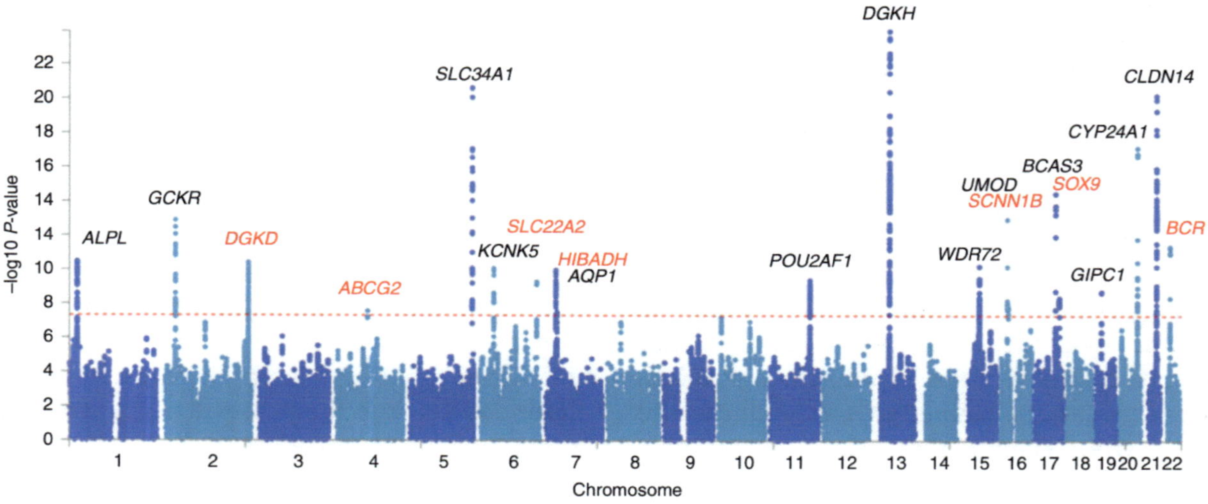

Figure 11.4. Mathematical models in epidemiology.

Source: By Sarah A. Howles, Akira Wiberg, Michelle Goldsworthy, Asha L. Bayliss, Anna K. Gluck, Michael Ng, Emily Grout, Chizu Tanikawa, Yoichiro Kamatani, Chikashi Terao, Atsushi Takahashi, Michiaki Kubo, Koichi Matsuda, Rajesh V. Thakker, Benjamin W. Turney & Dominic Furniss - Genetic variants of calcium and vitamin D metabolism in kidney stone disease. Nature Communications 10, 5175 (2019). https://doi.org/10.1038/s41467-019-13145-x, CC BY 4.0, https://commons.wikimedia.org/w/index.php?curid=110859268

11.2.1. Overview of Common Mathematical Models

Math modeling is a serious business when we attempt to understand how diseases spread, particularly for determining epidemic patterns. There's a whole range of models available, each with their own take on capturing real-world idiosyncrasies. The SIR (Susceptible-Infectious-Recovered) model, for instance, is used by many to divide people into three categories to monitor how a sickness spreads and dies down. And then you've got the SEIR (Susceptible-Exposed-Infectious-Recovered) model, which inserts that "Exposed" piece that is very crucial when a disease festers for a time before you see the symptoms. Broadly, all these approaches allow us to visualize how various interventions will alter the course of the outbreak and ultimately push public health actions one way or another. A completely different strand of these models begins considering space, which is especially valuable when addressing disease among poultry and livestock. Researchers require strong demographic data, so they tend to utilize models that map out where farms or facilities are. A useful tool is the Farm Location and Agricultural Production Simulator (FLAPS), which takes into account factors such as terrain and land use to draw a more realistic picture of how an infection could spread. Conversely, less sophisticated random methods may at times in excess the fine-grained dynamics, doing them a disservice in terms of the actual risk involved. In general, models that ace how premises group together demonstrate that how close they are can make all the difference when it comes to predicting outbreak locations. Next up is stochastic modeling—a true game breaker because it works with the day-to-day unpredictability of disease transmission. These models simulate a combination of what-if situations, gaining us a glimpse of just how dire or minor an outbreak might become under various conditions. In the case of nasty insects such as highly pathogenic avian influenza (HPAI), the call to urgent action is made loud and clear. For example, a study with H5N1 (introduced through wild birds) showed that reducing contact with domestic poultry and moving quickly with culling interventions can be a difference maker. By combining such random simulation techniques with firm, factual data, scientists can make more accurate predicts as to when an outbreak will strike, which allows public health interventions to be more effectively framed (Aly et al., 2013; Burdett et al., 2020).

11.2.2. The SIR Model: Susceptible, Infected, Recovered

Disease spread often gets reduced in such cases to models that unscramble complicated interactions into simpler bits. The SIR model, for instance, divides people into categories named Susceptible, Infected, and Recovered, and essentially is a simple mathematical device. Scientists apply it to trace how people move between these states along the course of time; it provides them with a glimpse of how infections spread through populations. Much of its strength relies on its understanding of the rates of transmission and recovery—essentially, the speed at which people acquire a disease and then recover. For the most part, fixing these rates allows for the prediction of when infection peaks will occur and approximately how long an outbreak will last, which in turn informs public health actions to contain it.

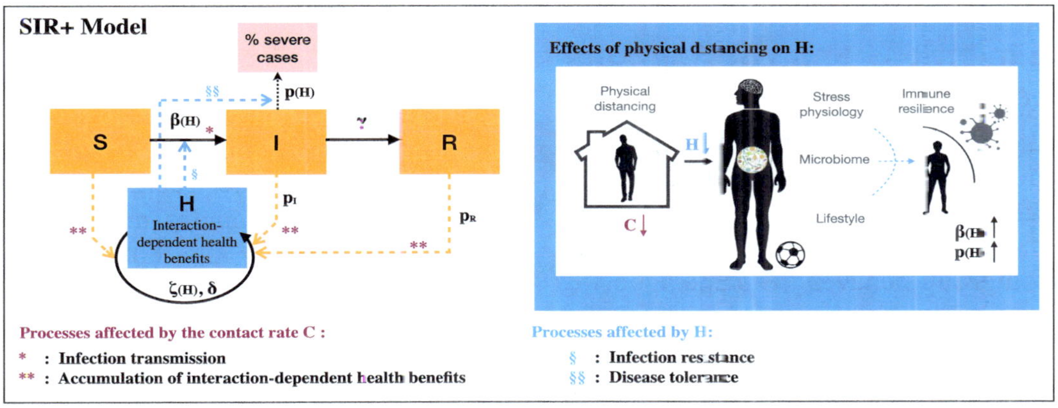

Figure 11.5. The SIR model: susceptible, infected, recovered.

Source: Gao, Y., Zhang, J., Chen, L., Li, H., & Wang, X. (2024). Figure 1 from "Estimation of disease burden of seasonal influenza in China from 2006 to 2019." *Scientific Reports*.

Basing the SIR model on math provides some nice insights into disease trends. One of the nice things is how it can approximate when an outbreak will get going—a quality that becomes even more cutting-edge once you add in how individuals interact in networks. Occasionally, researchers even rely on metapopulation models to prep for simulating pandemic spread under more difficult circumstances. Tossing in natural fluctuations further spices up the analysis, making risk estimates a bit more precise. In many cases, these ideas seem to match up nicely with percolation processes, building a sturdy framework for estimating pandemic thresholds across various networks, which in turn ups the SIR model's predictive chops (Barthelemy et al., 2010). Recent research, in general, has indicated that incorporating multilayer networks can enhance the SIR model's applicability in real-world scenarios. Such networks—social, geographical, even logistics-based interactions—have a massive impact on the way disease spreads through interlinked groups. How these layers integrate tends to elicit subtle characteristics and weak points that easier models may completely overlook. At other times, grasping these multi-level dynamics provides you with added perspective not just on disease transmission, but also on how important information travels, particularly public health information. When you bring all of these variables into the fold, the SIR model slowly transforms into a more holistic tool for predicting outbreaks, setting the stage for more intelligent interventions and policy-making (Magnani et al., 2014) (Figure 11.5).

11.2.3. Limitations and Assumptions of Mathematical Models

Modeling epidemics is not quite as simple as it would appear. Such analyses tend to rely on a few very general assumptions that can warp results. Models tend to assume everyone in the modeled group behaves the same, ignoring the real complexity of our social networks and heterogeneity in behavior. This method may be feasible on paper but tends to make predicts that don't exactly reflect what occurs on the ground. These models often ignore differences in the way people interact, age and background variations, and even how efficient interventions are across areas. Overall, relying solely on these clear, simplistic models risks a gross underestimation of disease unpredictability and the possibility of derailing public health responses and overall readiness (Davies et al., 2020). A second major challenge arises from the quality of the data upon which these models base their projections. Usually, they rely heavily on reported numbers of cases and fatalities—even though those figures can be tenuous due to underreporting or irregular data collection. This issue is especially evident in areas where healthcare systems and testing procedures are not all on the same level. For example, consider the models at the Institute for Health Metrics and Evaluation; they tend to rely on statistical projections based on mortality, without such a strong epidemiologic foundation. That approach invariably calls into question how solid those models are going to be (Jewell et al., 2020). In most instances, this may result in an unjustified feeling of certainty that ultimately directs policy and decision-making in an incorrect manner when it is most needed. There is also a measure of subtlety in the assumptions embedded in a lot of mathematical models. Very often, important elements, such as how quickly a disease spreads or the effectiveness of interventions—are tied to precise numbers. This inflexibility does not allow much space for surprises. When an epidemic takes a long time and public habits change or new variants appear, inflexible such models can make even more errors. Consider COVID-19: mortality and hospital demand estimates were repeatedly revised as more data emerged. These fluctuations remind us that although mathematical models may provide useful insights, their inherent assumptions and constraints deserve a cautious, near-skeptical examination when developing public health policies (Jewell et al., 2020).

11.3. Data Collection and Analysis

Successful epidemic modeling is heavily dependent upon the way data is obtained and how much detail it contains. Combining it all together risks overlooking the small nuances that arise in local areas. Burdett et al. (2020) demonstrated that when models of animal diseases were constructed using crisp spatial detail, the results did not correlate as well with random spot configurations as systems such as

FLAPS truly emphasize that realistic percepts of demographic spread are important. FLAPS clusters data in a manner that also helps pin down a more accurate basic reproductive number (R_0). That is not only the early estimates when an epidemic begins; it also influences what goes on later. With most cases, closely monitoring local specifics adds overall credibility to these models. Details of data also come into play in how vaccination strategies are implemented during an epidemic. Various approaches may have varying outcomes based on the reading and application of the numbers. As Pourbohloul et al. (2006) indicates, examining the variance between mortality-based and morbidity-based vaccine strategies for flu reveals that even minor changes in rates of viral transmission can make the difference.

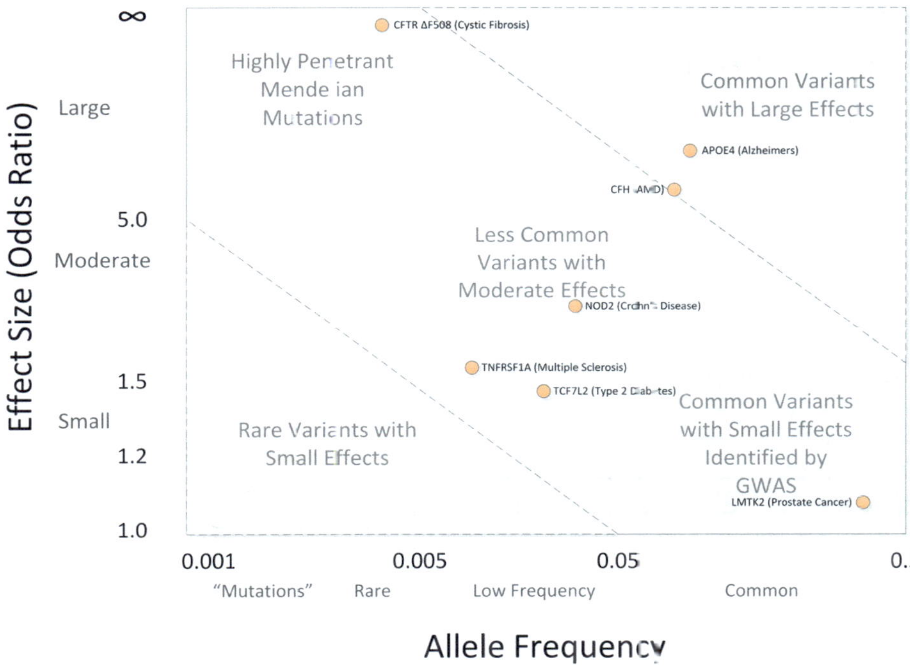

Figure 11.6. Data collection and analysis.

Source: By Bush WS and Moore JH - Bush WS, Moore JH (2012) Chapter 11: Genome-Wide Association Studies. PLoS Comput Biol 8(12): e1002822. doi:10.1371/journal.pcbi.1002822, CC BY 2.5, https://commons.wikimedia.org/w/index.php?curid=24121486

In general, the better you know your viral transmission rates, the more targeted strategies can be used to build up community immunity; if not, relying on mortality statistics may be the safer bet. This puts a premium on having good methods for collecting data which do not simply test current infection levels but attempt to predict what the future may hold. Lastly, overcoming the challenges in data gathering is not a solo activity—it requires individuals from various disciplines uniting. Merging conventional epidemiology and new data analytics creates a pathway to more robust models. The multiple reiteration of the need for fine-grained spatial and demographic data in Burdett et al. (2020) indicates that statisticians, epidemiologists, and even geographers must unite. Methods such as those utilized in contact network epidemiology can provide additional layers of understanding about how infection disease spreads and what risks are greatest, thereby opening the door for more targeted interventions during epidemics. As they expand, these collaborative projects will accumulate data sets that will be essential to make predictions about and manage future public health emergencies—even if sometimes the technique may be a little rough around the edges (Figure 11.6).

11.3.1. Sources of Epidemiological Data

Understanding how epidemics progress is not easy—it is a matter of having lots of solid data. Much of that information is collected by public health surveillance systems that monitor minute-by-minute data on rates of infection, who is falling ill, and where. Those systems, hectic as they are, provide information that influences fast-paced responses as well as longer-term strategy. At times, the figures they produce are plugged into elaborate time-series models that attempt to predict what will occur next with diseases. In a case study using actual infection records for Mumps and Chickenpox in Jordan, for instance, it was demonstrated that models constructed on data covering several years can make grave predictions regarding future outbreaks—essentially emphasizing the importance of good, well-rounded data gathering in epidemic predicting (Al-khateeb, 2024). A second prominent ingredient is provided by healthcare facilities and research organizations. Information drawn from clinical trials, observational studies, and a range of health surveys function similarly to the critical building blocks for a comprehension of disease transmission. These organizations tend to collaborate with global agencies in an effort to ensure the information is kept accurate and, more often than not, comprehensive. Just consider the 2014 Ebola outbreak—alerts from local Ministries of Health in various West African nations, combined with health surveys, provided a more detailed view of the drivers of infection rates and death. By examining the way that people act in conjunction with the raw figures, scientists can identify areas where interventions could reduce the transmission of disease, thus enhancing future outbreak responses (Leigh et al., 2024). It is not the traditional data alone; there are non-traditional sources entering into the mix as well. Social media sites and smartphone apps today provide a glimpse into actual-world behavior and attitudes, recording population health trends in a very immediate manner.

When you delve into such user-generated information, you tend to find public sentiment patterns and outbreak responses that allow officials to gauge the national mood—hence better communication. By combining these non-traditional pieces of evidence with traditional health indicators, it can provide a richer, more comprehensive picture of epidemic dynamics. Integrating social media metrics with traditional public health indicators might enhance predicting models, occasionally prompting action sooner. One study of outbreak responses even found that combining heterogeneous data streams improves the overall modeling process, providing researchers and health officials with a sort of balanced toolset for predicting and controlling epidemics (Al-khateeb, 2024).

11.3.2. Techniques for Data Analysis

Data analysis truly comes into its own when we attempt to get a handle on how epidemics behave, particularly when the outbreaks are surprise ones. In such rapid-paced health emergencies, reams of real-time data lead us to rely on robust, frequently confused analytic techniques. You may catch glimpses of raw descriptive figures, regressions run with models, or even Bayesian thought appended to the mix. Variables like congested neighborhoods, how residents get from place to place, and what local officials do all wind up playing off one another in a way that determines the course of an epidemic. Software like Comprehensive Meta-Analysis—yes, that one—assists in combining results from multiple studies, giving a type of rougher, richer image of public health challenges (Salari et al., 2020). It all winds up providing decision-makers with some pretty good clues for acting timely. In addition to those old-school statistics, predictive analytics comes into its own as an absolute essential for epidemic prediction. Consider, for instance, the time-series approach—algorithms such as the Prophet algorithm can detect regular patterns and surprise blips in the way infection spreads. Overall, this type of method was a lifesaver during COVID-19, when infections accelerated and models had to be as adaptable as possible (Mahalle et al., 2020).

By combining different sources of information—demographic information, medical capacity etc.—these predictive models have genuine potential to inform public health policy and direct resources to where they are needed. Ultimately, such sophisticated methods do more than superficially throw pretty numbers around; they enhance proactive measures to contain outbreaks before they runaway. Machine learning has been establishing itself in epidemic data analysis, too. Computations designed to process tremendous quantities of data can find knotty connections that older, more conventional techniques may miss. Clustering and classification, for example, are excellent at identifying high-risk groups and extracting the difficult variables responsible for disease transmission. Even models occasionally dip into social media buzz to pick up changes in public attitude and behavior that might trigger changes in outbreak patterns. By mixing various forms of data with some creative analytical methods, scientists end up with a better-rounded—but occasionally rather messy—picture of epidemic trends. This combination of new methods highlights the importance of continuing to mess around with our analysis methods as new public health issues continue to arise (Mahalle et al., 2020) (Figure 11.7).

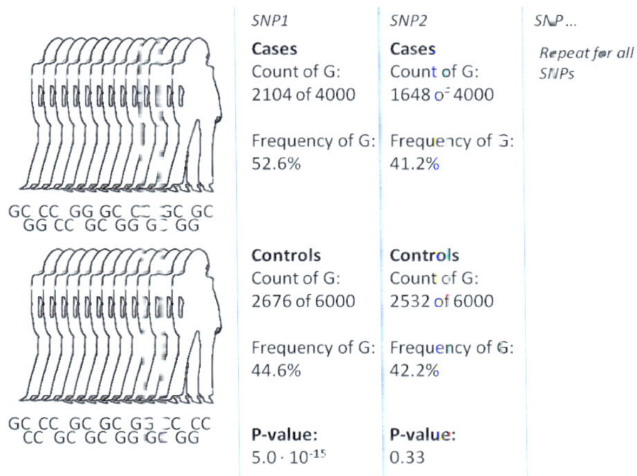

Figure 11.7. Techniques for data analysis.

Source: By Lasse Folkersen - Own work, CC BY 3.0, https://commons.wikimedia.org/w/index.php?curid=18062562

11.3.3. Challenges in Data Accuracy and Reliability

Obtaining accurate predictions regarding epidemics begins with having high-quality, trusted data. Without such information, models attempting to chart disease transmission easily will mislead you and make it difficult to guide public health interventions in the right direction. Recent research highlights that whenever diseases such as polio and measles return, it is not only health threats that escalate—logistical problems tend to add up as well, particularly if the data is not precise.

Real-time monitoring is very important; however, if the information brought in from the internet fails to prove reliable or capriciously unpredictable, the severity of an outbreak could get misconstrued. How the online buzz circulates also mirrors the true disease transmission and the exaggerated public responses, which tend to confuse how we perceive the trends. For most scenarios, keeping the data up to date is significant for devising useful interventions and managing healthcare resources effectively (Chen et al., 2019). Collecting the data itself is yet another tricky problem that can add additional complexities to the equation. Watching events such as Ebola or H1N1 teach us that our established notions of managing epidemics may not hold when surprise strikes. Models must balance a multitude of variables - from people's behavior and demographic oddities to surprise logistical hitches - each contributing unwanted layers to a problem that was already tricky to begin with. Some ethnographic research even indicates that if we rely too much on simplistic models, we may overlook the most important aspects of how diseases spread, potentially making unanticipated mistakes. In general terms, there is a requirement for a more expansive, flexible framework that reveals these subtleties while remaining robust to random data blips (Brown et al., 2017).

Contemporary epidemic modeling does not only involve just balancing variables—it also struggles with some substantial computational burdens. Mixing large, diverse datasets with handling the underlying uncertainties of both the figures and the unpredictable nature of illnesses is by no means easy. High-dimensional data compels us to adopt sophisticated processing techniques that could raise error probabilities and even bring down those precious response times. Although plunging into predictive analytics and machine learning can increase accuracy, they have their own uncertainties and thus the balance between cutting-edge developments and workability becomes an easily upset one. In most instances, public health authorities need to straddle such sophisticated models with good statistical procedures and local knowledge to maintain outbreak predictions in line and protect communities (Brown et al., 2017; Chen et al., 2019).

11.4. Predictive Modeling Techniques

Predicting epidemics has also experienced a spate of innovative methods that reflect how outbreaks emerge. One approach that has been gaining traction is the application of artificial neural networks (ANN); these networks sort through disorganized, complicated data and provide predicts that tend to awe. Many studies, in most instances, indicate that when you fine-tune these ANN-based models with past data—even in challenging instances like COVID-19—they often perform better than traditional math methods. For instance, Indian researchers recently enhanced their case predictions by including an about 14-day incubation period, an adjustment that enhanced real-time decision-making in public health (Manohar et al., 2022). This result highlights, all too well, that the selection of the appropriate model—one that captures time-based trends exhibited by such measures as mean square error and mean absolute percent error—can truly inform improved response strategies in the public. There is also increasing excitement about complicated network theory as another method to gaze into epidemic transmission. Instead of holding firm only to neural routes, this method traces out entwined relationships between individuals, groups, and even diseases, and shows how diseases can inch along social and transport networks. Researchers generally resort to link prediction methods—which are sort of like predicting the next link—to identify potential areas of outbreak before they fully emerge. This approach does not only deal with the structure of the network but also considers how the entities involved naturally act, presenting a sort of double vision. A closer examination of different datasets reveals that network embedding, especially using graph neural networks, has a propensity to improve link prediction accuracy, contributing a good piece to the epidemic modeling jigsaw puzzle

(Wu et al., 2022). Combining different predictive approaches is another area that provides a better picture of epidemic trends. Scientists combining the power of ANN with knowledge from complex network analysis can construct models that range from the fine – grain details of individual epidemics to the overall pattern of social contacts. Hybrid models are very convenient to use when it comes to simulating scenarios, allowing policymakers to try out the potential impact of interventions before implementing them. With data-driven adjustments continually fine-tuning these methods, the entire epidemic modeling paradigm is increasingly changing. With improved technology and data gathering in most instances, such predicting techniques are likely to become even more adept at detecting and containing outbreaks—assuming an important role in public health readiness and response (Manohar et al., 2022; Wu et al., 2022) (Figure 11.8).

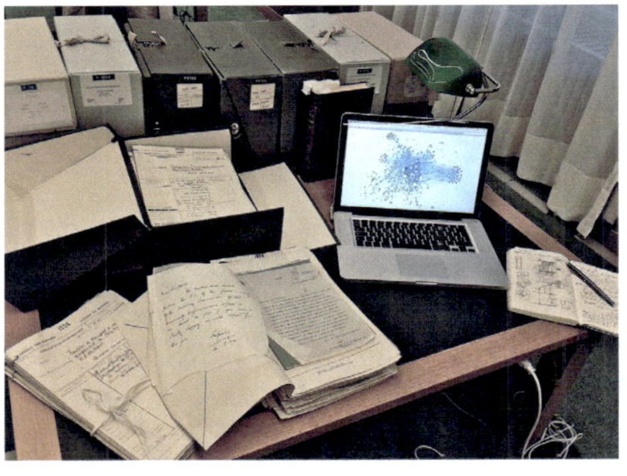

Figure 11.8. Predictive modeling techniques.

Source: By Calvinius - Own work : http://www.martingrandjean.ch/wp-content/uploads/2013/10/HumanitesNumeriques.jpg, CC BY-SA 3.0, https://commons.wikimedia.org/w/index.php?curid=29275453

11.4.1. Statistical Methods for Outbreak Prediction

Epidemics are difficult business—some serious heavy-duty, highly refined statistical machinery is needed to make things right, as we learned in recent Ebola outbreaks. Experts tended to employ a random branching model to get a rough estimate of how large an outbreak would be and how long it would last, combining various vaccination scenarios in the process. They employed today's counts along with historic outbreak records and made predictions that reflect the inherent randomness of the course of an epidemic. For instance; according to one study, when the suspected cases and high vaccine coverage were included, the median outbreak sizes resulted in what occurred These sophisticated techniques in most cases represent a true step ahead in outbreak predicting, providing real-time insights for public health interventions (Ackley et al., 2018). Statistical methods involved here are far from merely branching models. Recently, new approaches have emerged to reinforce epidemic control, as the classic models frequently ignore the messy realities of life. In general, evidence these days suggests that traditional epidemic theory tends to be somewhat too clear, so researchers have started combining with it longer models that address several practical frictions. Adding some risk and robustness factors provides a better vision of potential outcomes, even if—fairly candidly—the added complexity makes it harder to optimize management. These changes reflect the increasing demand for intelligent, adaptive analytical tools to maneuver today's complex epidemic landscape (Brown et al., 2017). Predictive approaches and epidemic control go hand in glove when it comes to making sound public health decisions. It is not just about unearthing past data; it also requires up-to-the-minute support and scenario checks that include varying public reactions. Advanced methods, such as Thiel-Sen regression, assist in projecting outbreaks more precisely from case counts seen, improving predictive impact overall. Several studies indicate that these hybrid methods not only assist in directing response actions, but also inform resource allocation and risk communication. Finally, as statistical methods continue to improve, they provide the foundation for our attempts to predict and control outbreaks, keeping public health measures grounded in actual evidence while navigating the idiosyncrasies of disease transmission (Ackley et al., 2018).

11.4.2. Machine Learning Applications in Epidemiology

Epidemics can spiral out of control quickly—public health infrastructure feels the pinch when disease rates skyrocket unexpectedly. It's no wonder that rapid ways to apprehend these outbreaks early become imperative. Tools such as EPIWATCH, for instance, draw on machine learning to analyze mountains of data and identify early signs of distress.

This is not a matter of gathering numbers; it is a matter of predicting when a small flare may instantly turn into a huge crisis. In most instances, combining open-source intelligence with these instruments enables governments and hospitals to act immediately, which can maintain both health and economic repercussions under control (MacIntyre et al., 2022). Social media has also become a significant hotspot for monitoring health data, particularly in times of crisis such as the COVID-19 days. Individuals are communicating online, and machine learning explores this noise in real-time—not just providing a sense of public mood but even assisting in tracking how diseases could be spreading. Some studies indicate these models are quite effective at indicating infodemics and identifying misinformation (sometimes twice, strangely enough), which in turn influences improved, accelerated health communication.

Furthermore, by monitoring the way governments react and the way people respond to health policies, these methods provide another component to our general strategy for pinning down outbreak dynamics (Shu-Tsao et al., 2021). It is sensible, therefore, to incorporate machine learning into public health education. In general, if tomorrow's epidemiologists are to manage real-world emergencies, they must have a working knowledge of such contemporary tools. Educational programs should be directed toward pragmatic uses, instructing experts in reading and understanding data—even when data arrive in odd, unforeseen formats. As the discipline evolves and expands, developing digital know-how and familiarity with these systems not only simplifies how we identify outbreaks but also refines our general readiness. By incorporating this type of instruction into the standard curriculum, we can aspire to meet epidemic threats head-on, tempering the severity of subsequent outbreaks and making our health systems more resilient overall (MacIntyre et al., 2022).

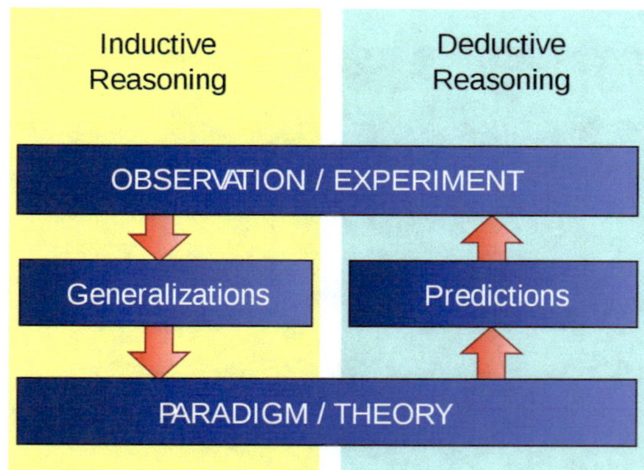

Source: By Brian Brondel at English Wikibooks, CC BY-SA 2.5, https://commons.wikimedia.org/w/index.php?curid=61793556

11.4.3. Case Studies of Successful Predictions

Outbreak prediction has become much smarter in recent times, with good examples combining old data with what is still arriving on a fresh basis. When the 2018–2019 Ebola outbreak occurred in the Democratic Republic of Congo, scientists employed techniques that mimic random spread in combination with traditional regression methods to map out short-term as well as subsequent courses. They married these methods—mixing historical figures with contemporary case counts—in some sort of ensemble prediction that suggested scales occasionally surpassing totals previously attained. In most instances, this model demonstrated just how important timely data is, particularly when disease spread leaps unpredictably in volatile, war-torn parts of the world (Hoff et al., 2019). Another instance is the CDC's 2013-14 U.S. flu season influenza predicting challenge. Many teams put their money where their mouth was by providing fortnightly predictions on when the flu would peak and how severe it would be. Success was varied, but some projections nailed it within roughly a week of the milestone's actual occurrence—perhaps demonstrating that experience is crucial to honing models. In all but one case, the changing competition highlighted a clear correlation between practice and enhanced precision. In general, this challenge calls for improving predicting tools in such a way that real-time data and changing environmental information directly enter public health planning (Allen et al., 2016). Collectively, these illustrations indicate an emerging trend where combining traditional statistics with dynamic, iterative processes truly comes through in predicting epidemic outbreaks. Officials, by comparing model predicts to what occurs, can refine their reactions and stay ahead of impending threats, even when sometimes the process is not entirely streamlined. There also appears to be a natural back-and-forth here: dissemination of insights—albeit with some rough edges—enables everyone to learn a little more every time. Effectively, this mutual learning not only constructs a blueprint for managing outbreaks at the local and global levels but also facilitates some of the uncertainty associated with monitoring infectious diseases (Allen et al., 2016; Hoff et al., 2019).

11.5. Role of Technology in Epidemic Modeling

New technology has transformed the way we think about epidemic modeling, disrupting old public health practices. A set of computational tools—from machine learning to AI—now sift through huge quantities of data to assist us in determining how diseases spread and evolve. Deep learning, for instance, has been able to detect outbreak signs such as COVID-19, flu, and even Ebola by reviewing past records and identifying patterns that could go unnoticed by a human eye. In general, these tools enable researchers to catch emerging health dangers a little earlier, so resources could be reallocated more rapidly. And with the assistance of AI in predicting likely future conditions, interventions can target the hotspots—as particularly required within the rapid spike of SARS-CoV-2 (Bhattamisra et al., 2023). Individuals are increasingly relying on digital information, which reminds us why combining technology with epidemic modeling is so essential. Mobile apps and web platforms introduce real-time insights of human mobility—information that is integral in deciphering how infection spreads. When modelers incorporate such information, they can deduce how interventions such as physical distancing function. For example, at the beginning of the COVID-19 days, mobile data proved to be a breakthrough by suggesting how behavior changed once lockdowns began. This type of diverse information allows scientists to gain a richer, if sometimes gruesome, picture of the course of an outbreak and provide policymakers with some useful guidance on control interventions. In most instances, combining several datasets merely makes models more acutely defined, filling in gaps in real-time tracking with wiser public-health action (Poletto et al., 2020) As health emergencies intensify, the need for more sophisticated epidemic models becomes more insistent. Doubt about disease transmission means that predicting tools are indispensable for planning—if not infallible, at least extremely helpful. Connecting these models to real field data serves to bring out critical pieces of information such as clandestine chains of transmission or those with no symptoms. However, one must acknowledge these models have limitations, especially when the data available are patchy. During the early phases of an outbreak, incomplete data may cause misestimated levels of risk, and therefore some advocate national centers dedicated to disease predicting and informing decision-makers. Overall, combining cutting-edge tech with epidemic modeling is not only essential for rapid workarounds; it also provides foundations for long-term preparedness against potential future outbreaks (Bhattamisra et al., 2023) (Figure 11.9).

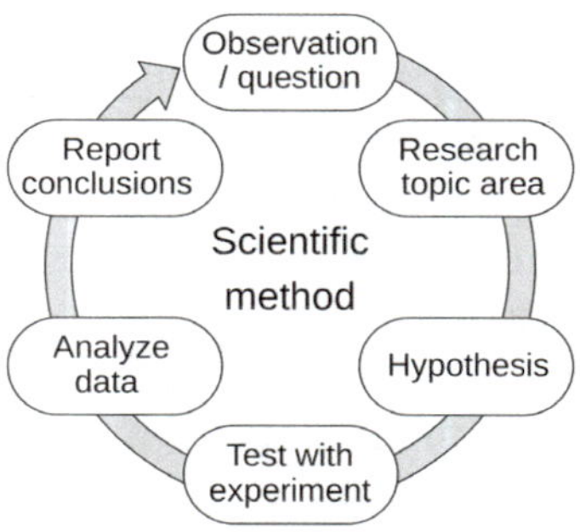

Figure 11.9. New technology has changed the way we look at epidemic modeling.

Source: By Efbrazil - Own work, CC BY-SA 4.0, https://commons.wikimedia.org/w/index.php?curid=102392470

11.5.1. Use of Simulations and Computational Models

Recently, computational models and simulations have truly become big business in international health. Government health officials now combine big data with intelligent algorithms to predict epidemic patterns in ways heretofore unseen. Scientists simulate various what-if scenarios—everything from testing diverse intervention srategies to analyze how individuals could respond, even adjusting variables such as viral transmission. This interactive method, even incorporating such measures as the effective reproduction number as a central indicator of control, has become paramount. You can observe this shift in full effect in cases such as the monkeypox outbreak, where these virtual experiments were crucial in determining vaccination strategies and overall responses (Khan et al., 2022). The COVID-19 experience, in large part, taught us how important such models are when informing policy and making decisions about resource allocation. Early on, during initial waves, scientists modeled statistical models onto not-so-apparent trends buried deep within epidemiological figures, such as hospitalization and death rates—that required real-time adjustments as conditions changed. This agile evolution is particularly significant when novel diseases break out and the traditional streams of data simply do not compute within the traditional frameworks (Keeling et al., 2022). It is not an abstract concept; these models have a hands-on function in crisis management by assisting policy-makers in forming decisions in times of uncertainty, which influences the way that health systems prepare and react. Apart from that, novel computational methods are revealing new avenues to explore new pathogens. By simulating molecular docking, researchers are mimicking the way potential vaccines may bind with immune receptors, essentially predicting what types of immune reactions we would see. For example, in the case of the monkeypox outbreak, the methods even assisted in developing a multi-epitope vaccine; researchers simulated how various components of the vaccine could induce immunity in different populations. Not only does this accelerate the process of designing the vaccine but also reduces the time for the long laboratory tests by providing early hints of efficacy (Khan et al., 2022). In several senses, the intertwining of such simulations with the actual experiments constitutes a fundamental change—one that is increasingly becoming an integral part of contemporary methodologies in public health policy.

11.5.2. Geographic Information Systems (GIS) in Tracking Outbreaks

GIS have become a genuine game-changer in epidemic modeling and outbreak predictions. They provide us with specific tools to show and dissect spatial information, and it becomes simpler for us to visualize the way diseases spread and assist those who manage public health in making quicker decisions. When disease spreads, the "where" is important—a reality GIS clarifies by allowing researchers and healthcare people to examine population patterns, weather anomalies, and even availability of care. This configuration paid off during a crisis like the pandemic of COVID-19, when real-time mapping of disease and hot spots for death allowed targeting interventions and shipping supplies to where they were most needed. When examining the spread of disease throughout various regions, GIS does not have a single-track approach. Rather, it blends a variety of techniques to make patterns and improbable associations stand out. For instance, during the COVID peak, health geographers used GIS to analyze how contagion changed over time as well as space and found dangerous areas and what drove them. By combining number-crunching and earth-based tech, scientists started developing theories of how spatial elements were influencing outbreaks, which tended to result in better crisis planning. These ideas, while applied in short-term fixes, also inform long-term plans by sketching out potential future situations through the interactive effects of social and environmental variables (Benitez-Valerio et al., 2024). GIS also elevates outbreak management with convenient surveillance and tracking features. Its ability to process tons of location-associated data makes it useful for public health officials to compare various means of disease control—sometimes even in situations such as veterinary outbreaks, demonstrating its wide applicability. Features such as map analysis and the unification of different types of data enable decision-makers to instantly verify what is effective and what isn't, even though the punctuation of ideas often comes across as slightly uneven. Ultimately, GIS is a key tool for knowing disease patterns, bringing health workers together to collaborate in predicting and suppressing future outbreaks (Haile et al., 2017) (Figure 11.10).

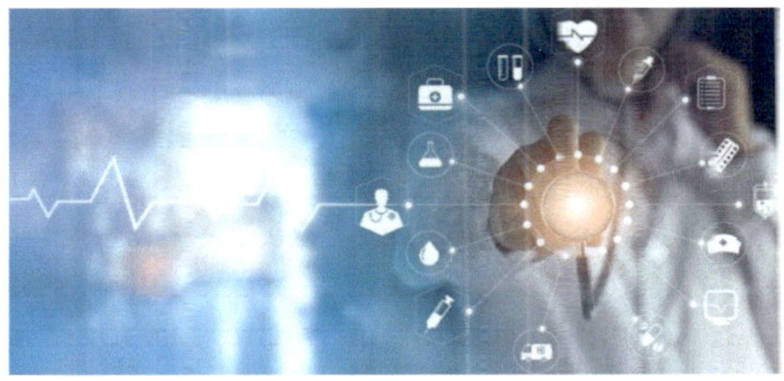

Figure 11.10. Geographic information systems (GIS) in tracking outbreaks.

Source: Elets Technomedia Pvt Ltd. (2019). Healthcare. *Elets eHealth*.

11.5.3. Mobile Technology and Real-Time Data Collection

Mobile tech is turning epidemiology on its head these days. Phones and tablets, which are a part of our daily lives now, capture every minute contact that we have, and that provides scientists with a means to see our social behavior like never before. Monitoring who gets close to whom—even for a minute—unveils concealed patterns that may be pivotal in knowing how diseases hop around (Lehmann et al., 2015). Catching this immediate buzz assists with creating models that are attuned to even the smallest things, and in most instances, this means that interventions can be more directly targeted to prevent an outbreak before it can get a foothold. Recent breakthroughs also enable data not simply bulked together but able to distinguish merely being in the same room from having a face-to-face chat. This type of subtle distinction makes a difference when creating disease risk maps because it can shift the way transmission is considered. Researchers blend high-resolution data on both types of interaction and then sometimes test techniques that generate surrogate contact networks—they match these against what occurs. As problematic as they can be, these sly data-gathering tactics provide an added layer of confidence to predictions regarding the ways that infections may spread (Barrat et al., 2017). Live data collection combined with mobile tech is not only opening doors, but also raising new questions in epidemiology. Detailed portraits of how individuals interact provide new information about the transmission of diseases, but relying too heavily on data-based approaches requires a close examination of how the numbers are collected. Since sampling methods can be good one day and not so good the next, researchers tend to have to adjust their approach based on context, local dynamics, and the purposes of their study. In general, maintaining an open line of communication between technological innovations and actualized difficulties allows our models to remain connected to the ground level but still inform timely public health actions.

11.6. Public Health Implications

Epidemic modeling isn't some theoretical concept—it has real stakes for public health as cities grow and our weather changes. Outdated predicting techniques tend to be off the mark when quick population increases and greater mobility obscure the boundaries of old-style predictions. Artificial intelligence is filling the gap today; with machine-learning algorithms, it is analyzing enormous piles of data to identify outbreak trends we never could before. In most instances, this new development not only increases our preparedness but also serves to more effectively target resources in times of disease when they strike hard (Nassimbwa, 2024). Climate change's influence on health is no trivial consideration. Climbing temps and changing rain habits are pushing mosquitoes, ticks, and other vectors to evolve in unexpected ways. Diseases such as malaria and dengue are appearing in regions previously considered to be safe – an indication that these pathogens are becoming smarter while their carriers expand their scope.

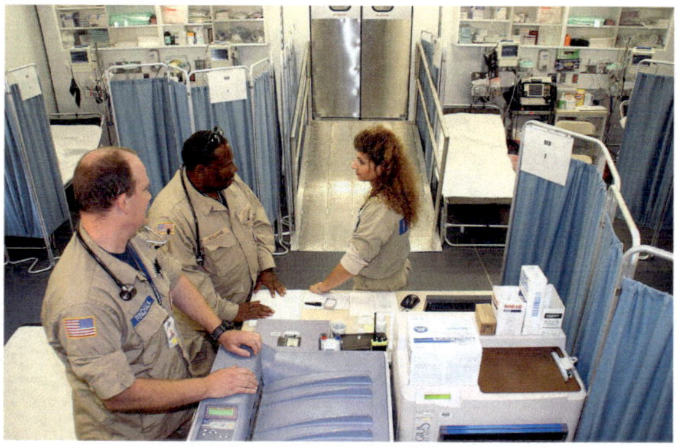

Source: By Robert Kaufmann - This image is from the FEMA Photo Library (obsolete as of 2019). An archived copy may be found at the Wayback Machine (note: link may be permanently dead, as not all photos were backed up in this way).If the FEMA link is permanently dead, the photo can be found at NARA Access to Archival Databases (only works if photo was taken between 1989 and October 2004), or at City-data.com., Public Domain, https://commons.wikimedia.org/w/index.php?curid=8085463

Frequent integration of genome-based tracing with predictive modeling provides us with a multi-layered safety net and head start on timely interventions (Pavia et al., 2024). It is important to know what these developments mean to enhance our health systems. As climate-informed predicts and AI continue to improve, it is increasingly apparent that the world needs global cooperation – no nation should be alone in the task of sharing information or best practices. It is not simply a matter of battling current outbreaks; investing in strong, climate-resilient health networks is about preparing for long-term challenges too. Overall, when the world unites in concerted action, public health programs are stronger to address both disease outbreaks and climate change, making communities safer as a whole (Nassimbwa, 2024; Pavia et al., 2024).

11.6.1. Policy-Making Informed by Epidemic Models

Urban disease control depends heavily on combining epidemic models with public policy, particularly in congested city centers. Computer-based and mathematical models thrown together assist us in getting a glimpse of how diseases spread; these findings—albeit somewhat sloppy at times—provide policymakers with some kind of prediction of what will occur. For instance, when policymakers model various types of intervention, they sort of have a preview of the results. Consider dengue fever: crunching data on different control measures allows experts to compare efficacy, which then informs decisions. This not only refines interventions but also ensures resources are allocated wisely so that health systems can pounce on burgeoning threats early. Epidemic models in most instances are viewed as a strategic evidence-based strategy that maintains policies as flexible and sensitive to shifting disease patterns. Some of the epidemic modeling methods, such as stability analysis and numerical simulation, tend to highlight just how sensitive and delicate disease dynamics can be. Examination of the models tends to reveal that relatively small variations in initial conditions have a great effect on the way an outbreak develops. For example, science tends to highlight that getting the numbers right—estimating how many will recover or, sadly, not survive—is quite important when it comes to dengue fever. And as policymakers do their best to design public health responses, incorporating these analysis insights, even though it's a little tricky, turns out to be essential.

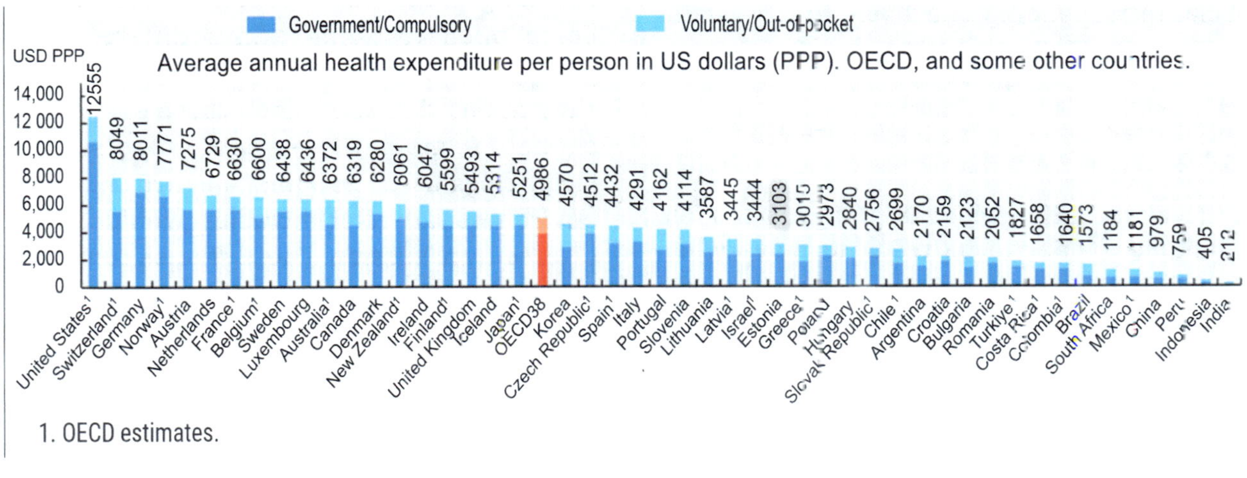

Figure 11.11. Policy-making informed by epidemic models.

Source: By OECD. Also, text was added via an image editor such as freeware IrfanView. - https://www.oecd-ilibrary.org/sites/7a7afb35-en/1/3/7/2/index.html?itemId=/content/publication/7a7afb35-en&_csp_=6cf33e24b6584414b81774026d82a571&itemIGO=oecd&itemContentType=book StatLink: https://stat.link/m6pzqb, Public Domain, https://commons.wikimedia.org/w/index.php?curid=126701185

With advanced modeling methods at their disposal, they stand a better chance of navigating the uncertainties that always seem to follow in the wake of any epidemic predict, finally creating policies that weigh prevention and control measures for diverse epidemiological settings. Charting the risk of diseases such as dengue fever in cities is another vital piece of the jigsaw. Careful spatial analysis of outbreak data can identify high-risk areas where immediate action must be taken—sometimes uncovering patterns that aren't at first apparent. When big data is combined with clever algorithms, you can identify nuanced spatial differences in disease transmission, informing targeted strategies designed to interrupt the transmission chains. It happens that adding socio-economic variables to the mix tends to fortify these risk assessments by identifying vulnerabilities spread out across various urban hotspots. Overall, linking epidemic models tightly with empirical data allows policymakers to construct public health policies that are not only medically valid, but also socially conscious and equitable, which is crucial in responding effectively to city health emergencies (Figure 11.11).

11.6.2. Community Preparedness and Response Strategies

In the world today, which is always in motion, communities have to be ready to move when epidemics strike unexpectedly. Being prepared is not only about establishing hospitals—it is also about combining genetic monitoring with boots-on-the-ground health care. In general, if you combine genomic data with little pieces of information about who is on the move and who is potentially at risk, it becomes a lot easier to identify the people requiring special attention. Sometimes, in a sudden epidemic, local health staff can take a glimpse at early warning indicators using these findings, which—if taken promptly—reduce how quickly an infection spreads. These pre-emptive measures, in most instances, assist in directing where funds are allocated and enhance a community's overall capacity to recover (Hill et al., 2021). Community engagement truly underlies the entire concept of being ready; it is not merely a catch-all phrase. Quite often, the magic ingredient is merely to tell people about potential health threats and what easy changes they can make. This type of clear-cut education has a way of establishing trust between the public health officials and the folks in the trenches—trust that pays off when the rumors begin to circulate. Neighborhood groups, in some cases even a combination of volunteers and neighbors who have learned rudimentary health expertise, create the foundation for a collective type of responsibility. Not only does this grassroots collaboration raise the pace at which a society can respond, it also provides people with a feeling of control of their own well-being.

And, to be honest, that additional line of communication tends to make sure vital news doesn't fall through the cracks when things are chaotic (Tao et al., 2021). Ultimately, having a community prepared is all about checking what has worked previously and being open to doing things differently. By glancing over previous outbreaks—usually in simulations that seize upon those ephemerals, changing moments—epidemiologists can glean clues as to how humans act and which environmental idiosyncrasies would compel disease transmission. These studies sometimes reveal that temporary variables, such as how groups roam or abrupt weather changes, can increase a community's risk. This blend of information allows administrators to create adaptable, adaptive plans that address the inescapable uncertainty of epidemics. In reality, by integrating these observations into long-term planning, communities are not merely responding—They are staying ahead, which can come a long way in terms of modeling and warding off future outbreaks (Hill et al., 2021; Tao et al., 2021).

11.6.3. Ethical Considerations in Modeling and Predictions

Epidemic models raise some serious ethical questions, and there is no simple recipe for solving them. Those constructing and applying these models—whether scientists or policymakers—tend to rely on neat assumptions that avoid the messy complexity of everyday life. Some of those models are based on a sort of ideal world, a world in which human responses and social fault lines simply do not appear, and that sometimes means that the strategies end up unfairly targeting people who are already disadvantaged. It is as if the models cut corners, and those simplifications can ultimately blow up in terms of policies that do not protect the weakest. To handle disease outbreaks better, one needs to loop in how management is practiced and account for the small snags that come along the way. Including methods of measuring risk and robustness can assist in bringing out the ethical consequences of various approaches so that the models are not only number-crunching devices but also socially aware (Brown et al., 2017). Individuals also encounter ethical dilemmas regarding how we pool our individual resources during epidemics. When people are being encouraged to alter daily routines for the public good, it's sort of like the classic prisoner's dilemma—where acting in your own best interest may conflict with acting in everyone's best interest. Whereas if everyone working in conjunction brings infections down, questions regarding individual sacrifice and collective responsibility necessarily arise. Understanding how cooperation adapts and forms itself in accordance with actual human behavior is central to creating public health policy that works. And when simulations demonstrate that just a bit more cooperation can reduce the spread of disease, they can support policies that reward civic cohesion and mutual responsibility, enhancing overall health gain (Karlsson et al., 2020). In the end, blurring ethical issues into the very center of epidemic modeling creates a sort of template for combating outbreaks better. The unpredictable side of human behavior reminds modelers to keep ethics in mind along with the data, even if that means juggling some messy details. Being clear about what assumptions are in play and what results are expected can do wonders for public trust, which is crucial during a health crisis. As models begin to incorporate more of the social and cultural idiosyncrasies that influence actual life, they should necessarily adopt a broader range of perspectives while advocating for equity in health measures. By incorporating ethical issues into the model-building process, scientists are not only able to target more accurate predictions but also assist in initiating the sort of cooperation and unity required to address infectious diseases, strengthening public health measures that much further (Brown et al., 2017; Karlsson et al., 2020).

CLOSER LOOK

Stochastic

Stochasticity in its most general definition is the nature of randomness or unpredictability in a process. It is a mathematically defined term closely analogous to randomness and probabilistic events as opposed to deterministic processes. Stochastic models are deployed to describe and analyze systems whose outcomes are determined by chance and uncertainty.

Core Concepts

- **Randomness and Uncertainty:** Stochastic processes naturally involve randomness, in the sense that the result of a specific event is not fixed.
- **Probabilistic Nature:** Rather than predicting with accuracy, stochastic models center on the probability of various outcomes happening.
- **Evolution over Time:** Stochastic models generally explain how systems evolve over time, with the evolution being determined by random events.

SUMMARY

Epidemic modeling is not merely keeping tabs on the transmission of diseases—it hugely influences public health decisions and directs intervention to combat outbreaks. COVID-19 reminded us, in most instances, that models (even compartmental ones) were able to provide profound insights into transmission rates and possible death counts under different circumstances. Scientists, relying on good data, tended to make fairly decent predictions with a rather astounding level of accuracy. These models, for example, note that interventions such as quarantine and contact tracing can significantly alter the course of an outbreak, making early data collection and analysis even more important (Duan et al., 2021).

Briefly, refining these strategies appears to be the key to being better prepared for future pandemics. Risk factors added into the equation complicate the issues even more. Some recent research observed that day-to-day stuff, such as stress levels, screen use and even sex—contributed to the surge of smartphone addiction during the pandemic (Duan et al., 2021). It is almost like mental health and epidemic results cross paths unobtrusively. Underlying social and behavioral conditions, as it happens, can increase the likelihood of disease susceptibility. So, as the models lead us to interventions that fight the epidemic in direct ways, they also suggest we tackle those additional psychosocial issues. In combining varied forms of data, epidemic modeling can develop public health measures that are far more holistic when an epidemic strikes. Data-based models and actions on the ground must unite if we are to prevail against future epidemics. The COVID-19 lessons were that timely, informed reactions—grounded in sound predicts—can quite significantly reduce cases and deaths. Indeed, many studies have demonstrated that certain strategic actions precipitated steep reductions in case rates (Zu et al., 2020). This quite strongly reinforces, for the most part, why it is so vital to invest in continuous research and allocate funds to improve epidemic modeling. Even as new infectious dangers emerge, drawing on lessons learned may prove to offer a more energetic, if somewhat imperfect, answer for protecting public health in the long term.

Modeling epidemics isn't easy—it tells us a lot about how disease spreads and how effective public interventions are. Consider the Oxford COVID-19 Government Response Tracker (OxCGRT); it is a useful tool that monitors from lockdowns to healthcare increases and watches how these actions inform a pandemic. They tally these steps through nearly 180 nations, allowing researchers to spot odd trends between state action and outbreaks. This continuous data set, which sort of never ends, not only tracks shifting measures but also allows for comparisons of the effectiveness of various strategies in slowing spread (Hale et al., 2021). In many instances, these observations bleed well beyond mere health issues, influencing both government and healthcare leaders in their decision-making. What occurs in financial markets is equally as important when crises such as COVID-19 arise.

The pandemic demonstrated, quite literally, that economic influences and the actions of companies are thoroughly entangled with public health. As the virus spread, globally interconnected firms, particularly those relying on trade with China—had significant declines in their stock prices. And then, as markets became unstable, becoming preoccupied with corporate debt management and cash hoards became almost essential to company survival. This combination demonstrates that under a genuine health shock, its money ripple effects can have serious implications for broad economic well-being (Ramelli et al., 2020). To summarize, incorporating economic indicators into epidemic models provides us with a wider, multilayered perspective, which can in general serve to predict what may happen next. Based on human behavior, no epidemic model can truly be complete without considering the ways people act during it all. Plain old trends, like people observing social distancing or wearing masks, heavily steer the progression of a virus's spread. Government policies and how individuals respond to them can affect the effectiveness of these public health interventions, so it is nearly imperative for scientists to account for social routines. Observe carefully and you will notice that policy changes tend to accompany changes in how the populace behaves—this ongoing cycle provides us with important windows into human conduct during epidemic eruptions. Overall, combining behavioral signals with hard epidemiological information equips public health communities with improved solutions for the next crisis, providing a more, well, holistic view of how epidemics transpire (Hale et al., 2021).

KEY TERMS FROM THIS CHAPTER

- Agent-based model
- Stochastic model
- Incubation period
- Herd immunity threshold
- Parameter estimation
- Calibration
- Forecasting
- Outbreak threshold
- Surveillance data
- Non-pharmaceutical interventions (NPIs)
- Deterministic model
- Latent period
- Population immunity
- Disease dynamics
- Sensitivity analysis
- Validation
- Scenario analysis
- Spatiotemporal modeling
- Real-time modeling
- Superspreading event

REFERENCES

1. Allen, C., Alper, D., Aman, S., Kumar, A., et al. (2016). Results from the Centers for Disease Control and Prevention's predict the 2013–2014 Influenza Season Challenge. *BMC Infectious Diseases, 16*, 357. https://core.ac.uk/download/98348865.pdf (accessed on 6 May 2025).
2. Barrat, A., & Génois, M. (2017). Can co-location be used as a proxy for face-to-face contacts? *EPJ Data Science, 7*, 1–18. https://core.ac.uk/download/343334871.pdf (accessed on 6 May 2025).
3. Barthelemy, M., Godreche, C., & Luck, J. M. (2010). Fluctuation effects in metapopulation models: Percolation and pandemic threshold. *Journal of Theoretical Biology, 267*(4), 554. Elsevier. https://core.ac.uk/download/52690458.pdf (accessed on 6 May 2025).
4. Benitez-Valerio, V. S., & Juárez, M. V. S. (2024). The challenges of the COVID-19 pandemic in geographic science. *Brazilian Journal of Health Review, 7*(2), 1–17. https://core.ac.uk/download/611862922.pdf (accessed on 6 May 2025).
5. Bhattamisra, S. K., Banerjee, P., Gupta, P., Mayuren, J., Patra, S., & Candasamy, M. (2023). Artificial intelligence in pharmaceutical and healthcare research. *Big Data and Cognitive Computing, 7*, 10. https://doi.org/10.3390/bdcc7010010.
6. Chen, K., Shrivastava, U., & Tindol, B. (2019). The dynamics of real-time online information and disease progression: Understanding spatial heterogeneity in the relationship. *Transactions of the International Conference on Health Information Technology Advancement, 4*(1). https://core.ac.uk/download/289123789.pdf (accessed on 6 May 2025).
7. Cinelli, M., Quattrociocchi, W., Galeazzi, A., Valensise, C. M., Brugnoli, E., Schmidt, A. L., Zola, P., et al. (2020). The COVID-19 social media infodemic. *Scientific Reports, 10*. https://doi.org/10.1038/s41598-020-73510-5.
8. Forgoston, E., & Schwartz, I. B. (2013). Predicting unobserved exposures from seasonal epidemic data. *Department of Applied Mathematics and Statistics Faculty Scholarship and Creative Works*, 105. https://core.ac.uk/download/386152033.pdf (accessed on 6 May 2025).
9. Gorbalenya, A. E., Baker, S. C., Baric, R. S., de Groot, R. J., Drosten, C., Gulyaeva, A., Haagmans, B. L., et al. (2020). The species severe acute respiratory syndrome-related coronavirus: Classifying 2019-nCoV and naming it SARS-CoV-2. *Nature Microbiology, 5*, 536–544. https://doi.org/10.1038/s41564-020-0695-z.
10. Gralinski, L. E., & Menachery, V. D. (2020). Return of the coronavirus: 2019-nCoV. *Viruses, 12*, 135. https://doi.org/10.3390/v12020135.
11. Guma, F. E. L., Badawy, O. M., Berir, M., & Abdoon, M. A. (2023). Numerical analysis of fractional-order dynamic dengue disease epidemic in Sudan. *Journal of the Nigerian Society of Physical Sciences, 5*(2), 1464. https://doi.org/10.46481/jnsps.2023.1464.
12. Haile, A. W., & Mengistu, T. S. (2017). Review on the application of geographical information systems (GIS) in veterinary medicine. *International Journal of Veterinary Health Science and Research, 5*(4), 176–182. https://core.ac.uk/download/pdf/144828117.pdf (accessed on 6 May 2025).
13. Hale, T., Angrist, N., Goldszmidt, R., Kira, B., Petherick, A., Phillips, T., Webster, S., et al. (2021). A global panel database of pandemic policies (Oxford COVID-19 Government Response Tracker). *Nature Human Behavior, 5*, 529–538. https://doi.org/10.1038/s41562-021-01079-8.

14. Jewell, N. P., Lewnard, J. A., & Jewell, B. L. (2020). Caution warranted: Using the Institute for Health Metrics and Evaluation model for predicting the course of the COVID-19 pandemic. *Annals of Internal Medicine, 173*, 226–227. https://doi.org/10.7326/m20-1565.

15. Karlsson, C. J., & Rowlett, J. (2020). Decisions and disease: A mechanism for the evolution of cooperation. *Scientific Reports, 10*(1). https://core.ac.uk/download/347172518.pdf (accessed on 6 May 2025).

16. Lehmann, S., Pentland, A. 'Sandy,' Sapiezynski, P., Stopczynski, et al. (2015). Temporal fidelity in dynamic social networks. *European Physical Journal B: Condensed Matter and Complex Systems, 88*(10), 249. https://core.ac.uk/download/43252555.pdf (accessed on 6 May 2025).

17. Leigh, L., Taylor, C., & Sheu, J. (2024). Path modeling of socioeconomic, behavioral, and environmental attributes of the Ebola epidemic in West Africa. *Global Health Economics and Sustainability*. https://www.semanticscholar.org/paper/57facdbc2e2c5134dea6c0f94feb366f87aaf101 (accessed on 6 May 2025).

18. MacIntyre, C. R., Lim, S., & Quigley, A. (2022). Preventing the next pandemic: Use of artificial intelligence for epidemic monitoring and alerts. *Cell Reports Medicine, 3*, 100867. https://doi.org/10.1016/j.xcrm.2022.100867.

19. Magnani, M., Marzolla, M., Montesi, D., Salehi, et al. (2014). Spreading processes in multilayer networks. *IEEE Transactions on Network Science and Engineering, 2*(2), 65–83. https://core.ac.uk/download/226199524.pdf (accessed on 6 May 2025).

20. Mahalle, P. N., Sable, N. P., Mahalle, N., & Shinde, G. R. (2020). Data analytics: COVID-19 prediction using multimodal data. https://doi.org/10.20944/preprints202004.0257.v2.

21. Mustafa, N., Rahman, J., Ishtiaq, U., & Popa, I. L. (2025). Artificial neural network-based approach for dynamic analysis and modeling of Marburg virus epidemics for health care. *Symmetry*. https://www.semanticscholar.org/paper/b2046ab2850097ad7eec8495755baf84c0cec7b6 (accessed on 6 May 2025).

22. Pavia, G., Branda, F., Ciccozzi, A., Romano, C., Locci, C., Azzena, I., Pascale, N., et al. (2024). The issue of climate change and the spread of tropical diseases in Europe and Italy: Vector biology, disease transmission, genome-based monitoring, and public health implications. *Infectious Diseases*. https://www.semanticscholar.org/paper/8db2bec1b4609afedf77a3db10f406c77958f40b (accessed on 6 May 2025).

23. Petersen, E., Koopmans, M., Go, U., Hamer, D. H., Petrosillo, N., Castelli, F., Storgaard, M., et al. (2020). Comparing SARS-CoV-2 with SARS-CoV and influenza pandemics. *The Lancet Infectious Diseases, 20*, e238–e244. https://doi.org/10.1016/s1473-3099(20)30484-9.

24. Poletto, C., Scarpino, S. V., & Volz, E. (2020). Applications of predictive modelling early in the COVID-19 epidemic. *The Lancet Digital Health, 2*, e498–e499. https://doi.org/10.1016/s2589-7500(20)30196-5.

25. Tao, Y., Hite, J. L., Lafferty, K. D., Earn, D. J. D., & Bharti, N. (2021). Transient disease dynamics across ecological scales. *Theoretical Ecology, 14*, 625–640. https://doi.org/10.1007/s12080-021-00514-w.

26. Tsao, S. F., Chen, H., Tisseverasinghe, T., Yang, Y., Li, L., & Butt, Z. A. (2021). What social media told us in the time of COVID-19: A scoping review. *The Lancet Digital Health, 3*, e175–e194. https://doi.org/10.1016/s2589-7500(20)30315-0.

27. Wu, H., Song, C., Ge, Y., & Ge, T. (2022). Link prediction on complex networks: An experimental survey. *Data Science and Engineering, 7*, 253–278. https://doi.org/10.1007/s41019-022-00188-2.

28. Yang, P., Qi, J., Zhang, S., Wang, X., Bi, G., Yang, Y., Sheng, B., et al. (2020). Feasibility study of mitigation and suppression strategies for controlling COVID-19 outbreaks in London and Wuhan. *PLoS ONE, 15*, e0236857. https://doi.org/10.1371/journal.pone.0236857.

29. Yin, S., Ren, C., Shi, Y., Hua, J., Yuan, H. Y., & Tian, L. (2022). A systematic review on modeling methods and influential factors for mapping dengue-related risk in urban settings. *International Journal of Environmental Research and Public Health, 19*, 15265–15265. https://doi.org/10.3390/ijerph192215265.

30. Zu, J., Li, M., Li, Z., Shen, M., Xiao, Y., & Ji, F. (2020). Transmission patterns of COVID-19 in the mainland of China and the efficacy of different control strategies: A data- and model-driven study. *Infectious Diseases of Poverty, 9*. https://doi.org/10.1186/s40249-020-00709-z.

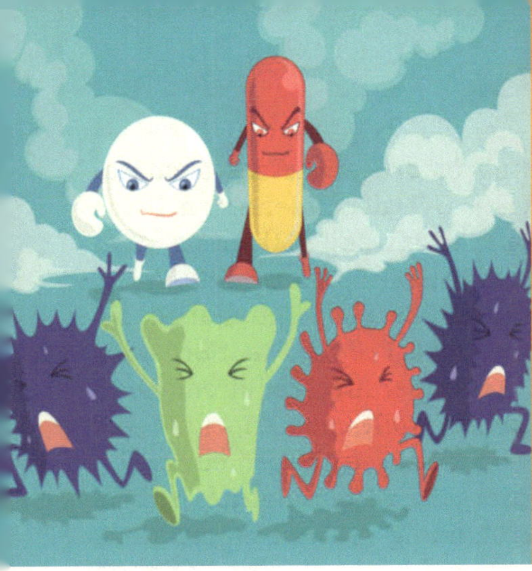

Chapter 12

ANTIMICROBIALS AND RESISTANCE

Contents

Introduction

Antimicrobial resistance (AMR) is a very dangerous public health and contemporary medical practice threat, as it has the potential to turn otherwise curable infections lethal. That is, AMR happens when microorganisms acquire resistance to the action of antimicrobial medicines, such as antibiotics, antivirals, antifungals, and antiparasitic. Adaptation not only reduces the effectiveness of such critical drugs but also leads to prolonged disease, higher healthcare expenditure, and increased mortality rates. The reach of AMR is vast and extends beyond human health to livestock and crops, thus compromising ecosystems and food security. Complete comprehension of AMR entails etiology analysis of its, evolution history, and the impact of AMR on contemporary medicine, which confirms the requirement of developing effective prevention and treatment strategies. The evolution history of antimicrobials is one of the most groundbreaking improvements in medicine, considerably lowering infectious disease morbidity and mortality. The discovery of the first antibiotic, penicillin, was in 1928 and ushered in a new era in the history of medicine. Yet, the following decades witnessed the widespread misuse of antibiotics, resulting in the alarming finding of drug-resistant bacterial strains, including Methicillin-resistant *Staphylococcus aureus* (MRSA). Overdependence on these drugs coupled with inefficient regulating structures has brought about the existing AMR crisis. With once-easily-treated infections growing harder and harder to treat, the healthcare community is confronted with the formidable task of holding on to its effective antibiotics while simultaneously working to develop new drug therapies all the while. It is such a chronological context that provides the setting for the appreciation of how complicated AMR is and the imperative requirement of responsible stewardship of antimicrobial drugs. As a result of growing AMR concern, there has been a universal push worldwide toward awareness and sensitization, and also toward education campaigns targeting healthcare professionals (HCPs) alongside the general population. Efforts by organizations like the WHO identify the necessity for an understanding of AMR implications and the need for concerted efforts toward fighting it. Training is critical in the practice of good prescribing and judicious use of antimicrobials, particularly in settings like agriculture where antibiotics are generally misused. Besides this, health education campaigns ensure that people are well aware of the risks of self-medication and the importance of following prescribed treatment courses. With a better understanding of AMR and its implications, society can start to address the complex challenge of this phenomenon with improved health outcomes and maintain future medicines' effectiveness (Figure 12.1).

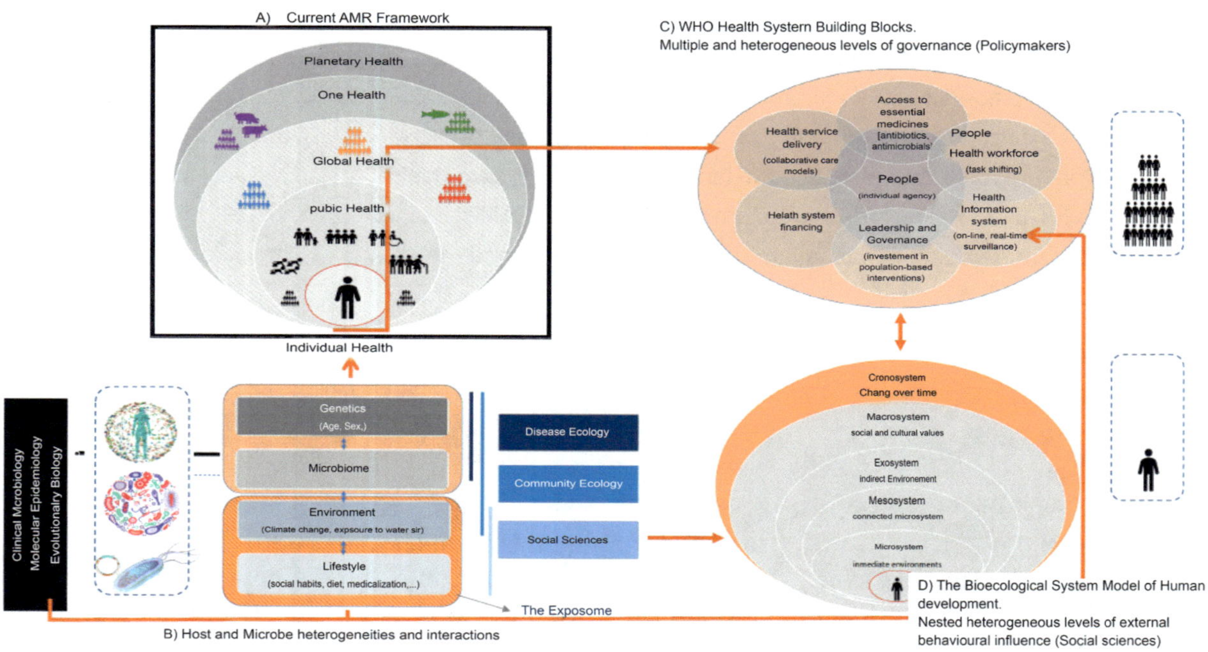

Figure 12.1. Antimicrobial resistance (AMR) poses a significant threat to public health and modern medical practices.

Source: Coque TM, Cantón R, Pérez-Cobas AE, Fernández-de-Bobadilla MD, Baquero F. Antimicrobial Resistance in the Global Health Network: Known Unknowns and Challenges for Efficient Responses in the 21st Century. Microorganisms. 2023; 11(4):1050. https://doi.org/10.3390/microorganisms11041050

Definition and Scope

The problem of AMR involves intricate interactions among microbial pathogens, medical procedures, and population behaviors. Essentially, AMR is the phenomenon where microorganisms—bacteria, fungi, viruses, and parasites—can resist the actions of drugs that previously treated them. It is a serious public health concern, making infection treatment difficult and resulting in high morbidity and mortality rates worldwide. As outlined in current publications, the reaction to AMR has been lacking, most especially in low- and middle-income nations (LMICs), in which the necessity for bespoke, context-based, and sustainable approaches is paramount (Khurana et al., 2023). As such, an overarching understanding of AMRs definition and broad scope is required to tackle the multi-dimensional challenges it poses to healthcare systems and beyond. To forestall the accelerating threat posed by AMR, a multi-professional effort is necessary. That includes harmonizing evidence-based information and locally tuned interventions for their application to varied epidemiological circumstances at local levels. AMR's impact does not weigh across the world even; rather it varies drastically, based on location and socio-economy. For example, coverage of new antibiotics and monitoring infrastructure are scarce in most areas, as the evidence from European surveillance systems (Evaluation et al., 2023) points out. This lack of monitoring and real-time tracking of resistance illustrates the imperative to ensure comprehensive data collection and institutionalize national action plans (NAPs) to combat AMR. Thus, the ambit of AMR is not limited to clinical issues, and efforts have to be made cooperatively involving HCPs, policymakers, researchers, and communities. Familiarizing oneself with the definition and ambit of AMR provides ways of focused interventions and policy changes. Under this scheme of things, the role of education and awareness programs cannot be overemphasized since they increase public knowledge of judicious antimicrobial use. By developing well-informed communities that understand the consequences of abuse, we can encourage practices that help maintain the effectiveness of currently available antimicrobial agents. In addition, continued research and the creation of new innovative strategies to track and respond to developing patterns of resistance are key to maintaining therapeutic choices (Khurana et al., 2023). Finally, resolution of the definition and scope of AMR is critical to maintaining safe healthcare procedures and protecting future generations from the effects of inefficient treatments.

Historical Background

The path to comprehension of AMR has its origins in the triumphant and tormented history of medical science. The discovery of penicillin in the late 1920s was a public health revolution, the first secure cure for bacterial diseases. It was greeted for its power to cut mortality from hitherto always lethal disease by miraculously depleted proportions. But with the emergence of the mid-20th century antibiotics, news of bacterial resistance spread, signaling the start of a sophisticated and consistent war between microbial adaptation and medical innovation. With every newly discovered antibiotic came the appalling increase in resistance, documenting the urgent necessity of learning more about the activity of bacteria and how it affects human health. The last few decades have seen the rise of multidrug-resistant strains fueling the interest in AMR history. The study data revealing antimicrobial susceptibility patterns in animals and humans accounts for the ever-changing landscapes of bacterial populations. For example, a study of urinary tract infections in canine patients revealed a concerning trend toward increased resistance to usual antimicrobials, especially with complicated infections. These results reveal not just the extent of problems but also the impact of previous antimicrobial utilization, possibly creating a cycle of increasing levels of resistance (Epstein et al., 2015). This situation highlights the need for continuous surveillance and investigation to support effective public health interventions and antibiotic stewardship. The complex interaction of microbe and human activity is described further through epidemic evidence in infection episodes in the past. The outcome of Salmonella outbreaks defines the contribution of subtyping techniques and their efficacy in the tracking of infection source. The dependence on whole genome sequencing has developed as an imperative tool for the investigation of such outbreaks, with an enhanced insight into the epidemiology of drug-resistant bacteria. The intricacies of foodborne pathogens demonstrate the broader situation of AMR for food safety and public health (Mohammed et al., 2020). The historical context of resistance development and epidemics of disease shed light on the necessity of adopting interdisciplinary measures to combat AMR, so that history would not repeat itself against new threats (Figure 12.2).

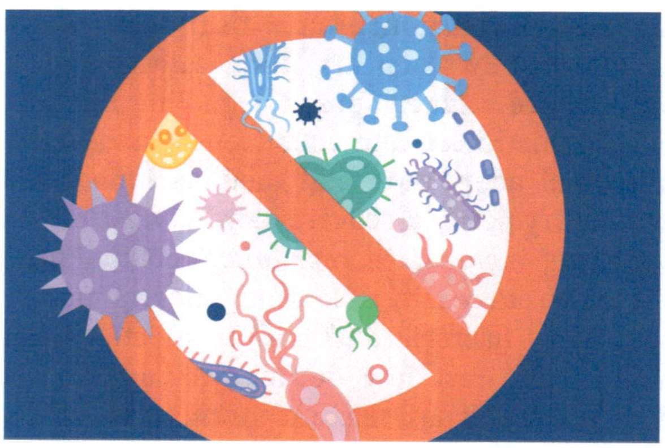

Figure 12.2. The journey toward understanding antimicrobial resistance (AMR).

Source: Union for International Cancer Control. (2023). *Artboard 981440*.

Importance in Modern Medicine

The evolution of antimicrobial agents marks a transformative milestone in the realm of modern medicine, underscoring the critical role these tools play in combatting infectious diseases. Historically, the introduction of β-lactam antibiotics, such as penicillin, revolutionized treatment options for bacterial infections. This pivotal moment provided a newfound ability to address previously dreaded ailments, drastically reducing mortality rates and shaping healthcare paradigms globally. Yet, as their unveiling has been fast followed by the fast-growing rise of resistance, misuse and overuse of these antimicrobials have muddled this early victory. This explains why responsible use must be supported by a balanced strategy ensuring a constant promotion of drug development progress, ensuring their effective control and prevention of AMR (Rathinavelu et al., 2024)). Comprehensive strategies and interdisciplinary collaboration are central in tackling the challenges of the new world of AMR. As observed, there is an urgent call for professionals in different sectors such as health, agriculture, and technology to come together and come up with innovative approaches. Through convergence of disparate views and competencies, healthcare systems can create environments that are supportive to integrated patient care while limiting the environmental implications of antimicrobial consumption. The interconnection of human and animal health, as well as the environment, as highlighted in contemporary discussion, necessitates an integrated methodology that goes beyond conventional biomedical thinking (Bandura et al., 2018). It is only through such cooperation that we can possibly try to curtail AMRs effects and, ultimately, ensure that life-saving treatments continue to be viable for generations to come. Worldwide acknowledgment and education about AMR are essential in assuring the future of contemporary medicine. The quick expansion of AMR is not only a national issue but a global crisis, as it impacts health systems across the world. Training healthcare workers and the public on the consequences of antimicrobial misuse and overuse can trigger large-scale behavior change among prescribing habits and personal decisions. In addition, encouraging sustainable agricultural practices to minimize antibiotic use in animals is a fundamental part of the overall strategy to stop resistance. As AMR continues to burden increasing numbers, high-priority efforts can inform future healthcare policy and practice, reinforcing the important role of education to ensure public health protection and the effectiveness of existing and future antimicrobial therapies.

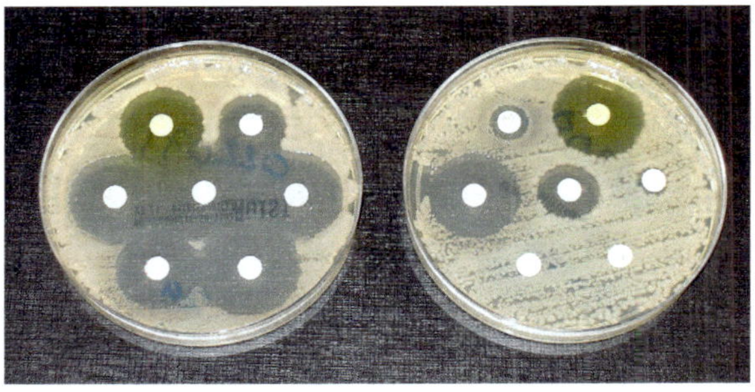

Source: By Dr Graham Beards at en.wikipedia, CC BY-SA 4.0, https://commons.wikimedia.org/w/index.php?curid=25206097

12.1. Types of Antimicrobial Agents

The antimicrobial armory includes a wide range of compounds active against a wide range of microorganisms, each tailored to treat infections, say, of a certain type. Antibiotics, say, are employed for the most part, to combat bacterial infections and operate through various mechanisms, say, by preventing cell wall formation or protein synthesis. They can be termed narrow-spectrum or broad-spectrum depending on the spectrum of their activity. Such differentiation is crucial since the overuse of broad-spectrum antibiotics can lead to antimicrobial resistance (AMR), and therefore there is a critical need to use these drugs judiciously. Recent studies, such as the evaluation of *Clostridioides difficile* isolate resistance profile, pose a critical necessity to determine what kind of antibiotic to use because rising numbers of resistant strains are being reported globally, making treatments less effective (Allerberger et al., 2022). In addition to antibiotics, antiviral drugs are also crucial in the treatment of viral infections, which are targeted toward specific stages of the life cycles of viruses.

In contrast to antibiotics, which target bacterial function, antivirals function to inhibit the release and replication of viruses. Their varied classifications, including nucleoside analogs and protease inhibitors, reflect the specific strategy needed for different viruses, such as HIV or influenza. Increasing viral resistance is also challenging the efficacy of antiviral therapy. For instance, some *Escherichia coli* O157 strains are reported to possess AMR, highlighting that the evolution of resistance is not an exclusive phenomenon of bacteria but a complex issue on the entire microbial front (Boyen et al., 2011).

Antiparasitic and antifungal medications also have a central role in treating parasitic and fungal infections, respectively. Antifungals such as azoles and echinocandins, for instance, disrupt cell membrane architecture or cell wall formation in fungi, whereas antiparasitic such as metronidazole act on select protozoal infections. Both types of resistances, when established, are a threat to public health, as witnessed in the emergences of multiple resistances for antimicrobials simultaneously. This is even more somber given the prevalence of resistant *Clostridioides difficile* organisms, which points to the paramount need for demystifying the resistance patterns in various microbial pathogens. Without addressing the looming threat to the effectiveness of the agents, the health crisis posed to the world by AMR may escalate (Allerberger et al., 2022) (Figure 12.3).

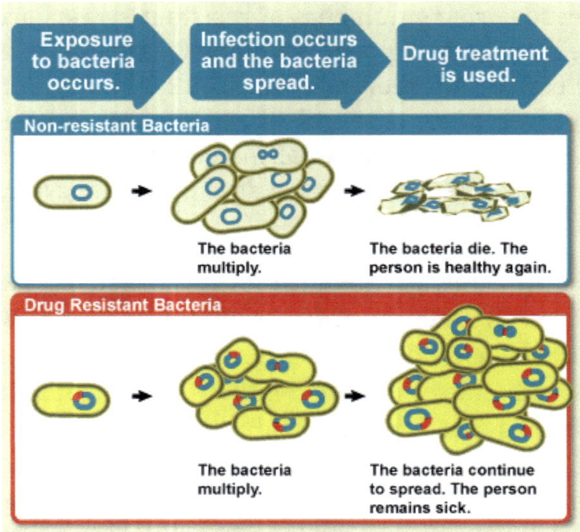

Figure 12.3. Overview of antimicrobial agents

Source: By NIAID – NIH - http://www.niaid.nih.gov/topics/antimicrobialResistance/Understanding/Pages/drugResistanceDefinition.aspx, Public Domain, https://commons.wikimedia.org/w/index.php?curid=41858152

12.1.1. Antibiotics

Alexander Fleming's discovery of penicillin was a watershed moment, dramatically lowering deaths from infection and transforming the management of infectious disease. With more use of these powerful drugs, so too did the development of AMR accelerate. The ready availability and frequent misapplication of antibiotics in medicine and agriculture were significant factors precipitating the spread of resistant microbes.

According to recent studies, bacterial resistance more and more undermines the effectiveness of such once-relied-upon therapies, leading to a startling rise in infection cases that are resistant to treatment. The process not only underpins clinical outcome but also drives healthcare costs upward, and therefore it is imperative that healthcare providers as well as the public be alerted to the importance of judicious use of antibiotics. Over the last few decades, the stark rise in AMR has made the issue need to be investigated again for its underlying mechanisms. Among the mechanisms involved, genetic mutations, horizontal gene transfer (HGT), and efflux pumps are all pivotal in the ability of bacteria to resist antibiotic action. Efflux pumps, for instance, are shown to be a huge factor in resistance development, enabling bacteria to efflux antibiotics before they can exert their effects (Zhang et al., 2024). Biofilm formation also presents additional problems, with bacteria within biofilms generally more resistant to antimicrobials. Any effort to counteract resistance therefore must consider these mechanisms as the foundation upon which successful interventions can be formulated. It can be seen that the problem of AMR calls for a multifaceted solution that is both scientific innovation and public health campaigns. Stopping the development of antibiotic resistance means not only improving prescribing habits but also reassessing the general social impacts of antibiotic consumption. The overuse of these drugs, particularly in agriculture to facilitate growth of livestock, has sustained a cycle of resistance that undermines their potency in human medicine (Sahgal et al., 2024). Additionally, unsanitary infection management in hospitals and communities can also stimulate the propagation of resistant bacteria. As the public continues to become more aware, it is becoming increasingly important to implement education campaigns to encourage prudent use of antibiotics. Through collaboration between healthcare providers, policymakers, and the public, we can enhance the perceptibility of AMR and provide sustainable measures that preserve the effectiveness of antibiotics for generations to come (Figure 12.4).

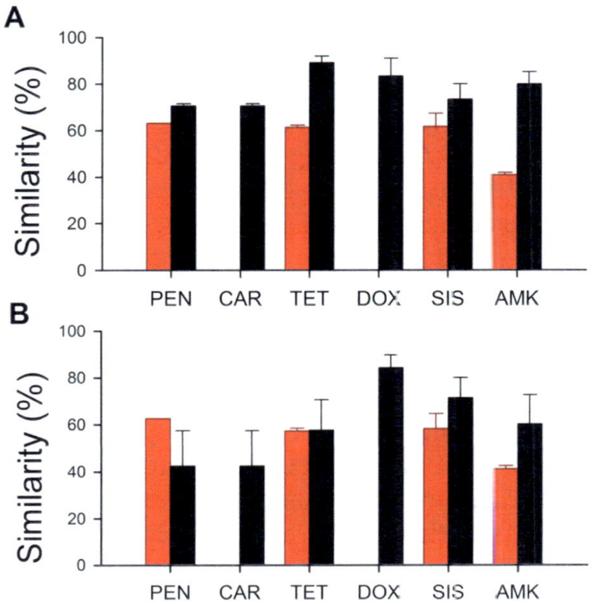

Figure 12.4. The introduction of antibiotics revolutionized modern medicine, providing effective treatments for bacterial infections that were once considered fatal.

Source: CC BY 4.0, https://commons.wikimedia.org/w/index.php?curid=148493512

12.1.2. Antivirals

Antivirals attack targeted sites in the virus lifecycle, blocking reproduction and facilitating recovery. The drugs lose potency over time because the virus can mutate and developresistance. As the case of the research on ribosomally synthesized and post-translationally modified peptides (RiPPs) has demonstrated, there is an expanding horizon that focuses on their promise as antiviral drugs. RiPPs possess strong antiviral activity against enveloped viruses, which are generally harder to treat effectively. The potential for engineering such peptides can create candidates with improved viral target affinities, thereby addressing the urgent demand for alternatives in antiviral therapy due to growing resistance concerns (Fu et al., 2021). The clinical profile of antiviral therapy is further confounded by emerging viral strains that are resistant to available drugs. Predominantly, viruses such as influenza A have increasingly developed resistance to commonly prescribed antivirals, emphasizing an important area of public health concern. Direct-acting antivirals (DAAs) have been very successful in the treatment of chronic viral infections, but their long-term effectiveness is threatened by the threat of resistance emergence. Notably, combination regimens have also shown great promise in averting resistance threats through the simultaneous administration of several agents against multiple viral mechanisms (Lackenby et al., 2009).

Such a multifaceted approach not only discourages adaptation by the virus but also optimizes overall treatment efficacy. In this respect, studies on novel combination therapies should be the priority area of antiviral research to fight the scourge of resistance. A world call for greater awareness and education concerning antiviral resistance is more pressing than ever before, driven by an appreciation of its implication in modern medicine and public health. Greater awareness of antiviral resistance necessitates a collaborative effort among HCPs, scientists, and policymakers to curtail its transmission. Education programs need to put greater stress on good prescribing practices and the implications of misuse of antiviral medication. Moreover, ongoing surveillance of antiviral effectiveness and resistance patterns can inform clinical guidelines so that clinicians are ever ready to give their best. Sustaining awareness about these issues and having an ongoing research program on novel antiviral approaches such as RiPPs is a critical pathway to maintaining the effectiveness of antiviral treatments in an evolving environment of resistance (Rathinavelu et al., 2024) (Figure 12.5).

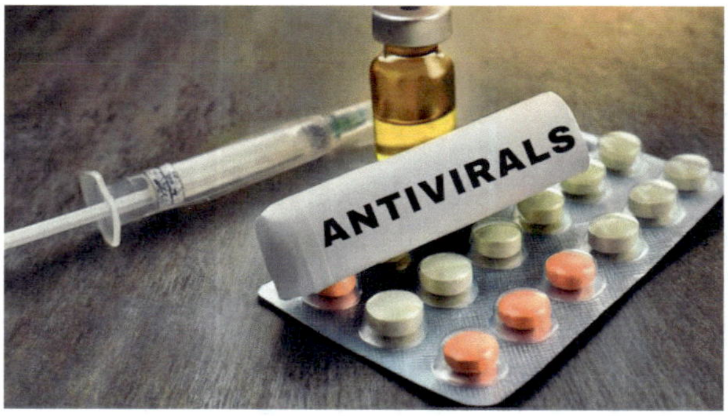

Figure 12.5. Advancements in antiviral research have increasingly highlighted the need for innovative therapeutic options to combat viral infections.

Source: Freepik. (n.d.). Antivirals_818056-5082. *Freepik.*

12.1.3. Antifungals

Antifungal resistance has become a cause of concern in the larger perspective of AMR due to several reasons. Among these are the overdose and inappropriately unwarranted administration of antifungal drugs, most of which takes place in the hospital setting as well as in agriculture. Since there is a limited number of antifungals, overdependence on certain groups of these drugs can result in selective pressure. This, in turn, favors the development of resistant strains. Indeed, fungi like Candida species become more resistant to typically employed antifungals, making treatment more complex and increasing health expenses. These phenomena further highlight the necessity of continuous monitoring and research activities to further elucidate and overcome antifungal resistance. In recent years, novel approaches are being investigated to overcome the challenges of antifungal resistance. For instance, new compounds with dual action potential are under investigation to address not just the fungal infection but even the inflammation that attends it. Investigation into agents such as Myriocin and Fulvic Acid has yielded their potential to inhibit fungal growth simultaneously with their anti-inflammatory activity (Borghi et al., 2015). This interaction is of paramount importance since chronic inflammation tends to be aggravated by biofilm growth, a typical feature of opportunistic infections. By designing such dual-functioning therapies, therapeutic effectiveness is hoped to be maximized and the swift development of resistance so frequently seen with conventional antifungal drugs minimized. Antifungal resistance awareness is also important to combat this chronic public health challenge. Training in proper antimicrobial stewardship (AMS) and the need to follow rigidly prescribed regimens of treatment becomes critical for both healthcare professionals (HCPs) and patients. Raising worldwide awareness regarding the limitations of current antifungal treatments and the possible effects of their improper use can give birth to a shared responsibility toward more responsible usage. In addition, delving into latest research that examines the metabolic processes employed by fungi in developing resistance to antifungal drugs will shed light on possible weaknesses (Kamat et al., 2010). Through fostering an educated society, we will all be able to encourage improved practice, ultimately curbing the spread of resistant fungal strains and guaranteeing successful treatment for susceptible groups.

12.2. Mechanisms of Resistance Development

These mutations could modify the shape of target proteins, making them ineffective against antibiotics, or alter metabolic pathways so that bacteria can circumvent the specific activity of drugs. For instance, a mutation could lead to a modified antibiotic target that does not bind to the drug anymore, thereby canceling its effects. In addition, the high rate of bacterial reproduction implies that these mutations can spread rapidly throughout a population. The contribution of genetic mutations to resistance highlights the importance of careful use of antibiotics, as the selective pressure from antibiotic exposure can hasten the emergence of resistant strains. It is important to understand the effects of these genetic changes to formulate measures to counteract AMR and guide antibiotic stewardship strategies. Other than genetic mutations, HGT is another important process by which bacteria inherit resistance characteristics from each other. This involves transformation, transduction, and conjugation, which enable the quick spread of resistance genes, even between different species. An example is plasmids, small DNA molecules found in bacteria, that tend to carry several resistance genes and can be transferred from one bacterium to another during conjugation. This enables the transmission of multidrug-resistant characteristics within hours or days, which is a major threat to public health. As mentioned, the irrational application of antibiotics increases the possibility of such mechanisms leading to the development of resistant strains. Therefore, the comprehension of HGT is crucial for the introduction of efficient measures to prevent the dissemination of AMR and makes the current antimicrobials effective. Some of the bacterial characteristics, including efflux pumps and biofilm development, also play a vital role in the emergence of resistance. Efflux pumps are dedicated proteins that actively remove antibiotics from bacterial cells, in effect reducing drug levels to below the lethal threshold. Not only does this system confer resistance, but it can also confer cross-resistance, where bacteria are resistant to more than one drug. Biofilms, organized communities of bacteria within a protective matrix, also enable survival in greater numbers against antibiotic therapy. Biofilm-dwelling bacteria can grow in a dormant state, making eradication even more challenging. The convergence of these mechanisms of resistance paints a picture of a complex environment where bacteria are constantly evolving to persist against challenges of therapeutics, warranting the importance of novel strategies in the fight against AMR, as highlighted in the literature identifying ways of evading these challenges (Busscher et al., 2020) (Figure 12.6).

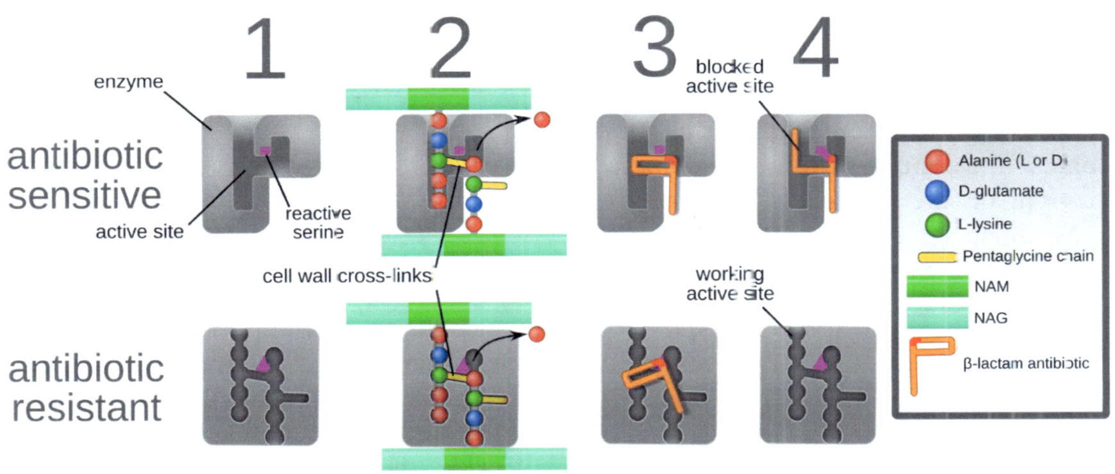

Figure 12.6. The emergence of resistance in bacterial populations is primarily facilitated by genetic mutations, which can occur spontaneously during bacterial replication.

Source: By Mcstrother - Own work, CC BY 3.0, https://commons.wikimedia.org/w/index.php?curid=14742117

12.2.1. Genetic Mutations

The development of AMR is closely associated with genetic mutations that allow the pathogens to survive under adverse conditions. Mutations could be due to spontaneous alteration during DNA replication or may occur as a response toward environmental stress, like exposure to antibiotics. The mutations could result in alterations of protein conformation and function in the bacteria, which allows them to become resistant to antimicrobial action. For example, the physiological reaction to elevated temperatures can cause stress in bacterial cells, leading to mutations that result in antibiotic tolerance. As such species evolve to handle such stress, resistance strains become more common, undermining effective treatment and public health (Cruz-Loya et al., 2020). Such adaptability advantage granted to mutant strains is a testament to the need to know how genetic change is involved in the processes of AMR and treatment. The processes of such genetic mutation are exceedingly intricate. Besides the spontaneous nature of mutations, HGT is also responsible for the rapid dissemination of AMR. Microorganisms can develop resistance through the inheritance of genes from the environment or from other microbial populations, further hindering travel through a more resistant microbial world. The emergence of new technologies like whole genome sequencing has shed light on the particular mutations to AMR in *Neisseria gonorrhoeae*, which is also critical information on how resistance develops and moves. It stresses the need for constant observation and research in determining mechanisms of resistance required for the design of new antimicrobial drugs and vaccines to control resistant pathogens (Bristow et al., 2019). An understanding of these complex interactions between genetic mutations and AMR will become essential in the battle against infectious diseases. The repercussions of genetic mutations do not stay confined to the lab bench but also reach clinical practice where the realities of AMR are harshly experienced in the real world. With the transmission of drug-resistant strains out of control, treatment outcomes cannot be anticipated as reliably, resulting in extended illness and higher healthcare costs. The problem is compounded further in poor-resource environments, where bacteria get the chance to become more susceptible to evolving and gaining resistance genes as they lack access to effective antimicrobial products. To combat the dynamics of genetic mutations driving AMR, a unified international effort has to be made involving public health campaigns, research funding support, and educational efforts. Approaches to addressing the phenomenon of AMR need to take into consideration not only the biological processes underlying resistance generation but also those socio-economic drivers of its emergence and propagation to ensure prevention and management strategies that are effective and evidence-based.

12.2.2. Horizontal Gene Transfer (HGT)

The exchange of genetic material among microbes is an important factor in the spread of AMR and essentially changes the behavior of microbial populations. HGT, as this process is termed, allows bacteria to pick up resistance mechanisms from their surroundings instead of just inheriting them. Environmental pressures and selection, including antibiotic usage, for example, increase the incidence of HGT. In situations where resistance genes to antibiotics are common in a population, resistant strains may arise and grow more quickly, thus making treatment more difficult. The capacity of bacteria to exchange genetic material ensures that they quickly develop adaptations to therapeutic measures, usually resulting in failures in the treatment process in medical contexts. This highlights the importance of comprehending HGT in the management of AMR. Experimental evidence shows that the association between antibiotic therapy and HGT is most significant in aquaculture and agriculture, where antimicrobial selective pressure promotes the dissemination of resistance genes. Treatment with florfenicol in catfish production systems was reported to not only alter the microbial community structure but also allow the propagation of florfenicol-resistant genes through both HGT and mutations (Liao et al., 2019). Equally, environmental engineering and science circles debate the contribution of HGT to environmental mechanisms that enable the evolution of antibiotic resistance (Alcalde et al., 2018).

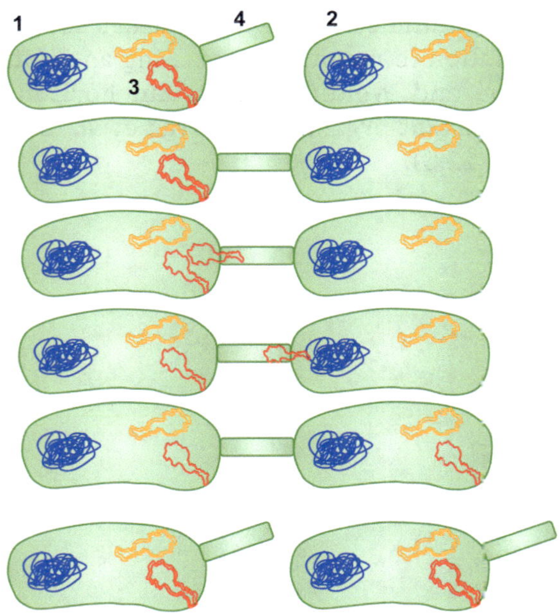

Figure 12.7. Horizontal gene transfer

Source: By KeeperGirl12 - Own work, CC BY-SA 4.0, https://commons.wikimedia.org/w/index.php?curid=59292718

This implies that resistance is not just a clinical issue, but also an environmental issue for which an effective management strategy involves inter-disciplinary engagement. Management of the spread of AMR requires addressing mechanisms of HGT to be effective. Strategies that reduce selective pressure with judicious use of antibiotics, and strong monitoring systems for following resistance patterns, are essential. The understanding of certain paths of gene transfer, along with the inferences derived from the dynamics of aquatic ecosystems, assists in anticipating and controlling outbreaks of resistant strains. Additionally, intersectoral cooperation among environmental scientists, agricultural experts, and medical practitioners will reinforce the measures to combat the emergence of resistant bacteria, eventually conserving the efficacy of existing antimicrobial agents for generations to come. Therefore, recognizing and managing HGT in microbial communities is central to formulating well-rounded strategies to address the growing issue of AMR (Figure 12.7)

12.2.3. Efflux Pumps

One of the numerous ways bacteria resist antimicrobial compounds is perhaps most significant when an efflux pump exists. These proteins are designed to act as a defense mechanism by actively removing a range of different substances, including antibiotics, from bacterial cells. This removal can lead to lower intracellular concentrations of antimicrobial compounds, allowing the bacteria to live concentrations that would otherwise be lethal. The sophisticated nature of such pumps, especially the ones belonging to the major facilitator superfamily (MFS), displays their ability to eject not only antibiotics but also other organic compounds, contributing to the complexity of the interaction between bacteria and the external environment. The significance of efflux pumps is not only resistance but also influences virulence, biofilm formation, and the capacity of the bacteria to colonize host cells, which shows how significant they are in the larger context of AMR (Barras et al., 2019). Experiments illustrate how these mechanisms of efflux can completely transform the efficacy of normal antibiotics and thereby present an issue in clinical conditions. In particular, studies have revealed that exposure to a specific chemical, for instance, sodium benzoate, can lead to increased resistance in *Salmonella typhi* bacteria. Sodium benzoate and chloramphenicol sensitivity is indicative of the dual function of external force in determining bacterial action. This process explores how the environmental stress can enhance already resistant traits or even create new ones, thereby making treatment options more complex and necessitating close monitoring of this antimicrobial usage (Anand et al., 2016). Further, the ability of efflux pumps to extrude a diverse range of substrates means that resistance can be multifaceted in nature. This necessitates gaining better insight into their mechanisms to facilitate effective countermeasures. Efflux pumps are not inert components of an antimicrobial resistant phenotype; they are active contributors to the evolutionary game of cat and mouse between bacteria and antimicrobials. Their function is inextricably entwined with the genes and regulatory systems that exist to control their expression, and these can be influenced by an enormous array of environmental stimuli. This interaction produces very plastic response to antimicrobial pressure, forestalling cuts to simplistic models of bacterial resistance. As we move deeper into the complexity of AMR, we discover that solving efflux pump mechanisms will be the solution to formulating new therapeutic strategies. Their resolution through multidisciplinary approaches could be the solution to maintaining existing antibiotics effective and avoiding the distant horizon of drug-resistant organisms (Barras et al., 2019) (Figure 12.8).

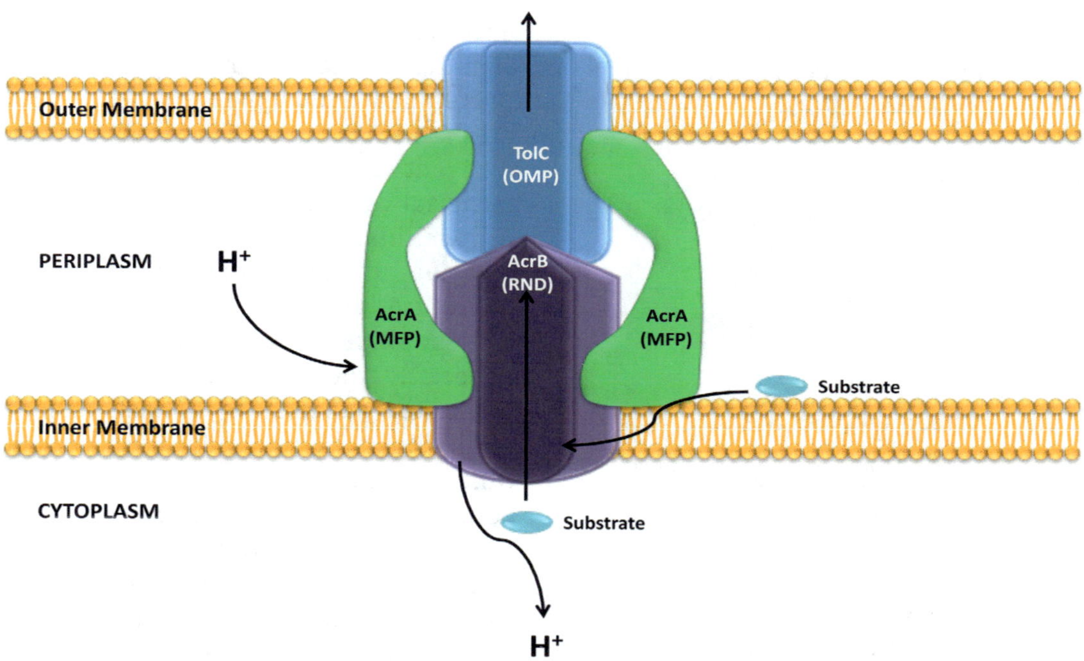

Figure 12.8. Efflux pumps.

Source: Li, X.-Z., Plésiat, P., & Nikaido, H. (2015). Efflux pumps. In The challenge of efflux-mediated antibiotic resistance in gram-negative bacteria. *Frontiers in Microbiology, 4*, Article 7.

12.3. Factors Contributing to Antimicrobial Resistance (AMR)

AMR is increasingly seen as a serious global health emergency fueled by different human activities and institutional practices. The most notable drivers of AMR are the misuse of antimicrobial drugs in both medicine and agriculture. In medicine, overprescription of antibiotics for illnesses that do not necessarily call for them leads to unnecessary pathogen exposure to the drugs. This repeated exposure imposes selective pressure, which enables resistant strains to develop and amplify. Likewise, in farming settings, the regular use of antibiotics for animal growth promotion or disease prevention in animals exacerbates the problem by enabling the transfer of resistance from animals to humans. This interrelation between human and animal health serves to validate the compelling necessity of responsible AMS in all aspects of society. Poor prescribing habits are also central to the emergence of AMR, which commonly results from the lack of systemic education for clinicians regarding proper use of antimicrobials. Physicians will occasionally prescribe broad-spectrum antibiotics rather than pathogen-directed treatment, fostering the growth of drug resistance. Compounding the problem are the pressures from patients requesting antibiotics even when not clinically warranted. This interaction between patient and provider dynamics results in unnecessary antimicrobials being prescribed, exacerbating the resistance issue. With patient satisfaction being at the forefront of healthcare systems, the need to ensure that prescriptions are warranted and useful can become secondary, showing the necessity of improved education and guidelines that prioritize responsible prescribing practices. Beyond prescribing practices, the use of antibiotics in agriculture is another major contributor to the encouragement of AMR. The use of antibiotics in agriculture, especially among livestock and poultry, is geared mainly toward increasing growth and keeping disease at bay in densely populated farming environments. The practice is not only risky from a health perspective for food consumed but also promotes the ideal environment for developing resistant bacteria. These resistant populations, once they are established, can be transferred to humans by the food chain, direct contact, or environmental routes. Dealing with AMR thus requires holistic strategies involving both the human and animal health branches, adequate regulatory practices with respect to agricultural use of antibiotics, and concerted efforts to induce sustainable practices. It is only through such holistic efforts that effective strides are made toward fighting the accelerated development of AMR.

12.3.1. Overuse of Antimicrobials

The effects of the overuse of antimicrobials are not limited to individual patients but also impact public health globally. The use of antibiotics without reservations has resulted in a staggering escalation of AMR, threatening to render these vital medicines ineffective. Research shows that inappropriate prescribing patterns, whether due to patient pressure or clinician insistence, play a key role in the development of AMR. Most of the time, patients anticipate the use of antibiotics even when they are not warranted, indicative of a deep-seated misapprehension about what these drugs do. In addition, healthcare settings need to institute effective surveillance measures to track prescribing and infection control practices, as described in Aarestrup et al. (2015). Failure to appreciate these subtleties accentuates the problem, making it a priority for both patients and providers to adopt judicious use of antibiotics for public health benefits. Patient education becomes an indispensable element in solving antimicrobial overuse. Programs that improve awareness among people on the use of antibiotics can encourage a better-informed patient population that appreciates the need to stick to prescribed medications and the risks associated with misuse. It has been documented that a well-written patient leaflet can enhance comprehension and acceptance of the "review & revise" strategy of antibiotic prescribing among hospitals, enhancing patient-HCP communication, thereby encouraging open communication among patients and HCPs (McCullough et al., 2020).

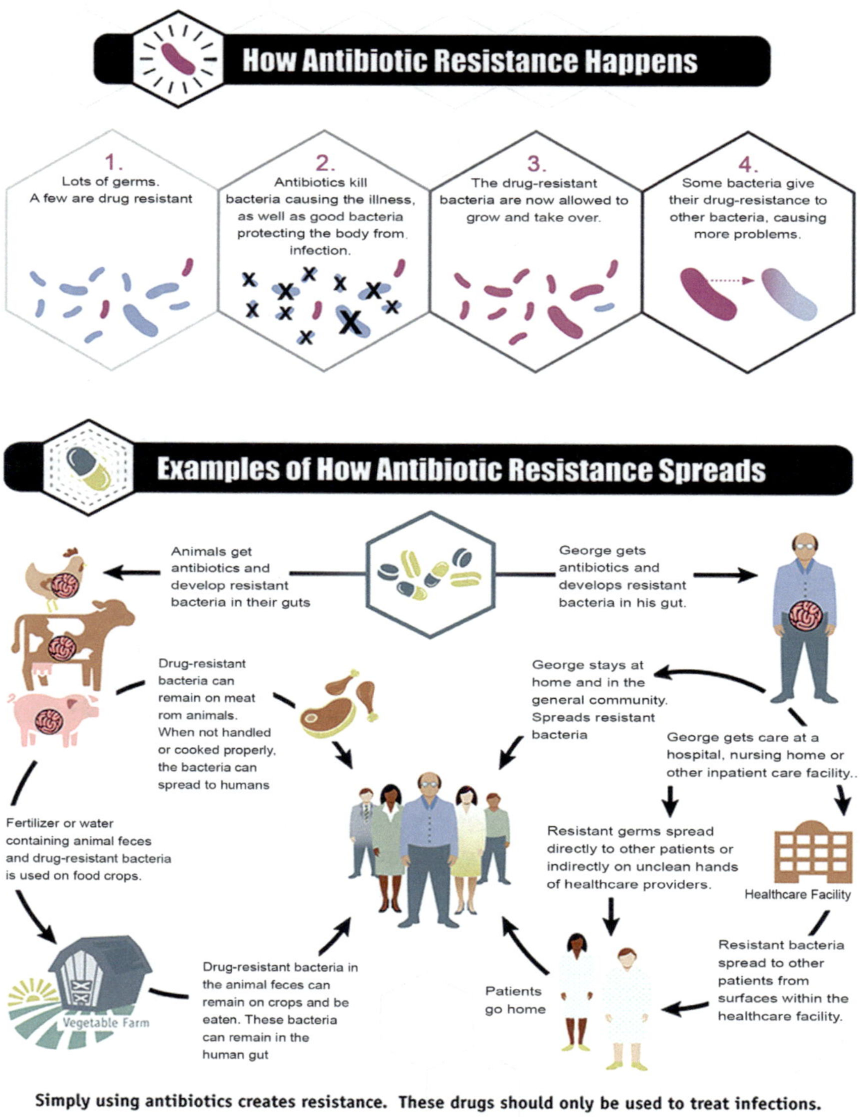

Figure 12.9. Overuse of antimicrobials.

Source: By CDC - https://www.cdc.gov/narms/faq.html, Public Domain, https://commons.wikimedia.org/w/index.php?curid=87884522

By encouraging trust and openness, patients can be made partners in decision-making about their treatment, thereby supporting better use of antimicrobials. Therefore, improving patient knowledge through educational tools and conversation can have a revolutionary impact in reducing the misuse of these valuable drugs. An approach that deals with the misuse of antimicrobials must be multi-faceted and involve policy modifications and One Health consideration. Bringing human, animal, and environmental health approaches together can combine to form a broader solution in fighting AMR (Aarestrup et al., 2015). Successful policies must be tailored to the specific demands of heterogenous populations and include strong surveillance networks that allow for effective responses to antibiotic resistance trends. Such policies must be advocated for, especially in low- and middle-income countries, where healthcare resources are not always available and awareness of AMR is low. Collaborative action across various sectors can facilitate magnifying the effect of educational programs and enhancing total management of antimicrobial usage. Relieving the AMR burden depends on our capacity to rally all stakeholders—clinicians, patients, and policymakers—toward one shared objective of responsible AMS (Figure 12.9).

12.3.2. Inadequate Prescribing Practices

Inadequate prescribing is a major driver of the overall problem of AMR. In many cases, physicians are under great pressure to promptly treat patient's requirements, and this may result in the indiscriminate choice of antimicrobials without careful consideration of previous resistance patterns. A study showed that inadequate empiric therapy is common, especially in septic shock patients with pneumonia who were given inappropriate antibiotics, leading to additional complications and longer recovery. Where clinicians fail to conduct a proper review of a patient's history, including prior antimicrobial use, there is enhanced risk of suboptimal prescribing, which promotes resistant organisms to grow and multiply. Therefore, it is essential to enhance awareness and training for physicians on best prescribing behavior in reducing the development of AMR. Furthermore, poor antimicrobial prescribing has far-reaching effects beyond individual patient results, affecting healthcare systems as a whole. Evidence in the research points out that insufficient treatment not only is associated with longer Intensive Care Unit (ICU) stays but also increases healthcare expenditure related to long-term antibiotic treatment and possible complications due to resistant pathogens. In one study, up to 70.5% of patients had received inappropriate therapy, pointing to the high frequency of this in clinics. The inability to start correct treatment may result in sustained illness and increased mortality, requiring a systemic change in the way clinicians' deal with antimicrobial treatment. Institutions are required to adopt stringent protocols that reinforce clinical decision-making procedures and highlight the significance of effective antimicrobial prescribing. Solutions to the problem of suboptimal prescribing practice require multiple strategies involving individual healthcare professionals as well as systematic organizational change. Successful interventions must involve extended training programs distinguishing between appropriate and inappropriate use of antibiotics, and electronic reminders in electronic health records encouraging clinicians to be mindful of possible resistance patterns. Additionally, hospital guidelines must promote teamwork between interdisciplinary teams to review antibiotic prescriptions on a regular basis to ensure that they are up to date with current clinical guidelines. By focusing on these strategies first, healthcare facilities can effectively tackle the emergence of AMR, thus protecting patient health and ensuring successful therapeutic results. The plight of AMR will keep mounting unless bold measures are taken to reform prescribing practices currently based on systemic shortcomings.

12.3.3. Agricultural Use of Antibiotics

In modern farming, routine administration of antibiotics in animals has become a key player in the alarming problem of AMR. Although antibiotics have played a pivotal role in improving animal health and productivity, their application as growth promoters, especially in pig farming, has drawn attention. Research has shown that the withdrawal of antibiotics for growth promotion could result in a huge reduction in producer profits, raising the economic cost of bans. The perceived advantages, though, have to be set against the threat to public health from rising antibiotic resistance. The pressure for selection created by subtherapeutic antibiotic use can promote the emergence and dissemination of resistant bacterial strains, which represents a grave danger to both human and animal health. The economic basis for the use of antibiotics in agriculture—i.e., for growth promotion—represents a multifaceted interaction between public health responsibility and agricultural productivity. Producers have observed that antibiotics have the potential to contribute to increased feed efficiency and total productivity, with a corresponding effect on profits. On the other hand, the long-term impact of this practice highlights the need for alternative methods that do not compromise antibiotic effectiveness. The reasons in support of agricultural antibiotics tend to discount the risks to public health involved, such as potential resistant organisms contaminating food supplies and the human population. Regulatory frameworks must evolve to balance these competing interests, ensuring that agricultural practices do not inadvertently contribute to the broader AMR crisis (Hollis et al., 2014). A multifaceted approach is essential for addressing the agricultural use of antibiotics and its implications for AMR. Efforts to reduce the overuse of such compounds may be complemented by education campaigns to educate producers on sustainable methods of producing more productively while not depending on antibiotics. The strategies can involve better animal husbandry, vaccination practices, and new farm technologies emphasizing animal welfare and health. Additionally, imposing user charges on non-essential antibiotic uses, as proposed in some current research, may discourage low-value uses while raising revenues for new antibiotic development. This would not only increase the sustainability of farming practices but also balance them with international health priorities, ultimately leading to a healthier food supply and better public health outcomes (Hollis et al., 2014).

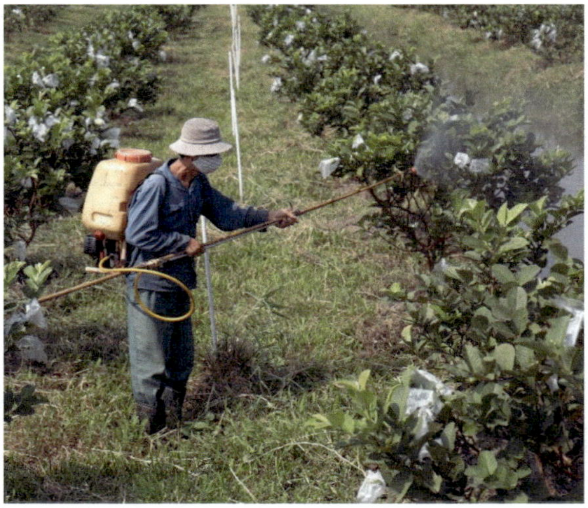

Source: CABI. (n.d.). *Spraying Antibiotics in Agriculture.*

12.4. Impact of Antimicrobial Resistance (AMR) on Public Health

The emergence of AMR presents huge challenges to public health systems across the world. When pathogens adapt and create mechanisms of resistance, the effectiveness of conventional treatments is lost, and the duration of illness is extended, medical expenses rise, and the healthcare resource burden is increased. Salger's in-depth research explains the need to comprehend the drivers of AMR, including the excessive use and misuse of antimicrobials among the susceptible population. Patient demand tends to place additional pressure on medical professionals to prescribe antibiotics, even in the case of viral infections where they are useless (Kostkova et al., 2004). This not only encourages resistance but also highlights the importance of public education and awareness campaigns to change perceptions about antibiotic use. Finally, AMR risks rolling back decades of medical advancement in treating infectious diseases, illustrating the critical nature of this crisis as it must be met through education and prudent prescribing. Not less troubling is the effect of AMR on the most vulnerable populations, including the elderly and immunocompromised patients. These individuals are at greater risk for infections that will become increasingly tougher to treat because of resistant bacteria. The trend toward an aging population, which is increased by chronic diseases, worsens this problem, leading to increased nosocomial infections within hospitals and long-term care facilities. The application of antimicrobials in agriculture for promoting growth has also added to the problem, such that resistant bacteria have entered the food chain and have consequently impacted human health (Tassew et al., 2016). Human health, food production, and public health interplay can no longer be ignored, and therefore an interdisciplinary strategy to fight AMR must be adopted. Enhancing infection control practices and ensuring the judicious use of antibiotics in all sectors are essential steps required to limit these threats. The public health dimension of AMR needs to be addressed with concerted actions to establish long-lasting solutions. Heightened surveillance of resistant infections, enhanced diagnostics, and the introduction of new antimicrobial agents must come together to win back control over infectious diseases. In addition, public health measures designed to encourage the prudent use of antibiotics can also play a major role in reducing resistance. There is evidence that education can change public perceptions of antibiotic expectations (Kostkova et al., 2004); such programs are needed to create a culture of responsibility for antibiotic prescribing. Finally, the fight against AMR will depend on an integrated strategy that both involves individual behavior and institutional modifications in healthcare, agriculture, and community culture. Through concerted efforts on all fronts, it becomes possible to mitigate the burden of AMR and maintain the effectiveness of these lifesaving drugs for generations to come.

12.4.1. Increased Morbidity and Mortality

The relationship between AMR and rising morbidity and mortality is intricate and alarming. When ordinary pathogens develop resistance to routine treatment, the outcomes for patients can be catastrophic. Not only does this make infection management more difficult, but it also increases hospital stays, healthcare costs, and severe complications. For example, surgical site infections (SSI) represent a particular concern here since they can occur where infection rates are increased by resistant organisms.

These microorganisms, most notably *Staphylococcus aureus* and *S. epidermidis*, have the potential to cause fatal diseases, most notably in the patient who has an implanted device, where a small infection can become dramatically severe (Chetter et al., 2015). Additionally, the economic cost of AMR must not be overlooked, as it significantly elevates the economic cost of dealing with resistant infections. The extra expenses due to longer hospital stays, greater intensive care needs, and requirements for more costly alternatives are among the factors contributing to this trend. It is estimated that AMR may cause thousands of deaths each year and have a huge impact on individual and public health systems. Malta, where resistance rates are the highest in Europe, has an urgent need to counteract this crisis (Borg et al., 2009).

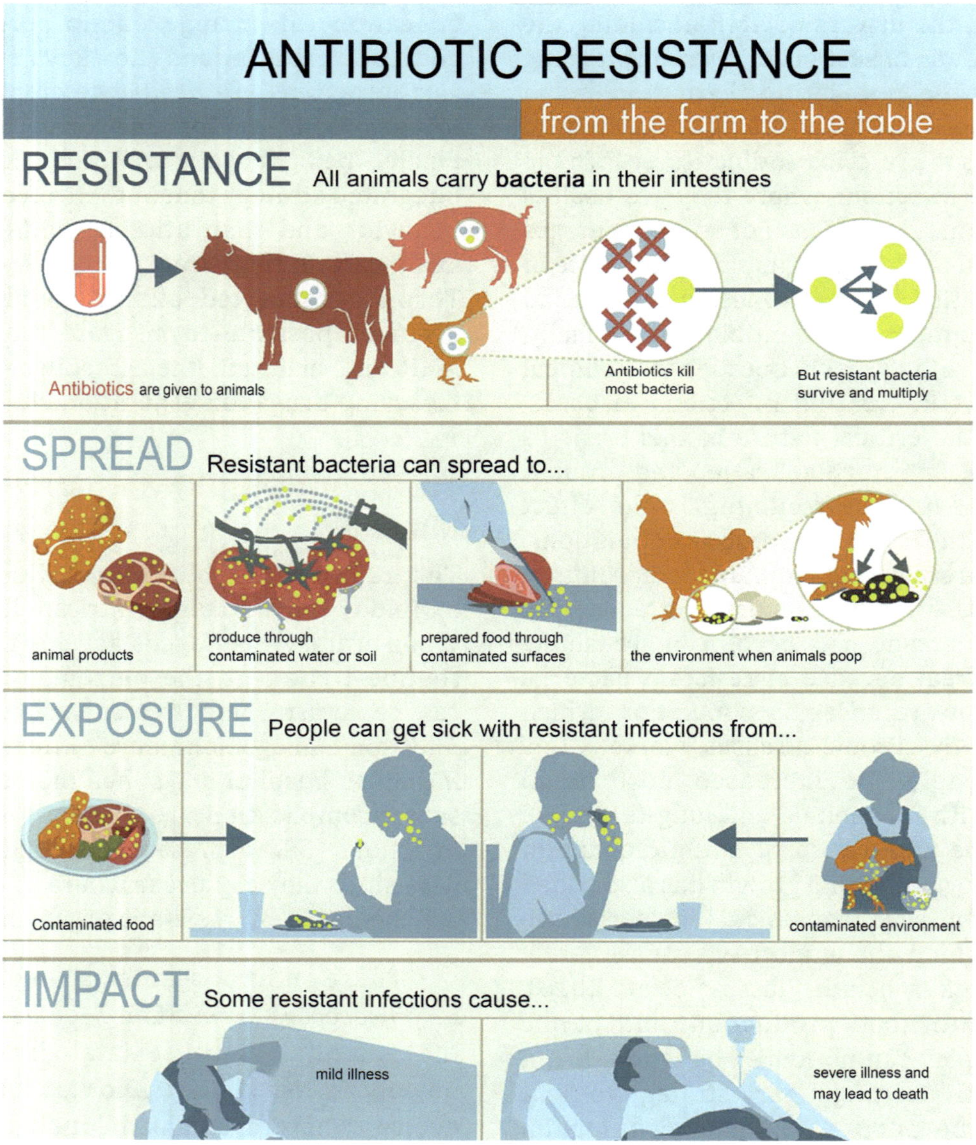

Figure 12.10. Increased morbidity and mortality.

Source: By CDC - https://www.cdc.gov/foodsafety/from-farm-to-table.html, Public Domain, https://commons.wikimedia.org/w/index.php?curid=41858460

The consequences of increasing morbidity and mortality highlight the urgency for active measures to control AMR by way of effective stewardship interventions and public health measures.

Efforts to address the increasing menace of AMR need to be multifaceted in nature with two-pronged goals of preventing infections as well as rational use of antimicrobials. This involves not just optimizing prescribing behavior but also operating effective infection control and strengthening patient education on how to properly use antibiotics. Having healthcare professionals who are careful in their prescribing helps decrease the threat of resistant infection, and therefore potentially reduce related morbidity and mortality. In addition, joint efforts between healthcare systems and farming industries can result in a major reduction in unjustified antibiotic use. It is only using a global strategy that the blighting trends in rising morbidity and mortality associated with AMR can be controlled effectively, thus protecting public health for generations to come (Figure 12.10).

12.4.2. Economic Burden on Healthcare Systems

The economic impact of AMR to healthcare systems is significant and far-reaching. With the rise in infections caused by antibiotic-resistant bacteria, the costs linked to longer hospital stays, intensified care, and higher technologies rise appreciably. The European Union and European Economic Area accounted for an estimated 671,689 infections caused by antibiotic-resistant pathogens in a single year alone, resulting in a staggering 33,110 attributable deaths and significant disability-adjusted life-years (DALYs) lost (Aarestrup et al., 2015). All of these numbers reflect not only the immediate health costs of care but also the economic burden on productivity and health resource expenditure in the long term. Policymakers must prioritize AMR concerns, as the rising financial strain threatens to overwhelm healthcare infrastructures, particularly in low and middle-income regions where resources are already stretched. Managing infections stemming from AMR necessitates intricate coordination across various healthcare sectors, creating additional financial challenges. Implementation of effective policies, such as responsible antimicrobial use, robust surveillance systems, and enhanced infection prevention protocols—is critical yet often expensive (Aarestrup et al., 2015). The absence of coherent strategies can lead to the ineffective delivery of resources, which heightens financial pressures on healthcare systems. Additionally, poor intervention enhances the economic loss of extensive infection transmission, which adds to complexity in outcome measures. By taking a One Health strategy that integrates human, animal, and environmental perspectives, public health agencies can formulate strategic interventions that reduce costs while improving health outcomes in communities. The economic importance of tackling the economic burden of AMR reaches beyond the immediate healthcare expenditure, influencing larger economic stability and health equity. The growth in infections caused by antibiotic resistance is disproportionally affecting susceptible populations, such as the elderly and infants, who tend to suffer from increased mortality rates and complex health issues (Sin et al., 2018). This population change calls attention to the necessity for adequately funded interventions that guarantee equal access to therapies and preventive interventions through socio-economic strata. Inaction in resolving the economic impacts of AMR may continue to fuel poverty cycles and medical ineffectiveness, affecting disproportionately those who least can afford it and subjecting already strained health systems and economies to further burdens.

12.4.3. Challenges in Treatment Options

The increasingly problematic case of AMR poses a significant challenge in the field of medical therapy. Through overprescription and abuse of current antibiotics, traditional therapies have become increasingly powerless against resistant bacteria strains. As noted in a WIPO Global Challenges Report, there exists an inadequate inventory of new diagnostics and medicines to combat the increase of multidrug resistance (MDR) (Bhagwandin et al., 2017). This is further compounded by an unawareness and failure to exercise proper antibiotic stewardship among patients and healthcare professionals. Additionally, the imbalance of investment in research and development for new antimicrobial agents creates a large gap between the clinical demands and the existing treatments. It is thus essential to develop a strong strategy that fills these gaps to ensure protection of existing medical practice and public health. To best fight AMR, it is important to realize the complex character of the factors underlying the problem.

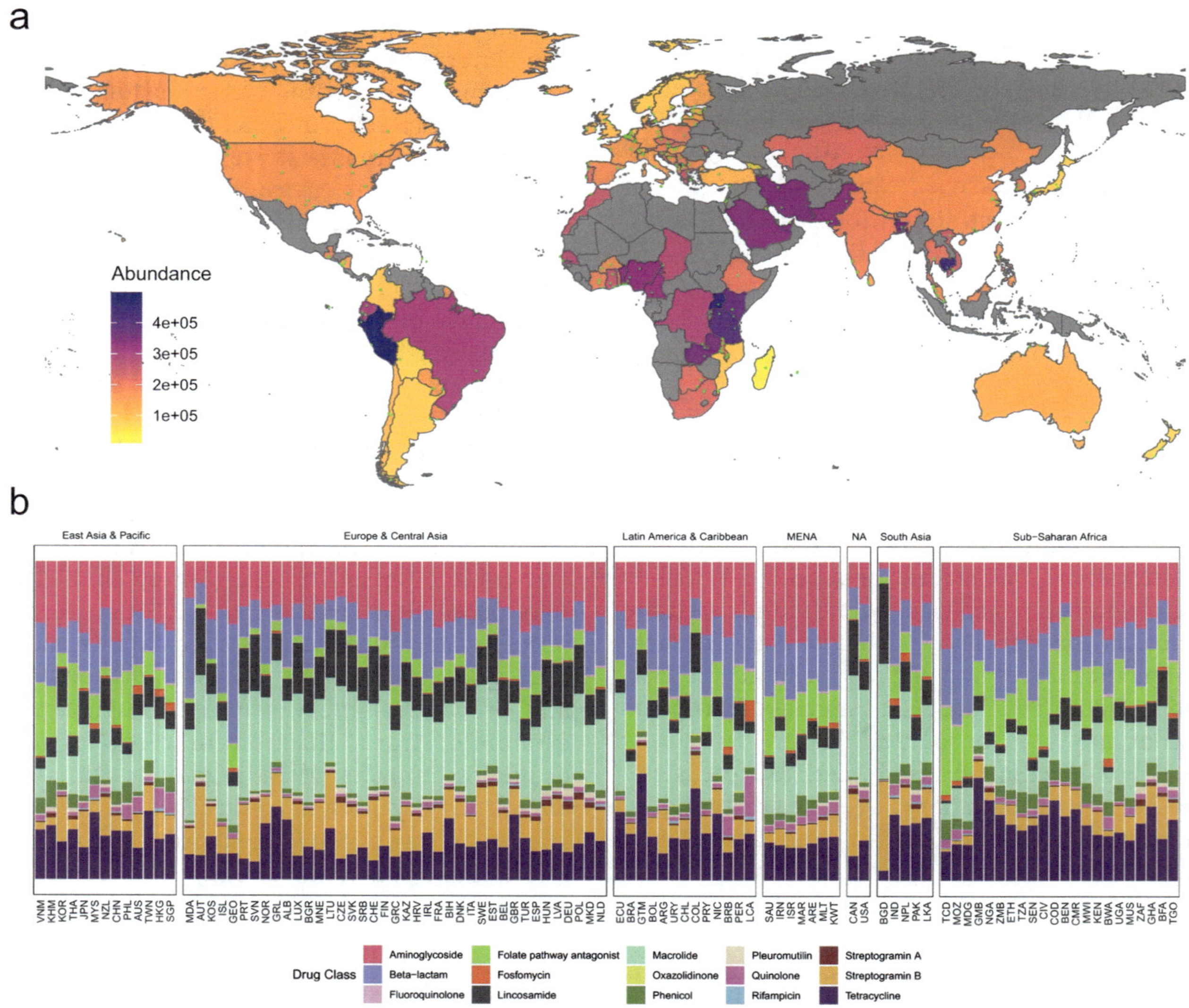

Source: By Authors of the study: Patrick Munk, Christian Brinch, Frederik Duus Møller, Thomas N. Petersen, Rene S. Hendriksen, Anne Mette Seyfarth, Jette S. Kjeldgaard, Christina Aaby Svendsen, Bram van Bunnik, Fanny Berglund, Global Sewage Surveillance Consortium, D. G. Joakim Larsson, Marion Koopmans, Mark Woolhouse & Frank M. Aarestrup - https://www.nature.com/articles/s41467-022-34312-7, CC BY 4.0, https://commons.wikimedia.org/w/index.php?curid=128336975

The growth in AMR can be explained by the presence of multiple factors, such as poor prescribing behavior and the extensive use of antibiotics on the agricultural sector (Aarestrup et al., 2015). This calls for a united and integrated policy framework that goes beyond single sectors. Taking a One Health perspective—where human, animal, and environmental health are interconnected—can stimulate the formulation of sensitive policies that are suited to the unique requirements and challenges of each sector. By constantly evaluating the efficacy and cost-effectiveness of these policies, stakeholders can guarantee that interventions are evidence-based and responsive to differing conditions in different regions and income levels. Ultimately, the solution to the challenges in treatment lies in a concerted global approach to promoting innovation in antimicrobial research and development. The stakeholders need to address the specific market issues of developing new treatments and diagnostics, as existing methods are found wanting (Bhagwandin et al., 2017). This involves looking at new incentives for the pharmaceutical industry and researchers, possibly using intellectual property rights constructively to promote development. In addition, it is imperative to ensure that effective innovations are accessible and implementable in all parts of the world, especially low- and middle-income countries (LMICs), where the burden of resistant infections tends to be most significant. A well-designed global framework that promotes both research initiatives and effective local application is critical to mitigating the effect of AMR and ensuring public health in the future.

12.5. Global Response to Antimicrobial Resistance (AMR)

Fighting AMR demands a coordinated international response involving intergovernmental, HCP, and public cooperation. Misuse and misuse of antimicrobial medications have exacerbated the AMR situation, especially in nations such as Mexico, where poor hygiene and lack of awareness are additional contributing factors (Acevedo et al., 2024). Campaigns of education are a necessary component of tackling AMR that must enlighten HCPs and the public about using antimicrobials responsibly. Through promoting a culture of awareness and prudent prescribing, the stakeholders can adequately curtail the development rate of resistance. Improved surveillance is critical in monitoring trends and insight into the process of resistance, which can facilitate timely and effective interventions to new threats. This collective effort will form the foundation for an enhanced global response to the AMR threat. Integrating a One Health approach is crucial to successfully addressing AMR in human, animal, and environmental health fields. These fields being interconnected in nature imply that resistance does not observe borders, which necessitates coordinated strategies to achieve effectiveness (Aarestrup et al., 2015). It calls for policies to ensure prudent use of antibiotics in human medicine and veterinary sectors, as well as strict controls on antibiotic use in agriculture Different countries with different levels of income experience unique challenges; therefore, personalized policy strategies are essential. Consistent evaluation of how these policies perform will guarantee that they address the individualized needs of all parts of the country and all groups of people. By focusing on infection prevention and control, the risk of resistance development can be reduced to assist overall public health and security. Last but not least, a strong international platform for research and development of novel antimicrobial drugs is critical in our efforts against AMR. Innovation has been hampered in recent years by economic constraints and regulatory barriers, which have left us with a declining pool of effective medicines. Investing in research that investigates new therapeutic alternatives—like bacteriophages, novel antibiotics, and immunotherapies—is crucial to reverse resistance (Acevedo et al., 2024). Improved collaborative networks between pharmaceutical firms, academia, and government can strengthen the development and delivery of new antimicrobials. Leverage of real-time information from international surveillance systems will enable swift action against new resistance patterns. Through a culture of collaboration and investment in research and development, the international community can reflate the war on AMR, ultimately safeguarding public health for generations to come.

12.5.1. World Health Organization (WHO) Initiatives

The complex nature of challenges presented by AMR has necessitated the WHO to undertake many initiatives to combat this increasing menace. Among them, the Global Antimicrobial Resistance Surveillance System (GLASS) was adopted to enable standardized collection and analysis of data on antimicrobial susceptibility. In addition to aiming to gain better insight into resistance patterns in different parts of the world, it underscores the important need for evidence-based intervention approaches. Research has established that patient demand for antibiotics is a key driver of their inappropriate use, highlighting the value of efforts targeted toward education and behavior modification in patients as well as healthcare professionals (Maher et al., 2024). Through the establishment of a centralized database, the WHO hopes to not only monitor AMR trends but also inform policymakers in designing effective responses specific to their local settings. Alongside GLASS, the WHO has prioritized solving the problem of patient expectations that unnecessarily prompt the use of inappropriate antibiotics, especially in primary healthcare. The importance of having strong behavior change interventions is important since there is evidence that antibiotic overestimation significantly leads to AMR (Maher et al., 2024). Public education campaigns addressing what antibiotics are needed and when they are warranted can alter community attitudes. The inclusion of training programs for both HCPs and patients provides a platform to encourage responsible antibiotic use, hence resulting in lower rates of resistance. Through the active involvement of communities in debate regarding antibiotics and their limitations, the WHO hopes to establish a better-informed public that is aware of the dangers of misuse and thus advancing the global front against AMR. In addition, WHOs commitment to addressing AMR also includes helping LMICs that carry the majority of the resistance burden and are frequently plagued by weak healthcare systems. The roll-out of GLASS guidelines for antimicrobial susceptibility testing (AST) is specifically important in these settings, as it brings order to best practices and enhances data collection. This initiative not only shapes local health policies but also ensures global efforts to monitor and control AMR are more effective. Through noting areas of improvement and highlighting the role of local context in AMR surveillance, the WHO seeks to develop actionable strategies that suit the specific needs of individual countries. These efforts highlight the WHOs role as a key player in coordinating international initiatives, thus enhancing collective actions against the pervasive threat of AMR (Figure 12.11).

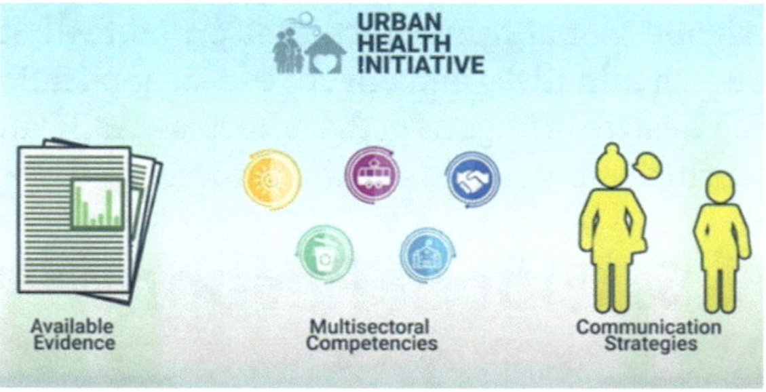

Figure 12.11. World Health Organization (WHO) initiatives.

Source: World Health Organization. (n.d.). *Urban Health Initiative: Available Evidence, Multisectoral Competencies, Communication Strategies.*

12.5.2. National Action Plans (NAPs)

In view of the increasing threat posed by AMR, numerous nations have established NAPs with the purpose of building capacity in their healthcare systems and reducing the risk of resistant infections. These strategic plans are crucial for creating a common approach to AMR, involving stakeholders at various levels, and encouraging the proper use of antimicrobials. A holistic NAP would thus include not just healthcare but also veterinary medicine and agricultural interventions, acknowledging human-animal health interdependencies. For example, the use of systematic situation analyses in current studies reflects a paramount necessity for such measures, particularly since the majority of reports stress political and legislative backing as critical to AMR fighting (Ahmad et al., 2019). Still, the discussion also identifies gaps, including the absence of industry and technology assessments, which lay out areas where NAPs can be improved to approach this pressing public health concern holistically. Stakeholder coordination is a foundation of effective NAPs, through which duties are distributed and efforts consolidated. The engagement of various groups, such as HCPs, researchers, and policymakers, promotes innovation and boosts resource mobilization. Effective NAPs have been able to build on the knowledge of various stakeholders to address the intricacies of AMR, a point that is supported by international activities like the International Dog Health Workshops (Bartels et al., 2017). During such sessions, members from diverse backgrounds come together and discuss particular needs and steps aimed at enhancing health outcomes, highlighting the importance of multilateral collaboration.

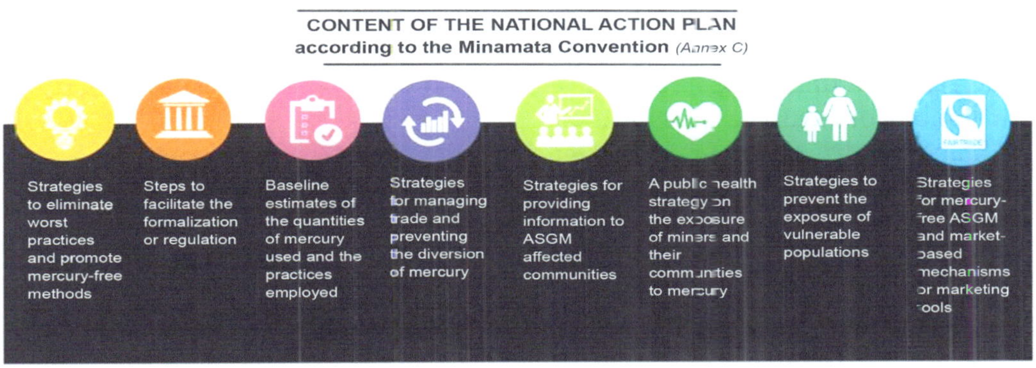

Figure 12.12. National action plans (NAPs).

Source: United Nations Environment Program. (n.d.). *National Action Plans (NAPs)*.

Through discussion and collaboration, NAPs can create a strong platform addressing not just the medical and scientific facets of AMR but also the social impact, opening the doors to holistic solutions. Monitoring and evaluation of NAP outcomes are essential for the effectiveness and responsiveness to evolving situations. Constant scrutiny enables policymakers to recognize challenges, monitor progress, and institute required adjustments. Effective implementation necessitates the development of measurable indicators and open reporting tools that stakeholders can apply for evaluating the effect of their interventions. The experience of previous initiatives indicates that in the absence of continuous assessment, NAPs are unlikely to meet their purpose or even neglect significant aspects of AMR control. Through the incorporation of systematic evaluative tools within

NAPs, nations can be responsive to new threats as they emerge while providing a culture of innovation and adaptability in addressing AMR (Ahmad et al., 2019). Finally, rigorous evaluation practices strengthen accountability and promote long-term action to address AMR effectively (Figure 12.12).

12.5.3. Role of Healthcare Professionals (HCP)

HCPs are at the forefront of the fight against AMR, having a crucial influence on prescribing behavior and patient education. As the first point of contact, HCPs have a responsibility to ensure that antibiotics are used wisely with the potential for resistance reduced to a bare minimum. There is a need for effective AMS strategies, with these influencing HCPs in the selection of therapies and dosages while acknowledging the imperative for prevention strategies. This is following research that has shown that combining AMS programs among health sectors can result in decreased antimicrobial prescribing and fewer instances of healthcare-associated infections (Ahmad et al., 2019). By following these recommendations, professionals can assist in reducing unnecessary drug exposure, leading to preventing the development of resistant strains. Within the surgical process, the HCPs' role becomes more than that of prescribing to cover an entire continuum of preoperative, intraoperative, and postoperative management. Inadequate antibiotic prophylaxis might yield adverse effects such as SSIs, which highlight the significance of accurate and proper administration of antibiotics (Ahmad et al., 2017). It is being increasingly acknowledged that healthcare professionals must not only direct their attention toward short-term clinical results but must also look toward the long-term consequences of the antibiotics they are choosing. Observations indicate that maximizing antibiotic therapy along the surgical continuum can notably reduce the incidence of SSIs, clearly reflecting a relationship between prescribed procedures and rates of resistance. Therefore, HCPs need to continually learn and assess to broaden their insight into the intricacies of antibiotic utilization. In addition, coordination between HCPs is essential in rolling out effective AMS programs and combating the multi-faceted problem of AMR. A multi-sectoral strategy involving physicians, pharmacists, nurses, and public health professionals has the potential to bring about a stronger response to the problem of rising resistance. Ongoing research into AMS programs integrated into healthcare settings emphasizes the beneficial consequences resulting from collaboration and communication among various settings of healthcare (Ahmad et al., 2019). In developing a culture of joint responsibility and accountability, professionals can design systems that place infection prevention and optimal antibiotic use at the forefront. Finally, a concerted reaction among health sectors will not only fight AMR but also enhance patient outcomes and protect the effectiveness of present antimicrobials for generations to come.

12.6. Strategies for Combating Antimicrobial Resistance (AMR)

Fighting AMR calls for a cross-cutting strategy that incorporates scientific discovery, good governance, and public mobilization. An important strategy is the improvement in the development of new diagnostics, vaccines, and therapies that can effectively tackle resistant infections. Public-private collaborations, as enumerated in Bhagwandin et al. (2017), are important in this endeavor, as partnerships bring the identification of priority research areas and the ability to steer funding to potential technologies. In addition, it is crucial to implement these innovations within the local healthcare infrastructure to make them accessible and operational. This response not only manages the current health requirements but also establishes a viable system to inhibit the development of additional resistance. Awareness and education play a crucial role in combatting AMR, highlighting the complexity of the problems and the necessity for action.

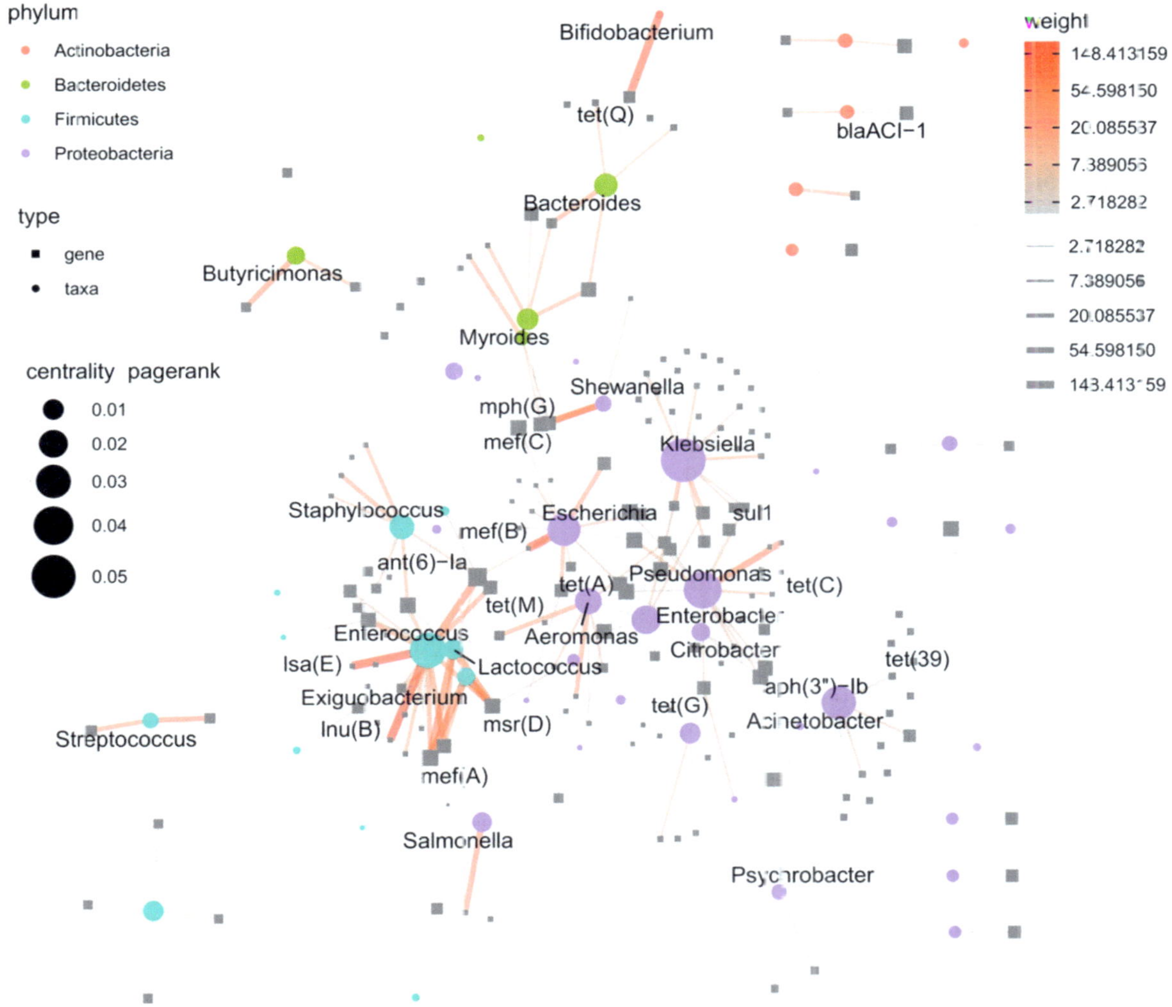

Figure 12.13. Strategies for combating antimicrobial resistance (AMR).

Source: By Authors of the study: Patrick Munk, Christian Brinch Frederik Duus Møller, Thomas N. Petersen, Rene S. Hendriksen, Anne Mette Seyfarth, Jette S. Kjeldgaard, Christina Aaby Svendsen, Bram van Bunnik, Fanny Berglund, Global Sewage Surveillance Consortium, D. G. Joakim Larsson, Marion Koopmans, Mark Woolhouse & Frank M. Aarestrup - https://www.nature.com/articles/s41467-022-34312-7, CC BY 4.0, https://commons.wikimedia.org/w/index.php?curid=128336969

Healthcare professionals, patients, and the public need to be aware of the consequences of antibiotic abuse and the need for appropriate infection control. Measures that support responsible antimicrobial use in both human medicine and agriculture are crucial. For example, as stated by Bristow et al. (2019), existing surveillance schemes for *Neisseria gonorrhoeae* infections demonstrate the significance of global awareness campaigns in monitoring resistance patterns. These initiatives provide health agencies with the data they need to make informed policy, research, and community engagement, thus creating a culture of responsibility around antimicrobial drugs. Finally, successful stewardship and governance are essential for reducing the development of resistance on an international level. This involves applying good governance initiatives that mobilize political will as well as promote global cooperation. As noted by Bhagwandin et al. (2017), there is a need for the creation of an international framework that promotes innovation while ensuring strong local stewardship. An integrated strategy could also include the possible leveraging of intellectual property as a reward system to act as an incentive for the research and development of novel antimicrobial agents. Using these governance frameworks has the potential to greatly improve collective capacity to solve the urgent problems of AMR, providing present and future generations with access to necessary medical treatments (Figure 12.13).

12.6.1. Stewardship Programs

This growing rate of AMR has led healthcare systems globally to adopt formalized systems for optimizing antimicrobial use. In this regard, stewardship programs have become crucial strategies that encourage the judicious use of antimicrobials in different healthcare settings. The focus of these programs lies in informing healthcare providers about proper prescribing, surveillance of antibiotic use, and adherence to treatment guidelines. The Society of Healthcare Epidemiology of America and the Centers for Disease Control and Prevention emphasize the importance of such programs, noting their contribution to the fight against emerging AMR danger with far-reaching repercussions for patient treatment as well as public health (Bucheit et al., 2017). Through the development of cooperation between HCPs, stewardship programs establish a framework that supports the reduction of unnecessary misuse of antibiotics, thus improving outcomes for the patient and lowering the rate of resistant infections. Assessing the impact of stewardship programs is important in determining their influence on AMR. Studies have shown there exists a direct link between the implementation of these programs and patient safety outcomes, with a significant decline seen in the case of multidrug-resistant infections in medical facilities. Literature review conducted between 2008 and 2018 showed that those institutions with these programs in place saw significant reductions in AMR rates, though not without difficulty (Funes et al., 2019). Significantly, all such studies point to the fact that compliance among healthcare providers is a major challenge, as many are concerned with the limitation on their prescribing practices. Thus, increased education and awareness are required to counteract false assumptions regarding stewardship initiatives so that medical practitioners can accept such important initiatives as means to augment their practice while also joining the general fight against AMR. Overall, stewardship programs are a keystone of the strategies to combat the impact of AMR in modern healthcare. Their creation and deployment are not so much reactive measures to the escalating specter of AMR as they are proactive steps toward changing prescribing practices and maximizing patient outcomes. In spite of the challenges in achieving widespread adoption by healthcare professionals, the large body of evidence testifying to the value of these programs attests to their significance in creating a culture of prudent antimicrobial use. Finally, stewardship program success relies on teamwork between HCPs, educational efforts, and persistent commitment to changing practice to focus on patient safety and prevent the development of resistant pathogens (Bucheit et al., 2017; Funes et al., 2019).

12.6.2. Research and Development of New Antimicrobials

The persistent threat of AMR has intensified interest in the research and development of novel antimicrobial agents. This is a priority because the prevalence of resistant infections continues to escalate with high morbidity and mortality rates worldwide. Developing new antimicrobials is a sophisticated process that calls for multidisciplinary approaches and the integration of new technologies and innovative strategies. Studies have largely focused on redirecting currently known compounds, especially ones previously discontinued due to safety concerns, e.g., colistin (Chivu et al., 2019). Such an approach offers a chance to build on current knowledge while avoiding long and expensive processes involved in discovering brand-new drugs. Nevertheless, the demand for truly new classes of antimicrobials is still critical, as the use of older drugs may further aggravate resistance instead of solving it. Attempts at devising synthetic materials with antimicrobial activity are gaining favor as traditional avenues cut back on returns. The use of polymers that possess intrinsic antimicrobial properties may revolutionize therapeutic applications as well as the efficiency of medical devices. Many polymer subgroups based on natural peptides and organometallic blends are being investigated for their ability to fight ESKAPE pathogens—*Enterococcus faecium*, *Staphylococcus aureus*, *Klebsiella pneumoniae*, *Acinetobacter baumannii*, *Pseudomonas aeruginosa*, and Enterobacter spp. (Chivu et al., 2019). Since these pathogens are known to acquire resistance against traditional therapy, knowing how new polymers can block their growth is critical. This innovative research pathway not only addresses immediate clinical needs but also aligns with a longer-term vision for sustainable antibiotic use. Despite the promising advances in research and development, significant gaps remain in our understanding of the economic implications of antimicrobial use in both human and animal health sectors. The decision-making frameworks surrounding antimicrobial applications require comprehensive data collection to evaluate trade-offs more effectively. Existing practices should take into account how antimicrobial usage in animals affects the emergence of resistance, since this directly affects human health. Higher price signals for antimicrobial drugs used in animals need to be true representations of production costs as well as resistance externalities. By developing a strong data-based strategy, stakeholders are then in a better position to deal with the AMR complexities and enhance the results for public health and agriculture approaches, thereby creating an integrated strategy for antimicrobial use and development.

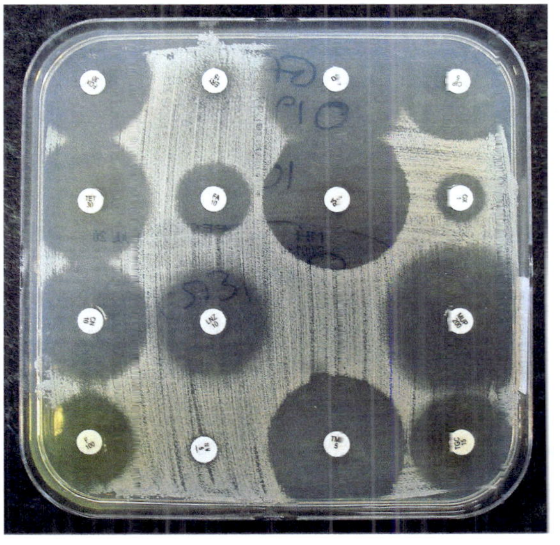

Source: By Dr Graham Beards - Own work, CC BY-SA 4.0, https://commons.wikimedia.org/w/index.php?curid=91284633

12.6.3. Public Awareness Campaigns

Creating awareness on AMR is essential, particularly in a time when effective antibiotics are becoming harder to find. Public awareness campaigns act as the liaison between sophisticated scientific principles and day-to-day practices. They seek to inform the general public on the effects of misusing antibiotics, hence promoting responsible action. By emphasizing the interlinkage between antibiotic misuse in human medicine and agriculture, these campaigns aim to change norms of behavior and develop a culture of vigilance around antimicrobial use. For example, recognizing key drivers of AMR, such as poor prescribing and agricultural antibiotic use, can be well conveyed through multimedia channels to mobilize different populations. This training ultimately plays a central role in encouraging a proactive resp nse to healthcare and environmental conservation, critical to an effective battle against AMR. In combating AMR, public awareness campaigns also look to promote community involvement and cooperation among stakeholders. Using local health organizations, schools, and community groups ensures that the message becomes embedded within the different populations. Tactics can involve workshops, social media campaigns, and educational pamphlets to make content available and engaging. These activities can result in ground-level movements that get community members to campaign for the responsible use of antimicrobials, increasing the campaign's reach even further. Of note, public awareness campaigns are not only directed at common citizens; they are also aimed at healthcare providers to trigger a rethinking of prescription practices. As exhibited in the different contexts covered by the European Commission, collaboration of all stakeholders can lead to more efficient handling of AMR. This interrelatedness points to the significance of awareness campaigns as windows of opportunity through which to share essential information about shaping individual and systemic antimicrobial behaviors (Brand et al., 2023). Finally, the effectiveness of public awareness campaigns depends on how they can translate knowledge into action. As people become knowledgeable about AMR consequences, they are most likely to embrace responsible practices, e.g., finishing prescribed courses of antibiotics and refraining from the pressure to insist on antibiotics for viral diseases. In addition, when education produces more public dialogue regarding AMR, it can provoke policy shifts and encourage additional research. Securing public backing for legislation regulating antibiotic utilization in agriculture, for example, can be driven by successful educational engagement. Combining science communication with community participation creates a context in which the public feels empowered to become responsible for making their own health choices. Facilitating this degree of awareness eventually leads to a joint effort in preventing the AMR crisis, so that future generations can depend on potent antimicrobial treatments (Brand et al., 2023).

CLOSER LOOK

Stewardship

Stewardship in its widest meaning is responsible stewardship and care of something that has been left in one's hands, whether it is a personal resource, a natural resource, or even a company. It is about acknowledging that one has been entrusted with something valuable and exercising duty and generosity in using and taking care of it. Stewardship can be applied in different settings, such as in business, environmental conservation, and even in personal life.

Here is a closer examination of various aspects of stewardship:

1. Stewardship in Business
   - **Stewardship Theory:** This theory asserts that executives are tasked with behaving in the best interests of shareholders and stakeholders, serving as protectors of the organization.
   - **Corporate Stewardship:** This framework focuses on accountable decision-making and value creation based on multiple factors such as performance, protection, people, purpose, and the planet.
   - **Servant Leadership:** This leadership style is concerned with taking responsibility for constituents, the organization, and its behavior, being accountable to oneself and others.
2. Stewardship in Environmental Protection
   - **Natural Resource Management:** Stewardship means utilizing natural resources responsibly, being mindful of ecosystems, and encouraging conservation activities.
   - **Product Stewardship:** This is concerned with reducing the environmental impact of a product over its life cycle, from design to end-of-life disposal, as described on Saint-Gobain Tape Solutions website.
   - **Stewardship Science:** This entails gathering and reporting information to guide management decisions about natural resources.
3. Stewardship in Personal Life
   - Biblical Stewardship: This focuses on being good stewards of all that God has given, including finances, environmental stewardship, and personal life, as detailed by Paybee.
   - Sense of Place: This is an individual's or community's worldview and how this relates to his/her stewardship actions in a specific location, as given by ScienceDirect.com.
   - Responsibility of Stewardship: This involves employing materials which are safe to biodegrade, minimizing waste through recycling and taking into account the environmental impact of infrastructure and inventions.

SUMMARY

The problem of AMR is a paramount public health concern that necessitates keen observation and swift action. The finding from a Scotland national point prevalence survey shows a high rate of healthcare-associated infections as well as a high rate of prescribing antimicrobials, affirming the urgency of this public health problem (Cairns et al., 2018). The persistence of such infections as urinary tract infections and pneumonia despite the antibiotics indicates that specific intervention measures need to be more followed and points out the necessity for increased awareness among medical practitioners. Additionally, the intricacies of biofilm development by pathogens such as *Burkholderia cepacia*, particularly among susceptible populations, show how complex and deep-seated AMR can be (Coenye et al., 2010). This scenario sheds light on the need for holistic strategies that include not just treatment but upstream interventions to tackle the causative factors of infection. Combating AMR requires a multidisciplinary effort, and this involves cooperation across different fields such as healthcare, agriculture, and public health policies. Education and awareness are crucial in addressing AMR; better educational programs for prescribers can lead to more cautious and responsible antimicrobial prescription. The historical background of AMR development indicates that it is not only a modern phenomenon but an accumulation of decades of practices. Hence, having a profound understanding of how resistance develops, such as genetic mutation and HGT, provides greater insight into developing effective measures to prevent and control AMR in clinical practice (Cairns et al., 2018). Ultimately, combat of AMR is not merely a matter of changing the way in which we prescribe antibiotics; it requires a change in paradigm on how we deal with infection control and prevention on a wider level. Incorporating emerging scientific knowledge on the formation of biofilms, as seen in the complexities of *B. cepacia* complex, underscores the need for new research and development in antimicrobial therapy (Coenye et al., 2010). An integrated approach that involves education, judicious use of antibiotics, and effective policy-making will be vital in reducing the emergence and spread of resistant strains and thus safeguarding public health as well as ensuring the efficacy of current antimicrobial agents in the future. Hence, though the challenge is steep, coordinated action at present can make a substantial impact on combatting AMR.

The issue of AMR is a serious concern in healthcare, extending to human and veterinary medicine. It is crucial to realize the interconnection of antimicrobial use in humans and animals, as noted by the WHO, which underscores the significance of AMR as a foremost global health risk (Speksnijder et al., 2017). This complex link necessitates thorough monitoring and controlling of antimicrobials in various sectors. Nation-states are increasingly appreciating the need for methodologies to be harmonized in antimicrobial use reporting, even if efforts toward this are still largely voluntary. Lack of compulsory compliance may derail the success of policies meant to contain AMR. It becomes necessary to campaign for more stringent, enforceable guidelines that can guarantee a systemic approach to monitoring and controlling antibiotic use within healthcare facilities and agricultural production. In addition, incorporating a One Health strategy into surveillance is crucial for managing this complex problem. Existing resistance monitoring systems primarily target food animal species based on fecal samples, with a lack of attention to key elements such as companion animals (Speksnijder et al., 2017). This omission supports the argument that a more comprehensive approach is needed to determine the extent of AMR. To apply effective interventions, there is a need to consider the effects of resistance on human health, animal welfare, and ecosystem stability. Emphasizing the interlinked nature of these spheres may potentially reinforce the arguments for all-encompassing surveillance systems and inter-stakeholder cooperation that is required for effective public health interventions against AMR. Lastly, analyzing the economic consequences of AMR shows how there are enormous long-term expenses from its uncontrolled development. Resistance may cause higher healthcare costs and lost productivity as patients with resistant infections take more time in hospitalization and more elaborate treatments. Furthermore, the agricultural industry has its own economic consequences with lower efficiency in food production and poorer animal health. Supporting One Health surveillance infrastructure, as highlighted in findings of importance, enables us to respond to the different economic effects of AMR in an overall way. Applying sound, concerted policies not only holds potential for health advantage but also achieves economic efficiencies that benefit society at large. Recognizing such considerations makes clear the need for a broad, concerted war against AMR, requiring cooperation among human health, veterinary medicine, and environmental conservation.

KEY TERMS FROM THIS CHAPTER

- Antimicrobial
- Antiviral
- Antiparasitic
- Narrow-spectrum
- Resistance
- Multidrug resistance (MDR)
- Pan-drug-resistant (PDR)
- Plasmid-mediated resistance
- Mutation
- Resistance gene
- Antibiotic
- Antifungal
- Broad-spectrum
- Minimum inhibitory concentration (MIC)
- Antimicrobial resistance (AMR)
- Extensively drug-resistant (XDR)
- Superbug
- Horizontal gene transfer
- Selective pressure
- Efflux pump

REFERENCES

1. Ahmad, R., Birgand, G., Charani, E., Holmes, A., Leather, A., Mendelson, M., Moonesinghe, S. R., Sevdalis, N., Singh, S., & Tarrant, C. (2017). Opportunities for system-level improvement in antibiotic use across the surgical pathway. *International Journal of Infectious Diseases, 60*, 29-34. Elsevier BV. https://core.ac.uk/download/323057621.pdf (accessed on 6 May 2025).
2. Ahmad, R., Ferlie, E., Holmes, A., Leather, A. J. M., & Zhu, N. J. (2019). Strengthening strategic management approaches to address antimicrobial resistance in global human health: A scoping review. *BMJ Global Health, 4*, e001730. https://core.ac.uk/download/323057623.pdf (accessed on 6 May 2025).
3. Ahmad, R., Holmes, A., McLeod, M., Micallef, C., Shebl, N. A., & Sim, F. (2019). A whole-health-economy approach to antimicrobial stewardship: Analysis of current models and future direction. *PLOS Medicine, 16*(3), e1002774. https://core.ac.uk/download/323306206.pdf (accessed on 6 May 2025).
4. Bhagwandin, N., Jenner, A., & Kowalski, S. P. (2017). Antimicrobial resistance (AMR) and multidrug resistance (MDR): Overview of current approaches, consortia, and intellectual property issues. *University of New Hampshire Scholars' Repository*. https://core.ac.uk/download/215505935.pdf (accessed on 6 May 2025).
5. Borg, M. A. (2009). Addressing the challenge of antibiotic resistance in Maltese healthcare settings. *Malta Medical Journal, 21*(2), 7–12. https://core.ac.uk/download/46602217.pdf (accessed on 6 May 2025).
6. Borghi, E., Borgo, F., Morace, G., Nile, C., Rajendran, R., Ramage, G., & Sherry, L. (2015). New strategic insights into managing fungal biofilms. *Frontiers Media SA*. https://core.ac.uk/download/42365456.pdf (accessed on 6 May 2025).
7. Boyen, F., Cobbaut, K., De Zutter, L., Haesebrouck, F., & Houf, K. (2011). Genotyping and antimicrobial resistance patterns of *Escherichia coli* O157 originating from cattle farms. *Mary Ann Liebert Inc, 8*(6), 719–724. https://core.ac.uk/download/55843227.pdf (accessed on 6 May 2025).
8. Brand, H., García, L. P. O., Kaur, K., & Schröder-Bäck, P. (2023). Scenario planning: An alternative approach to European Commission for combating antimicrobial resistance by 2050. *South Eastern European Journal of Public Health*. https://core.ac.uk/download/553169603.pdf (accessed on 6 May 2025).
9. García, L. P. O., Kaur, K., Brand, H., & Schröder-Bäck, P. (2023). Scenario planning: An alternative approach to European Commission for combating antimicrobial resistance by 2050. *South Eastern European Journal of Public Health*. https://doi.org/10.70135/seejph.vi.186Bucheit, J., Collins, R., Lee, K. B., Ramirez, J. A., Sanogo, K., & Stevens, M. P. (2017). Antimicrobial stewardship practices in Virginia. *VCU Scholars Compass*. https://core.ac.uk/download/84402996.pdf (accessed on 6 May 2025).
10. Cairns, S., Gibbons, C., King, H., Llano, M., MacDonald, L., Malcolm, W., Milne, A., Reilly, J., Robertson, C., Sneddon, J., & Weir, J. (2018). Results from the third Scottish National Prevalence Survey: Is a population health approach now needed to prevent healthcare-associated infections? *Journal of Hospital Infection, 99*(3), 312–317. https://doi.org/10.1016/j.jhin.2018.03.038.

11. Chivu, A., Choong, S. S., De Fatima Pina, M., Gibson, A. J., Hamdan, R. H., Kamaruzzaman, N. F., Tan, L. P., & Wong, W. K. (2019). Antimicrobial polymers: The potential replacement of existing antibiotics? *International Journal of Molecular Sciences, 20*(11), 2747. https://doi.org/10.3390/ijms20112747.

12. Coenye, T. (2010). Social interactions in the *Burkholderia cepacia* complex: Biofilm formation and quorum sensing. *Future Microbiology, 5*, 1087–1099. https://core.ac.uk/download/55759389.pdf (accessed on 6 May 2025).

13. Cruz-Loya, M., Lozano-Huntelman, N., Rodríguez-Verdugo, A., Savage, V., & Yeh, P. (2020). Compounding effects of climate warming and antibiotic resistance. *iScience, 23*(4), 101024. https://doi.org/10.1016/j.isci.2020.101024.

14. Eichenfield, L. F., & Nguyen, T. A. (2015). Profile of clindamycin phosphate 1.2%/benzoyl peroxide 3.75% aqueous gel for the treatment of acne vulgaris. *Clinical, Cosmetic and Investigational Dermatology, 8*, 549–554. https://doi.org/10.2147/CCID.S79628.

15. Epstein, S. E., Westropp, J. L., & Wong, C. (2015). Antimicrobial susceptibility patterns in urinary tract infections in dogs (2010–2013). *Journal of Veterinary Internal Medicine, 29*(4), 1045–1052. https://doi.org/10.1111/jvim.13571.

16. Florez, K., & Sullano, C. (2020). Probiotic biotherapy: Discussing its influential role in oral health. *VCU Scholars Compass*. https://core.ac.uk/download/322936745.pdf (accessed on 6 May 2025).

17. Funes, V. (2019). Implementation of stewardship programs in hospitals: Systematic review. *eScholarship, University of California*. https://core.ac.uk/download/484272122.pdf (accessed on 6 May 2025).

18. Häsler, B., Queenan, K., & Rushton, J. (2016). A One Health approach to antimicrobial resistance surveillance: Is there a business case for it? *International Journal of Antimicrobial Agents, 48*(4), 422–427. https://doi.org/10.1016/j.ijantimicag.2016.06.001.

19. Kamat, N. M., & Velho-Pereira, S. (2010). Exploring hidden dimensions of soil fungal biodiversity: A simple technique to detect soil fungi resistant to antifungal compounds. https://core.ac.uk/download/pdf/289013.pdf (accessed on 6 May 2025).

20. Kostkova, P., Madle, G., Mani-Saada, J., Weinberg, J., & Williams, P. (2004). Changing public attitudes to antibiotic prescribing: Can the internet help? https://core.ac.uk/download/323199986.pdf (accessed on 6 May 2025).

21. Kreft, J. U., Nambi, I. M., Rathinavelu, S., Sonkar, V., Thatikonda, S., & Uluseker, C. (2024). Mapping the scarcity of data on antibiotics in natural and engineered water environments across India. https://core.ac.uk/download/603468660.pdf Rathinavelu, S., Uluseker, C., Sonkar, V., Thatikonda, S., Nambi, I. M., & Kreft, J. U. (2024). Mapping the scarcity of data on antibiotics in natural and engineered water environments across India. *Frontiers in antibiotics, 3*, 1337261. https://doi.org/10.3389/frabi.2024.1337261 (accessed on 6 May 2025).

22. Mohammed, M., & Thapa, S. (2020). Evaluation of WGS-subtyping methods for epidemiological surveillance of foodborne salmonellosis. *One health outlook, 2*, 13. https://doi.org/10.1186/s42522-020-00016-5Mustafa, B. E., Rehman, S. U., Ashraf M., Ashraf, M. A., & Bashir, M. K. (2019). Emergence of antimicrobial resistance, causes, molecular mechanisms, and prevention strategies: A bovine perspective. *IntechOpen*. https://core.ac.uk/download/322438439.pdf (accessed on 6 May 2025).

23. Sahgal, S., & Srivastava, D. (2024). Antimicrobial resistance and innovation in the development of antimicrobial reagents. *Semantic Scholar*. https://www.semanticscholar.org/paper/17d28f47ab918cb904223a352a4a6673fbc26d72 (accessed on 6 May 2025).
24. Tassew, A. (2016). An overview on the rise of antimicrobial resistance and its potential threat in the control of diseases in developing countries. *The International Institute for Science, Technology and Education (IISTE)*. https://core.ac.uk/download/234687431.pdf (accessed on 6 May 2025).

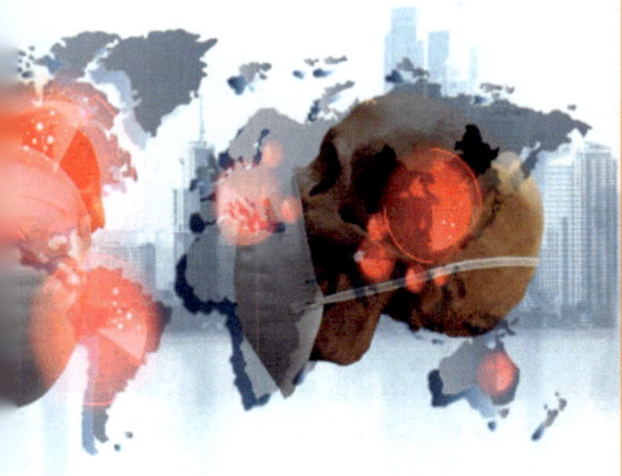

Chapter 13

GLOBAL HEALTH AND EMERGING INFECTIOUS DISEASES

Contents

Introduction

Our interconnected world has brought tremendous public health advances—but it has also made it simpler for new microbes to make the leap across borders. New diseases emerge suddenly, leaving us to grapple with problems that do not recognize national boundaries. The World Health Organization (WHO) continues to say that keeping an eye on things and developing smart solutions is the way forward, particularly when you note that antibiotic resistance—a continually increasing issue—has become a real headache. For the most part, this resistance accounted for approximately 4.95 million deaths by 2019, an incredible indicator of just how much it is disrupting our progress (Murray et al., 2022). Understanding how these diseases function is not only a matter of safeguarding our well-being—it is also important in the pursuit of sustainable development goals. When COVID-19 arrived, it was not only our physical health that suffered; our mental wellbeing suffered also. The pandemic exacerbated old mental issues even further—problems already a heavy burden on the global health burden. Other research even estimates that approximately 53.2 million additional cases of major depressive disorder arose globally in 2020, thanks solely to stress and the uncertainty of the times (Santomauro et al., 2021). This connection of mind to body issues indicates to us, in no uncertain terms, that mental health has a rightful place in any sound global health plan. With physical and mental challenges appearing at the same time, it stands to reason that our response to health emergencies has to be as comprehensive as we can make it. And on top of that, intelligent policy must address both sides if we are going to create communities capable of recovering from whatever is on the horizon. Examining these new diseases shows a complex blend of problems, with socioeconomic factors, such as income and access to care—having a gigantic impact. In many cases, poorer, underserved populations wind up receiving the worst blows, which merely exacerbates existing disparities. Greater access to healthcare, vaccination campaigns, and improved education are all essential if we are to prevent new infections from getting out of hand. The WHO has always emphasized that equitable access to care is an absolute necessity for any sustainable strategy for world health. And as the climates change and the cities grow, new and unpredictable patterns for spreading disease keep arising. These evolving circumstances require us continually to study, keep our information current, and adapt our tactics to the particular demands of each location. Ultimately, a forward-looking strategy which merges understanding from all kinds of specialists is truly critical to establish an enduring health system tomorrow.

Definition of Global Health

Health determinants globally blend together in ways that obscure national borders—health soon becomes a community problem, not an issue of personal circumstances. Global health encompasses far more than merely not being ill; it is also about biology, our daily environment, and even socio-political idiosyncracies that all affect how well individuals get along. More often than not, this concept extends beyond the lack of illness, suggesting fairness in the care of health for all. New contagious diseases that unexpectedly spread from border to border merely increase the requirement for good, unified systems. Research such as the Global Burden of Diseases indicates non-fatal illness on the rise, demonstrating different populations struggle with different issues. Overall, all of these put into perspective the fact that it is the responsibility of countries to tackle inequalities and improve general well-being (James et al., 2018). Looking at how health systems need to change, particularly in LMICs (low-income and middle-income countries), there is genuine pressure for a radical overhaul. In general terms, such countries require a strategic plan that not only addresses the healthcare needs of today but also prepares for surprises such as unexpected disease outbreaks. Individuals expect quality and accessible care anywhere, an objective that can be monitored by establishing clear indicators of what constitutes a robust health system. The unequal distribution of disease in these areas—magnified by a shortage of resources—truly illustrates where there are gaps in care, and why it's so critical to invest in improved systems, especially for vulnerable populations (Kruk et al., 2018). If you move over to the ethics side, global health is inextricably linked with social justice and human rights. Sustained health inequalities across different populations require interventions that make all communities benefit from enhanced policies. As infectious diseases keep appearing and persisting, public health action must be equitable, prioritizing extra attention for those most affected. Sharing information and coordination at the global level can take us a long way in constructing resilience to new threats. In the end, international health is not simply a technical or scientific problem—it also has a moral dimension, challenging us to collaborate ethically while promoting health equity in the global arena (Kruk et al., 2018) (Figure 13.1).

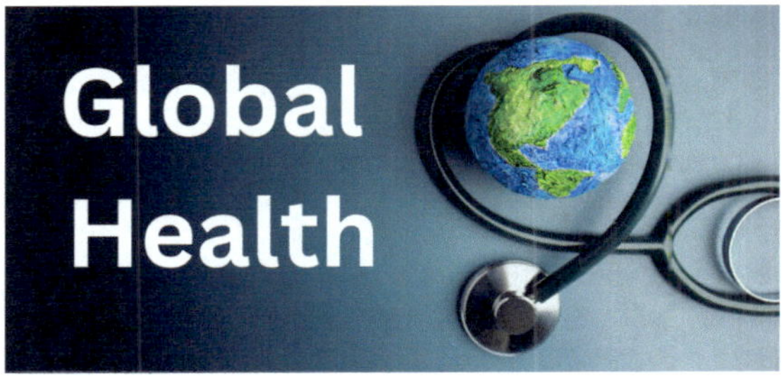

Figure 13.1. The global health.

Source: Arya, N. (2024). Global health 3. *Neil Arya.*

Overview of Emerging Infectious Diseases

Ecological, social, and biological pressures continue to shift, remodeling the world of infections in ways we never quite anticipate. As humans move into places that used to seem so wild and untouched, the possibility of contracting disease from animals begins to rise—diseases that, in a very straightforward way, travel from animals to humans. SACIDS, the Southern African Centre for Infectious Disease Surveillance, leaps in here with a One Health strategy that attempts to weave together animal, human, and natural health.

Reviews tend to indicate there is potential in these initiatives but issues in sharing resources and country cooperation continue to exist, revealing just how complicated the battle against emerging diseases can be (Anderson et al., 2018). As more new infectious diseases emerge, the practice of keeping things the same just isn't going to cut it anymore. In Southeast Asia, individuals have been experimenting with what they refer to as Ecohealth—a concept that bridges the gap between our day-to-day living environments and the biological one—to gain a better understanding of how urbanization and agricultural practices factor into disease risk. When One Health strategies are combined with Ecohealth concepts, researchers begin to notice patterns and linkages that would otherwise be invisible. Certainly, this integration requires an expansive, holistic perspective on health, but it also reveals persistent challenges in creating well-designed projects and in coordinating various institutions. It appears to shift ahead not merely to overcome ingrained research behaviors but to recast training and policy in ways that truly meet the local terrain (Doria et al., 2015). To face these tough, new diseases implies that we need to hybridize solutions—anything from following trends in diseases to taking the natural world into account, through socio-economic profiling. Globalization accelerates travel and commerce in a manner that makes infections have more paths to follow, so vigilance becomes nearly imperative. What may begin as a local problem of health can—if not checked—fast turn into a world crisis. It is for this reason that all attempts at bridging worlds between countries and generating a common understanding of the dangers inherent are so crucial. By combining approaches such as those of SACIDS with Southeast Asia's hands-on Ecohealth, global society can hopefully enhance its capacity for tackling these dynamic threats and ensuring public health on a large scale (Doria et al., 2015; Anderson et al., 2018).

Importance of Studying the Intersection of Global Health and Infectious Diseases

Health sectors blend in ways not expected when dealing with infectious diseases. Trade and travel continue to expand due to globalization, so disease does not remain tied to one nation but leap across borders nearly by default. The One Health Initiative demonstrates this by combining human, animal, and environmental specialists in a very pragmatic manner. Considering zoonotic disease from this combined perspective usually tells us something about how infections get transmitted and what they can do. Most of the time, this broad approach aids in developing strategies that reduce risk – since human, animal, and environmental health are married together in ways that truly require a collaborative effort (Pearsall et al., 2019).

History has taught us that we have been pushed to learn about infectious diseases in a global health context for a long time. With incidents such as the 2009 H1N1 pandemic, governments all over the world began to stock up on medicines as a kind of contingency measure. In general, the allure of medicines such as Tamiflu is not only in defeating one type of virus but also in preventing society from collapsing in the tough times. There has been considerable controversy—at times heated—about whether these stockpiles are worth it and in what way they fit into a broader public health strategy. Understanding that political and economic forces drive health policies, in most instances, enables us to view how to adjust our responses in the best way (Roemer-Mahler et al., 2014).

Pumping health and infectious disease research into the same room stimulates the development of more just health systems, ones that are able to respond when emergencies strike. Researchers and policymakers, through learning about these intersections, can identify soft spots in existing configurations, and then collaborate on improved readiness and response strategies. Research that takes the social aspect of health into account sometimes uncovers inequalities that get in the way of disease management. An all-out effort allows us to frame policies that prioritize health equity, building world health infrastructure piece by piece. Ultimately, such mixed study not only enhances our understanding of infectious diseases but also sets the foundation for durable, equitable solutions in today's globalized world (Figure 13.2).

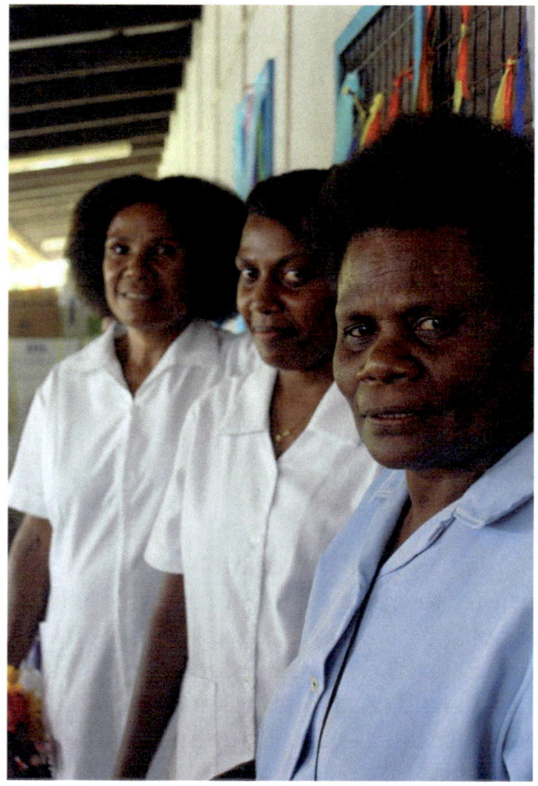

Figure 13.2. The intersection of global health and infectious diseases.

Source: By Department of Foreign Affairs and Trade - Nurses at Butawin Urban Clinic, PNG, CC BY 2.0, https://commons.wikimedia.org/w/index.php?curid=32165874

13.1. Historical Context of Infectious Diseases

Historically, infectious diseases have tended to appear in tandem with changes in society, economy, and even the environment. Human behavior, such as humans packing into cities with no sanitary measures in place during the Industrial Revolution—can truly whip things into a frenzy. Altering agriculture practices, a warmer climate, and increased urbanization all tend to co-mingle, producing exactly the right kind of perfect storm for epidemics. In retrospect, one could say that developing an understanding of why and how diseases arise makes it easier for us to design improved systems for tracking and addressing them, particularly in areas where health systems are weaker (Cleaveland et al., 2017). The legacy of colonialism still resonates in the way we do global health. Then, exploitation and marginalization of local communities left scars that still influence health conditions and disturb institutional trust. Today, increasing numbers of researchers are looking to decolonization theories, in a broad sense, to unpick how those historical abuses still resonate. If you look at the histories of traditional and new global health alliances, it is apparent that justice and respect for local social and cultural context are the fundamental elements of any long-term solution. Public health responses have evolved significantly over time as well. Earlier measures, such as those of quarantines back in the 14th century, and subsequently additional steps, like the creation of the World Health Organization (WHO) during World War II times, underscore how heightened consciousness in our society increased since the world connected increasingly. Recent crises, though, remind one that there were gaps still far from being fulfilled, particularly in lower-resource settings. It is certain that buckling down and building up these systems is essential as these regions are usually at the forefront of new disease threats. By learning from the past and refining existing approaches, global health efforts can be more ready to meet emerging infectious diseases (Cleaveland et al., 2017).

13.1.1. Major Pandemics in History

In the 20th century, pandemics upended global health—take the 1918 influenza outbreak, for example, which folks still remember as one of the deadliest ever. That H1N1 strain spread with startling speed, infecting around one-third of the world's people and, by most estimates, taking roughly 50 million lives. It hit in three distinct waves, each one pushing medical facilities to their limits and shaking up the public health response. This terrible episode tended to reveal how vulnerable societies are to infectious diseases and pushed the development of concerted responses, such as mass vaccination campaigns and fundamental infection prevention practices—into mainstream health policy. The consequences of that experience, with their long-term repercussions, have continued to influence public health policy through the decades, underlining how urgently well-preparedness for the pandemic is (Miranda et al., 2022). HIV/AIDS, which erupted in the latter part of the 20th century, took international health into uncharted territory, revolutionizing the way we conceptualize and address infection fundamentally. Initially identified in the early 1980s the virus rapidly became a full-blown crisis characterized by mortality rates, particularly among populations such as men who have sex with men and intravenous drug users. Most often, it revealed some underlying societal prejudices and injustices which, in turn, influenced both healthcare access and quality, with sub-Saharan Africa suffering the most. Gradually, the dual pressure for treatments and knowledge resulted in breakthroughs—antiretroviral therapy, for example—turning HIV/AIDS from a virtual death sentence into a disease that, though serious, is manageable. In the end, this international battle highlighted that to combat a multifaceted disease, one needs sound medical treatment alongside strong public health education (Miranda et al., 2022). In COVID-19, precipitated by the SARS-CoV-2 virus, the globe was threatened with difficulties it had never seen, showing us how intricately connected our societies are. Identified in the final weeks of 2019, the virus spread so rapidly that governments around the globe scrambled, trying everything from lockdowns to restrictions on travel in an attempt to stem its tide. There has been a definite ripple effect on mental health as well; incidences of significant depressive and anxiety disorders increased, fueled by months of isolation and economic instability. It sort of fell into place that a robust mental health support mechanism was a critical component of any pandemic response plan. When communities are attempting to piece themselves back together, the learnings from COVID-19 could potentially be the fulcrum for shaping future strategies for confronting new diseases, assisting in forging a more resilient global health architecture (Miranda et al., 2022) (Figure 13.3).

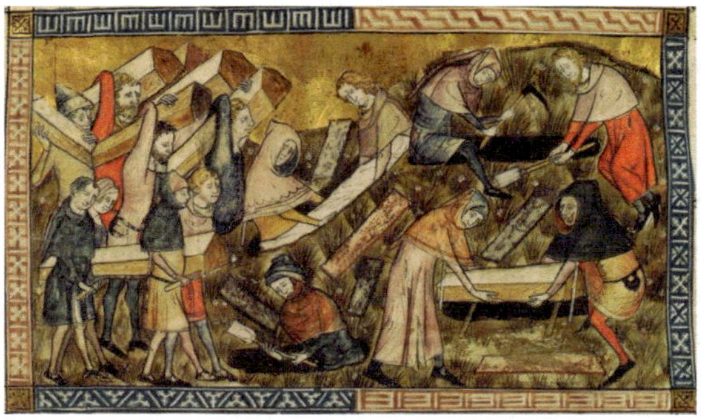

Figure 13.3. Major pandemics in history.

By Pierart dou Tielt (fl. 1340-1360) - http://balat.kikirpa.be/photo.php?path=X004175&objnr=20049662, Public Domain, https://commons.wikimedia.org/w/index.php?curid=64384803

13.1.2. Evolution of Public Health Responses

Reflecting on history's pandemics tells us quite well how public health struggles are organized. It is not solely the tale of scientific miracles; politics and society complicate the narrative as well. Consider it—those initial reactions to the Black Death and Spanish flu, respectively, resulted in our very first disease outbreak manual for today. One of the largest takeaways, in broad terms, was that there was an immediate requirement for mechanisms that were capable of rapidly identifying and tracing infections. History, in all its lessons, keeps us one step ahead of time, ever prepared for new microbes to emerge and compels everyone—from lab workers to local officials—to unite in creating stronger defenses (Dias, 2024). The COVID-19 crisis, in a way, hammered home many of these lessons, especially around gearing up vaccines and earning people's trust. Vaccine hesitancy hit high during the global emergency, showing that communicating about health is not as simple as it sounds. Groups of different backgrounds, swayed by everything from misinformation to deep-rooted cultural beliefs, made the whole vaccination push even trickier. It soon became apparent that our health plans must address individually what each community is concerned about. Online educational campaigns have filled the gap, dispelled misinformation and increasing confidence, although mandates and reluctance controversy continues to distort the discussion, reminding us that policies must adapt as circumstances evolve (Waitzberg et al., 2024).

This all this talk is in the process of developing strategies that not just protect us but also sew communities together when there is a crisis. Combining technology into public health response is another step forward. New equipment that captures real-time information now allows us to trace outbreaks in real time and respond quickly, even if at times the pieces get a little mixed up. Initiatives such as immunization data systems and other technology-based solutions have a significant role to play in soothing vaccine anxieties and boosting coverage rates. While we attempt to make sense of why individuals choose to get vaccinated or not, public health interventions are beginning to integrate knowledge regarding human behavior—a solution as pragmatic as it is required. By combining learnings from the past with modern-day technology magic, bureaucrats can construct strategies that resonate with the dynamics of society today. Ultimately, all these innovations highlight the need for a system of health that is not just resilient against diseases in the present but capable of shifting when fresh challenges call at our door (Dias, 2024; Waitzberg et al., 2024) (Figure 13.4).

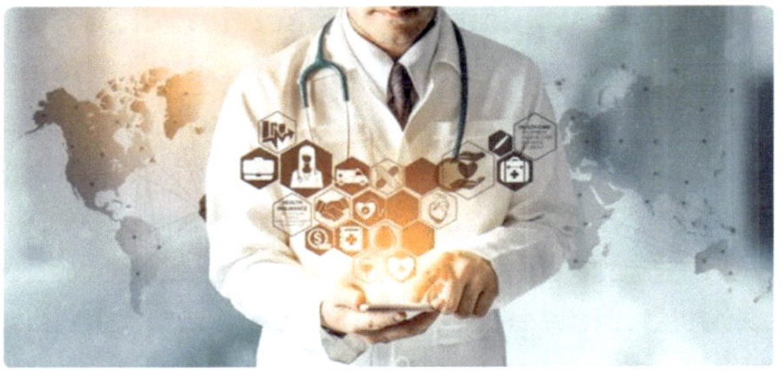

Figure 13.4. Evolution of public health responses.

Source: Shutterstock. (2021). *Image of a Person Holding a Smartphone in a Medical Setting.*

13.1.3. Lessons Learned from Past Outbreaks

Previous outbreaks have taught us a lot about preparing for future threats. We witnessed it during the Ebola outbreak in West Africa and saw it again with COVID-19, when having robust health facilities and genuine community buy-in proved to be instrumental. In COVID-19, for example, having sufficient community health facilities and adequate funding made all the difference – demonstrating that public health systems need to align with local requirements. Stakeholders, by being committed to local problems and collaborating closely with city governments, can stay ahead of future risks, with responses being swift and effective (Lee et al., 2024). It is also important to observe that our healthcare workers, particularly those who are front line, have their own vulnerabilities. History keeps reminding us that failure to provide adequate support to these crucial people has a dire cost. Consider what occurred with nurses in COVID-19 – they experienced the largest proportion of losses among healthcare providers, indicating a dire need for reform. They are worth not just sufficient personal protective equipment but also strong mental healthcare and rapid emergency education. Shortages will simply worsen in most situations unless systemic reforms prioritize the safety and retention of front-line workers (Strasser, 2024). Willingness to keep on learning and a pinch of innovation in health prep are things you simply cannot do without. Florence Nightingale's trailblazing tells us history about why community-centered care is so important. Looking back at epidemic responses, we see that remaining adaptable—incorporating new technology concepts and innovative methods—is always what works when a new illness emerges. Investment in R&D for improved protective equipment, hardened supply lines, and hands-on drills constructs a system that can get through emergencies. If we remember these lessons, not only does it enhance our preparedness but also showcases the irreplaceable value of community outreach in ensuring public health safe from future dangers (Lee et al., 2024; Strasser, 2024).

13.2. Factors Contributing to Emerging Infectious Diseases

New diseases tend to arise from a knotted combination of environmental and social transformations. Climate change—use it as a case in point—alters environments and pushes people and wildlife into closer, sometimes unanticipated, proximity. Increased heat and erratic weather events, such as floods or droughts, increase the likelihood of diseases jumping from animals to humans. In a lot of regions that are seeing huge shifts, rudimentary monitoring networks simply do not exist, so identifying outbreaks early is very difficult. In all but a few instances, managing these intersecting challenges is critical if we hope to avoid pandemics in the future and safeguard those at greatest risk (Moslehi et al., 2025). Urban areas, also, have a significant role in how new infections establish themselves. As more people migrate to urban areas, the places are hotspots for germs, partially due to crowded conditions that favor disease spread. This trend appears most prominently in poor locations where there is poor infrastructure and lacking healthcare measures. With individuals crammed together, infection can travel at high speed, whereas the deteriorating condition of some cities further exacerbates health disparities. Residing nearby also increases the likelihood of contact with disease carriers such as mosquitoes that carry malaria or dengue fever along with them.

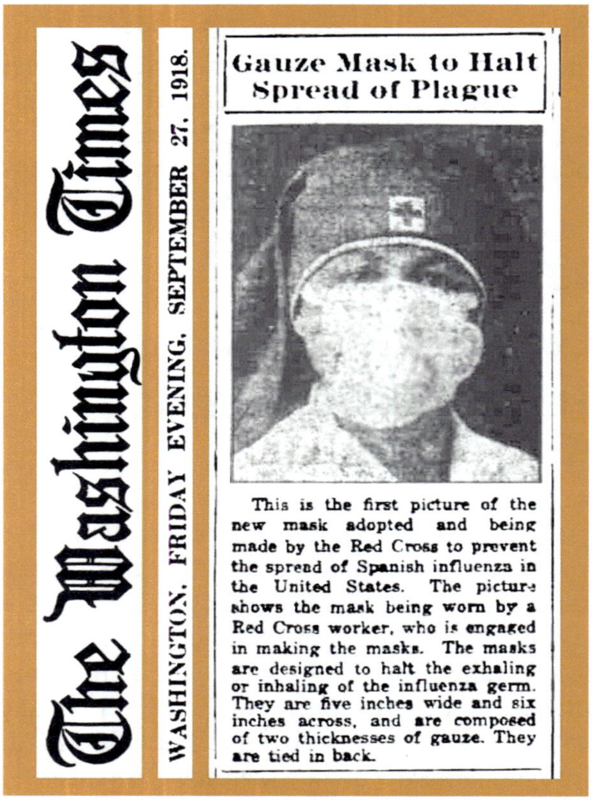
The Washington Times

WASHINGTON, FRIDAY EVENING, SEPTEMBER 27, 1918.

Gauze Mask to Halt Spread of Plague

This is the first picture of the new mask adopted and being made by the Red Cross to prevent the spread of Spanish influenza in the United States. The picture shows the mask being worn by a Red Cross worker, who is engaged in making the masks. The masks are designed to halt the exhaling or inhaling of the influenza germ. They are five inches wide and six inches across, and are composed of two thicknesses of gauze. They are tied in back.

Figure 13.5. Factors contributing to emerging infectious diseases.

Source: By The Washington Times (newspaper, Washington, D.C., U.S., September 27, 1918) - https://newspaperarchive.com/washington-times-sep-27-1918-p-3/, Public Domain, https://commons.wikimedia.org/w/index.php?curid=94760795

Evidently, planning smart for cities and implementing more effective public health measures can travel a long way toward alleviating these risks (Rampedi et al., 2024). International travel and commerce also mix the pot where outbreaks are concerned. Modern transportation networks allow people and products to zip from one continent to another, compressing distance in a way that sometimes provides pathogens with an easy ride. The rapid spread of H1N1 and COVID-19 demonstrated how quickly a virus can propagate when borders are hardly a hindrance. Even wildlife or agricultural product trades can unknowingly introduce insects borne by animals into new areas. In the majority of instances, collaboration globally and adherence to stringent health regulations is necessary; creating an enhanced and responsive global health system with enhanced monitoring and rapid response plans can prevent these dangers from looming (Moslehi et al., 2025) (Figure 13.5).

13.2.1. Climate Change and Its Impact on Disease Spread

Climate and public health are getting increasingly entwined in ways that are not difficult to observe today. The warming of the planet is not merely a statistic—it promotes comfortable conditions for nuisance animals such as mosquitoes and ticks. Urbanization and other human migrations disrupt natural habitats and ultimately push us toward zoonotic insects. Deforestation, for example, does not just remove trees—it forces people into more frequent, sometimes messy, encounters with wildlife, letting germs slip out from where they used to hide. Places like East Africa feel this double whammy especially, with illnesses like leishmaniasis putting a strain on local health efforts. Clearly, ramping up monitoring and control is needed to keep these new threats at bay (Jones &Welburn, 2021). Aside from these biting insects, climate change draws on a wider array of emerging infections.

Human activities are disrupting nature's balance and increasing the chances that diseases cross the species barrier. Consider COVID-19—a stark reminder that when the environment changes, the old protection barriers fall short. As environments shift, those natural barriers that historically maintained the pathogens under control begin to break down, leading to an actual need to dig deep into the mechanics of how these barriers function. In studying the complex connection between wildlife, human societies, and their environments, it is revealed that climate change flips everything around in ways beyond anticipation (Zhang et al., 2021). With these fast-changing issues, it is quite apparent that proactive strategies need to be at the forefront. We require interventions not only responding to climate change but also addressing its ripple effects on the spread of disease as well. Increased investment in healthcare, particularly in low- and middle-income regions—is essential. This involves improved control of disease vectors, accelerated reporting, and rapid turnaround interventions for diseases such as leishmaniasis. And, quite simply, global collaboration is imperative; the exchange of ideas and resources can strengthen our collective response. Only by combining these strategies together can we aspire to traverse the increasing intersections of public health and climate change, striving toward a healthier world for communities across the globe (Jones & Welburn, 2021).

13.2.2. Urbanization and Population Density

Urban areas are growing at a fast pace, and this boom has created agitations in the way individuals inhabit and connect with nature—frequently in unforeseen manners. In much of the Global South, for instance, neighborhoods are bursting with people, which occasionally provides a sort of breeding ground for disease. Over half the inhabitants of the planet live in cities now, a transformation that, for the most part, has been associated with a surge in both brand-new cases as well as the resurgence of established ones, not to mention a plethora of chronic ailments. Economic disparities, which tend to add to these challenges, make things even more difficult for the most at-risk populations in poorer regions. In some sense, delving into these urban health mysteries, particularly in the less-frequently observed peri-urban enclaves (Dorsey, 2024)—appears more important than ever. Large cities, expanding unevenly as it may appear, tend to grapple with antiquated or incomplete infrastructure, and that can wreak havoc on our capacity to manage public health emergencies. Dense populations, as one might observe, can speed up the spread of diseases that jump from animals to people, a trend that now marks a sizable share of new threats. Add a bit of climate change and the ongoing loss of biodiversity into the mix, and the results can be especially worrisome. The COVID-19 pandemic, for example, uncovered the dangers of living shoulder-to-shoulder in densely populated city areas—something most healthcare units had not fully prepared for until then. Such challenges in the healthcare of city residents are not merely concerned with the delivery of medical interventions; they intertwine closely with social and economic issues, tending to require a much wider, population-based care approach (Burkle, 2020). We simply cannot overestimate how much urban development affects world health, and most would say that action from health professionals and policy-makers alike is required immediately. Further examination of how people live in cities creates a complex knot of environmental and socio-political processes that determine health outcomes; overall, a biocultural approach may be our best option in this case. This kind of strategy could open the way for interventions attuned to the particular needs of urban populations, particularly those on the periphery. And ramping up global cooperation in the face of new infectious dangers may well strengthen our overall public health resilience. Ultimately, as much as it may sound somewhat scholarly, how our urban spaces have come to be is central to designing effective systems of health for our increasingly complex world (Dorsey, 2024).

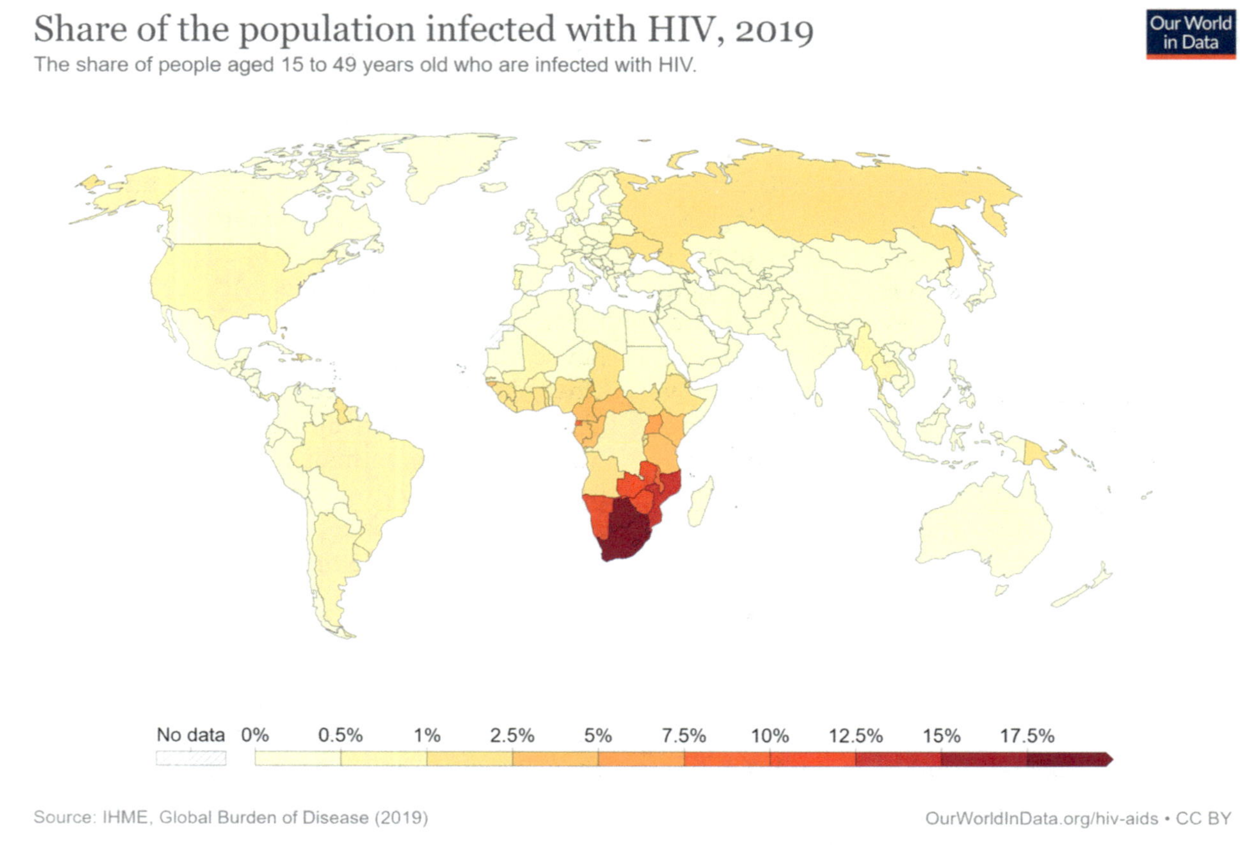

Source: By Our world in data - https://ourworldindata.org/hiv-aids, CC BY-SA 4.0, https://commons.wikimedia.org/w/index.php?curid=135466504.

13.2.3. Global Travel and Trade Dynamics

International travel combined with contemporary commerce can shake up the propagation of fresh disease, making health measures that much more complicated to cope with. Millions take on journeys across frontiers daily — to take a brief holiday or for a business trip — and, for the most part, such mobility provides microorganisms with a chance to travel across communities nearly imperceptibly. A small epidemic can quickly whip up into a global issue, as we experienced with SARS, which demonstrated that our interconnected world can turn a local problem into a global crisis. The sudden spreading of diseases somehow compels us to develop cutting-edge health measures that are not only about looking for signs but also about blocking problems before they even develop at global borders (Azzam, 2024). All things being equal, as travel and trade patterns continue to change, learning about the way these systems function becomes critical to informing wise public health policy. Trade has a sneaky way of making the mess deeper. It is not just about humans on the move – transporting products, ranging from foodstuffs to live animals, occasionally finds its way in with sneaky infectious agents without so much as a ceremony. When zoonotic disease epidemics compel trade restrictions, it highlights how economic activity and health issues are strangely linked. Oftentimes, such newfound diseases can have their origins in common farming practices or the high-density wildlife markets where humans and animals converge too frequently. For instance, the development of the wild meat business has clearly increased human exposure to zoonoses, raising legitimate health concerns (Azzam, 2024). This leaves us at a juncture where economic needs and health security have to be weighed to prevent small eruptions from growing into full-blown epidemics. One Health isn't merely a slogan—it provides a good approach to addressing these multi-faceted issues. It unites human, animal, and environmental health, illustrating that these are knotted together with one another in ways more than one. By partnering with government public health agencies, veterinarians, and environmental scientists, we can stay in front of conditions that have a propensity to create outbreaks. International collaboration, through collaborative data-sharing and even halting but genuine resource sharing, strengthens early detection mechanisms so that nations can react when things begin to go off the rails. The experience gained from recent epidemics readily demonstrates that collaboration is not only essential during a crisis; it is equally as vital in preventing international travel and commerce from fueling the fire of new health crises (Galvani, 2004).

13.3. Case Studies of Emerging Infectious Diseases

Emerging infectious diseases continue to increase, the trend influenced by environmental change, social changes, and even the uniqueness of biology. Zika and Ebola, for example, have revealed evident weak points in our global health infrastructure that occasion closer, collaborative watchful efforts. A review by Onyebuchi et al. (2025) indicates that we tend to miss early warning signals and adequate sharing of data – both important when these epidemics begin rolling in. With climate change tweaking ecosystems in ways, we often do not expect, these illnesses are likely to show up or come back when least anticipated, throwing a wrench in planned health strategies. Some case studies, repeated over time, indicate that flexible, adaptive methods are needed, while the lessons of past outbreaks remind us, albeit imperfectly, to boost our overall preparedness. Healthcare administrators, in so many words, occupy the center of addressing these disease challenges – particularly where resources are tight.

Mobarak et al., (2024) inform us that managing outbreaks is not merely a matter of strict infection screening; it is also providing much-needed psychosocial support to medical professionals who truly carry the burden. Training sessions that combine various fields assist in creating a more secure culture among hospitals, although the process at times appears a bit awkward. The COVID-19 pandemic, for example, varied local responses resulted in patchy outcomes, demonstrating the point that local contexts matter. As a general rule, when health authorities make investments in ongoing surveillance and rapid data checks, they can stem the harm from these pathogens and gradually develop a system resilient to unforeseen shocks. Technology and innovative solutions are moving ahead as prominent warriors in our struggle against such problematic outbreaks. Onyebuchi et al. (2025) indicate that coming to terms with technology has seriously the ability to enhance responses all over the globe, despite resources still existing on the ground. Collaboration—governments, community members, or medical practitioners—increases our combined ability to respond accordingly. Various case studies reveal that when communities lean into collaboration and forward-thinking leadership, they will adapt faster when things go wrong. As our world becomes increasingly interconnected (with all its kinks), advocating for policies that combine tech integration with mental healthcare appears to be more essential than ever. Ultimately, future studies and interventions must address all these intersecting corners if we are to have a well-fortified global health strategy against EIDs (Figure 13.6).

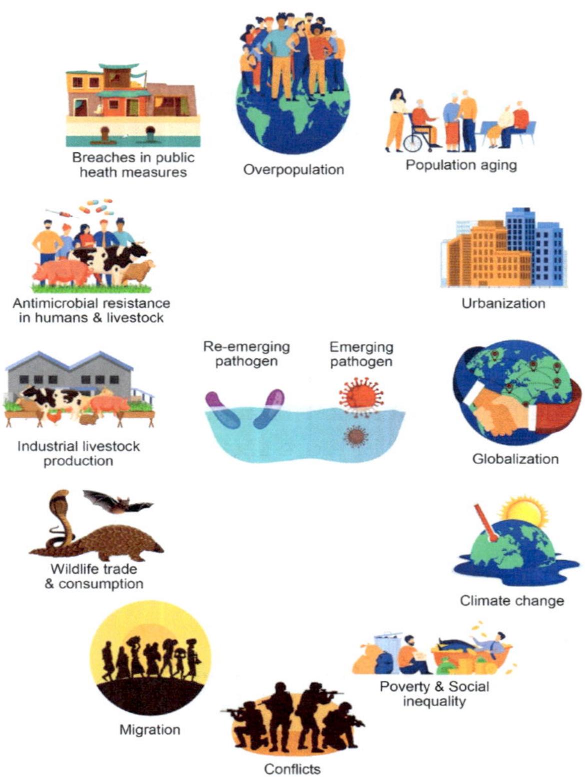

Figure 13.6. Case studies of emerging infectious diseases.

Source: MDPI. (2021). Factors that precipitate the occurrence and transmission of emerging and re-emerging infectious diseases. *Microorganisms, 10,* 98.

13.3.1. Ebola Virus Outbreak in West Africa

Between 2014 and 2016, Ebola struck hard in West Africa and disclosed much about our world's preparedness for epidemics. It all began in Guinea and then quickly crossed over to Liberia and Sierra Leone – an epidemic that demonstrated just how fragile health systems are in low-resource settings when surveillance mechanisms are not satisfactory and there is no prior experience with such outbreaks. Local hospitals were overwhelmed by mounting caseloads and complicated logistics and made it evident that we not only needed improved response plans but an organized international push as well. In the majority of instances, lessons realized at the time go on to inform subsequent public health efforts and governing globally. The crisis also made evident the need for a more dynamic research and development environment focused uniquely on infectious diseases. While the world frantically searched during the Ebola crisis, the best talents were mobilized to accelerate vaccines and medicines, although development was repeatedly stymied by rare investments and cumbersome administration. A responsive public health system – one that seizes on scientific studies as soon as trouble begins – may be precisely what is required to accelerate interventions the next time around. Strategies must also ensure equitable access to treatments, as the existing R&D environment is at times uneven and supply-led. Constructing partnerships between governments, academia, and business accelerated innovation during the Ebola epidemic, and these partnerships might enhance health outcomes in the future (Olliaro & Torreele, 2022). The emergence of Ebola also reminds us of the sloppy connection between animal-transmitted diseases that leap across species and human well-being, particularly where there is a hub of biodiversity. In West Africa, intimate contact between wildlife and humans – from hunting bushmeat to the frequency of live animal markets – provides the ideal setting for viruses to jump. With different species that co-exist together, there is ample scope for these spillover events to happen, as many of the Ebola epidemics have already demonstrated. Continued efforts to redesign the regulation of live and wet markets, along with heightened biosecurity protocols, are necessary to slice future risks. Furthermore, increasing public awareness and education on zoonotic diseases can minimize opportunities for transmission, which in turn will help strengthen global health security against possible epidemics (Naguib et al., 2021).

13.3.2. Zika Virus and Its Global Implications

New infections remind us how important it is not to lose sight of how diseases can transfer from animals to humans—zoonotic transmissions are very important to public health. Consider the Zika virus, for example; it travels primarily on Aedes mosquitoes, and you can observe that our changing environment as well as our daily human activities tend to drive these diseases into new areas. Global warming and urban sprawl at a breakneck pace combine to expand the playing field for these loathsome vectors and expose more people to harm. Travel today—so networked and so quick—allows the virus to whizz around borders in an eyeblink, transforming what would otherwise have been a small-time problem into an issue that commands international attention. It is nearly as though the knowledge of how exactly these transmission routes operate is as valuable as a cure, and that is the reason why health systems today lean into new solutions for controlling mosquitoes and improved community advice. Nature, society, and health issues all merge in unimagined fashions to inform our reaction to threats such as Zika. If you take a closer look, Zika's effect goes deeper than the direct illness; it interferes with maternal and infant health, as well. Most studies tend to state that if a pregnant woman becomes infected, it may cause severe birth defects—microcephaly being one of them—that ultimately affect a child in the long term and, consequently, the entire household. These perinatal issues are not random events; they reflect larger, sometimes careless, systemic challenges that health organizations across the globe must contend with. Even a single lag in implementing safeguards or vaccines can amplify the risk for expectant mothers and their unborn children. It appears fairly obvious that initiatives designed to improve maternal health must take a lesson from earlier outbreaks and truly concentrate on collecting good data on pregnancy outcomes. After all, when the effects of Zika appear in so many layers, a holistic approach to maternal care and illness surveillance becomes necessary, particularly in outbreak-prone locations (Malange et al., 2023). Taking the larger picture into account, how Zika exploded is a reminder that global health initiatives have to be a group effort supported by significant research investments. Yes, its sudden outbreak made headlines, but in the majority of instances, what matters most are the long-term solutions—prevention measures, better vaccines, and fresh medicines. The rapid, nearly pandemic-level dissemination of Zika only demonstrates how close-knit our global health is: a small problem can propagate quickly to disturb us all. Greater cooperation between nations, health organizations, and research institutions is more of a necessity than an option now; improved tests, intelligent treatments, and increased grassroots action all depend on this cooperation. And incidentally, more recent research with blood tests has indicated some promise in distinguishing Zika from other flaviviruses, which might be a game-changer in controlling outbreaks. Perhaps spending money on a more robust global health infrastructure and building lasting international collaborations is our best hope to control Zika—and to prepare for whatever new disease comes along next (Bombaci et al., 2024) (Figure 13.7).

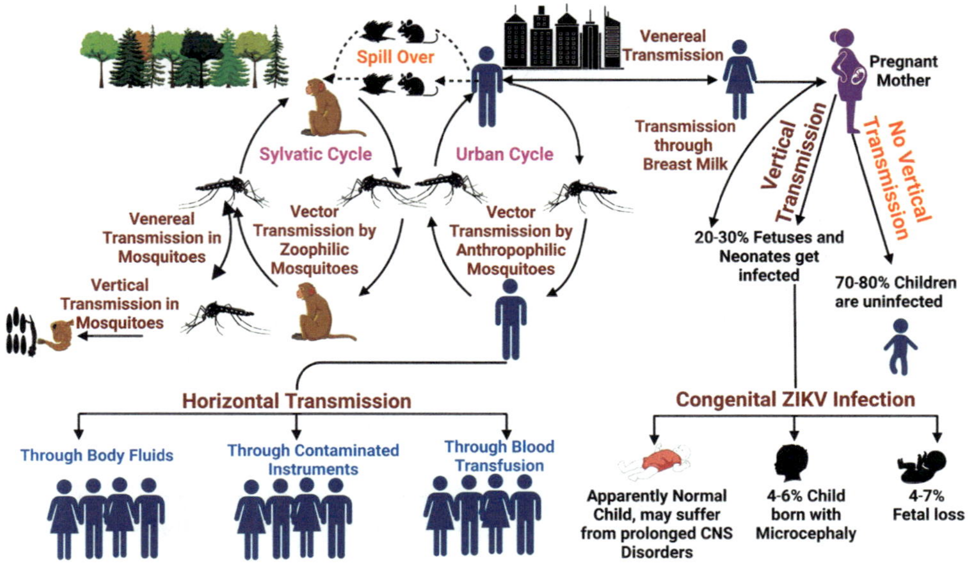

Figure 13.7. Zika virus and its global implications.

Source: Wahaab A, Mustafa BE, Hameed M, Batool H, Tran Nguyen Minh H, Tawaab A, Shoaib A, Wei J, Rasgon JL. An Overview of Zika Virus and Zika Virus Induced Neuropathies. International Journal of Molecular Sciences. 2025; 26(1):47. https://doi.org/10.3390/ijms26010047

13.3.3. COVID-19 Pandemic and Its Effects on Global Health Systems

OVID-19 came on the scene and ripped off the veil hiding our global health systems' vulnerabilities—shortcomings that had been well-concealed for much too long. Physicians, nurses, and other healthcare professionals in high-risk positions found themselves struggling with unforeseen challenges; many believed their risk level was quite close to that of emergency personnel. In one survey, almost half of Bulgaria's otorhinolaryngologists confessed that their risk of contamination ended up equaling that of emergency responders and that they experienced not just sharp financial losses but also severe psychological distress (Milcheva et al., 2025). These scenes, in some ways, tell more than individual struggles; they indicate the pressing need to upend the way our health systems are organized so that frontline workers receive the assistance they require, even when outbreaks become sudden and unannounced. One of the pandemic's wider lessons is the need to consider public health as an integrated thing, not in clear little boxes. The One Health system—a pragmatic concept bringing together human, animal, and environmental health—has gained prominence since COVID-19 affected nearly every aspect of our existence. Some research, in general, points out that bridging how ecological changes result in the emergence of infectious diseases is fairly important when it comes to preventing and combatting outbreaks (Zyoud, 2024). This entire experience opened a defining door, incentivizing further investment in One Health initiatives and challenging scientists from various disciplines (at times in unusual combinations) to collaborate and develop more robust defenses against future pandemics. The financial aspects of the pandemic have been tough, as well. Many healthcare institutions have been squeezed financially; reports show that hospital-based specialists in busy, high-contact areas saw their incomes drop dramatically – a situation that only added to the toll on their mental well-being (Milcheva et al., 2025). And then there is the knock-on economic impact, which has cut back much-needed funding for public health programs, leaving us less prepared for whatever comes next. More often than not, global health systems must acknowledge these fiscal barriers and begin shifting toward long-term funding frameworks, frameworks designed for long-term sustainability. Fortifying fiscal support will not only bolster existing infrastructures—it will also enable communities to test and implement more efficient methods to keep diseases in check (Zyoud, 2024).

13.4. Role of Global Health Organizations

Global health has its own cutthroat network of groups that confront emerging infectious diseases in methods that are not necessarily by the book. Most of these organizations, as frontline sentinels, blend innovative resource maneuvers with raw collaboration to keep dangers at bay. You can view this in the DSN Initiative—a scheme that, as per an assessment by the Rockefeller Foundation, advocates for robust, cross-border networks to enhance disease surveillance and rapid responses (Kimball et al., 2011). In general terms, the notion is that doing a little bit of everything and doing it together makes disease management much more efficient even when, sometimes, nothing necessarily goes according to a script. Aside from coordinating, these health organizations go into research and innovation, particularly when there emerge new infectious issues out of nowhere. Clinical Trials Organizations (CTOs) and Public-Private Partnerships are excellent models of this mixed bag strategy: they come together in unpredictable ways to hasten the discovery of new drugs. Such action is so important in low-resource regions—the very places where infections tend to strike hardest. Research indicates that understanding how these groups grapple and give each other support, with all their small sustainability oddities, could well kick next steps in health (Brown et al., 2009). It seems that a small ongoing collaboration can culminate in larger, more creative leaps. The global health world is not static; it's always changing, so these institutions must constantly adapt if they're going to stay one step ahead of new pathogens.

New germs don't wait, so it is a matter of developing plans for quick response while also developing systems that persist over time. Organizations ultimately operate on a cycle of trial and (occasionally) error—learning from success and failure, but with some minor bumps along the road. For example, re-reading the DSN Initiative's management strategies has illustrated the worth of accountability and savvy, sometimes even unique , investments in health philanthropy. In most cases, putting a premium on these evaluations not only sharpens their own next moves but also adds to the larger conversation about keeping the spread of diseases in check (Kimball et al., 2011) (Figure 13.8).

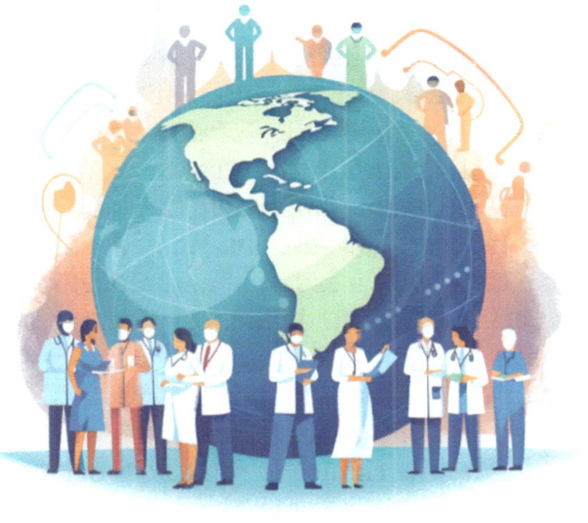

Figure 13.8. Role of global health organizations.

Source: International Hospital Federation. (2023). *Young Executive Leaders 2023 Program Poster.*

13.4.1. World Health Organization (WHO) Initiatives

When confronted with new infectious diseases, strong teaming up among nations proves to be the key. Receiving consistent funding alongside down-to-earth, hands-on involvement truly matters. The WHO is among the lead players in this regard, forcing initiatives that improve global health infrastructures, particularly in countries with lower and middle incomes. U.S. efforts, directing funds through several programs, contribute toward filling gaps that usually hinder the responses. In effect, the employment of American resources in support of improved observation and rapid response in at-risk areas has become a cornerstone for hardening healthcare systems. At the core of WHO's activities is the effort to enhance the speed at which we can detect and address infection. Their response is not merely about responding to emergencies immediately but also about developing sustainable health capacities in areas that typically bear the burden of these epidemics, such as most LMICs. Local healthcare systems' strengthening assists nations in being able to monitor disease patterns better and respond more quickly, as Cleaveland et al. (2017) indicate, action that reduces health disparities and even improves local economies. Through the adaptability of strategies to suit what local communities require, a better-balanced, equitable approach to global health comes into effect. Another major emphasis is on scaling up research and development for vaccines and medicines to combat these diseases. Collaborating with pharmaceutical companies and researchers, WHO facilitates an environment where innovative ideas in science have the chance to rapidly translate into workable solutions to public health emergencies. This strategy is important because it not only provides countries with the immediate tools, they need for emergencies but also establishes overall readiness for what lies ahead. And, by engaging local communities in the process, those most impacted have a voice—helping to create ownership and accountability that are hallmarks of sustainable health gains over the long term.

13.4.2. Centers for Disease Control and Prevention (CDC) Contributions

Easing many of the challenges that emerging infectious diseases present, the Centers for Disease Control and Prevention (CDC) has had a fairly significant role to play. In the majority of instances, they have established surveillance systems that monitor outbreaks and changing trends, which in turn allows them to respond rapidly to health threats. Their studies delve deep into infection transmission—advocating intervention based on firm evidence and attuned to various communities. For example, their research into vaccine strategies, particularly for kids, truly demonstrates a commitment to preventing disease before it gets around. Occasionally, by trawling through trends over time and offering local outreach programs, the CDC ensures communities receive valuable health advice that enhances both national and international security. The COVID-19 pandemic, quite literally, drove home the importance of teamwork and comprehensive health planning—with the CDC in the thick of it. Their leadership at the time paved the way for guidelines that not only addressed the short-term health hazards but also skirted the larger social and economic waves. It could be argued their participation in One Health initiatives highlights a dedication to a balanced strategy that connects human, animal, and environmental health. Combining applied multidisciplinary research with collaborative models, the CDC has, in most instances, become a major force against infectious diseases—keeping efforts on track and effective globally (Zyoud, 2024). Outside U.S. territories, the CDC's work is not limited at all; they leap into global health programs designed to ward off threats worldwide. They have supported innumerable initiatives intended to build stronger health infrastructure in developing countries, which, in the majority of instances, serves to increase global preparedness and resilience upon the occurrence of outbreaks. Their aptitude for outbreak response clearly manifests through backing for sturdy surveillance networks and lab facilities—occasionally even with minor discrepancies in the way things are being presented—around the world. Through information sharing and cooperative resourcefulness, the CDC forms alliances that are crucial in reducing risks associated with emerging infectious diseases. Overall, their sweeping strategy indicates that addressing global health issues does require concerted, evidence-based, and coordinated action in multiple sectors.

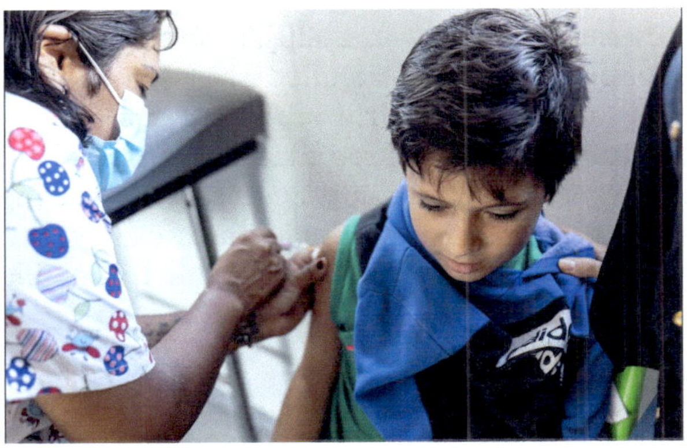

Source: Pan American Health Organization. (2023). *Child Receiving Vaccination.*

13.4.3. Non-Governmental Organizations (NGOs) and Their Impact

The global health issues of today require innovative responses beyond traditional government action, particularly in the face of emerging infectious diseases. NGOs, with their agile organizational structures and strong links with communities, have assumed leadership roles in such initiatives. They initiate diverse Digital Social Innovation initiatives that leverage technology for disseminating critical health information, mapping disease outbreaks, and creating avenues toward healthcare access for marginalized communities. These organizations often collaborate directly with local communities—developing interventions that fit individual circumstances. Such collaboration illustrates how NGOs can step in where traditional public health systems leave gaps and an important role that has increased even in crises like the COVID-19 pandemic (Qureshi et al., 2021). NGOs do not only leap into action when a threat is imminent; they also make investments in projects that are long-term, fostering more robust and resilient local health systems. They prepare communities for upcoming challenges by providing essential information on disease prevalence and accessible services. They enable locals to take control of their own health by establishing digital platforms for knowledge sharing and resource mobilization. This strategy, in the vast majority of instances, is consonant with the Sustainable Development Goals by ensuring health equity and incorporating members of the community into important decision-making. This forward-thinking action is particularly crucial when conventional healthcare systems first experience difficulties under unprecedented stress (Budd et al., 2020). Continued change in global health necessitates a renewed consideration of how all stakeholders, including NGOs, frame health emergencies. More and more, these organizations are forming alliances across multiple sectors—partnering with technology companies and academic institutions to apply digital innovations in innovative ways. Through their collaborative efforts, they aim toward a holistic approach to preventing and managing disease outbreaks, identifying the strength that comes from cooperation. NGOs are leading the way on applying digital health solutions that address pressing needs while also paving the way for long-term gains. This combination of social innovation and technological advancement evidently indicates how greatly they are shaping the future of public health (Qureshi et al., 2021).

13.5. Strategies for Prevention and Control

Emerging diseases hit hard, and handling them is not as cut-and-dry as it might seem. Prevention and control are not part of some magic formula but rather a bundle of public health moves. Think about beefing up surveillance so that outbreaks can be spotted early, giving authorities a chance to jump in quickly. NCEZID, the National Center for Emerging and Zoonotic Infectious Diseases, invests a lot of effort in making sure we track outbreaks better and raise local health capacity. Their emphasis on transparency and regular updates creates a sort of public trust. And when technology enters the picture—making it better how data is gathered and read—it enables health teams to act before things get out of hand (Center N for Emerging and Diseases ZI (US). We also cannot discount that health is a global concern. The coronavirus pandemic reminded us, in the majority of instances, that no nation is an island in the matter of disease threats. Policies now have to think not merely locally but at a greater level as well. When communities make a difference and every individual has equal access to healthcare, the battle against disease becomes more resilient. The pandemic demonstrated that when the government is complacent and not adequately prepared, the loopholes exacerbate inequalities. In the end, ethics do matter, and future strategies have to adopt inclusivity and delve into vulnerability's deeper causes (Gellert et al., 2020). Frontline worker training and enhancing public health systems are equally important. A skilled staff can be the pillar in the event of an outbreak—this is why ongoing training and drill readiness are crucial. At the same time, investing in robust public health infrastructure ensures that our systems can weather threats more consistently. National and international collaboration is necessary, as sharing resources and expertise can fill in those all-too-gaping holes. NCEZID strategic plans clarify that only such collaborations can result in scaling-up interventions that can bring about a tangible impact on health outcomes (Center N for Emerging and Diseases ZI (US)) (Figure 13.9).

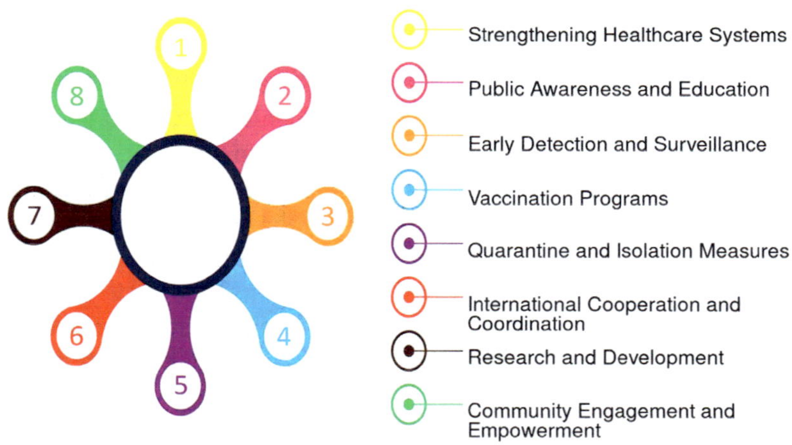

Figure 13.9. Strategies for prevention and control.

Source: FasterCapital. (n.d.). *Global Health Crisis: Veba—A Global Health Crisis Demanding Urgent Action: Strategies for Prevention and Control.*

13.5.1. Vaccination Programs and Their Effectiveness

In most communities, childhood vaccinations determine our overall health globally. Research indicates that when vaccines are implemented effectively, they tend to decrease the prevalence of infectious diseases in children. For example, extensive immunization campaigns usually reduce cases of measles, pneumococcal pneumonia, and Hib drastically—even some records indicate declines of over 90% in high-coverage areas. Conversely, areas with low vaccination rates continue to experience outbreaks, suggesting that there is a definite need to extend these programs. Overall, continuing these vaccination programs is important in ensuring public health and generations to come remain safe from preventable diseases (Karaut, 2024). Aside from pediatric care, immunization campaigns are important in combating emergent infectious threats. With the increasing new health dangers, as well as problems such as antimicrobial resistance (AMR) making things more difficult, new public health concepts are essential. Vaccines benefit not only by preventing illness but also by reducing the severity of drug-resistant bacteria. New reviews indicate that vaccines can reduce both the incidence and severity of diseases such as tuberculosis (TB) and malaria. Add to that, new vaccine technologies and immunotherapy products—new strategies for augmenting our body's own defenses—provide promising methods to combat these challenges, particularly in areas hardest struck by new diseases (Alnakhli et al., 2024). Ultimately, the success of vaccination programs relies on more than meticulous planning—it falls on how well informed the public becomes and can access these shots. As long as communities know why vaccines are important, more people can get vaccinated, strengthening the process of herd immunity along the way. Vaccine hesitancy campaigns that address misconceptions and clarify things are crucial, especially for those populations that have been left behind. In addition, even striving to improve healthcare infrastructure so that vaccines are more accessible remains imperative for vulnerable populations. Considering how diseases can evolve us, investing in vaccine programs all the time is a stone foundation for a healthful future for all (Alnakhli et al., 2024; Karaut, 2024).

13.5.2. Surveillance and Early Detection Systems

Speed is important in containing emerging infectious diseases in their infancy. Rapid detection and response to outbreaks are a big deal, and sophisticated monitoring systems—ones that provide us real-time on-the-spot data—are instrumental in helping us make split-second decisions. Food markets, for instance, where domestic and wild animals rub shoulders, do not always have credible checks in place even though They are hotspots for zoonotic dangers. The idea of intelligent markets—melding routine environmental inspections with new detection technologies—is full of potential. When public health teams deploy such advanced systems, they can typically anticipate danger before it erupts, safeguarding humans and animals alike (Sievers et al., 2024). Early warning systems (EWS), likewise, are important, although their approaches sometimes may appear a little scatterbrained. Typically, these systems are designed to detect faint cues in clinical data that suggest patients deteriorating, triggering interventions at the earliest opportunity. Many studies on the models have uncovered a range of methods for picking up on the likes of acute respiratory infections. Across remote villages to humming cities, communities pass on pieces of information, admittedly in ways that are not necessarily specific, that contribute toward better overall surveillance. By making good use of hospital and emergency room info, these systems tend to catch outbreaks quickly. In most cases, their flexibility is what keeps them effective in dealing with ever-changing health threats (Patel et al., 2024). Mixing traditional surveillance with modern tech brings a fresh spin to our approach against emerging diseases. New sampling concepts like testing wastewater or monitoring air quality have opened up our capacity to track down pathogens—enhancing not just data quality, but also giving clues on environmental drivers of outbreaks. Multimodal setups that integrate these different methods can enhance early detection and rapid responses. And as communities become more connected—sometimes in complicated, unpredictable ways—the demand for global collaboration becomes increasingly clear. Collaboration can ultimately result in mutual best practices and harder, more resilient systems that raise the game of public health reactions to new threats (Patel et al., 2024; Sievers et al., 2024) (Figure 13.10).

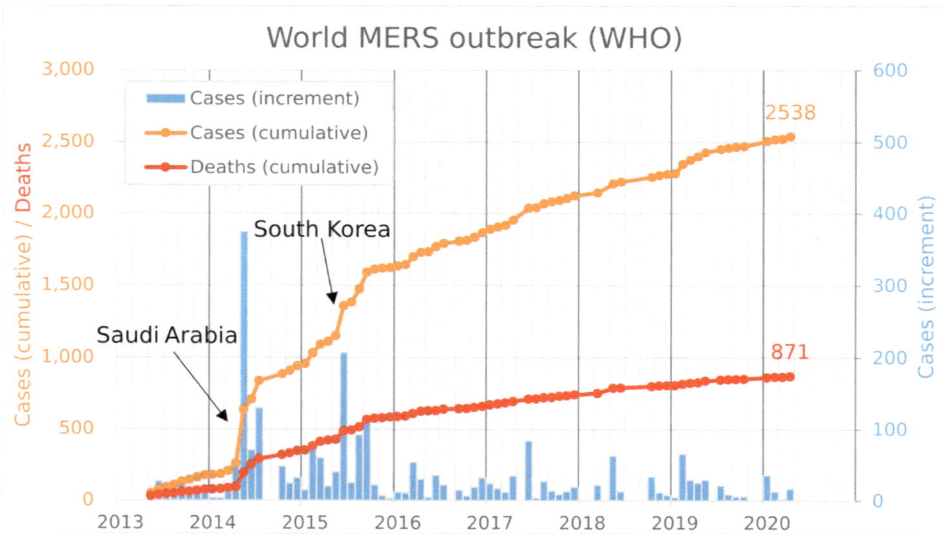

Figure 13.10. Surveillance and early detection systems.

Source: By Phoenix7777 - Own workData source: MERS-CoV - Disease outbreak news. World Health Organization., CC BY-SA 4.0, https://commons.wikimedia.org/w/index.php?curid=40913864

13.5.3. Public Health Education and Community Engagement

Groups are now the key to public health initiatives; when new infectious illnesses strike with all their sneaky complications, local action becomes more than a good thing—it's almost necessary. When neighbors collaborate, trust is developed automatically and individuals, in most instances, begin to take their health into their own hands. During epidemics, for instance, getting clear, timely information out can soothe panic and dispel out-of-control rumors. Local education campaigns—even those that may use simple language—can make it simpler to understand how diseases spread and how to stay safe. Studies even indicate that increased public learning facilitates emergency responses and coordination with health authorities during large infectious outbreaks (Wei et al., 2025). In total, prioritizing public health education leads communities to make wiser decisions and prepare themselves for upcoming difficulties. The advantages of public health education extend to our mental health as well. Reflect on how the COVID-19 pandemic made several individuals feel like they were stuck in an uneasy, unpredictable situation where depression and fear could gain a foothold (Omoregie, 2024). By integrating mental health education into wider health drives, communities can assist people in coming to terms with the psychological impact of emerging diseases, like Mpox, without it feeling too clinical. Outreach work—albeit sometimes a bit ad hoc or patchy—helps reduce stigma and enhance mental health understanding, coaxing people gently toward a solution before things get bad, and ultimately reducing the pressure on health services. And when cases emerge, community champions inevitably step forward, clarifying messages and minimizing biases and calling for everyone to adhere to health guidelines.

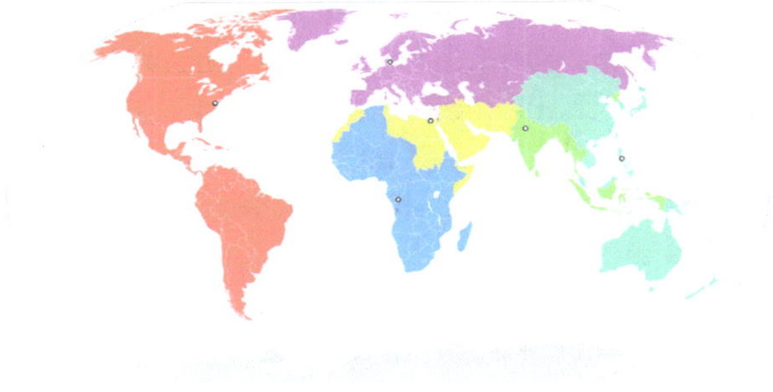

Figure 13.11. Public health education and community engagement.

Source: By Derfel73; Canuckguy et al. - This file was derived from: BlankMap-World6.svg, Public Domain, https://commons.wikimedia.org/w/index.php?curid=17152682

13.6. Ethical Considerations in Global Health

Global health is changing so rapidly these days, particularly with the emergence of new infectious diseases all the time. AI and machine learning are combining into work on vaccines and disrupting immunological research in ways we never imagined, opening new doors that increase speed as well as precision. But with each advance comes a thorny question—who exactly gets the benefits? Although tech can refine vaccines and expand healthcare, the best of it keeps ending up in the hands of wealthier countries. Obviously, we require some flexible ethical rules of thumb so everyone is kept informed, ensuring low- and middle-income countries (LMICs) are not left behind. Parallel to this, these concerns are not merely over who gets to use technology; these bleed into concerns over privacy and good consent when treatments are implemented.

As AI mines enormous sets of data to dial in disease control and develop treatments that are just right, the potential for patient privacy to become muddled grows. When you begin to use genomic information to customize treatments, even when it sounds quite thrilling-it also raises the kinds of debate surrounding who owns that genetic information. Addressing those kinds of issues highlights the value of having proper data ethics frameworks in place to develop trust among all parties. Srivastava et al. (2024) point out how intelligent guidelines are capable of snuffing out future ethical mishaps before they arise when diagnostics go into the nitty-gritty of infectious diseases. Otherwise, consider the greater picture: the globe is not constructed on a level playing field, particularly when disasters threaten and pandemic preparation becomes a race. New diseases will strike the most susceptible quite forcefully, so any reaction—ranging from detecting an outbreak to implementing vaccines—must intersect with fairness at every level. The moral aspect of such worldwide disparities must be a point of burning debate, demanding policies that enhance accessibility and increase preventives. National governments and global organizations do have a role to play in establishing fundamental practices that promote ethical behavior in health care, and the framework they establish today will reverberate into how we manage future pandemics and epidemics.

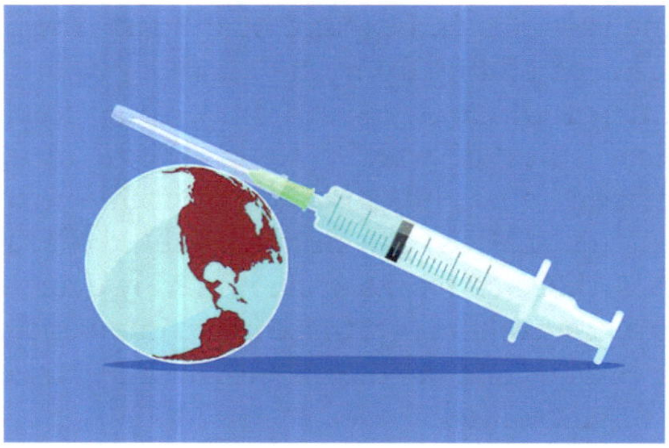

Source: University of Washington. (n.d.). *Vaccine Ethics.*

13.6.1. Equity in Access to Healthcare Resources

Around the globe, the uneven dispersal of health resources is a gigantic headache. In most places—consider areas in India, for instance—public health infrastructure is collapsing, putting communities at risk, particularly when it comes to diseases like TB. When such persistent strains as multidrug-resistant TB arise, it greatly reflects how precarious healthcare can be, frequently because of weak access and uneven treatment follow-through. You can find another image in places with agile public health systems that ace early detection and receive quality medication on schedule. In the majority of scenarios, overhauling and remodeling such systems to reflect strategies in places with fewer MDR-TB problems is essential (Gamon et al., 2013). Equitable access to healthcare is not only a moral virtue; it is crucial to preventing epidemics of new illness.

The Ebola outbreak in West Africa—of countries such as Sierra Leone, Liberia, and Guinea—identified just how bad vulnerable systems can become. It appears to spiral out of control when response expense rises to around $4.3 billion, well over the approx. $1.58 billion that experts calculated would be needed to reinforce these systems beforehand. Overall, investing in prevention, albeit it may seem a lot today, will prove to be much more worthwhile than playing catch-up later. This strategy keeps the short-term threats in check and lays the foundation for more robust long-term community health (Hanna et al., 2015). Getting everyone a fair shot at actual healthcare requires making some big, big policy adjustments. It involves increasing health literacy and providing care that suits various cultural requirements. Local leaders collaborating with government agencies—and sometimes even competing with one another—can create real transformations in the way we monitor and respond to health threats. The painful lessons of Ebola and the persistent challenges of MDR-TB compel us to be proactive instead of merely responding after crises occur. Practically, this means deploying rapid diagnostic kits and adaptable treatment protocols that accommodate every community's idiosyncrasies - similar to what has been seen in some regions of India. Overall, these actions could set the stage for improved results and a safer international health future (Gamon et al., 2013).

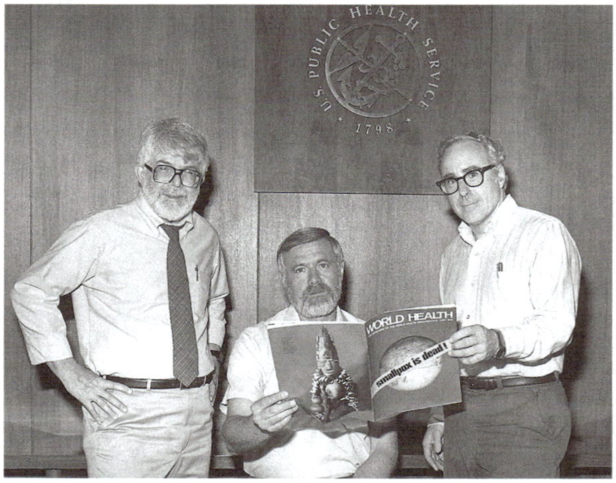

Source: By Photo Credit:Content Providers(s): CDC - This media comes from the Centers for Disease Control and Prevention's Public Health Image Library (PHIL), with identification number #7079.Note: https://commons.wikimedia.org/w/index.php?curid=3156882

13.6.2. Balancing Individual Rights with Public Health Needs

Pandemics ignite a chaotic mix of concerns where safeguarding public health and preserving individual liberties come into conflict. Reflecting on experiences such as the 1918 flu pandemic, we can notice how state actions rewrote health reactions and, in so doing, ignited debates regarding individual autonomy—raising issues that continue to reverberate now. When the danger level increases, authorities may suddenly implement practices such as quarantine, enforced vaccinations, or even travel bans, all of which are intended to nip the infections in the bud—though, in the majority of instances, these measures are not devoid of controversy. At times, the very strategies designed to protect us end up undermining our rights, eventually representing a hybrid of societal values connected with freedom and mutual care (Berkman & Gostin, 2007). In our hyper-connected world, diseases can zip aross borders with lightning speed, forcing authorities to move quickly—yes, even at the cost of trampling on individual freedoms. Health authorities, normally motivated by a desire to save the many, could inadvertently tread on privacy rights; consider contact tracing, which sometimes feels a bit too intrusive. The rules of law that authorize the state during emergencies tend not to be accompanied by defined playbooks, which usually leaves leeway for overstepping and disrupts public trust. Briefly, the constant tug-of-war between maintaining public safety and respecting individual rights necessitates seeking a middle path that is just and reasonable (Gostin et al., 2003). Ethical dilemmas also arise when policies put in place to protect the population erode personal rights. It is not at all surprising for policymakers to become entwined in decisions that, though enhancing aggregate health, have a disproportionate impact on those who are already marginalized. In times of scarcity, dispersing them thinly may leave some particular demands unrealized—an arrangement that does little to satisfy our need for equity. Both a healthy society and the rights of every individual are important, so that the only sensible thing is for solutions to tilt toward justice and equilibrium. While nations adapt their strategies, maintaining the dialogue open, albeit somewhat messy from time to time, could be the way to stitch together ethical principles with collective and individual dignity in hard times (Berkman & Gostin, 2007).

13.6.3. Ethical Dilemmas in Vaccine Distribution

Rollouts of vaccines duringa pandemic never go smoothly. Health workers are always grappling with ethical dilemmas that impact the health of the population. Which group receives the vaccine first? Usually, the priority goes to groups such as the elderly and frontline health workers because they are most likely to contract serious illness. Still, this approach sometimes leaves behind other communities who may not get the attention they need, and in most cases, fairness is supposed to be the watchword guiding these decisions. When fairness is skipped, trust takes a hit and health gaps only widen—a problem that can spiral into a persistent cycle, further complicating how the world deals with new outbreaks. The logistical aspect of vaccine administration creates a further level of complication. Logistics problems, such as getting shots into people when infrastructures are in disrepair, or when transportation is limited—combine with the difficulty of rampant disinformation, which spreads fast and, in some cases, plants seed of doubt among already marginalized groups. For example, availability of nearby facilities can result in some individuals being denied timely immunizations. Meanwhile, as stated by Muteeb et al. (2023), falsehood and rumors tend to create suspicion among those historically felt marginalized, necessitating education and outreach. Public health initiatives tend to have to double down on attempts to dispel myths and build confidence, and that includes the ethical obligation beyond merely distributing vaccines—it requires a real, continuous conversation regarding needs and access, even if it gets a little messy. The controversy regarding vaccine patents and intellectual property rights still rages across the globe. Pharmaceutical companies' patents can restrict the manufacture of cheaper, generic vaccines that could otherwise benefit low- and middle-income countries, posing some uncomfortable moral questions regarding profiteering from life-saving medicines in times of crisis. As highlighted by Malik et al. (2023), cutting-edge solutions such as nanomedicine and innovative vaccine delivery mechanisms hold potential, but issues around who gains from these advances persist. Most experts indicate that relaxing patent laws for a brief period during crises can provide a window of opportunity for increased production and availability. In the end, solving these complex ethical dilemmas not only defines our response now but also sets the stage for a more equitable strategy in the future—one that ideally prioritizes public welfare over raw profit, even if the way is never clearly defined (Figure 13.12).

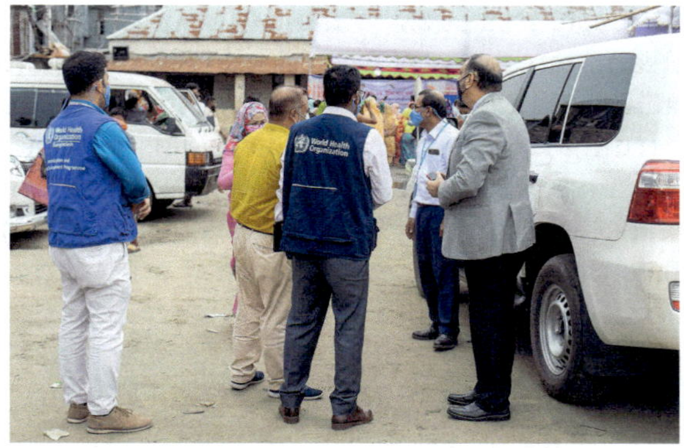

Figure 13.12. Ethical dilemmas in vaccine distribution.

Source: By Jubair Bin Iqbal - Own work, CC BY-SA 4.0, https://commons.wikimedia.org/w/index.php?curid=132893668

CLOSER LOOK

Infectious Diseases

Infectious diseases are diseases that occur when small living things enter the body and increase in number. Bacteria, viruses, fungi, and parasites are some of the organisms that cause disease. Most organisms exist within and on our bodies. They are too microscopic to be detected by the eyes. And they are usually harmless or even beneficial. However, under specific circumstances, some organisms cause disease. Some disease-causing germs are infectious. Some can be transmitted from person to person. Some are spread by insects or other animals. You might acquire others by ingesting contaminated food or water. Or you might be exposed to germs in your surroundings, like those on surfaces.

Symptoms of infectious diseases depend on the cause of the infection. But usually, they include fever and fatigue. Rest and home treatment may resolve mild infections. However, other infections can be fatal, and treatment might include hospitalization. Numerous infectious diseases, like measles and chickenpox, may be averted by vaccines. And other diseases, like COVID-19, may make you less ill if you receive the vaccine. Regular and proper hand-washing also prevents you from most infectious diseases.

SUMMARY

Global health has become more complicated these days—new illnesses keep cropping up in surprising manners. The COVID-19 debacle, for instance, demonstrated how our lives are interconnected throughout the world and exposed some vulnerabilities in our healthcare systems. You can observe it in the shifting trends of respiratory diseases in children, which informs us that we may have to adjust our public health actions not only for the short term but deep into the future. New disease agents emerge all too frequently, so in much of what we do, our system must balance pressing necessities with longer-term security strategies. Simple, preventive measures such as better tracking and transmitting simple health advice can stem the tide of outbreaks and keep vulnerable populations slightly safer. Ensuring that everyone has equal access to healthcare is equally vital, particularly when you think about how the ups and downs of daily life contribute to our health. Not all of us wind up with the same outcomes—the striking increase in dental issues in disadvantaged communities emphasizes the point. Applying such interventions as fluoride treatments regularly tends to be a wise, budget-friendly means of improving the oral health of those who truly need it. When neighbors contribute and share knowledge locally, it creates a sort of communal resilience against emerging threats of disease. Ultimately, closing these gaps benefits not only individuals but also whole communities by demonstrating that equity in treatment does make a difference. At the end of the day, recent medical crises remind us that teamwork and innovation are essential when new challenges emerge. New obstacles appear, and Overall, the intersection of modern technology, sound health numbers, and common cultural wisdom appears to be the path forward. This involves collecting pieces of information from everywhere and allowing that info to guide real-world decisions, as well as calling for improved health know-how in individuals. With all-round plans that address each level of our health concerns—as some recent research suggests—we are positioning ourselves to manage upcoming pandemics and create a world both more resilient and a little more equitable for all.

Global health is struggling with some formidable challenges with the emergence of infectious diseases. Closely studied explorations of several pathogens and their injurious characteristics have established that these infections are no trifling thing. In the vast majority of instances, new RNA viruses exhibit a remarkable diversity in the harm they can cause—a factor that truly counts when determining their prospective public health impact. Researchers, employing machine learning techniques, have mined fundamental ecological features, such as how a virus replicates and on which tissues it has a predilection for—to gain insight into its virulence. We find that a virus's ability to infect several organ systems, and how it's transmitted, contribute significantly to how bad the disease gets, and this highlights our requirement for sound prevention strategies and public health preparedness (Brierley et al., 2019). Another giant puzzle piece is recognizing that most chronic diseases can indeed have infectious causes. Over time, the views have changed significantly; what was waved away earlier often tends to be confirmed by research nowadays. As an instance, Human papillomavirus was revealed to play a significant role in cervical cancer causation. Institute of Medicine-conducted workshops have fueled these discussions, outlining the promising study possibilities as well as the remaining barriers. In general, specialists concur that identifying the precise infectious perpetrators would alter clinical practice and inform health interventions, particularly in alleviating long-term health loads for industrialized countries (O'Connor et al., 2002). The effect of infectious pathogens doesn't end with long-term ailments—it also complicates public health mechanisms, particularly for poorer nations. As more people suffer from chronic illnesses, we cannot overlook how infections, such as those that co-occur (co-infections), tend to degrade general health. Latest discussions have even pointed to the fact that constant infections from diseases such as malaria can result in lasting complications. Solving these multifaceted issues requires an actual team effort, focusing on sound research approaches merged with collaborative efforts between scientists and healthcare practitioners. By maintaining close observation of how infectious agents and chronic diseases interact, we have a greater opportunity to design public health interventions that address the varied needs of populations globally (O'Connor et al., 2002).

KEY TERMS FROM THIS CHAPTER

Global health	Emerging infectious disease (EID)
Re-emerging disease	Zoonosis
Spillover event	International Health Regulations (IHR)
Surveillance systems	Health systems strengthening
Public health infrastructure	Cross-border health threats
Travel medicine	Vector-borne disease
Antimicrobial resistance (AMR)	Climate change
Urbanization	Population mobility
Resource-limited settings	Non-governmental organization (NGO)
Centers for Disease Control and Prevention (CDC)	Global health security

REFERENCES

1. Alnakhli, R. H., Nagei, S. H. A., Alotaibi, A. S., Ataifi, H. I. Y., Almutairi, M. B. K. B. H., Al Mutairi, M. S., Ghashum, R. Q. A., et al. (2024). The significance of vaccines in mitigating emerging infectious diseases: A comprehensive review. *Journal of Ecohumanism*. https://www.semanticscholar.org/paper/e85382ce8a86ec2a6df84b65901749a7cd309528 (accessed on 6 May 2025).

2. Anderson, B., Aragrande, M., Argyris, Y., Chomel, B., Coker, R., Epstein, J., Gibbs, E., et al. (2018). A One Health evaluation of the Southern African Centre for Infectious Disease Surveillance. *Frontiers in Veterinary Science, 5*, Article 33. https://core.ac.uk/download/159106431.pdf (accessed on 6 May 2025).

3. Gostin, Lawrence O. and Berkman, Benjamin E., "Pandemic Influenza: Ethics, Law, and the Public's Health" (2007). Georgetown Law Faculty Publications and Other Works. 449. https://scholarship.law.georgetown.edu/facpub/449 (accessed on 6 May 2025).

4. Brown, C. J., & Frame, P. (2009). Communities of practice in the public-private-partnership sector for neglected diseases drug development: The importance of mindset mapping. https://core.ac.uk/download/1639972.pdf (accessed on 6 May 2025).

5. Budd, J., Miller, B. S., Manning, E., Lampos, V., Zhuang, M., Edelstein, M., Rees, G., et al. (2020). Digital technologies in the public-health response to COVID-19. *Nature Medicine, 26*, 1183–1192. https://doi.org/10.1038/s41591-020-1011-4.

6. Burkle, F. (2020). Political intrusions into the International Health Regulations Treaty and its impact on management of rapidly emerging zoonotic pandemics: What history tells us. *Prehospital and Disaster Medicine*. https://www.semanticscholar.org/paper/77cf67ae595f5a54df0394ea8d0e350bd2528b5a (accessed on 6 May 2025).

7. Doria, S., Grace, D., Mallee, H., Nguyen-Viet, H., et al. (2015). Ecohealth research in Southeast Asia: Past, present and the way forward. *Infectious Diseases of Poverty, 4*, Article 5. https://core.ac.uk/download/33300685.pdf (accessed on 6 May 2025).

8. Dorsey, F. (2024). Urbanization and infectious disease. *American Journal of Human Biology*. https://www.semanticscholar.org/paper/6ff9dfd18157423bb018e2da6b4df7deef549bd5 (accessed on 6 May 2025).

9. Gamon, M. (2013). *Multidrug-Resistant Tuberculosis in India: Solving A Problem by Reconstructing the Public Health Infrastructure* (Ronald E. McNair Scholars Program 2013, Book 12). https://core.ac.uk/download/67755957.pdf (accessed on 6 May 2025).

10. Gellert, G. A. (2020). Ethical imperatives critical to effective disease control in the coronavirus pandemic: Recognition of global health interdependence as a driver of health and social equity. *Online Journal of Health Ethics, 16*(1). https://core.ac.uk/download/301300518.pdf (accessed on 6 May 2025).

11. Gostin, L. O. (2003). When terrorism threatens health: How far are limitations on personal and economic liberties justified? https://core.ac.uk/download/70375715.pdf (accessed on 6 May 2025).

12. Hanna, L., Mailfert, M., & Wright, S. (2015). *A Wake-Up Call: Lessons from Ebola for The World's Health Systems*. https://core.ac.uk/download/75780901.pdf (accessed on 6 May 2025).

13. Jones, C., & Welburn, S. C. (2021). Leishmaniasis beyond East Africa. *Frontiers in Veterinary Science, 8*, Article 618766. https://doi.org/10.3389/fvets.2021.618766.

14. Kimball, A. M., Gugerty, M. K., Abernethy, N., & Curran, S. (2011). *Disease Surveillance Networks Initiative Global: Final Evaluation*. https://core.ac.uk/download/86445037.pdf (accessed on 6 May 2025).

15. Kruk, M. E., Gage, A., Arsenault, C., Jordan, K., Leslie, H. H., Roder-DeWan, S., Adeyi, O., et al. (2018). High-quality health systems in the Sustainable Development Goals era: Time for a revolution. *The Lancet Global Health, 6*(11), e1196–e1252. https://doi.org/10.1016/s2214-109x(18)30386-3.

16. Lee, J., & Lee, S. (2024). Spatial analysis of health system factors in infectious disease management: Lessons learned from the COVID-19 pandemic in Korea. *Healthcare, 12*. https://www.semanticscholar.org/paper/dc2cbf143f48cb3942b6570baceae9ee1552aaeb (accessed on 6 May 2025).

17. Malik, S., Muhammad, K., & Waheed, Y. (2023). Emerging applications of nanotechnology in healthcare and medicine. *Molecules, 28*(18), 6624. https://doi.org/10.3390/molecules28186624.

18. Miranda, M., Pingarilho, M., Pimentel, V., Torneri, A., Seabra, S. G., Libin, P., & Abecasis, A. (2022). A tale of three recent pandemics: Influenza, HIV and SARS-CoV-2. *Frontiers in Microbiology, 13*, Article 889643. https://doi.org/10.3389/fmicb.2022.889643.

19. Murray, C. J. L., Ikuta, K. S., Sharara, F., Swetschinski, L. R., Robles Aguilar, G., Gray, A. P., Han, C., et al. (2022). Global burden of bacterial antimicrobial resistance in 2019: A systematic analysis. *The Lancet, 399*, 629–655. https://doi.org/10.1016/s0140-6736(21)02724-0.

20. Muteeb, G., Rehman, M. T., Shahwan, M., & Aatif, M. (2023). Origin of antibiotics and antibiotic resistance, and their impacts on drug development: A narrative review. *Pharmaceuticals, 16*(11), 1615. https://doi.org/10.3390/ph16111615.

21. Naguib, M. M., Li, R., Ling, J., Grace, D., Nguyen-Viet, H., & Lindahl, J. F. (2021). Live and wet markets: Food access versus the risk of disease emergence. *Trends in Microbiology, 29*(6), 573–581. https://doi.org/10.1016/j.tim.2021.02.007.

22. O'Connor, S., Shinnick, T., & Taylor, C. E. (2002). Institute of Medicine Forum on Emerging Infections: Linking infectious agents and chronic diseases. *Emerging Infectious Diseases, 8*(12), 1529–1530. https://www.semanticscholar.org/paper/88e7080821a1107b7b5ebe2bcd2f280cdcc5cf39 (accessed on 6 May 2025).

23. Olliaro, P., & Torreele, E. (2022). Global challenges in preparedness and response to epidemic infectious diseases. *Molecular Therapy, 30*(6), 1801–1809. https://doi.org/10.1016/j.ymthe.2022.02.022.

24. Pearsall, M. E. (2019). The One Health initiative: The intersection of human, animal, and environmental health. *Senior Honors Projects, 2010-Current, 705*. https://core.ac.uk/download/223058966.pdf (accessed on 6 May 2025).

25. Rampedi, P. N., Ogunrombi, M. O., & Adeleke, O. A. (2024). Leading paediatric infectious diseases—Current trends, gaps, and future prospects in oral pharmacotherapeutic interventions. *Pharmaceutics, 16*(1). https://www.semanticscholar.org/paper/d5a3942f82dd8344d4f663571e536423354c24e7 (accessed on 6 May 2025).

26. Roemer-Mahler, A., Long, C., Clarke, A., Cooper, M., & Elbe, S. (2014). Securing circulation pharmaceutically: Antiviral stockpiling and pandemic preparedness in the European Union. *Security Dialogue, 45*(5), 440–457. https://doi.org/10.1177/0967010614530072.

27. Srivastava, V., Kumar, R., Wani, M. Y., Robinson, K., & Ahmad, A. (2024). Role of artificial intelligence in early diagnosis and treatment of infectious diseases. *Infectious Diseases*. https://www.semanticscholar.org/paper/778e1cc1cce627e48a9d9c5aa1b6cf844be68b94 (accessed on 6 May 2025).

28. Strasser, S. (2024). Protecting frontline nurses: What will it take? A review of policy, practice and lessons learned from high consequence infectious diseases like Ebola and COVID-19. *Medical Research Archives*. https://www.semanticscholar.org/paper/c9163733c7da15522289c39bdce6e387437f9165 (accessed on 6 May 2025).

29. Waitzberg, R., Spatayev, Y., Atanasova, S., & Zapata, T. (2024). 2.I. Scientific session: Addressing vaccine hesitancy: From understanding determinants to implementing targeted strategies. *The European Journal of Public Health, 34*(Supplement 1). https://www.semanticscholar.org/paper/dab2dcc1651a9f6b963fe993353655da99fd8e56 (accessed on 6 May 2025).

30. Zhang, D., Yang, Y., Li, M., Lu, Y., Liu, Y., Jiang, J., Liu, R., et al. (2021). Ecological barrier deterioration driven by human activities poses fatal threats to public health due to emerging infectious diseases. *Engineering, 10*, 155–166. https://doi.org/10.1016/j.eng.2020.11.002.

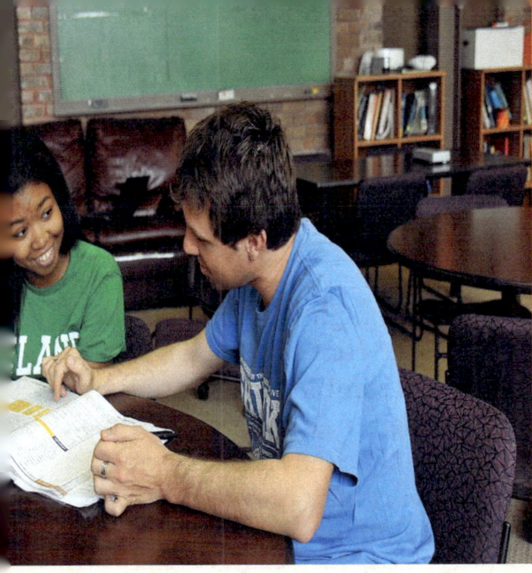

Chapter 14

SOCIOECONOMIC AND BEHAVIORAL FACTORS

Contents

Introduction

Socioeconomic status and the way individuals act determine health outcomes, particularly for drug use. According to research, an individual's wealth can influence daily decisions, such as whether they should smoke. This is rather obvious for lower- to middle-income nations, where education and healthcare are less accessible. For instance, during the time of COVID-19, some qualitative studies observed huge changes in smoking behavior and questioned why some continue smoking and others attempt to quit. It is worth mentioning that individuals having harder economic times tend to encounter additional barriers—habitual and psychological hurdles that public health interventions don't always address effectively. When you peer closer, you notice how what people understand and perceive about health hazards can influence their behavior. During crises such as the COVID pandemic, knowledge of the risks associated with smoking can differ significantly based on one's economic status. Most studies uncover that while individuals know tobacco is bad for them, it is hard to alter habits that have been around for decades due to a combination of factors—from financial difficulties to lacking the necessary assistance from friends or relatives. In most instances, combining findings on behavior, attitudes, and financial burdens is essential in creating health initiatives that succeed. All of these interconnected factors require approaches that combine individual experiences with the general social environment to provide improved smoking cessation opportunities. Another compelling approach relates to the new application of machine learning to the study of high blood pressure and its accompanying risk—a place where behavior and economic influences converge. Scientists, in their efforts to enhance heart health, are discovering machine learning can combine conventional risk factors with information on economic and behavioral drivers, providing a new perspective in managing health. This technological enhancement is not only useful for diagnosis and treatment strategies but also illustrates the reasons why we need to include all the various determinants of health. When these factors cross, researchers can construct intricate, occasionally odd, predicting models that lay the groundwork for tailored treatments, ultimately seeking to enhance health equity and outcomes among individuals from diverse economic backgrounds.

Definition of Socioeconomic Factors

Individuals' activities are difficult to pinpoint without considering where they reside and what they encounter on a daily basis. More often than not, you will discover that social and economic circumstances—the kind some refer to as socioeconomic factors—have a tremendous role in determining daily life. Consider things such as how much someone is paid, what education they receive, what work they do, and even what society perceives them to be; all of these determine who gets superior care, access to valuable resources, or just a generally easier life. These factors aren't background noise, however—they cause behavior we observe in domains such as health, academic achievement, and mobility. More often than not, individuals of varying financial or societal standings do end up existing in distinct worlds, which then influences how they make choices, handle stress, and take care of overall health. Looking a little deeper, you can find that these conditions based on socioeconomic status are ingrained within the very fabric of society. Economic security, for example, frequently sets the stage for improved education and, subsequently, more professional opportunities. To illustrate, those brought up in affluent households typically have significantly greater access to high-quality healthcare and schooling, which predisposes them to more positive circumstances in virtually all aspects of life. Conversely, individuals who are in worse economic positions may struggle with something like food instability or spotty access to healthcare—problems that tend to increase levels of stress and hinder individual development. In a lot of situations, this tends to create some sort of vicious cycle where negative factors feed upon themselves, rendering it even more difficult for the individual to overcome the limitations of their situation. Ultimately, the effects of these social and economic issues extend far beyond individual existence—they have ripples that reach throughout communities overall. Poor neighborhoods frequently struggle with a concentration of issues like increased crime, lack of healthy food sources, and inferior healthcare services, which merely exacerbates both individual and community issues. In such settings, survival tends to take center stage over personal advancement, eroding the social connections and support systems that can promote individuals. Obviously, this combination of difficulties requires holistic interventions that address both personal behaviors and the underlying economic circumstances. By understanding how all these pieces fit together, public health experts and policymakers can design strategies that not only boost individual outcomes but also help build healthier, more equitable communities overall (Lai et al., 2021; Lovallo, 2016) (Figure 14.1).

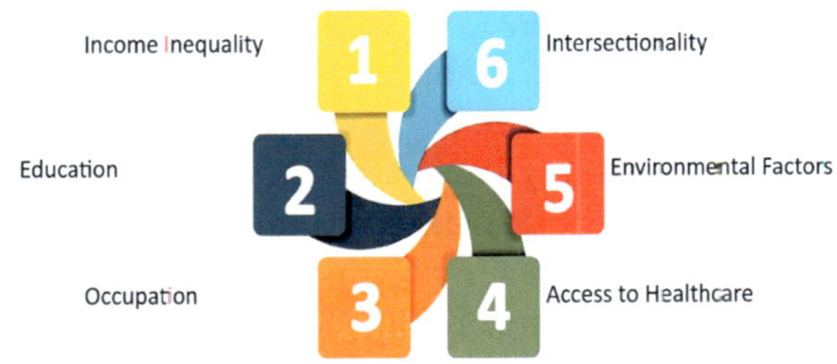
Income Inequality
1
6
Intersectionality
Education
2
5
Environmental Factors
Occupation
3
4
Access to Healthcare

Figure 14.1. The socioeconomic factors.

Source: FasterCapital. (n.d.). *Mortality Differentials: Investigating Disparities in Mortality Table Data—Analyzing Socioeconomic Factors and Mortality Rates.*

Definition of Behavioral Factors

Examining what influences our health, daily habits take center stage. Individuals' habits—maintaining personal hygiene, deciding what to eat, and being active—have a direct influence on their overall well-being. Even the speed at which one rushes to visit a doctor or continues with their treatment can change the trajectory of an illness. Most of the time, such daily decisions become the foundation of public health policies that respond to local demands and attempt to fill gaps in treatment, particularly infections (Alam et al., 2024; Shaheen et al., 2025). It is a testament that what we do on a daily basis is far from insignificant. The contribution of such behaviors becomes evident if we study how diseases propagate and exacerbate in populations. For instance, irregular usage of protective equipment, such as not using bed nets for protection against mosquito-borne diseases—can result in increased infection rates. Where economic and educational hurdles are genuine, individuals might be unable to implement healthier habits merely because they do not have the means. Research tends to indicate that greater awareness and proactiveness toward healthcare correlate closely with improved results, connecting behavior with socioeconomic conditions. By considering the backgrounds of victims, experts emphasize that we must have interventions specifically designed to promote healthier habits among our most vulnerable members (Alam et al., 2024; Shaheen et al., 2025). When day-to-day behaviors combine with economic difficulties, the scene becomes fairly muddled. Individuals in lower-income communities tend to experience more illnesses—not only due to insufficient access to resources, but also because they don't always engage in the healthiest habits. There is usually a glaring knowledge gap regarding how to avoid illness, and this lack can hinder preventive action, perpetuating the cycle of unhealthy status. At times, these cross-cutting issues of economics and behavior even feed into one another, creating continuing problems. Public health initiatives must thus aim to increase education and make resources more accessible, emphasizing just how important it is for all to attempt to adopt healthier lifestyles (Alam et al., 2024; Shaheen et al., 2025).

Importance of Studying the Interplay Between These Factors

Socioeconomic conditions and daily routines blend together in interesting combinations when it comes to health concerns such as obesity, particularly in individuals who are already predisposed. It is fascinating to see how, in many instances, an individual's financial situation can influence decisions such as what one eats or the amount of activity they engage in. For example, the Longitudinal Study of Australian Children indicates that biological factors account for approximately 29% of obesity variation—while family income appears to contribute more than 49% (Gautam et al., 2025). That emphasizes that health outcomes do not solely depend on personal decisions; They also closely relate to broader, sometimes nearly invisible, economic determinants. Essentially, in designing targeted interventions, we must remember such conflating influences, particularly for individuals trapped in strained economic situations. Occasionally the combination of behavior and economic strain creates an even more messy scenario—specifically when considering mental health. Stress, for example, in pressure situations such as immediately before surgery, has a tendency to confuse how individuals perceive pain and cope with stress (Padhy et al., 2023). And when times get tough economically, people may find themselves with coping strategies that are doing more harm than good—if not exacerbating general health problems. For the most part, this interaction highlights the importance of health policies addressing socioeconomic and psychological issues as elements of one confused knot, not as discrete issues. Knowing these interwoven factors can go a very long way toward improved, more responsive interventions across different communities. Examining more closely how our economic realities influence behaviors transcend merely impacting health—it permeates the very essence of society. Knowing that what we make (or don't) can direct our everyday habits lays down a sort of foundation for more equitable resource distribution and wiser policies. It's the same with obesity, for instance. Plugging only the behavioral gap without sorting out economic stress is like trying to fight windmills. Even evidence from the LSAC suggests we could make a significant impact on obesity levels among children and adolescents if we concentrate on closing income disparities (Gautam et al., 2025). Thus, while it may begin as an intellectual question, these findings necessitate actual action in policy and community initiatives—propelling us toward a future where health equity is not only a pleasant notion, but a reality.

14.1. Overview of Socioeconomic Factors

Different components of the socioeconomic puzzle—whom wealth is held by, what education is offered, and what type of job prospects there are—can determine how individuals and communities behave. In most instances, they influence health, civic engagement, and quality of life. When there are big gaps in money, people sometimes struggle to access basic goods, which ultimately decreases school success and reduces community involvement. There is this notion, highlighted in Thelma (2024), that being informed as a citizen is an important driver of social advancement. All of this encourages us to support policies that reduce these economic inequalities, eventually creating more room for democratic rule. Culture also enters the fray with economic issues, intertwining a very knotty social landscape. Individuals' ethnic origins and distinct cultural histories frequently dictate the way they perceive and address common challenges even mental health issues. A portion of research indicates that what clinicians gain from the history of a client can modify how treatment is managed and the outcome that it achieves.

In research featured by Addo (2018), one gets the feeling that a lack of cultural sensitivity by healthcare workers can fuel additional misunderstandings, leaving certain communities feeling further marginalized. This kind of goes to show why incorporating cultural understandings into services and curriculum plans could be so beneficial in responding to these challenges. When considering socioeconomic issues, it is impossible not to notice the obstinate structural hurdles that continue to keep inequality on life support. Systemic prejudice and restricted access to quality healthcare and education affect marginal groups the most. Civic education—in line with Thelma (2024)—tends to raise awareness regarding these discriminatory practices, and its inclusion in schools becomes even more imperative because of it. Even further, efforts to guarantee equal resource access, mobilizing community participation, and collaborating across groups could mitigate some of these ill effects. Overall, a mixed strategy that depends on both civic education and cultural awareness appears fairly central to braiding our society together tighter and increasing the prospects for long-term progress (Figure 14.2).

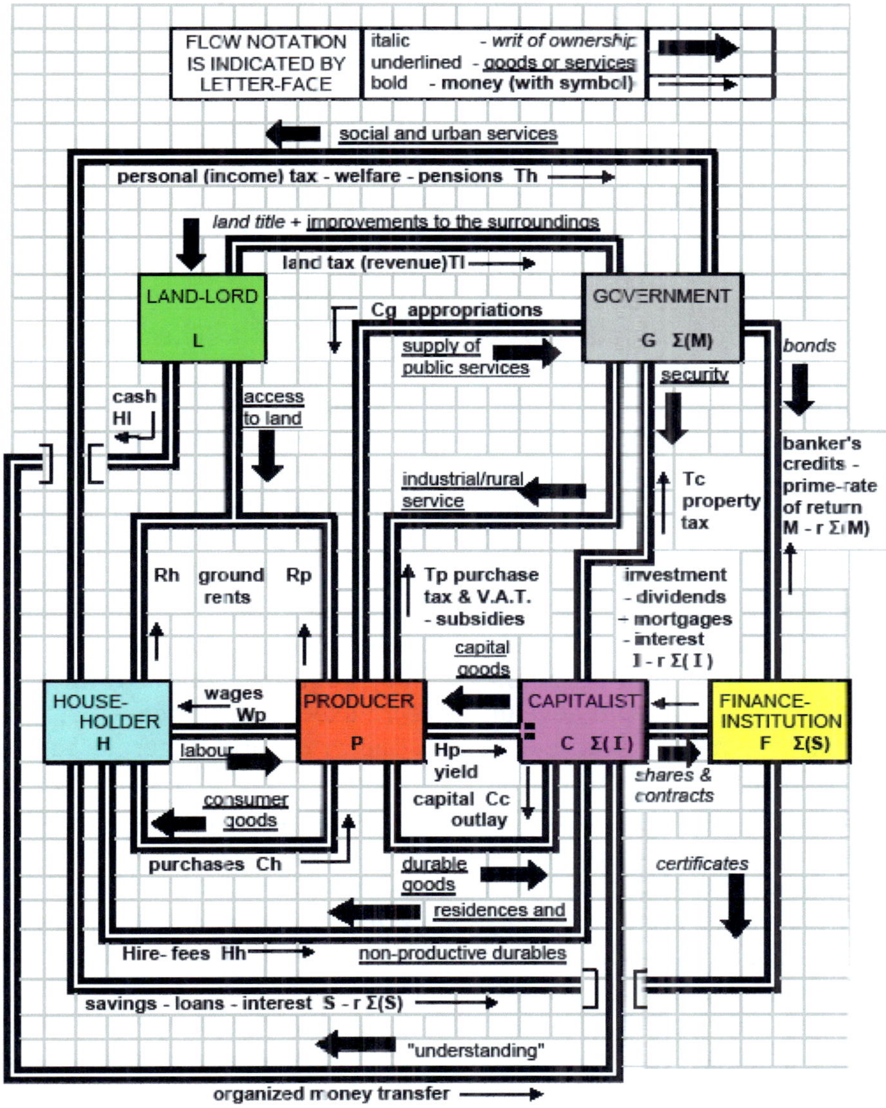

Figure 14.2. Overview of socioeconomic factors.

Source: https://en.wikipedia.org/wiki/File:DiagFuncMacroSyst.pdf

14.1.1. Income Levels and Economic Status

Income and economic circumstances tend to determine health results, particularly for individuals with more challenging situations. Studies indicate that individuals with less income sometimes cannot afford fresh, healthy food and find themselves relying on ultra-processed options that are not exactly healthy-friendly. Children and adolescents in these populations may be losing out on the advantages of a varied diet, which could even change the composition of gut bacteria they are dependent on—although strangely, some more recent studies have not found an apparent association between these foods and shifts in gut flora (Alves et al., 2025). In most instances, it appears that the relationship between what one eats and his or her overall economic status is more complicated than we initially believed, prompting us to extend research for it to deduce everything. Economic status is not only reflected in food choices; it also appears to influence how individuals cope with stress and make decisions during times of adversity. In the COVID-19 pandemic, for example, people in low and middle-income groups demonstrated changes in tobacco use—a messy combination of behavioral and emotional changes that at times is difficult to define with right-or-wrong data. Some even reported mixed emotions regarding stopping smoking or concerned about the danger the virus presented, showing a type of everyday battle that is not always easily contained within academic brackets. These diverse tales highlight how economic stress can at times drive individuals to develop habits that are detrimental to their well-being. Money concerns also have a long shadow over general health experiences, tending to reinforce disadvantage cycles. Individuals in lower-income environments are constantly battered by environmental stress, patchy access to quality healthcare, and scarce health know-how, all of which erode well-being. When you combine behavioral elements with economic pressures, you realize that focused policies must be put in place to alleviate such pressures. By addressing both lifestyle habits and economic issues, better support can be created for disadvantaged groups, increasing the overall quality of life and closing the health gaps observed between different income levels (Alves et al., 2025).

14.1.2. Education and Access to Resources

Socioeconomic status and education access mess with how people learn in real, sometimes surprising, ways. Income, schooling, and even what you eat all play into whether someone can tap into helpful resources like tech tools or nutritious food. For example, those with deeper pockets usually get healthier food options and can grab onto newer learning aids—generally speaking, these folks end up more proactive about their education. Even some studies indicate that the more money you have and the more educated you are, the less likely you are to engage in health-risk behaviors, which pretty much connects school participation and overall health. These findings suggest that focused assistance, particularly during times of adversity such as the COVID-19 pandemic when disparities become all too glaring—may indeed increase community health and resiliency (Chakraborty et al., 2025). Digital resources and online access are the big thing in today's learning environment, although the landscape isn't the same for all. Many lower-income students just don't have what they require—simple tech, good internet, or a relaxed study area—just exacerbating the cycle of disadvantage. Research indicates that without these digital fundamentals, learning participation can decline. For the most part, gaining a handle on device ownership and access to connect online is central to solving these problems (Joshi et al., 2024). Teachers and policymakers are now in search of new ideas that enhance access to technology and digital content, with a view to allowing underserved communities not only to keep pace academically but also to participate more deeply in society. If schools are going to equalize the playing field, they can't just disregard the way that culture and routine habits appear in a student's learning. Parenting, gender roles, and community values all find their way into the equation and alter the distribution of resources. Research tends to suggest that when learning strategies are collaborative and culturally receptive, students become more engaged and motivated. It is vital to recall that additional money and formal schooling don't act by themselves—they interact with social expectations and norms in complex ways. By understanding such interconnections, educators can modify strategies to serve varied needs, creating equitable opportunities for all. In general, achieving this type of equity involves taking a layered strategy that weaves together understanding of both resources and the day-to-day contexts of learning (Joshi et al., 2024; Chakraborty et al., 2025) (Figure 14.3).

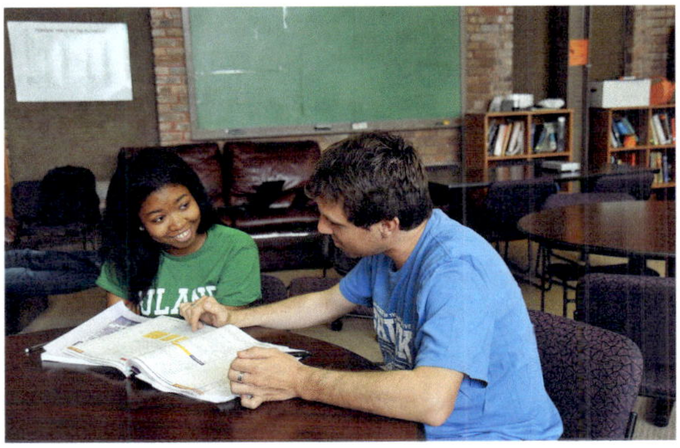

Figure 14.3. Education and access to resources.

Source: By Tulane Public Relations - Tutoring CenterUploaded by TulaneSally Tulane Public Relations, CC BY 2.0, https://commons.wikimedia.org/w/index.php?curid=29678987

14.1.3. Employment Opportunities and Job Stability

Socioeconomic determinants and career choices tend to become entangled in unforeseen manners. Individuals choose vocational training based on both interest and the fact that the near-by employment world—conditioned by their background—pushes them in particular directions. In Kenya's Taita Taveta County, research suggests that family businesses and good career guidance can influence trainees' decisions, implying that a dash of informed counsel does make a difference. Surprisingly enough, even where there are great expectations, the fact of job vacancies does not always guide an individual in a precise direction, which could indicate a disconnection between training selected and vacancies (Chola et al., 2025). Job security is intimately associated with having consistent employment, particularly in private consignment work environments. When people maintain a steady, even though perhaps irregular, upgrade of skills, they are more apt to remain in jobs securely. Research of employees at private employment agencies reveals that personal goals, income, and age contribute significantly to the way careers develop. In most instances, individuals who yearn for greater autonomy and some genuine power in the workplace are more likely to change jobs to find that elusive stability (Huh et al., 2024). All of this appears to emphasize the notion that tailored educational programs not only prepare individuals for employment but also assist in developing a sense of security in the workplace. Training and education, in general, are the very staples of increased employability and job security. The increasingly dynamic labor market of today compels employees to continually adjust and reskill, hence becoming better candidates for jobs. Experiments indicate that the combination of one's socioeconomic status with good training intricately outlines their professional journey. Institutions thus have a genuine mandate to introduce programs that address these imbalances, particularly in the marginalized communities. By emphasizing empowering individuals through specialized career guidance and hands-on learning programs, it is possible to improve both employment opportunities and long-term stability, creating a more robust economic base for individuals and society (Huh et al., 2024; Chola et al., 2025).

14.2. Overview of Behavioral Factors

Socioeconomic status and daily action intertwine, powerfully influencing the way individuals take care of their health and make decisions. People with lower incomes typically experience setbacks in attempting to obtain adequate medical care, technology, and simple advice on controlling ailments. For instance, continuous glucose monitoring (CGM) devices—essential for maintaining diabetes under control—rarely appear among these populations. And it has nothing to do with having money; even one's ethnicity and social life enter the picture. As a general rule, this chaotic problem is not only an issue of income but also of a entire range of system-level barriers curtailing access to new health technologies, which have direct ramifications in diabetes care outcomes, and indicating the necessity for targeted interventions (Been et al., 2024). Aside from individual health decisions, behavior also becomes shaped by how individuals perceive their environments and the communities they belong to. Occasionally, the narrative spills forth in unfamiliar form—when sports travelers engage in neighborhood activities, they find themselves constructing conclusions on the social and economic impacts they observe, which can even determine whether they choose to return. This type of interaction, where personal impressions and larger socioeconomic atmospheres blend, illustrates how choices aren't made in isolation. In most instances, picking up on these behavioral subtleties is very significant to establishing stronger community ties and even pushing economic development in small ways (Ramos et al., 2024). Stepping back, seeing behavior as an important piece of socioeconomic puzzles opens us up to a larger picture. Many of these psychological and social factors cut through our daily behaviors—influencing everything from what we consume to the way we access health care. Individuals in lower-income groups tend to fall into riskier behaviors sometimes simply because, literally, they don't have resources or good information, which only exacerbates cycles of bad health. That fact emphasizes why community-oriented approaches, ones that encourage healthier behaviors and increase overall health literacy, are so vital. Even educational initiatives that attempt to be culturally sensitive and cost-effective can go some way in reducing the gaps left by these social disparities. Overall, combining information regarding behavior with economic information is imperative for informing public health policy that is going to reduce health inequities (Figure 14.4).

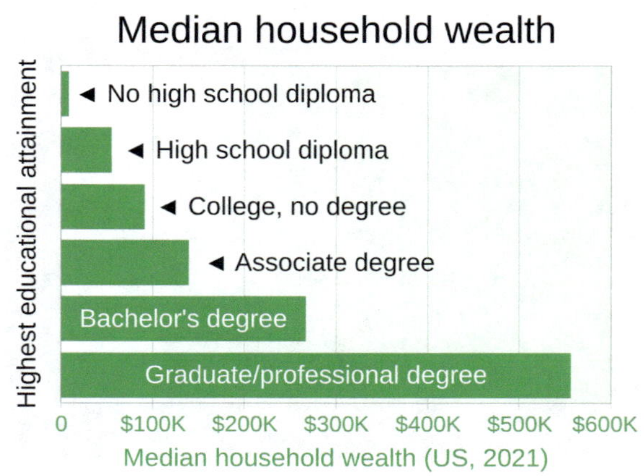

Figure 14.4. Overview of behavioral factors.

Source: By RCraig09 - Own work, CC BY-SA 4.0, https://commons.wikimedia.org/w/index.php?curid=149016754.

14.2.1. Lifestyle Choices and Health Behaviors

Many researchers have looked at how the economic status of an individual relates to daily choices and the influence on our health appears to be substantial. Consider, as an illustration, a study of Libyan undergraduates revealed an alarming trend—numerous female students, whose expenditure on food and income are strongly interrelated, have high levels of obesity. For the most part, having less money seems to go hand in hand with choosing poorer diets, which in turn increases the likelihood of obesity and all of its complications. The research even identifies variations in how men and women eat and exercise, suggesting that tailored measures should be adjusted to accommodate these discrepancies. To summarize, by focusing on these crossover issues, public health strategies could potentially further encourage healthier options among communities living in economic disadvantage (Lahter et al., 2025). Uncovering a bit more about the places where income and health converge, another study emphasizes that money concerns have a central role in activating threats of disease such as diabetes. Low-income individuals are more likely to demonstrate a greater prevalence of issues—primarily because they usually don't have convenient access to resources and adequate know-how regarding healthy living. Day-to-day decisions regarding food and physical activity are heavily influenced by one's financial status, so it is practically imperative to advocate for policies that close this gap. For example, programs that provide nutritional advice and low-cost access to healthier diets may empower people to make healthy choices about their food. In nearly every way, integrating economic conditions into health research provides policymakers with a better understanding of the origin of health inequities (Horestani et al., 2024).

Those observations extend far beyond personal behavior and require more expansive public health policies designed to create healthier communities. Economic conditions tend to lay the groundwork—either opening doors to healthy habits or putting up surprises in their path. It appears that initiatives encouraging greater exercise and improved diets, particularly in poor communities, could have profound impacts on overall health. Concurrently, a greater understanding of how different populations make practical, everyday decisions can assist in developing health campaigns that resonate with them. Overall, this multi-level strategy not only aims to reduce health threats but also pushes society toward being healthier and more proactive about health, eventually enhancing public results (Horestani et al., 2024; Lahter et al., 2025) (Figure 14.5).

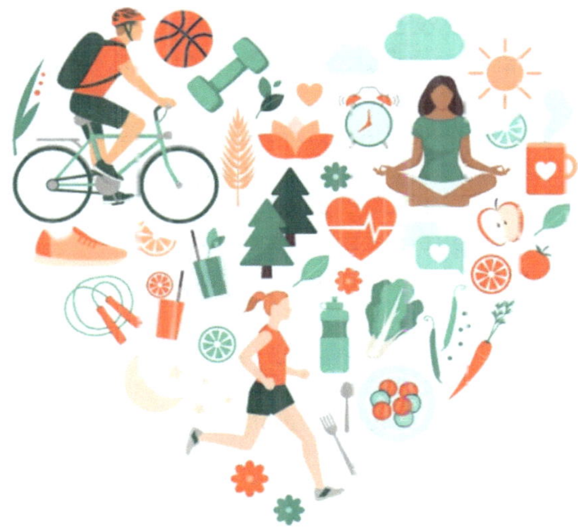

Figure 14.5. Lifestyle choices and health behaviors.

Source: https://static.wixstatic.com/media/25b00d_492547eb5017499c8e569d102b9f5350~mv2.png/v1/fill/w_568,h_524,al_c,lg_1,q_85,enc_avif,quality_auto/25b00d_492547eb5017499c8e569d102b9f5350~mv2.png

14.2.2. Social Norms and Peer Influences

Adolescence is complicated. Discovering who you are usually means maneuvering your internal self-concept among all manner of family, peer, and larger community expectations. Teens inadvertently adopt the general values of their communities—even if they do not realize it at first, community signals permeate. More often than not, the contemporary digital world, complete with the round-the-clock chattering on the topics of beauty and achievement, has much to say regarding how these concepts come to be formed. Typically, research finds that what society and cultural factors posit, combined with the hubbub of social media, informs teenagers' notions of beauty. This then goes on to impact their self-esteem and mental wellbeing. Knowing how all of these parts fit together can guide us toward more effective ways to assist youth in creating a healthier sense of self, one that resists too narrow, conventional expectations (Varghese & Akshaya, 2024). Peer influence is a big deal, particularly in fostering entrepreneurial aspirations among students. As it happens, the atmosphere emanating from friends and class settings has more influence than many would think. For the most part, students are inspired and directed by their peers, pushing them toward creative endeavors in subtle ways. Classrooms that fuse social and entrepreneurial concepts appear to generate interest, showing that having a positive role model can give a student confidence to handle future obstacles. Understanding these multi-layered influences may even give rise to adjustments in teaching strategies, inculcating an attitude of experimentation that carries throughout current days' changing economic reality (Khoirunisa et al., 2024). Naturally, the effect of social norms is not the same for all. Various collectives—divided by gender, ethnicity, or socioeconomic status—may discover Them to be differently expected. Overall, these differences imply that every teen's experience is different; the values and expectations they absorb can be different in unexpected ways. Scholars investigating these intersections tend to emphasize the importance of a more inclusive framework that takes into account diverse identities. Ultimately, actual progress in increasing self-esteem and mental health among youth comes from acknowledging that one-size-fits-all expectations simply do not work (Varghese & Akshaya, 2024).

14.2.3. Psychological Factors and Mental Health

Financial resources and social support make a significant difference in our mental health. People who lack more of it commonly struggle with day-to-day money concerns and restricted healthcare—problems that can drive rates of depression and anxiety, and even enhance the risk of heart issues (Abdullah et al., 2024). Public health interventions, in general, should be concerned about these intertwined causes instead of addressing them as individualized issues.

When you notice that lower socioeconomic status brings additional stress, it logically follows that one should incorporate mental healthcare into comprehensive care; after all, emotional and physical well-being go hand in hand. Childhood adversity, such as neglect or trauma, sometimes persists far into adulthood. In most marginalized groups, where economic setbacks render support systems weak, these initial difficulties become all too frequent, and they can slowly erode emotional strength. These repeated stresses tend to result in coping strategies that are not necessarily healthy—and even propagate these patterns through generations to come. Research, in general, indicates that assisting people and their families early on can slowly alleviate the long-term consequences of early difficulties (Alsughier, 2024). Establishing programs that target early mental healthcare may well lead to improved development and healthier community connections. Culture provides yet another dimension to how individuals cope with mental adversity. Different cultural tales and traditions at times tend to present mental health concerns in a negative way, which ultimately makes individuals reluctant to seek help. Such stigma, though subtle, tends to entrap individuals with chronic anguish and loneliness. Recognizing that mental health is not necessarily solely about individual issues—but also cultural and socioeconomic contexts—may be the secret to crafting services that truly benefit everyone (Abdullah et al., 2024; Alsughier, 2024). By thoughtfully crafting policies honoring these combined influences, we might find strategies that reduce stigma and promote overall wellness even if the process is not entirely seamless (Figure 14.6).

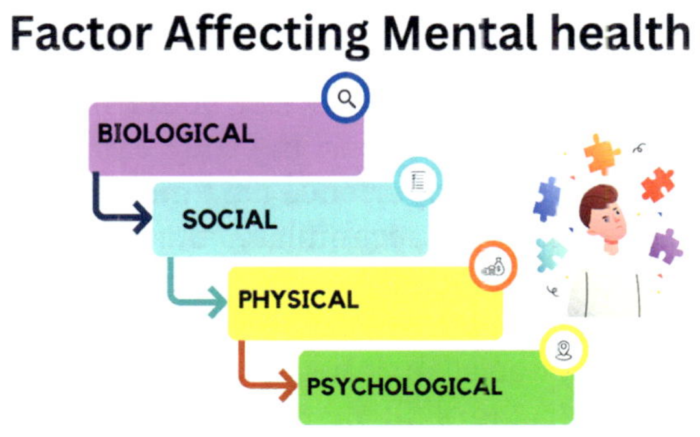

Figure 14.6. Psychological factors and mental health.

Source: Prep With Harshita. (2023). *Champagne and Colorful Step-By-Step Build Your Business Graph 4.*

14.3. Impact of Socioeconomic Status on Behavior

There is no shortage of surprises in how social status — or SES — interacts with everyday behaviors. The less well-funded are left with fewer opportunities to reach for health food, adequate care, even community programs that can help out. This type of deficit does not simply take its toll on the body; it can get at the mind as well, sometimes pushing people to turn to coping mechanisms such as more drinking or other less-than-optimal solutions. Studies, for the most part, indicate that when a person feels further down the social rung, they might begin to flaunt pricey things as a means of masking underlying insecurities (Yang et al., 2025). Effectively, they shed light on larger, messier trends in our own lives and society as a whole. Examining health behaviors more closely, the connection between SES and how we live isn't that difficult to see. Research into older adult memory and cognitive problems suggests lower SES is a large red flag: those with less often experience more cognitive issues than those in higher strata (Feng et al., 2024). Older adults in more affluent groups typically have a bit of a cushion against mental decay, particularly when consideration is given to lifestyle choices made as part of daily life. On the whole, the promotion of healthier lifestyles could smooth some of the harshest rough edges that exist between economic groups, eventually moving us toward a world where the burden of problems such as cognitive decline isn't so disproportionately borne. Social life also comes under the sway of economic factors, even on social media. There is a sense that merely browsing network pages can make individuals feel more excluded, which, paradoxically, may lead them to spend on flashier purchases to 'keep up' with others (Yang et al., 2025). This trend, whereby ostentatious consumption tends to dominate over true connection, results in a vicious cycle of overspending and dissatisfaction that exacerbates pre-existing problems. When you put all of this together, it is obvious that addressing SES is not merely about bank accounts; it also involves confronting the habits and emotions that accompany our station in life, leading to a more equitable, healthier future.

14.3.1. Correlation Between Income and Health Behaviors

If you look at society, you see that how much money someone has can determine how well people take care of themselves. Those who have more income get better access to primary health care—think checkups or mental health counseling—so they make decisions that result in healthier lives. Economic security, in the majority of instances, even appears to mitigate the sort of anxiety that frequently afflicts less affluent individuals, and research indicates that such anxiety if left unmitigated, can cause damage to health. The variation in how individuals eat, exercise, or adhere to medical guidance begins to become apparent, all intertwined with the general economic situation in which they reside (Murthy, 2017). So, comprehending that web of relationships between income and health is important to increasing community well-being. Individuals with less income tend to have their fair share of challenges to maintain good health. Tight budgets sometimes result in forgoing healthy food, and the endless struggle of day-to-day problems may leave one with no space for exercise—survival may be of higher priority. This cycle of struggle and poor habits appears to trap individuals in a spiral downward, which is reason enough to see why such support for these populations is imperative. The National Mental Health Survey even states that decreased income correlates with an increased risk of mental disorders (Murthy, 2017).

Overall, gaining control over these challenges is critical if we are going to construct health policies that bridge the gap between various income groups. From the perspective of considering the larger picture, these income-based variations in health extend well beyond the person themselves—they pose legitimate challenges for public health systems and policymakers. When communities are left trapped in unhealthy habits due to financial difficulties, it can exacerbate healthcare expenses and place additional strain on already stretched services. In general, this scenario requires thoughtful interventions that aim to enhance health literacy (HL), provide accessible care, and even integrate mental health services into community resources. Some recent writing has indicated that public health initiatives are most likely to be effective when they take into account the varied realities of individuals at all income levels. By combining approaches that meet economic challenges with daily decision-making about health, society may very well inch toward a more level and fair health playing field for all.

14.3.2. Influence of Education on Decision-Making

The people end up making wiser, better-informed decisions due to the learning they experience. A fine education experience isn't merely one of acquiring facts— it accumulates that gut feeling that serves well when things get complicated, be it coping with health issues, financial problems, or everyday social anxieties. On other occasions, it acquires the skill of reading numbers or understanding what risk is; in the majority of instances, individuals who have experienced a more wealthy educational life normally end up picking better things than those who lack this. In a kind of circuitous fashion, becoming accustomed to examining details has the real power to open doors, promoting overall health and even reducing some of the social and economic gaps we experience today. Education also operates more subtly by influencing the way that we perceive the world around us—our individual interpretation of the norms of society is refined as we are subjected to varied perspectives and viewpoints. When students interact with varying viewpoints, they end up thinking about their values, often repeatedly, which makes them better connected to their community. For instance, Sørensen et al. (2012) point out how health info knowledge is not just knowing a whole lot of facts; it is connected with being able to cope with the turns of complicated health systems. What that implies is that by having a firm handle on issues of health, people are better positioned to make decisions regarding preventive care or treatment. Education, in a very real sense, extends beyond imparting information—it shapes how we move through the greater fabric of society. Similarly, the power of education reaches into economic choices and planning for the long term. When individuals gain qualifications, they typically end up opening the doors to more favorable occupations and better-paying jobs, which in turn allows them to budget their spending, investment, and saving in a manner that may not have been available to them before. On the other hand, individuals with a little less formal education often tend to get entangled in responding to short-term needs and not planning long term—a fact well illustrated in certain studies on socioeconomic trajectories (see Riahi et al., 2016). If you step back and take a look, increasing education levels and promoting a sort of critical, reflective thought appears to set the stage for a future in which short-term decisions and long-term strategies are better aligned with the needs of the individual—although the process is not always squeaky clean.

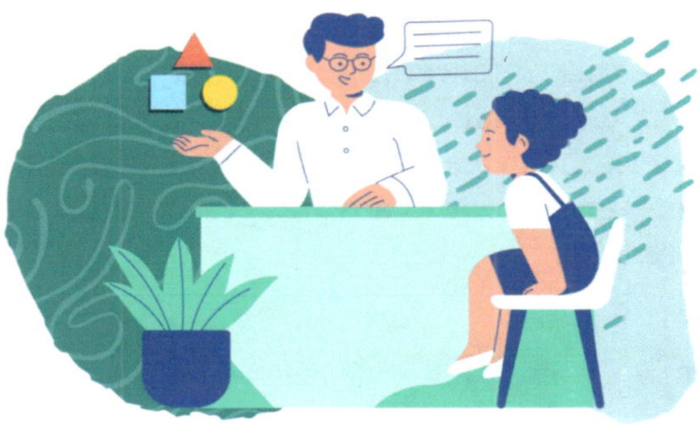

Source: Wellspring Center for Prevention. (2022). *Decision-Making Skills.*

14.3.3. Employment Status and Stress-Related Behaviors

Employment status is closely correlated with stress behaviors, and it reveals social inequities in surprising manners. When individuals are confronted with unemployment or precarious work arrangements, they experience a severe tension that can exacerbate chronic illnesses. A stable job is not merely a matter of bringing home a paycheck—job stability also provides an individual with a sense of identity and belonging. The loss of that anchor can lead to a sense of inadequacy and an increase in anxiety, which, as various studies in general observe, might lead individuals toward self-destructive behaviors like drug abuse or social withdrawal. The pattern itself is more common with communities that are already under the pressure of financial instability, where those added mental pressures tend to pile up. Understanding how employment mixes with stress, then, is pretty essential for crafting effective interventions (Rahmat & Sabila, 2024). Job security, or the lack thereof, plays a big role in shaping mental and physical well-being. Research suggests that feeling secure at work not only keeps one's finances steady but also builds up inner resilience, helping people develop coping skills to better tackle stress. Conversely, employees in short-term, high-stress occupations typically report increased stress levels—leading to conditions like missing appropriate meals or reducing exercise. It's fascinating how such early employment conditions might end up affecting long-term well-being, as well; indeed, the effects of transient work can carry well into the middle and beyond. Overall, these points highlight the necessity for considered workplace policies and improved mental health care, which are more or less necessary for a healthier workforce (Luc et al., 2024). To consider job status as a cause of stress is to take a wider perspective on the social organization we inhabit. Economic insecurity tends to be accompanied by restricted access to medical care, education, and supportive community services, and that combination can boost stress levels. For instance, individuals from lower-income backgrounds might find it hard to find steady work, which in turn fuels a self-perpetuating cycle of stress and ill health. If those conditions compound, it is easy to see why specific job-creation policies and enhanced mental health services are essential. By confronting these system-wide problems, we can begin to chip away at the dichotomy between precarious work and stress-related conduct. This multi-pronged method, according to Rahmat & Sabila (2024), provides a promising path toward improved health equity and an increased quality of life for those hardest struck by economic adversity.

14.4. Impact of Behavioral Factors on Socioeconomic Status

Behavior and social status contribute enormously to health and community outcomes. HL, for example, is frequently the pathway between socioeconomic status and the disparities we observe in health—studies tend to reveal that individuals with lower SES also have lower HL. This may, in turn, influence day-to-day health, quality of life, and even whether an individual utilizes preventive care. Increasing HL may indeed be viewed as a modifiable risk factor, one which may temper the adverse effects of low SES. By advocating for education to enhance HL, communities may ultimately promote healthier behaviors as well as push us toward equitable access to care (Stormacq et al., 2018). Earliest adversity, such as child abuse or neglect, puts another spin on this tale. Individuals exposed to excessive adverse childhood experiences (ACEs) tend to have trouble completing high school or going on protracted periods of unemployment. Such obstacles have a way of entrapping people in the poverty trap—when job and school setbacks compound, earning power decreases. As a rule, the comprehension of such setbacks reinforces that intervening early may be enough to change a person's life. In many instances, interventions to curtail ACEs may also have broader socioeconomic benefits, and they have the potential to break the cycle of poverty transmitted from one generation to another (Metzler et al., 2016). On a bigger scale, the advantages of addressing these behavioral factors extend well beyond individual results.

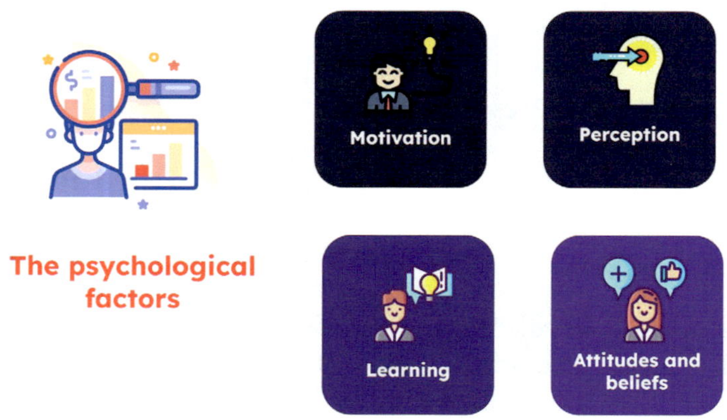

Figure 14.7. Impact of behavioral factors on socioeconomic status.

Source: https://cdn.prod.website-files.com/66dffa95f947b62fb545cc4d/671e4b72237cac00777cc431_AD_4nXddqWCa-TYcu-v-DJBBjHDIB75sS0v7tSp4WZxtUWPyll6tzbpYXalFjggndh4lqKQ4fFkF2UJmXj4nyVzjCihID2G6rUnTSMS8PJ5byiQo5TbwtuaeWWoD5f_F32Z-FTlLo5lcWRF1UL2sbhinZeMkNq0.jpeg

As public policy considers how factors such as HL and early life experiences mix with socioeconomic status, a more complete approach to combating inequality becomes apparent. Investment in community assets, such as early childhood education, mental health care, and programs that enhance HL—can incite healthier patterns and contribute to improved overall economic circumstances. These interventions not only empower individuals but also increase community resilience and, in the best cases, even decrease poverty levels and accompanying health problems. Overall, if societies are to provide authentic, fair opportunities, attention to trends in behavior and early-life problems is rather a necessity when designing sustainable solutions for both economic and health inequalities (Metzler et al., 2016; Stormacq et al., 2018) (Figure 14.7).

14.4.1. Health Behaviors Affecting Productivity

Individuals' daily health decisions have a significant influence on how well they perform—the issue is not merely about being good, but also about longer-term economic and social consequences. Cutting corners on adequate nutrition, regular exercise, or sufficient rest can cloud your mind and even result in additional lost work. This connection tends to arise even more so among individuals struggling with financial struggles and ongoing pressure, which can propel them deeper into poor habits. Consider, for example, groups such as the Gonds tribe where medical care and schooling are not always readily available; comprehending those habits in depth is imperative when attempting to devise solutions that increase productivity. When healthcare stakeholders address such particular issues, they may establish a setting that pushes individuals toward improved decisions, possibly increasing productivity in the process (Singh et al., 2024). Cultural norms also play an actual voice in how individuals manage their health, and this consequently impacts productivity across a range of social contexts. What we eat, how we respond when things go wrong, and even our views about exercise are usually laden with tradition. In many instances, traditional approaches prefer particular foods—even if they do not produce a balanced diet—reducing energy and compromising general health. Individuals in low-income positions, say, can find it difficult to place a value on preventive care during regular money matters, too frequently allowing regular checkups and inoculations go by, which could prevent subsequent issues from developing (Ranjan et al., 2024). These areas of lack of care eventually lead to further lost workdays and assist in perpetuating the cycle of poverty and ill health. To address these cultural influences, it is essential to blend in successful health programs that promote healthier habits and, ultimately, enhance productivity among economically disadvantaged groups (Ranjan et al., 2024). Education has a surprisingly close part in this entire picture as well. Most times, higher education accompanies an improved understanding of health information, which enables individuals to make better, more informed decisions about their health. This relationship is particularly clear where an education is not taken for granted; those with lower levels of schooling may have it difficult to make sense of health information, resulting in decisions that detract from their overall well-being. Again turning to the example of the Gonds tribe, targeted educational efforts, particularly for women's health at pivotal points such as menstruation and pregnancy—may tip the scale. Educational programs, being deeply integrated with the efforts of the community, tend to empower citizens, change day-to-day habits, and raise overall productivity. Any plan to promote health and productivity in most instances would need to consider education in addition to cultural and economic obstacles (Singh et al., 2024).

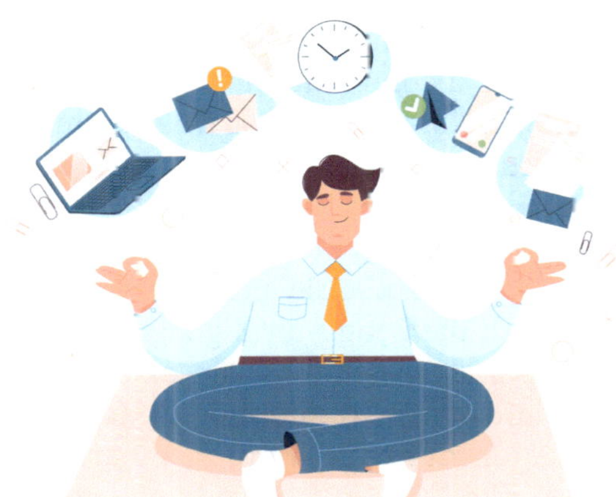

Source: Entrepreneur. (n.d.). *Image of Person Working on Project.*

14.4.2. Education and Its Role in Behavioral Choices

Education and behavior are intertwined in ways we may not realize. Learning determines how we make decisions on a day-to-day basis—whether that's balancing investment options, selecting a health plan, or even choosing life insurance. Individuals who have more education are better positioned to receive risk, and in the process, they find themselves taking up such decisions as the purchase of real estate; the nature of the schooling they do even alters their reading and processing of information. For instance, a general education enhances consumer competence—a decisive factor when resolving life insurance decisions—since research has indicated that income and availability of information can be used to predict the behavior of buying insurance (Methasani et al., 2025). If you look at things generally, education tends to be paired up with socioeconomic status, and that combination has its own influence on behavior. More often than not, higher levels of education lead to better career opportunities and higher wages, which can in turn influence investments or insurance decisions. Even some research goes so far as to identify that education is a key determinant of whether people go for investments such as REITs or other money tools. Nevertheless, pure traditional economic considerations alone cannot fully account for why individuals invest as they do—there is a combination of educational and psychological forces at play as well (Gothi, 2025). At the end of the day, learning is a powerful force behind major life choices. By nurturing critical thinking and boosting financial smarts, education helps people make decisions that line up with their long-term goals. Educational programs and institutions can also chip away at the confusion surrounding complex financial products, encouraging a broader participation in the market. Other studies have shown that people who have a full education will understand the repercussions of their financial decisions, whether in life insurance or other investments—who in most instances prove just how much education plays a role in influencing our daily decisions.

14.4.3. Social Networks and Economic Opportunities

Social connections can truly determine someone's economic prospects. Individuals tend to gain access to essential resources, good information, and a stable support group through their networks. It is not rare to notice that better-connected individuals, such as the presence of a mentor or an influential professional acquaintance—end up with enhanced employment leads and even higher salaries than others who are less connected. That kind of social advantage allows individuals to better find their way around the labor market, occasionally tipping the scales from stagnation to a decent career boost. For the most part, being in the know socially also means that you're better attuned to opportunities at school, and this can greatly influence academic and economic outcomes. It's also worth considering why students get discouraged from finishing at school. Daily realities such as tight funds and even unreliable family backing play a large role in whether the student remains or leaves. For instance, research conducted at Eloy Alfaro Lay University discovered that a large percentage of students cited financial deficiencies and work-related difficulties as the main explanations for leaving. Such evidence indicates that the presence of a strong, supportive network may be able to alleviate these issues, providing additional encouragement, means, or even alternative choices. Typically, the existence of supportive social connections can help increase a student's resolve to persevere, with just how closely tied social relationships and academic persistence are to one another. Examining further abroad, it appears that improved access to education may also assist with the reduction of crime. A study conducted in Abraka showed a significant correlation between quality education and reduced criminal activity (Agbamu & Irogbo, 2024). They discovered that when individuals disconnect from schooling, crime begins to creep in, a trend that emphasizes the importance of strong schools in keeping communities safe. Investing in schools—and by implication, in building social networks—can set the stage for spaces in which economic and social empowerment flourish. Ultimately, building improved educational opportunities with the support of solid connections to communities does not only lead to jobs; it can introduce a measure of security and satisfaction that serves entire communities (Figure 14.8).

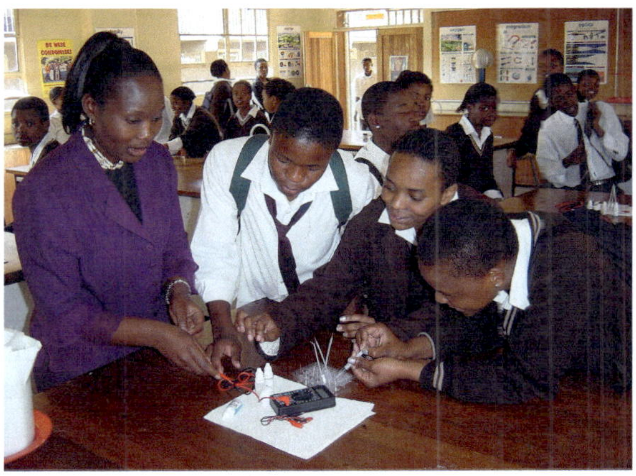

Figure 14.8. Social networks and economic opportunities.

Source: By USAID in Africa - Education in South Africa, Public Domain, https://commons.wikimedia.org/w/index.php?curid=70818192

14.5. Case Studies and Real-World Examples

Case studies demonstrate to us a complicated blend of socioeconomic and behavioral influences in action. Consider, for example, the treatment of head and neck cancer—delays in initiating postoperative radiotherapy (PORT) tend to leave a stark impression on patient results. Recent analyses largely cite that these delays usually arise from a mixture of patient barriers, including general health, comorbid illnesses, and socioeconomic issues that, frankly, stand in the way of getting treated in a timely manner. There are also institutional problems — consider short hospital resources and administrative holdups — that only feed the fire. Through these different considerations, healthcare teams can then organize interventions, eventually improving outcomes and survival rates for such vulnerable patients (Sharma et al., 2024). Another fascinating study examines how dynamic networks are utilized to address public health issues. Researchers, for example, have noted that when you look at the role of socioeconomic factors on network formation, you can observe how vital health information ends up getting disseminated throughout communities. Methods such as time-varying embeddings and dynamic network analysis provide insights into community activity and information transmission — particularly in the case of epidemics. These techniques not only appear to predict disease transmission but also inform interventions intended to enhance health outcomes. The disparity between theoretical models and what occurs on the ground, in a majority of instances, highlights the necessity for more robust frameworks considering behavior dynamics to aid social interventions (Tjøstheim et al., 2022). Health projects in communities also have a powerful narrative of converting socioeconomic issues into opportunities for resilience. For some low-income communities, initiatives centered around food security and nutrition education have yielded very encouraging outcomes. Easy concepts such as creating community plots and conducting workshops on nutrition play a long way in promoting better diets and in creating a community spirit among dwellers. Such a two-stroke strategy impacts both the socioeconomic and behavioral aspects of health—plainly revealing that cooperation among local stakeholders and health agencies benefits. Where socioeconomic obstacles are proactively addressed, the resultant positive, at times even cyclical, changes in behavior can create enduring health improvements in the community. Ultimately, these practical illustrations emphasize the imperative for a comprehensive approach that merges pragmatic behavioral strategies with socioeconomic understanding to realize health equity (Sharma et al., 2024) (Figure 14.9).

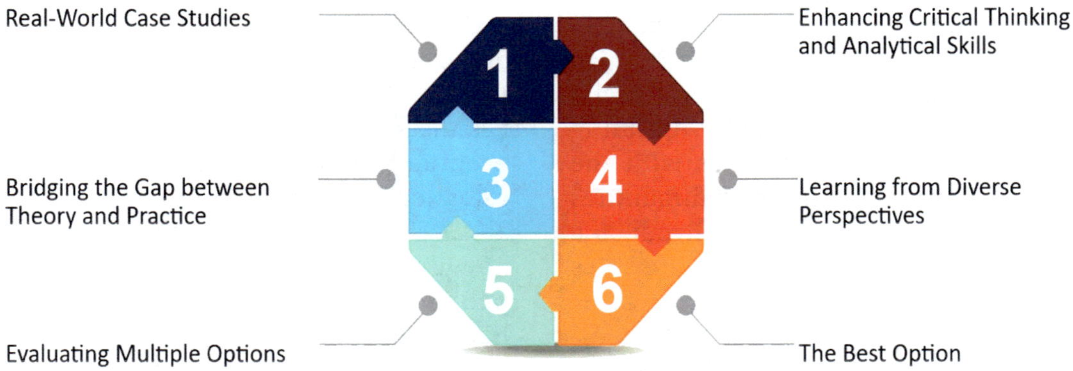

Figure 14.9. Case studies and real-world examples.

Source: FasterCapital. (n.d.). *Chapter9 Case Studies: Analyzing Real World Examples.*

14.5.1. Analysis of Low-Income Communities

Poor communities are confounding environments with a knotted combination of determinants that influence overall health—access to decent healthcare, say, is a genuine problem for mothers and children. Across much of the globe, such as coastal Bangladesh, pregnant working women encounter enormous obstacles when attempting to access even simple antenatal care (ANC) services. It is not merely a matter of access to a nearby clinic; occasionally, limited facilities and native cultural beliefs keep these women's chances of accessing appropriate care in check, which in the majority of situations could improve maternal health as well as child development. Consequences of unavailable maternal resources ultimately prove to be particularly acute in such environments, suggesting that there is a pressing need for interventions aimed at accessibility and community engagement (Al-Mamun & Uzzal, 2025). Consumption patterns in such places also speak of wider economic hardship. Plain simple meals turn out to become an indicator of deeper issues, as individuals sometimes end up with excess fat and inadequate intake of fruits and vegetables. Take the case of sickle cell disease (SCD), for instance—individuals fighting this disease in addition to struggling with economic woes often find their nutritional deficiencies exacerbating their condition. Studies tend to identify that where you live makes a big difference: residents of these economically stressed areas tend to have greater fat consumption and reduced intake of nutrient-dense foods, a pattern that further erodes health. Such link between finances and what ends up on the dinner table not only exposes significant vulnerabilities but also highlights the value of community-based nutritional programs (Ally et al., 2024). Addressing these problems requires a combination of strategies that address both the social and behavioral aspects of health. It is about increasing community awareness of existing health and nutrition services and making quality care an everybody affair in everyday life. In most instances, action-oriented, locally adapted interventions, such as those in coastal areas or among individuals with SCD—can bring significant changes. Policymakers, healthcare professionals, and community leaders must unite, each contributing a part of the puzzle, to create strategies that suit the individual needs of these groups. This type of collaboration could just lead to a healthier, more even community, even if the road there is a little lopsided at times.

14.5.2. Behavioral Interventions in Public Health

Cardiovascular disease and diabetes blend together in ways that require prevention measures attuned to daily habits and financial concerns. Public health campaigns, such as campaigns to quit smoking, eat healthier, and get more exercise, frequently hold hope even if the outcomes are not always simplistic. For instance, reaching out to older folks or those struggling financially, using ideas about how people change, can spark healthier routines in unexpected ways. Data keeps nudging us to note that lifestyle choices and socioeconomic hurdles both play a big part in these diseases, meaning successful interventions have to tackle personal actions along with bigger systemic issues (Amornortey et al., 2025). Income, in most instances, is a heavyweight determinant of how health outcomes unfold. During times of financial constraint, diabetes makes its presence known more frequently, with limited availability of care and health expertise lurking behind the lower-income populace. Public health policies are gradually married to the notion of addressing income as a key ingredient in their strategy. Initiatives that combine financial assistance or modest incentives with hands-on advice on prevention and nutrition appear to resonate with individuals experiencing economic difficulties—a strategy that addresses current needs while developing sustained resilience within populations (Horestani et al., 2024). Behavioral interventions in public health ought to remain adaptable rather than fixed. Local circumstances and specific anecdotes count a great deal, so making sense to create programs based on what particular neighborhoods require is reasonable. Consider low-income communities devastated by heart disease and diabetes—tailoring efforts there can bring about genuinely visible improvements. Engaging with community organizations frequently highlights actual local issues, organizing efforts that feel authentic and shifting over time. Ultimately, basing public health programs on both behavior change and economic facts is necessary to erode health disparities and improve the general well-being of communities (Amornortey et al., 2025; Horestani et al., 2024) (Figure 14.10).

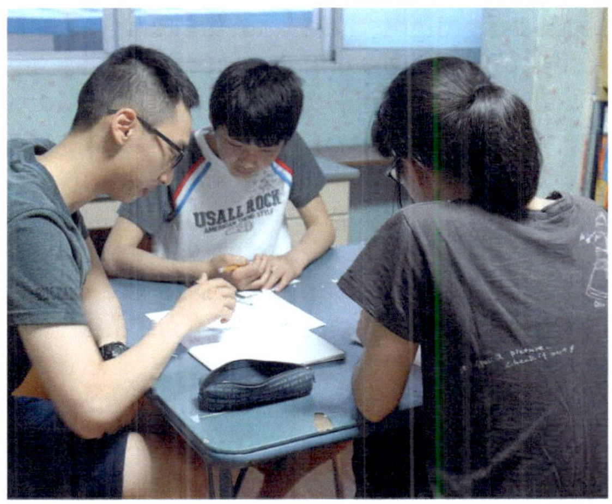

Figure 14.10. Behavioral interventions in public health.

Source: By Pfc. Sung-jun Lim - This image has been extracted from another file, Public Domain, https://commons.wikimedia.org/w/index.php?curid=139505283

14.5.3. Success Stories of Socioeconomic Mobility

Socioeconomic mobility is not just about individual determination—it illustrates how our decisions intersect with larger, sometimes messy, systems. Education is a case in point; success stories are often told of how children from disadvantaged backgrounds can rise out of poverty through determination and ingenuity. Jessica McCrory Calarco has examined how parenting practices, usually associated with class, influence children's school outcomes. Middle-class parents, whose individualistic strategies provide their children with an advantage in being able to navigate the world of academics, are a prime example. When school inequality remains in places, these dynamics make all the difference. Calarco's research indicates that if children are taught to advocate for themselves—a quality prevalent within most middle-class households—they fare better and increase their prospects of climbing up the social ladder (Foley, 2018). All of these episodes highlight the importance of parental involvement and resource access, and they emphasize the need for policies that can address these long-standing shortcomings. Migration throws another fascinating wrinkle into the narrative of social mobility. Recently, scholarship has been more interested in how transnational connections enable individuals to create both economic and social capital. Individuals who migrate tend to rely on their networks to find their way around, even while maintaining some connection to home. The two-way connections sometimes serve as a buffer—either through financial remittances or mutual cultural know-how—and assist them in settling down. Through exchanging resources across borders, such migrant networks tend to initiate perceptible steps up, illustrating that the gain made through worldwide connections can be quite large (Levitt et al., 2007). This combination of experiences illustrates that dealing with mobility entails both traditional and contemporary paths to economic success. In considering success in socioeconomic mobility, a variety of considerations come into consideration. The tales we tell—of people who were raised locally or of people who traveled abroad—emphasize the virtues of community support, a little grit, and intelligent use of resources. For many, those who make it rise have beaten long odds by drawing on both individuals will and wider social support. Looking ahead, it seems critical for policymakers and educators to consider these diverse elements that shape how people move forward. By building more inclusive spaces that emphasize both individual empowerment and needed systemic change, we can get closer to equalizing opportunities for everyone. Most times, current studies indicate that we have to continue grappling with the social and economic determinants that control our career and educational trajectories (Levitt et al., 2007; Foley, 2018).

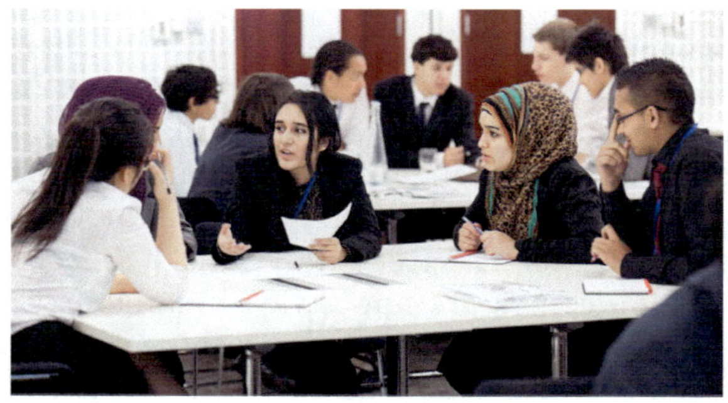

Source: https://media.licdn.com/dms/image/v2/D4E12AQHH1nQCoWJ59w/article-cover_image-shrink_720_1280/article-cover_image-shrink_720_1280/0/1688737324782?e=2147483647&v=beta&t=DiqKzmESAan-3Tan3IANFMup3uOBQ7xWpT3WAmb6bZo

14.6. Policy Implications

Electric cars have not taken off as immediately as one might anticipate, despite their potential to reduce emissions. Consumers' behaviors appear to be entwined with common issues such as how convenient it is to charge a vehicle, and environmental and technological concerns. It turns out that what people do when purchasing automobiles is intertwined with social and economic considerations. In general, policymakers have to be inventive, combining incentives such as subsidies with investment in charging infrastructure—to persuade individuals to opt for cleaner options. Redressing disparities between groups and sensitizing the population can progressively change public preference toward green rides, making cities greener and economically thriving (Gautam et al., 2024). The narrative is not limited to cars. When it comes to what ends up on our plates, the mix of cultural and economic influences calls for fresh thinking too. People are increasingly aware of the downsides of animal-based diets, so shifting toward plant-based proteins seems more sensible than ever. Generally speaking, as income grows, protein consumption tends to rise, but the pattern is not exactly identical all over Europe. Variations in regions, traditions, and economic conditions are all at play. It appears that public education and planned campaigns regarding the benefits of sustainable diets, as well as policies favoring plant-based alternatives, can go a long way in shifting consumer behaviors over time. Ultimately, combining regulations, education, and incentives for business can incite genuine change in the way we eat—making what we eat healthier and better for the planet for all (Prochazka et al., 2024). When it comes to both electric cars and what we eat, governments cannot simply solve the problem with simplistic economic solutions. Individuals make decisions based on an entire package of social and economic considerations. A combination of interesting publicity campaigns, directed subsidies, and supportive infrastructure can work, but the things need to be done subtly—sometimes rather unofficially, sometimes with a more official, measured approach. When data are used effectively, they enable these kinds of measures to be adapted to the changing economic context, so that policies become responsive and inclusive. The intent is to create systems that not only promote sustainable decisions but also provide equitable access to greener technology and healthier food; in so doing, governments can trigger a transformation that is good for the environment as well as society as a whole (Gautam et al., 2024; Prochazka et al., 2024).

14.6.1. Importance of Addressing Socioeconomic Disparities

Socioeconomic disparities truly make their presence known when it comes to health, particularly for those who are already vulnerable. Less advantaged individuals experiencing strokes and such are usually left with poorer recoveries and tragic higher mortality. A study in Los Angeles County indicates that when both income, education, and access to healthcare are all out of balance, recovery is truly a hill too steep to climb. Racial disparities then introduce a complicating factor, ensuring that specialized assistance must come into action earlier rather than later. For the most part, if healthcare systems can target those money and resource problems, they could just reduce those adverse results and ensure more leveling of the playing field (Mayorga et al., 2025). Financial woes don't merely play havoc with your body—these go deep into your mental and emotional life as well. Recent research examining the COVID-19 aftermath in Southeast Asia generally finds that more economically depressed regions have people reporting a lot more stress. Consider, for example, the stark contrast between stress levels in Brunei and Vietnam; it truly illustrates how weak economic foundations can set your mental balance askew. For the most part, that added stress will fuel additional mental health issues while eroding general resilience. Overall, more effort toward economic equity and increased access to mental health services may just be the answer to help communities create a stronger sense of well-being (Rahmat & Sabila, 2024). Often the solution for these economic challenges lies within policy, where policymakers must have an overall vision to address the source of the issue. Making sure people who have been excluded from the decision-making loop are well cared for, have decent jobs, and an opportunity at education appears to take care of both body and mind. There is a developing notion that investments in health clinics, schools, and steady employment—not to mention a wiser examination of how social circumstances impact health—can turn health around. When you combine these social and economic conditions, it is clear that addressing these imbalances is not merely a moral obligation; it is a necessity for creating a healthier, more equitable society for all (Mayorga et al., 2025; Rahmat & Sabila, 2024).

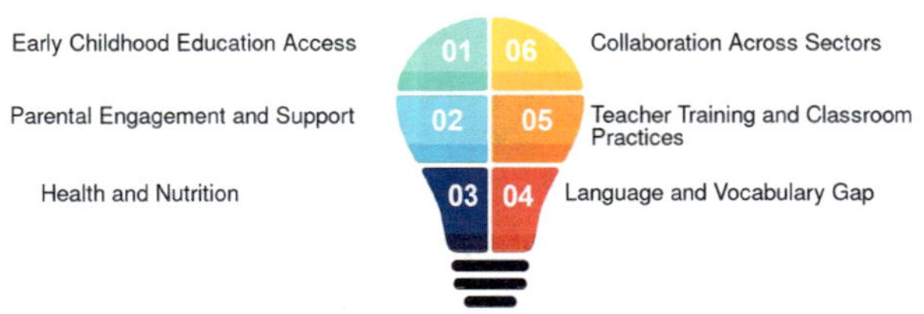
Early Childhood Education Access
Parental Engagement and Support
Health and Nutrition
01
02
03
04
05
06
Collaboration Across Sectors
Teacher Training and Classroom Practices
Language and Vocabulary Gap

Figure 14.11. Addressing socioeconomic disparities.

Source: FasterCapital. (n.d.). *Closing the Kindergarten Readiness Gap: Lessons for Startup Founders Addressing Socioeconomic Disparities.*

14.6.2. Behavioral Health Programs and Their Effectiveness

Socioeconomic challenges and behavioral health disorders blend together in complex ways that determine how successful mental health programs end up being. A lot of people stuck in these issues are confronted with a cluster of issues - such as unpredictable finances, loss of employment, and inadequate access to healthcare - and once those start to accumulate, stress and mental pressure tend to follow. Programs that address these actual life issues end up being more effective overall. For instance, those that combine direct mental aid with some kind of financial assistance not only calm the mind but also lift some of the heavy burden off worries about money. This type of brush-stroke thinking appears to create a welcoming environment where individuals just continue to return, and over time normally culminates in consistent gains in mental well-being (Yoshikawa et al., 2020). It's not all about the money, either; it's about finding a match between mental health programs and the cultural and daily lives of the people they're working with. Programs that draw on community strengths and respect local traditions tend to resonate more strongly. Such as, when services draw on well-established community values and leverage the natural communication patterns of people, confidence between those giving and receiving assistance increases - and that can significantly increase participation. This approach, in addition to engaging more participants, seems to open the way for improved overall health as well. Then, adding in peer support or advocacy provides individuals with an opportunity to rely on commonality, something particularly vital for populations with similar challenges (Volkow, 2020). At times how successfully these efforts pan out even hinges on how the programs approach technology, especially through tough times. Recall the days of COVID-19. When meetings in person decreased, telehealth came into play as an essential resource. Programs that switched quickly to online maintained many of their users, even in time of uncertainty. The transition to virtual formats dissolved physical barriers, opening access to mental healthcare for individuals who may otherwise have been denied it due to the fact that face-to-face sessions simply were not feasible. This flexible adjustment suggests a future model, one that prioritizes pliability and takes into account the varied levels of access to tech, particularly within poor communities (Yoshikawa et al., 2020). In numerous aspects, these changing tactics not only appear to enhance overall performance but also assist in making sure that mental health services remain present during both peaceful and turbulent times (Volkow, 2020) (Figure 14.12).

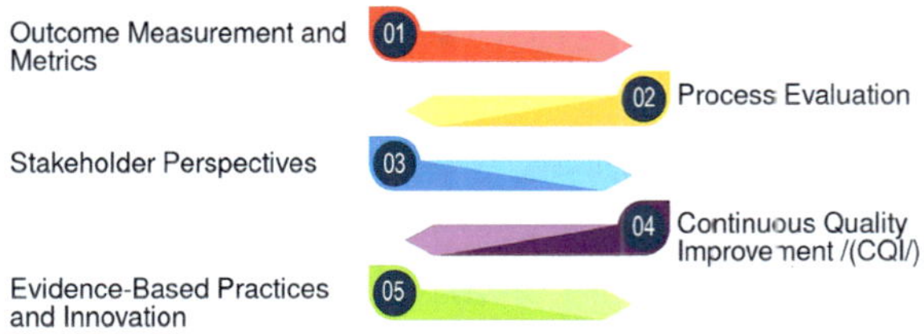
Outcome Measurement and Metrics
01
02
Process Evaluation
Stakeholder Perspectives
03
04
Continuous Quality Improvement /(CQI/)
Evidence-Based Practices and Innovation
05

Figure 14.12. Behavioral health programs and their effectiveness.

Source: FasterCapital. (n.d.). *Effective Strategies for Behavioral Health Management: Evaluating and Improving Behavioral Health Programs.*

14.6.3. Recommendations for Future Research and Policy

HL is evolving rapidly, and today more than ever before, research has to explore the ways in which individuals look for health information while balancing their financial realities. It is important to observe here that both mindset considerations and daily social factors subtly form these behaviors, something that truly counts when creating strong health policies. Applying models such as the Health Belief Model and even that Information-Motivation-Behavioral Skills arrangement provides one mechanism to deduce these complex dynamics. When you consider it, bringing libraries, community organizations, and health systems into a single effort can initiate solutions tailored to specific needs. That is particularly important in communities with low socioeconomic status. Minor investments in innovative HL programs through such collaborations will enable public health initiatives to more closely match the needs of various groups, ultimately improving outcomes and equity (Halder et al., 2024). Integrating technology into health initiatives is yet another new frontier for both policy and research. More and more, individuals are coming to see that Health Recommender Systems (HRS) could be the key to making health recommendations genuinely personal—they listen not just to what someone may prefer but also to the bigger social scene. In those socioecological models—Overall—are highlighting nested influences, there is a specific opportunity to design HRS that address structural challenges such as restricted access to high-quality care or even nutritional supplies. Policy-makers should support research that tests how well these systems work in different environments and ensure that they can access populations most affected by inequalities. When HRS data is involved, decision-makers might mold policies that prioritize accessibility and equity as the central concerns of health communication and intervention programs (Figueroa et al., 2024). Lastly, investing effort in interdisciplinary strategies appears to be the way to go if we are to make health interventions more effective. Future work should combine behavioral scientists, health practitioners, and policy analysts to work out evidence-based strategies that home in on the economic drivers of our health decisions. This combination can unravel the complex web of health inequities and provide a more accurate image of how mundane systemic barriers guide personal choices. There is also an effort to incorporate decolonial insights into health research and policy—a step that shakes up traditional notions that have long pushed aside the voices of the marginalized. Combining these various viewpoints may well redefine interventions to be culturally attuned and successful. Ultimately, future projects need to address not only individual health behaviors but also the larger structural conditions that underpin them; such a dual agenda is needed to generate lasting improvements in health outcomes (Figueroa et al., 2024; Halder et al., 2024).

CLOSER LOOK

Health Disparities

Health disparities are inequalities in health outcomes and access to care among varying population groups, specifically by race, ethnicity, and socioeconomic status. The disparities can be a result of numerous factors, such as socioeconomic status, lifestyle, age, and environmental factors. The two terms, "health disparities" and "health equity," are frequently used together, with the latter being the equitable and just distribution of health opportunities across all groups.

Key Aspects of Health Disparities

- **Definition:** Health disparities refer to the variations in health status or healthcare access that are causally linked to social and/or geographic factors and not biological differences.
- **Underlying Factors:** These differences may be affected by the intricate interaction of factors, such as socioeconomic status, education, and access to healthy food, safe shelter, and good healthcare.
- **Impact:** Health disparities can have a significant impact on individual health and well-being, as well as on the health of communities as a whole.
- **Equity vs. Equality:** Health equity seeks to provide a good opportunity to all individuals to attain their complete health potential, whereas equality tries to offer equal resources and opportunities to all, irrespective of their requirements.

SUMMARY

Socioeconomic and behavioral influences appear to intersect in complex ways that define our perception of public health. Emerging evidence indicates that variations in housing quality are associated with the frequency and severity of illness. Poor housing not only allows vector-borne disease to spread but can also worsen it, obviously calling for targeted public health interventions. Addressing these building issues could assist in reducing health hazards, resulting in improved outcomes for those most vulnerable.

If you take into account how our environment and lifestyle together, it describes a complicated but captivating picture of influencing health (Shaheen et al., 2025). Observing how individuals behave when coping with health adds another dimension to the equation. Too often, procrastination in seeking care and variable routines, such as not consistently using bed nets—reflect a definite need to increase active health practices. In most instances, waiting so long for treatment can alter the course of a disease, particularly with illnesses such as cutaneous leishmaniasis where timing is crucial. It appears that community-based initiatives, although not flawless, can promote improved health choices and enhance access to required services (Adugna et al., 2024). Overall, exploring socioeconomic and behavioral factors paints a complex, multifaceted picture that demands mixed methods. In general, addressing health disparities at their core involves better living conditions, heightened health awareness, and adherence to sustainable lifestyles that benefit communities. The messages emerging from research call policymakers and health professionals alike to prioritize these elements because addressing both the societal and individual aspects of health is pivotal to alleviating disease and enhancing overall community health (Adugna et al., 2024; Shaheen et al., 2025).

Socioeconomic realities and daily habits blend together in ways not always immediately apparent at first glance; comprehending how they combine is central to addressing education problems. The portrait is not yet complete without considering a range of perspectives—some based on empirical fact, some on more practical intuition. Historical anomalies and day-to-day circumstances, for instance, influence our schools and our practices more than we realize. In many instances, theories such as complexity and even context-first views allow us to deconstruct the ways in which these various pieces interact and show how measures such as grades and retention rates can be influenced.

Browsing through numerous studies, we can observe that academic success is often quantified by something as straightforward as the GPA of a student. It so happens that whereas the SAT and ACT, these standardized tests, have a more or less moderate correlation with GPA, qualities not necessarily based on raw intelligence—efficiency in school, how students organize their work, even goals set—also emerge as significant. Overall, strong self-efficacy belief is strongly related to GPA, and such combination of mental and motivational abilities demonstrates why any new pedagogy must address more than pure cognitive exercises (Richardson et al., 2012).

Overall, these findings indicate an involved connection where both economic status and individual routines contribute their share to learning. Comprehending that mix, on the whole, becomes critical when attempting to develop equitable and efficient school reform. How various life experiences and attitudes mix and mingle means a one-size-fits-all strategy just will not work. By looking back to familiar contexts and double-checking the most recent information, teachers and policymakers are better positioned—sometimes by a significant margin—to establish systems that serve the varied needs of students today (Foley, 2018).

KEY TERMS FROM THIS CHAPTER

- Socioeconomic status (SES)
- Income inequality
- Social determinants of health
- Access to healthcare
- Health-seeking behavior
- Discrimination
- Compliance
- Community engagement
- Misinformation
- Occupational exposure
- Migration
- Health inequities
- Education level
- Poverty
- Health literacy
- Cultural beliefs
- Stigma
- Behavior change
- Trust in healthcare system
- Social norms
- Vaccine hesitancy
- Overcrowding
- Urbanization
- Food insecurity

REFERENCES

1. Addo, M. E. (2018). Cultural influences on psychiatrists' constructions of mental health problems: A repertory grid study. *Semantic scholar*. https://www.semanticscholar.org/paper/6d8e0f5d60ca90821e36a94eb9bf54b811394ef1 (accessed on 6 May 2025).
2. Adugna, Y. M., Ayelign, A., & Zerfu, T. (2024). Suboptimal nutritional status of school-age children in Addis Ababa: Evidence from the analysis of socioeconomic, environmental, and behavioral factors. *Frontiers in Public Health, 12*. https://www.semanticscholar.org/paper/405ad994784908c1e3f42fe8b932e4ca28c8f55c (accessed on 6 May 2025).
3. Agbamu, M. E., & Irogbo, P. U. (2024). Socioeconomic factors as determinants of crime rates in Abraka, Delta State. *Gusau International Journal of Management and Social Sciences*. https://www.semanticscholar.org/paper/4e3cc5dfaeadd9b600441c965b2e26a406d52aa0 (accessed on 6 May 2025).
4. Ally, S. A., Han, J., Molokie, R., Ruiz, M. A., Gordeuk, V., Lash, J., & Saraf, S. (2024). Socioeconomic factors and dietary patterns in adults with sickle cell disease. *Journal of Sickle Cell Disease*. https://www.semanticscholar.org/paper/9d4c3706411d53df8ac79ec67ca612e376bf226e (accessed on 6 May 2025).
5. Al-Mamun, M., Kalam, A., & Uzzal, N. I. (2025). Factors affecting maternal health and antenatal care services of working mothers in southwestern coastal Bangladesh: A cross-sectional study. *Annals of Medicine and Surgery, 87*, 487–496. https://www.semanticscholar.org/paper/ad36f84b646fb83ecb53f61197079f221f6e7754 (accessed on 6 May 2025).
6. Been, R. A., Lameijer, A., Gans, R., van Beek, A. P., Kingsnorth, A. P., Choudhary, P., van Dijk, P. V. (2024). The impact of socioeconomic factors, social determinants, and ethnicity on the utilization of glucose sensor technology among persons with diabetes mellitus: A narrative review. *Therapeutic Advances in Endocrinology and Metabolism, 15*. https://www.semanticscholar.org/paper/32c924b7c6f548dfa7dae10b6a073f9ff89bda31 (accessed on 6 May 2025).
7. Chakraborty, A., & Shah, J. (2025). Assessing the role of socioeconomic factors—income, education, broadband access, and healthy foods on location-wise disparities in COVID-19 cases. *Archives of Public Health, 83*. https://www.semanticscholar.org/paper/f3401b93b5940e3db2fcb8b8a0ce76e121a0e042 (accessed on 6 May 2025).
8. Chola, R. M., Kiplagat, H., & Mubichakani, J. M. (2025). Influence of job opportunities on course choice in vocational training centers in Taita Taveta County, Kenya. *Saudi Journal of Engineering and Technology*. https://www.semanticscholar.org/paper/06cbc9102efe99360b00055b2e6e2a421cab0012 (accessed on 6 May 2025).
9. Foley, N. F. (2018). Negotiating opportunities: How the middle class secures advantages in school. *Harvard Educational Review, 88*(3), 407–411. https://doi.org/10.17763/1943-5045-88.3.407a.
10. Gautam, N., Chowdhury, A., Rahman, M. M., & Khanam, R. (2025). Socioeconomic inequalities in childhood and adolescent obesity in Australia: The role of behavioral and biological factors. *PloS one, 20*(4), e0321861. https://doi.org/10.1371/journal.pone.0321861 (accessed on 6 May 2025).

11. Gothi, V. (2025). Evaluating the socioeconomic determinants of REIT adoption in Mumbai: Behavioral barriers and drivers in investment decision-making. *International Scientific Journal of Engineering and Management*. https://www.semanticscholar.org/paper/5fb385e728639447ac28e12932b21d52aef52524 (accessed on 6 May 2025).

12. Henrich, J., Heine, S. J., & Norenzayan, A. (2010). The weirdest people in the world? *Behavioral and Brain Sciences, 33*, 61–83. https://doi.org/10.1017/s0140525x0999152x.

13. Huh, J. S., Choi, E., & Kim, J. (2024). Factors influencing career development of private consignment employment service career counselors. *The Korean Career, Entrepreneurship & Business Association*. https://www.semanticscholar.org/paper/6d92dc8e827e80c842e53457144f35eb9525053a (accessed on 6 May 2025).

14. Joshi, B. M., Khatiwada, S., & Pokhrel, R. K. (2024). Influence of socioeconomic factors on access to digital resources for education. *Rupantaran: A Multidisciplinary Journal*. https://www.semanticscholar.org/paper/c78a1e92273abf95370bb505637c49b14ab3ddd9 (accessed on 6 May 2025).

15. Khoirunisa, A., Fauzi, P., Fadillah, F., Azahra, S. A., & Santoso, A. M. (2024). Preparedness of students in social norms to entrepreneurial intentions (Case studies on students). *Linguanusa: Social Humanities, Education and Linguistic*. https://www.semanticscholar.org/paper/e93bd6d361dfd80d9b780b48f65fcab194691b4e (accessed on 6 May 2025).

16. Layton, A. T. (2024). AI, machine learning, and ChatGPT in hypertension. *Hypertension*. https://www.semanticscholar.org/paper/3e26e01a2f24aa88a56c56a88e1e557ee4e2879c (accessed on 6 May 2025).

17. Levitt, P., & Jaworsky, B. N. (2007). Transnational migration studies: Past developments and future trends. *Annual Review of Sociology, 33*, 129–156. https://doi.org/10.1146/annurev.soc.33.040406.131816.

18. Lovallo, W. R. (2016). *Stress and Health: Biological and Psychological Interactions*. SAGE Publications. https://doi.org/10.4135/9781071801390.

19. Methasani, J. L., Aliaj, A., & Tota, I. (2025). Understanding consumer perceptions and behavioral indicators in the life insurance market. *Journal of Educational and Social Research*. https://www.semanticscholar.org/paper/f85e7ddf797292b99ac21aa4f2bdaac6ed23ee7a (accessed on 6 May 2025).

20. Metzler, M., Merrick, M. T., Klevens, J., Ports, K. A., & Ford, D. (2016). Adverse childhood experiences and life opportunities: Shifting the narrative. *Children and Youth Services Review, 72*, 141–149. https://doi.org/10.1016/j.childyouth.2016.10.021.

21. Murthy, S. A. (2017). National mental health survey of India 2015–2016. *Indian Journal of Psychiatry, 59*, 21–21. https://doi.org/10.4103/psychiatry.indianjpsychiatry_102_17.

22. Padhy, S., Fatima, R., Jena, S., Kar, A., Durga, P., & Neeradi, V. K. (2023). Effect of stress on contextual pain sensitivity in the preoperative period- A proof of concept study. *Journal of Anesthesiology, Clinical Pharmacology, 39*, 603–608. https://www.semanticscholar.org/paper/9c20f6375cc16876eda1d9cce8cf815fc40cdf38 (accessed on 6 May 2025).

23. Prochazka, P., Soukupová, J., Abrhám, J., Mullen, K. J., Tomšík, K., Čechura, L., Čábelková, I., et al. (2024). Protein consumption in Europe: Sustainability, tradition, and policy implications. *Sustainable Development*. https://www.semanticscholar.org/paper/a7345b0193db70f6ec0c294f782d35680bd48e82 (accessed on 6 May 2025).

24. Rahmat, S. K., & Sabila, F. V. (2024). Exploring the impact of socioeconomic factors on stress levels using clustering in Southeast Asia during the COVID-19 pandemic. *Indonesian Journal of Applied Mathematics and Statistics*. https://www.semanticscholar.org/paper/aebbbf2b1d9a841faa153a6ee070154e273be79c (accessed on 6 May 2025).

25. Richardson, M., Abraham, C., & Bond, R. (2012). Psychological correlates of university students' academic performance: A systematic review and meta-analysis. *Psychological Bulletin, 138*(3), 353–387. https://doi.org/10.1037/a0026838.

26. Rojo Ramos, J., Gómez Paniagua, S., Guevara Pérez, J. C., & Morenas Martín, J. (2024). Validation of a scale on the perceptions of the socioeconomic impact of nature sports tourism. *e-Motion: Revita de Education, Matricidal e Investigation*. https://www.semanticscholar.org/paper/8acf760c5050596e17ee4bafc3bc90ad31e26b28 (accessed on 6 May 2025).

27. Sharma, A., Deshmukh, P. T., Jain, S., Gaurkar, S., & Sharma, A. (2024). Factors contributing to postoperative radiotherapy delays in head and neck cancer: A comprehensive review. *Cures, 16*. https://www.semanticscholar.org/paper/35a022e1459dc832facc5d9aa52b9893028cf11b (accessed on 6 May 2025).

28. Sørensen, K., Van den Broucke, S., Fullam, J., Doyle, G., Pelikan, J. M., Słońska, Z., & Brand, H. (2012). Health literacy and public health: A systematic review and integration of definitions and models. *BMC Public Health, 12*, 80. https://doi.org/10.1186/1471-2458-12-80.

29. Stormacq, C., Van den Broucke, S., & Wosinski, J. (2018). Does health literacy mediate the relationship between socioeconomic status and health disparities? *Health Promotion International, 34*(5), e1–e17. https://doi.org/10.1093/heapro/day062.

30. Varghese, A. A., & I, Akshaya. (2024). The perceptions of beauty among teenagers. *International Journal for Multidisciplinary Research*. https://www.semanticscholar.org/paper/1de58929578bfd3c56a54aafa58025bf55b93cf1 (accessed on 6 May 2025).

31. Yang, X., Wang, X., Yu, J., & Gao, J. (2025). Why does browsing social networking sites increase conspicuous consumption? The effects of relative deprivation and subjective socioeconomic status. *BMC Psychology, 13*. https://www.semanticscholar.org/paper/8082c22aa44ed5a3295a494c50d3e4355bed4d2b (accessed on 6 May 2025).

32. Yoshikawa, H., Wuermli, A. J., Rebello Britto, P., Dreyer, B. P., Leckman, J. F., Lye, S. J., Ponguta, L. A., et al. (2020). Effects of the global coronavirus disease-2019 pandemic on early childhood development: Short- and long-term risks and mitigating program and policy actions. *The Journal of Pediatrics, 223*, 188–193. https://doi.org/10.1016/j.jpeds.2020.05.020.

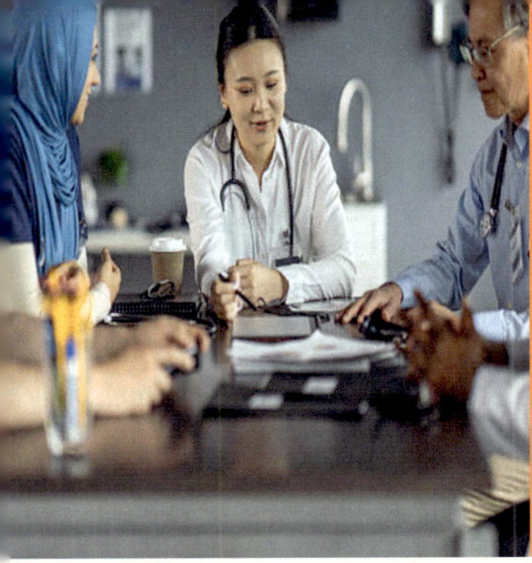

Chapter 15
PUBLIC HEALTH POLICY AND FUTURE DIRECTIONS

Contents

Introduction

With a more interconnected world, the role of global health policy and governance has become critical. The intricacies of international relationships require an intergovernmental approach to battle health issues that know no borders, like pandemics, infectious diseases, and antimicrobial resistance (AMR). Governance here is not just about coordination of the international community's response but about national policy harmonization with world health goals. This chapter is going to examine the processes by which global health policy is designed and implemented, their relative success, and the range of actors involved, including international institutions, nation states, and non-state players. Through case studies and existing frameworks, we hope to shed light on the complex and multifaceted nature of global health governance and its implications for policy. Finally, comprehension of these dynamics is critical to developing health equity and enhancing the health of populations globally in the context of future global health risks.

Definition of Global Health Governance

Global health governance includes the institutions, policies, and processes that design global action to respond to health threats, prioritizing co-operation among countries and organizations. It is primarily characterized by the cross-relationship of several actors, including governments, non-governmental organizations (NGO), and global organizations, all playing important roles in framing health policy and establishing standards. This multi-dimensional strategy is more and more pronounced in the actions of emerging powers, including the BRICS group of nations, which challenge dominant paradigms and emphasize more inclusive approaches to health security during international health crises, like the COVID-19 pandemic (Akbar, 2024). Besides, initiatives such as India's vaccine diplomacy highlight the ethical considerations inherent in the health governance that mirror the importance of moral solidarity and equity in global health policy agendas (Mondal, 2024). As a result, global health governance not only deals with present health challenges but also attempts to promote system-wide cooperation that enhances capacities to resist future threats (Figure 15.1).

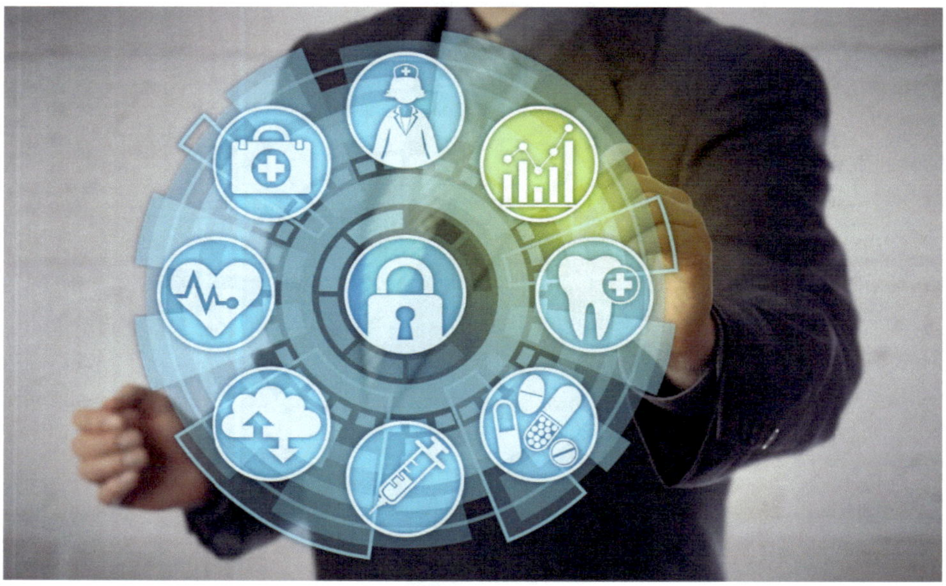

Figure 15.1. Global health governance.

Source: Global Governance Project. (2022). *Microscopic Organisms and Global Health Research.*

Importance of Global Health Policy

The importance of global health policy cannot be overemphasized, especially in the age of transnational health threats such as pandemics, climate change, and emerging infectious diseases. The call is for strong policies that will facilitate effective global health governance through international cooperation that promotes equitable access to resources and aid to the poor. For example, BRICS countries, particularly South Africa, together when dealing with health crises emphasizes the calls for flexibility and inclusivity in policy-making. Further, tackling environmental determinants like soil contamination emphasizes the intricacies of health policy where ecological balance is symbiotically mixed with public health outcomes. As countries race toward carbon neutrality under the threat of developing toxins, incorporating environmental health into global policy structures emerges as a critical agenda. Thus, broad health policies form the basis of collective action aimed at reducing risks to health and encouraging sustainable health globally.

Historical Context of Global Health Initiatives

The historical background of global health programs demonstrates a multifaceted interplay of social, political, and economic forces that have influenced modern health governance. In the last century, the development of international health organizations has created structures to address diseases that cross national borders. For example, the AIDS/HIV epidemic of the late 20th century spurred international cooperation and produced Community Advisory Boards (CABs) in trial sites, highlighting local initiative within health policy-making. Evidence has pointed to the requirement to comprehend socio-political environments as a means of integrating community input into international health policy (Upton et al., 2011). Additionally, the changing university role in regional integration in Southern Africa underscores the convergence of academic involvement with health programs, hence the fostering of informed action and discussion toward equitable access to health (Kotecha, 2011). Emphasizing these convergences is crucial for redressing historical injustices in global health governance (Figure 15.2).

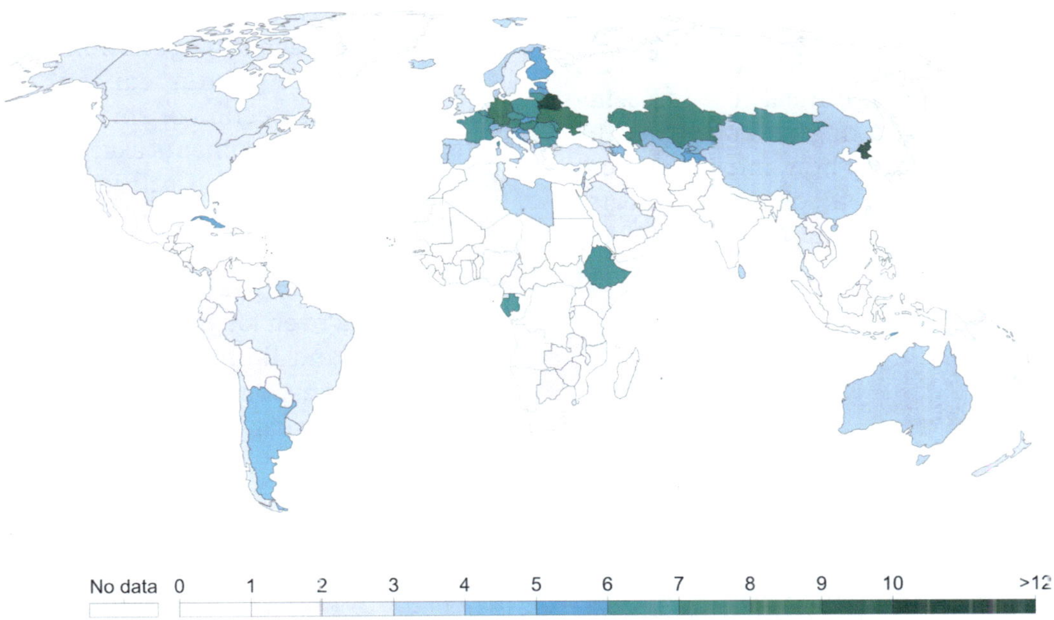

Figure 15.2. The historical context of global health initiatives.

Source: By Our World in Data - https://ourworldindata.org/grapher/hospital-beds-per-1000-people?year=2013, CC BY 4.0, https://commons.wikimedia.org/w/index.php?curid=87793883

Key Stakeholders in Global Health Governance

In global health governance, a wide range of stakeholders is involved in formulating health policies and responses to transnational health issues. Governments in individual countries have historically headed health programs; however, globalization has expanded roles to involve international organizations, nongovernmental organizations (NGOs), as well as the private sector. For example, the World Health Organization (WHO) is a focal point in convening global health action, with regional organizations such as the Association of Southeast Asian Nations (ASEAN) becoming better known for their ability to promote regional collaboration and effectively address regional health issues (Hong et al., 2012). Civil society organizations are also vital advocates who ensure that marginalized groups have their voices heard in policy development. This collaborative strategy is critical to addressing health equity and executing all-encompassing strategies, demonstrating how interdependent actors bring strength to a solid global health governance structure (Chaturvedi et al., 2015) (Figure 15.3).

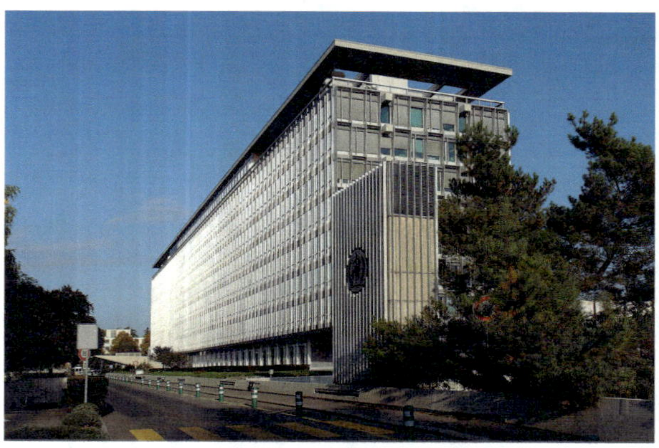

Figure 15.3. The stakeholders in global health governance.

Source: © Yann Forget / Wikimedia Commons, CC BY-SA 4.0, https://commons.wikimedia.org/w/index.php?curid=6661816

Twitter. (n.d.). *Health Governance Capacity Development Model.*

Overview of Global Health Challenges

Global health issues are also more integrated and interconnected, which requires unified action from everyone concerned, including governments, nongovernmental organizations (NGOs), and international agencies. Pandemics, non-communicable diseases (NCDs), and health inequalities are only a few of the issues that require an integrated strategy to policy and governance that transcends national frontiers. The post-2015 Development Agenda provides a unique opportunity to reaffirm commitment to such goals for these global health priorities, and to recognize the principle of the common but differentiated responsibilities, as articulated in recent negotiations on global health governance (Chaturvedi et al, 2015). In addition, the intersection of environmental and socioeconomic determinants exacerbates health inequities, highlighting a call for policies that consider underlying determinants of health within a unifying international development policy (Yeates et al., 2015). As such, in the future, there will be a need for the integration of varied perspectives and unified collaborative efforts to effectively respond to these global health challenges, eventually enhancing global health outcomes.

Significance of Effective Governance in Health

Good governance in health is essential in building a strong system that solves the complex problems within global health systems. This is ensured in that policies become evidence-based, equitable, and specific to the specific needs of populations, which contributes to better health outcomes and stronger system efficiency. The dynamics between state and non-state actors are central; states have classically wielded power, but with the advent of non-state players, the landscape of governance has been pluralized. Denationalization of political power has resulted in a complementing strategy in which states fill the gaps in non-state actors' capacities, all contributing their respective resources to public health measures (Genschel et al., 2008). Ultimately, successful governance not only encourages transparency and accountability but also generates public trust, which allows for an effective response to health emergencies and the facilitation of health equity throughout the world and hence highlights its pivotal position within the larger global health governance and policy framework.

15.1. Frameworks of Global Health Governance

In examining global health governance arrangements, it is clear that effective collaborative institutions are key to responding to health inequalities between countries. The post-2015 Development Agenda provides a critical platform for building international agreement on priority health issues, highlighting the importance of shared but differentiated responsibilities that promote differentiated national policies (Chaturvedi et al, 2015). This model not only considers various health environments but also provides an opportunity for countries to come up with measures that are suited to their own circumstances. Moreover, principles of aid effectiveness like harmonization and mutual accountability are required in improving the provision of health services while financing aligns with the priorities of the locals (Dennis, 2009). Through the alignment of these frameworks, global health governance can ensure integrated responses to future health hazards, thereby increasing the general effectiveness of policy response and ensuring fair health outcomes between populations (Figure 15.4).

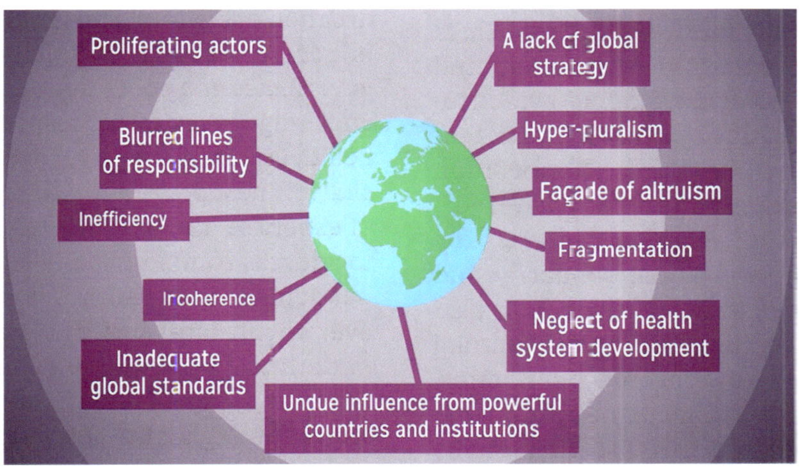

Figure 15.4. The frameworks of global health governance.

Source: Penn Today. (2021). *Global Health Governance Illustration.*

15.1.1. International Health Regulations (IHR)

The International Health Regulations (IHR) represent a key international health governance model intended to enhance the maximum level of international cooperation and action in response to public health emergencies. The most recent updates to the IHR, approved at the 77th World Health Assembly, broaden the scope of the regulations to include a concept of pandemic emergencies, thereby necessitating prompt and concerted international interventions during crisis situations such as pandemics. The reforms are equity-oriented in global health and mandate every nation to ensure access to health products as well as funding, especially for developing nations (Zidar et al., 2024). Further, the application of the IHR has been instrumental in managing vector-borne diseases (VBDs), thus the need for robust surveillance and epidemic intelligence systems varying significantly across countries (Subtil et al., 2024). This emphasizes the necessity for states to continue developing their strategies as per the lessons of the COVID-19 pandemic and thus build a more robust global health environment.

15.1.2. World Health Organization (WHO) Roles and Functions

For international health governance, the WHO is a core component of policy making and directing health interventions globally. The WHO functions as a central agency, which is responsible for stewardship of international health, and this involves developing evidence-informed recommendations as a means of addressing health emergencies. This position has been consolidated after the COVID-19 pandemic, when the WHO became a key player in advocating for global solidarity and cooperation among states. Additionally, it also enables resource mobilization toward funding health programs in low-income economies, thus helping in the attainment of sustainable development goals (Kibets-Pashutina et al., 2023). Though the organization has been able to maintain substantial influence on health agendas, its effectiveness is regularly being tested by the evolving context of global governance, calling for a reactive policy to stay abreast of the new challenges on the health horizon. This double role of setting norms and enabling global cooperation evidences the organizations' distinctive role in global health governance (Figure 15.5).

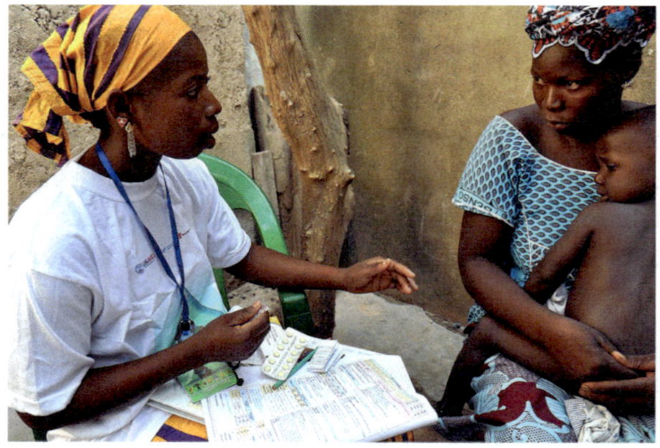

Figure 15.5. World health organization (WHO) roles and functions.

Source: By President's Malaria Initiative - Community Health Worker treats child, Public Domain, https://commons.wikimedia.org/w/index.php?curid=72085321

15.1.3. Bilateral and Multilateral Agreements

Creation of bilateral and multilateral frameworks is core under the authority of global health governance and policy because these frameworks encourage a worldwide response to transnational health crises. Through resource and information sharing, best practices exchange, and the sharing of expertise, these frameworks enable countries to address common health challenges, including pandemics and healthcare worker flight, that overwhelm local health systems. For instance, initiatives by multilateral institutions like the WHO and the International Organization for Migration highlight the call for collective policy actions to deal with the international migration of health professionals (Pilpersist et al., 2013). These agreements promote the development of healthy food systems and nutrition programs as an approach to solidifying the interdependence of health, development, and migration policies (Bruce et al., 2013). Lastly, bilateral, and multilateral agreements are at the forefront of strengthening global health security and improved health outcomes, depicting the centrality of international cooperation in health governance.

15.1.4. The Role of Non-Governmental Organizations (NGOs)

Non-governmental organizations (NGOs) play an important part in international health policy and governance by acting as key intermediaries among international agencies, governments, and impacted people. The advocacy efforts of NGOs facilitate the building of accountability and voice for marginalized communities in policy arenas. NGOs are helpful by establishing capacity-building programs to facilitate local people's active participation in decision-making on health, which enhances civic engagement and democratic government. The NGOs' heterogeneity also guarantees a dynamic cross-pollination of ideas and methods in health policy design, which results in creative solutions to emerging health crises. However, the variability in the definition and definition of civil society organizations makes their incorporation into governance systems challenging, as noted in research into the role of civil society within international organizations (Pedraza-Farina et al., 2013). Streamlining the infrastructure that engages NGOs in global governance could help foster cooperation and eventually yield improved health gains throughout the world (Peter Walkenhorst et al., 2011).

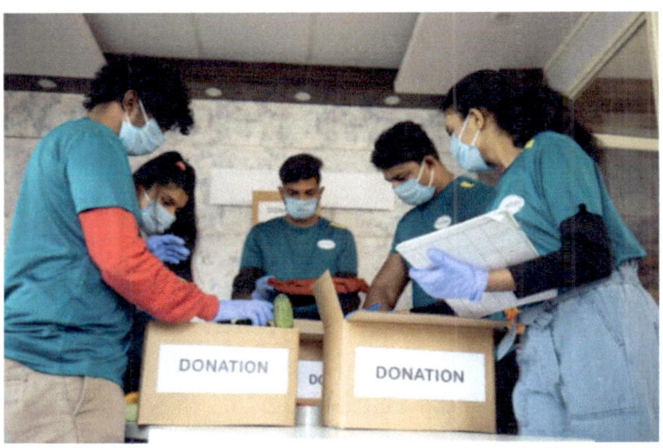

Source: Medium. (n.d.). *Global Health and Policy Concept Image.*

15.1.5. Public-Private Partnerships (PPPs) in Health

Public-private partnerships (PPPs) in health are a milestone in international health governance in which the capacities and resources of both sectors are utilized for achieving minimum health needs. But their success is still contingent upon the realization of a balance between the public sector health interests and profit-making interests. For instance, research indicates that although policy responses to obesity can be enhanced through collaboration with the food industry, they tend to tend of opening up problems of accountability such that commercial actors can deflect responsibility and undermine public health goals (Ralston et al., 2019). Similarly, entry of emerging market manufacturers into supply chains has enhanced access to vaccines and medicines while fueling concerns around the sustainability of such efforts under competing business interests (Roemer-Mahler et al., 2014). PPPs can end up initiating new health interventions but are sure to be successful only under constant surveillance and upholding public health above profit.

15.1.6. Regional Health Governance Structures

Regional health governance systems become more widely acknowledged as central to determining world health outcomes. Such systems, usually following frameworks created by organizations such as the WHO, enable transnational cooperation and policy formulation, as can be seen in varied contexts ranging from Norway to Cuba. For example, whereas Norway's public health policy is primarily following WHO policy significantly to a high extent of policy reproduction, Cubas strategy focuses more on local community participation and implementation of these directives according to local requirements (Schultz-Hardt et al., 2022) Furthermore, the increasing role of United Nations (UN) bodies in promoting human rights incorporation in health governance offers an imperative context for regional action. By mainstreaming human rights throughout different health programs, the UN shapes the way regional organizations react to public health issues, further entrenching the interdependence between local interventions and global priorities (Gostin et al., 2019). Effective regional governance is therefore not just underpinning national health plans but also congruent with global health goals.

15.1.7. The Impact of Global Health Governance on Local Policies

Global health governance has a direct impact on local policy by establishing frameworks that shape health interventions through both direct mandates and indirect incentives. In the instance of maternal and child health programs in different African countries, where different governance structures have produced different outcomes, this dynamic can be seen. Interestingly, Rwanda's strong health policy environment, with strong linkages between the local and central governments and innovative schemes such as community health insurance, demonstrates how good governance can drive improvement in the delivery of health services (Ntukanyagwe et al., 2020).

Conversely, Uganda's poor implementation of policies highlights the need for accountability and local leadership in the attainment of health objectives (Ntukanyagwe et al., 2020). In the same vein, international migration health policy has unveiled discrepancies between international research priorities and immediate migrant health concerns; hence, highlighting local responsive policy imperatives to fill those identified gaps. In the end, it is the interface of global health governance and local policy that determines the effectiveness of health interventions on the ground.

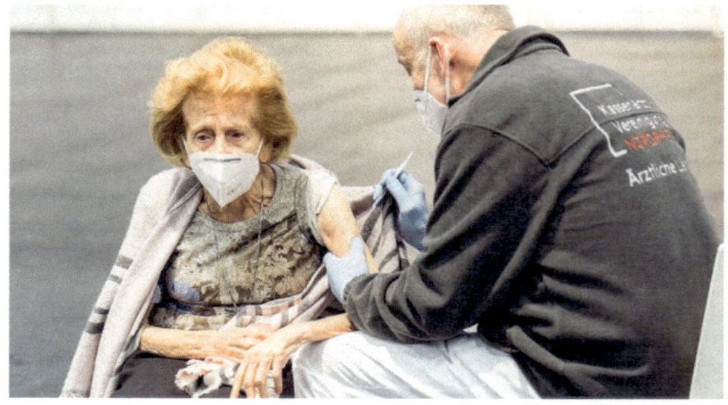

Source: By © Raimond Spekking / CC BY-SA 4.0 (via Wikimedia Commons), CC BY-SA 4.0, https://commons.wikimedia.org/w/index.php?curid=99676922

15.1.8. Accountability Mechanisms in Health Governance

Accountability mechanisms are central to health governance improvement and the effectiveness of global health policies. Transparent and responsive accountability enables health systems to fulfill their mandates as well as respond to inequities. If we look at Rwanda's case studies, we find that governance systems of clear ideological alignment and consistent participation on the part of health professionals in the community have significantly improved accountability in health results. The inclusion of local systems, for example, imihigo, highlights the need to position local governance toward higher ends in health so that the delivery of services is enhanced. Other nations, for example, Uganda, regardless of policy formation, are limited by inefficient implementation due to compromised local measures of accountability (March et al., 2021). Finally, integrating robust accountability mechanisms into health governance not only enhances performance but also entrenches the political commitment to health equity, which is key to advancing global health policy and programs (March et al., 2021).

15.1.9. Challenges in Implementing Governance Frameworks

Application of global health governance frameworks is riddled with a plethora of fundamental challenges that derail effective policy application. One such major challenge lies in the mismatch between political capacity and commitment at different countries, which typically creates irregular application of health policies (March et al., 2021). Additionally, isolation of health governance from other fields might weaken the impact of action taken for tackling health equity in a comprehensive manner, as fragmented policies overlook the interdependency of social determinants (March et al., 2021). Besides, accountability mechanisms are underdeveloped, and the institutions of governance lack proper capacity to strengthen compliance and implement rules. With weak institutional arrangements for social engagement, marginalized groups are likely to be excluded from decision-making, widening disparities. Addressing these issues demands collective effort to establish inclusive systems that promote equity and coherence and eventually result in a more robust global health governance system.

15.2. Global Health Policy Development

The creation of international health policy is now widely seen as central to responding to the complex issues raised by health disparities and new health challenges. As urbanization speeds up, cities are key battlefields for advancing health policies that foster social justice and advance public health results. Evidence indicates that successful urban governance can act as an agent for health equity by combining policy coherence, accountability, and social engagement in local health policy, as highlighted through the case study of urban cities such as Barcelona and Liverpool (March et al., 2021). Additionally, regional institutions like the Union of South American Nations (UNASUR) and the Southern African Development Community (SADC) are working to infuse pro-poor norms into national and global health agendas, therefore promoting policy advocacy for health rights and equity (Riggirozzi et al., 2015). This intersection of local and regional policy drives demonstrates the promise of collaborative governance arrangements in influencing comprehensive and efficient global health policy (Figure 15.6).

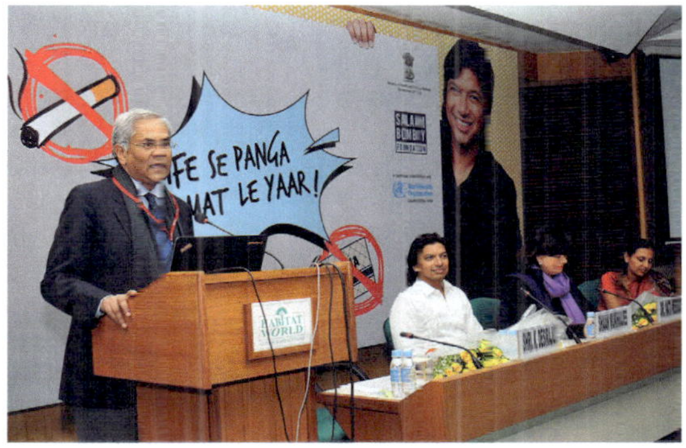

Figure 15.6. The impact of health policies and development policies on health status.

Source: By Ministry of Health and Family Welfare (GODL-India), GODL-India, https://commons.wikimedia.org/w/index.php?curid=71789278

15.2.1. The Policy-Making Process in Global Health

The process of policy-making in global health is marked by a complex interaction among stakeholders, evidence-based decision-making, and the need for accountability and transparency. With the development of global health challenges, the role of health policy and systems research (HPSR) becomes essential to guide the reforms under way to achieve universal health coverage (UHC). For example, strong evidence ecosystems should enable the free flow of information between evidence producers, synthesizers, and implementers so that policies can be guided by the highest level of available evidence (Mathews et al., 2019). In addition, the introduction of algorithmic systems into health decision-making has both opportunities and challenges, as these systems can handle complex data to improve efficiency in making decisions, but also bring very important concerns about transparency and human rights implications (Clifton et al., 2019). Accordingly, the effectiveness of global health governance does not only depend on sound utilization of data but also on promoting collaborative architectures that emphasize accountability within the policy-making process (Figure 15.7).

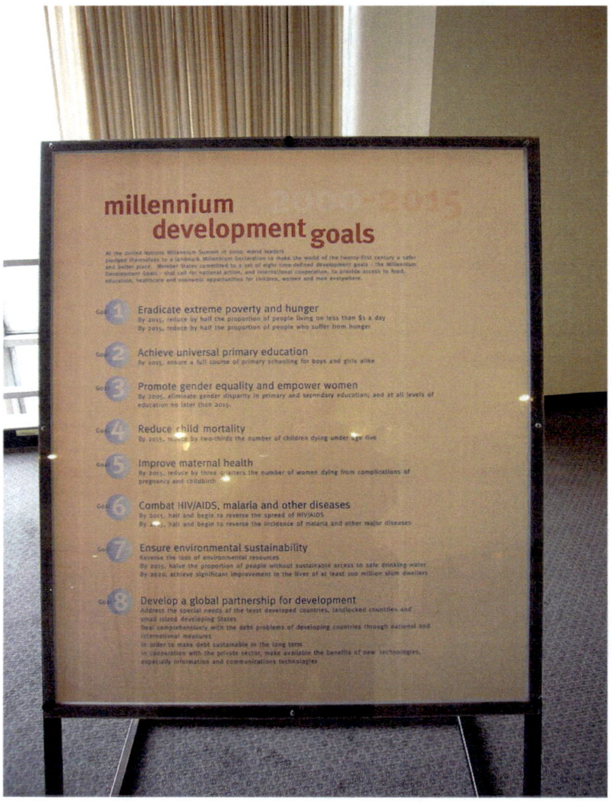
millennium development goals
Eradicate extreme poverty and hunger
Achieve universal primary education
Promote gender equality and empower women
Reduce child mortality
Improve maternal health
Combat HIV/AIDS, malaria and other diseases
Ensure environmental sustainability
Develop a global partnership for development

Figure 15.7. Proposed policy process cycle for developing health in all policies.

Source: By Babucke. - Own work., Public Domain, https://commons.wikimedia.org/w/index.php?curid=3970712

15.2.2. Evidence-Based Policy Formulation

In global health governance, evidence-based policymaking is a pivotal determinant of successful decision-making and resource deployment. This strategy leverages scientific studies and empirical evidence to inform policymakers on how to effectively solve intricate health problems, and therefore, build transparency and accountability in health systems. For example, the ASSAf consensus study panel highlights the importance of evidence integration in addressing governance failures in South Africa's health system and thus working toward quality UHC through well-established strategic visions and policy architectures (2024). In addition, combating the pressing crisis of the global care and health workforce requires a long-term commitment to evidence-based practice, to ensure that policies continue to be effective and applicable in fast-changing environments, like the period following the COVID-19 pandemic (Correia et al., 2024). Finally, adopting evidence in policy-making not only strengthens governance but also substantially improves health outcomes worldwide.

15.2.3. Stakeholder Engagement in Policy Development

Involvement of various stakeholders in policymaking is central to successful global health governance because it ensures that the policies are inclusive and allow for diverse views in addressing complex health issues. Multi-stakeholder strategies, as supported by the WHO, provide arenas for coordination among Member States, NGOs, and the private sector, thus resolving possible conflicts of interest (COI) inherent in health policy. Though NGOs and universities usually push for more sweeping limits on commercial participation to see that public health concerns take precedence, private sector representatives generally resist such frameworks, claiming current disclosure mechanisms are adequate. This tension highlights the need for sophisticated engagement approaches that can balance public health interests with private sector expertise to drive higher policy returns and keep governance frameworks relevant and effective for global health.

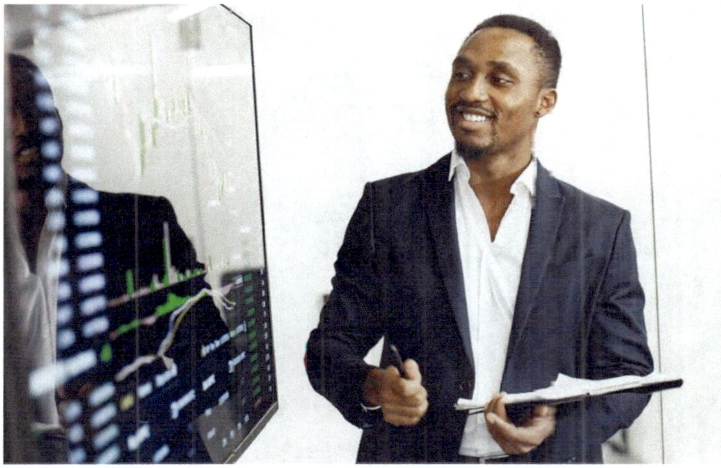

Source: Kajabi. (n.d.). *African Man in Black Suit Giving a Presentation on a Large Screen.*

15.2.4. The Role of Research and Data in Policy-Making

The incorporation of research and evidence is central in informing effective health policies in the context of global health governance. Such an evidence-based strategy allows policymakers to identify emerging health concerns and set priorities accordingly. For example, growing health complexities wrought by globalization demand strong data-gathering mechanisms that allow for sound decision-making (Hong et al., 2012). In addition, specially focused research efforts, like those investigating the potential of regional organizations such as the SADC and the UNASUR, highlight the significance of regional strategies in access to equitable health (Yeates et al., 2017). Through keen examination of healthcare measures and social determinants, actors can respond effectively to inequalities and improve public health outcomes. Therefore, the integration of data and research not only provides a basis for policy creation, but also acts as an agent for fostering social equity in health governance globally.

15.2.5. Policy Evaluation and Impact Assessment

Successful policy analysis and impact assessment are essential elements of global health governance because they offer a structured mechanism for comprehending the effects of health interventions. Through measures of the relevance, effectiveness, and efficiency of policy measures, stakeholders can ascertain whether programs achieve their envisaged objectives and make strategy adjustments accordingly. For example, the United Nations Development Assistance Framework (UNDAF) prioritizes alignment with government priorities and the inclusion of different stakeholder views, illustrating the value of collaborative results frameworks in the realization of health goals (Food and Agriculture Organization of the United Nations [FAO], 2014). In addition, assessments such as those done on the Disease Surveillance Networks (DSN) Initiative underscore the importance of examining multi-sectoral interventions in terms of improving capabilities in disease response (Kimball et al., 2011). In this manner, rigorous evaluation processes not only serve to strengthen accountability, but also to promote learning, allowing for more informed decision-making and ultimately leading to health improvement in the global governance environment (Figure 15.8).

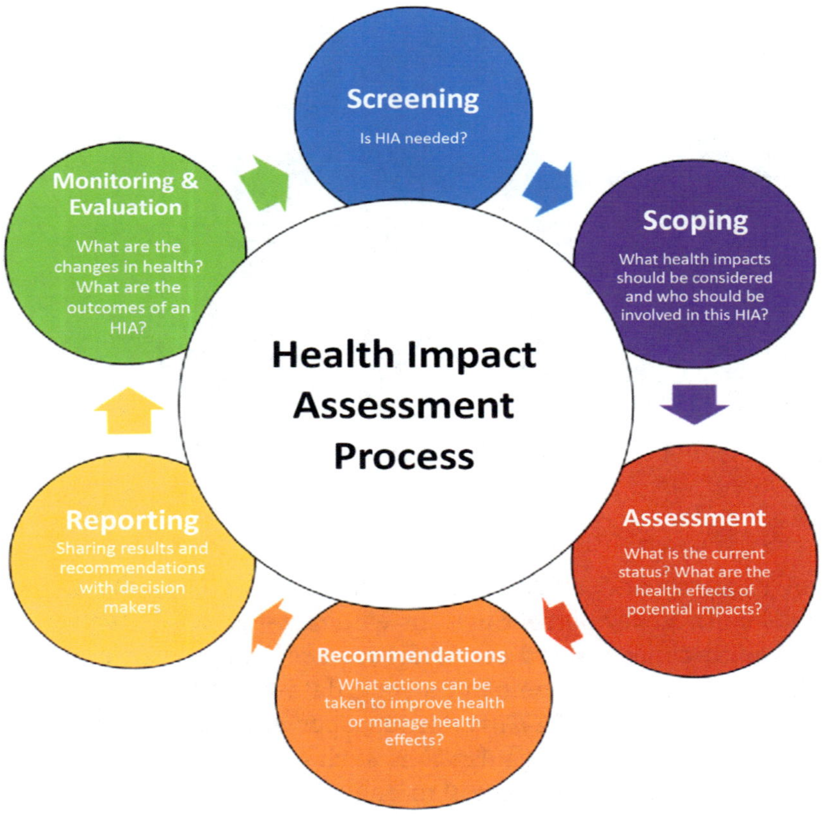
Health Impact Assessment Process
Screening
Is HIA needed?
Scoping
What health impacts should be considered and who should be involved in this HIA?
Assessment
What is the current status? What are the health effects of potential impacts?
Recommendations
What actions can be taken to improve health or manage health effects?
Reporting
Sharing results and recommendations with decision makers
Monitoring & Evaluation
What are the changes in health? What are the outcomes of an HIA?

Figure 15.8. Policy evaluation and impact assessment.

Source: Hilly Consult. (2023). *The Six Steps of the Health Impact Assessment Process.*

15.2.6. Case Studies of Successful Health Policies

By analyzing successful health policy case studies, the role of strategic governance and multi-stakeholder frameworks in ensuring successful outcomes is clear. The COVAX program, which was launched to promote global access to COVID-19 vaccines, is one prime example of the power of co-ordinated health policy in addressing a crisis (Pushkaran et al., 2023). In the face of challenges like vaccine nationalism, the initiative underscored the centrality of equity and accessibility in health governance. Additional scrutiny shows that the WHO has continued to play a central position in stewardship and policy generation, as revealed by its high degree and eigenvector centrality across different functions, reflecting the effectiveness of the organizations in worldwide health reaction. The case studies as a whole highlight the need for adaptive governing frameworks that advance solidarity and cooperation among states, increasing resilience to impending public health risk and solving current disparities within global health systems.

15.2.7. Barriers to Effective Policy Implementation

There are several barriers that confront the proper implementation of efficacious health policies, with an adverse impact on advancements in international health governance. The major deterrent is policy incoherence that typically arises as a consequence of dispersed healthcare structures and the insufficient synchronization between numerous organizational aims and health aims (March et al., 2021).

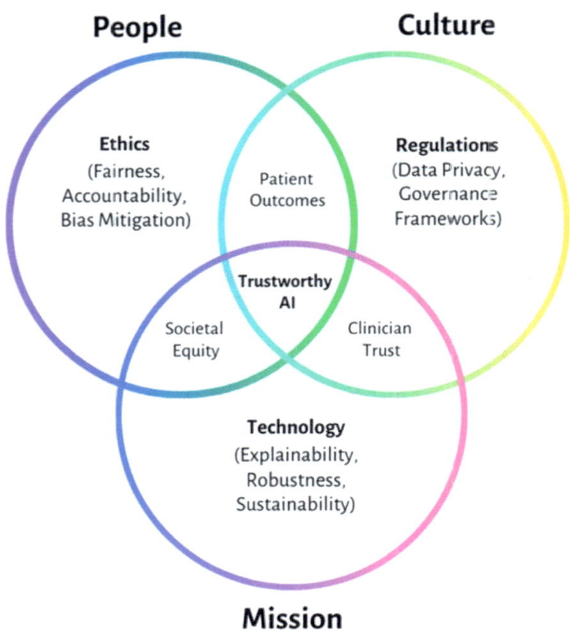

Figure 15.9. Barriers to effective policy implementation.

Source: Goktas P, Grzybowski A. Shaping the Future of Healthcare: Ethical Clinical Challenges and Pathways to Trustworthy AI. Journal of Clinical Medicine. 2025; 14(5):1605. https://doi.org/10.3390/jcm14051605

Further, weak accountability mechanisms also worsen these issues because most health programs lack effective oversight and adequate evaluation strategies, resulting in inefficient responses to health demands (Gatonga et al., 2013). Limited budgetary funds, including low budgetary expenditure for health programs, hinder the scale-up of key services, such as intermittent preventive treatment (IPTp) against malaria in pregnancy. In addition, human resource difficulties, including under-staffing and low motivation levels among health workers, result in reduced effectiveness in service delivery, affecting the overall impact of health policies. To counteract these challenges, an effective framework facilitating policy coherence, accountability, and proper resource allocation is necessary for better improving global health outcomes (Figure 15.9).

15.2.8. The Influence of Political Will on Health Policy

Political will is crucial to influencing health policy, especially within the realm of global health governance. The ability of governments to make health public initiatives a priority is also based on the convergence of political interests with health needs, indicative of a deeper realization of health as an integral aspect of national security and economic stability. Successful health policy formulation necessitates collective action by political leaders to prioritize resources, design holistic strategies, and ensure intersectoral coordination. The COVID-19 pandemic response is a prime example of how political determination can help expedite the mobilization of resources and health facilities onto the top of the political agenda (Aguanno et al., 2022). On the other hand, political unwillingness can retard progress, as it may fail to provide enough support for crucial public health interventions and sabotage the efforts aimed at reducing health disparities (Okumus et al., 2022). Thus, building strong political commitment is critical in progressing effective health policy and enhancing worldwide health outcomes.

15.2.9. Future Trends in Global Health Policy Development

As the global health issues change, future directions in the development of health policy will notably place great stress on collaborative governance and evidence-based decision-making. Emerging infectious diseases, climate change, and health disparities require an all-encompassing approach that goes beyond national borders. A trend worth observing is the augmented utilization of complex data analysis for guiding policy action, such as can be observed through initiatives like the Pardee Centers Searchlight project, that analyzes regional newsletters in a methodical way for revealing health patterns across varied environments (Gopal et al., 2012). In addition, conferences like Africa 2060 call attention to the need for the inclusion of local voices in global health discourse so that policies are both culturally appropriate and responsive to the needs of vulnerable groups (Clapp et al., 2010). Prioritizing coordination between international organizations, governments, and communities will enable future global health policies to build resilience and flexibility in response to continuing health emergencies and social determinants of health.

15.3. Health Equity and Access

Health equity and access are essential elements of global health policy and governance, especially in the context of recent public health emergencies such as the COVID-19 pandemic. The pandemic highlighted extreme inequalities in healthcare access, with richer countries quickly cornering vaccine supplies while low- and middle-income countries (LMICs) faced shortages, reflecting structural inequalities in global health systems. Efforts such as COVAX sought to counteract these inequities, but the inability to achieve global vaccine coverage exposed the fault lines in current structures. The exploitative tendencies of the pharmaceutical industry only make these problems worse, as seen in the increasing gap in access highlighted in Borges et al.'s review of vaccine rollout and global health diplomacy. In addition, fair access also requires not just monetary investments but thorough policy adjustments aligned with the individualized socioeconomic contexts of LMICs (Santangelo et al., 2024). Health equity must be met through synergistic efforts that cut across borders and place priority on healthcare access justice (Figure 15.10).

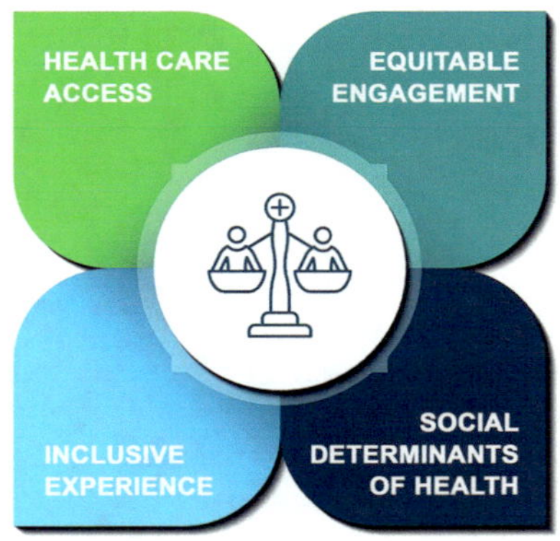

Figure 15.10. Health equity and access represent critical components of global health governance and policy.

Source: Business Group on Health. (2023). *Health Equity Infographic.*

15.3.1. Defining Health Equity in a Global Context

Global health equity requires an informed understanding of how structural inequities are expressed in health resource access across populations. The challenge is not just to respond to short-term healthcare needs but also to identify social determinants that complicate disparities, especially in poor environments.

Based on studies targeting regional health policies in low-income settings, it is essential that organizations such as the SADC and the NASUR create social policies that are inclusive and address the health issues of the world's poorest communities (Yeates et al., 2017). Enhancing regional collaboration and health programs can greatly propel poverty eradication and fair access to health commodities. In addition, encouraging participatory approaches in research and policy-making allows for the empowerment of marginalized voices, such that health equity programs reflect community demands and local knowledge, hence supporting the priority of local context in global health governance (Gagnon et al., 2017).

15.3.2. Social Determinants of Health

The social determinants of health concept is a range of many factors that have a significant impact on health outcomes at a population level, ranging from socioeconomic status and education to healthcare access. These determinants form the pillars of understanding global disparities in health, since they tend to intersect with environmental and cultural settings, determining people's trajectories in health. For example, local authorities are critical to the formulation of public health systems that can respond to these wider determinants effectively, leading to enhanced community resilience and health equity (Gamsu et al., 2014). In addition, globalization aggravates these problems by adding resource limitation that triggers the need for innovative measures, for example, sustainable eating habits, which not only intervene in nutritional well-being but also work toward environmental sustainability (Cogill et al., 2015). Therefore, global health governance needs to focus on ensuring the incorporation of social determinants into policy arenas to develop multi-faceted strategies that overcome inequalities and optimize overall public health (Figure 15.11).

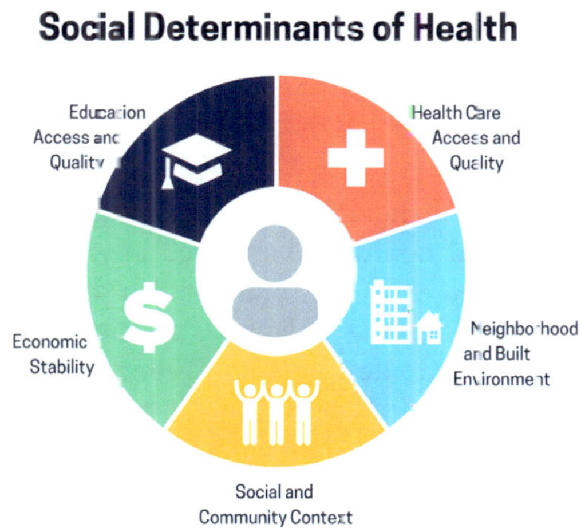

Figure 15.11. Social determinants of health.

Source: aTrain Education. (2023). *Healthy People 2030: Social Determinants of Health Graphic.*

15.3.3. Disparities in Health Access and Outcomes

Health access and outcome disparities are paramount issues in global health governance and policy, highlighting the disproportionate distribution of resources and services that have far-reaching impacts on marginalized groups. Such disparities tend to be rooted in socioeconomic status, geography, and institutional discrimination, which create unequal health outcomes across different population segments. For example, statistics documented in recent reports show low-income neighborhoods often have greater incidence rates of chronic diseases, compounded by the lack of preventive care and adequate treatment options (Birnbaum et al., 2011). Such a skewed environment highlights the need for interventions tailored toward advancing health equity as highlighted in the recommendations drafted by stakeholders (Birnbaum et al., 2011). By removing the systemic barriers that maintain these inequities, global health governance can not only enhance health outcomes but also promote increased social justice and equity among populations.

15.3.4. The Role of International Aid in Health Equity

Global assistance is key to furthering health equity through response to inequities in access to and quality of healthcare among various groups. Multilateral efforts, e.g., the UNDAF in Kenya, in the global health governance environment are good examples of how collective action can be synchronized with national health agendas to further service delivery. Such frameworks enable cooperation among various stakeholders, such as governments, civil society, and international organizations, to develop end-to-end solutions to health issues. Furthermore, the COVID-19 pandemic has emphasized the imperative need for equal access to vaccines, as inequalities can exacerbate the spread of the disease and cycles of poor health and poverty. Thus, global aid mechanisms not only deliver much-needed resources but also foster global solidarity in propelling progress toward health equity through strategic alliances and focused interventions that streamline the distinct needs of marginalized populations (Figure 15.12).

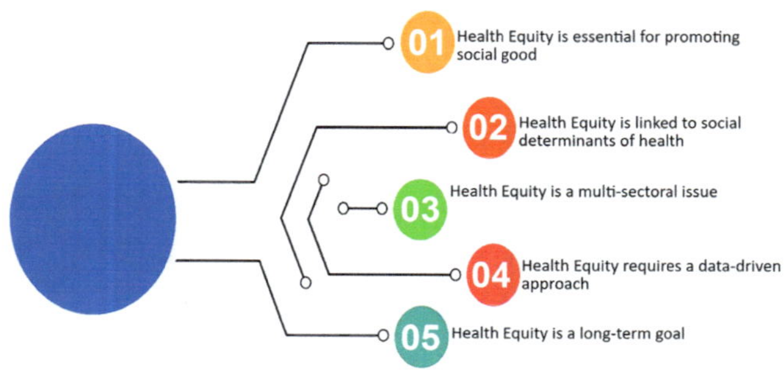

Figure 15.12. The importance of health equity.

Source: FasterCapital. (n.d.). *Striving for Health Equity: Promoting Social Good and Understanding the Importance of Health Equity.*

15.3.5. Strategies to Improve Access to Healthcare

Enhancing healthcare access is a complex issue that requires multifaceted approaches anchored in efficient global health policy and governance. At the core of this process is the development of equitable health systems that address the needs of different populations. This can be realized through improving infrastructure, especially in marginalized communities, as well as developing culturally appropriate services that honor local languages and practices. Efforts to strengthen the healthcare workforce, especially in low-income nations, should also be given high priority; as explained, multilateral agencies are working hard to identify ways to respond to health workforce migration, diminishing local healthcare access (Pilpersist et al., 2013). In addition, the post-2015 Development Agenda offers a vital forum to address structural inequities and call for ambitious national policies that take account of specific regional contexts while promoting mutual accountability across actors (Chaturvedi et al, 2015). Together, they provide a powerful set of options for improving healthcare access as an integral element of global equity in health.

15.3.6. The Impact of Globalization on Health Equity

The impact of globalization on health equity has become a pressing issue in global health governance and policy agendas. As countries get more connected, differences in health outcomes tend to reinforce existing inequalities, especially in LMICs. Globalization allows for easy dissemination of health technologies and innovations; yet, it can also lead to unequal access to these resources, resulting in a health divide. For example, advanced countries enjoy the benefits of state-of-the-art medical innovations, while marginalized groups can stick to old treatments, slowing health equity progress. In addition, the movement of goods and capital tends to favor profit more than health requirements, as exemplified through the governance issues with biopharmaceutical innovations where technology commercialization can overlook rural and poor communities (Chen & Ely, 2011). It demands policies that integrate equity, not only to advance sustainable development but also to provide equitable access to healthcare resources among populations (US Partnership for the Decade of Education for Sustainable Development, 2006) (Figure 15.13).

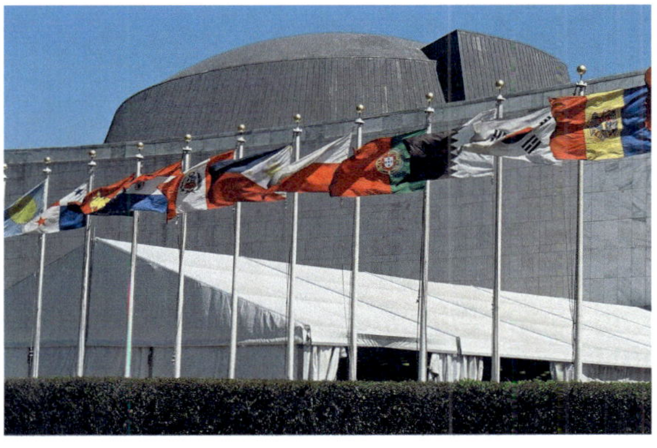

Figure 15.13. The impact of globalization on health equity.

Source: By I, Aotearoa, CC BY-SA 3.0, https://commons.wikimedia.org/w/index.php?curid=2284433

15.3.7. Gender and Health Disparities

Gender and health inequalities are such key determinants that have a great impact on the health outcomes at the global level, which calls for a focused strategy within health policy and governance structures. Women and vulnerable gender groups tend to suffer from systematic barriers that affect access to healthcare, education, and nutrition, thereby adding to existing inequalities. For example, evidence suggests that in numerous LMICs, some economic or social groups have declining health indicators, e.g., child mortality rates. Furthermore, addressing these inequalities is essential to obtain equitable health results; Rwanda and Bangladesh, for example, have shown that using inclusive policies, steep declines in child mortality are attainable, elevating whole populations instead of marginalizing vulnerable populations. This evidence highlights the importance of gender-based strategies being prioritized by global health efforts to ensure that everyone, with or without gender status, is given the care and resources to succeed.

15.3.8. Indigenous Health Issues and Governance

Indigenous health matters are closely interlinked with governance systems, and their importance underscores the policy imperative to reduce health inequalities within and among Indigenous populations. Governance systems that promote Indigenous self-determination allow communities to create culturally tailored health interventions that are vital to address core problems like access to health care, mental health, and health outcomes affected by climate change. Vulnerable groups, such as Indigenous peoples, tend to experience magnified health threats because of insufficient reactions from current policy systems, which tend to ignore traditional knowledge and practices (Otorkpa et al., 2024). Effective health governance should include collective strategies involving Indigenous leadership to ensure that health policies are not only inclusive but also derived from the social determinants of health unique to these populations (Kilibarda, 2024). Strengthening governance arrangements demonstrates a commitment to health equity while promoting resilience and sustainability in Indigenous health practices in the face of changing global health issues.

15.3.9. Ethical Considerations in Health Equity

In global health governance, ethical implications of health equity issues are essential for making inclusive and equitable health systems. The differences in health outcomes between populations usually represent underlying inequalities in society and necessitate that policymakers recognize and act on these ethical dimensions. Efficient governance requires the inclusion of ethical principles that prioritize equity and support the moral imperative to address vulnerable groups first. Of particular interest is the introduction of ethics into science and technology policy, highlighted in current literature, which promotes a strong emphasis on understanding dominant systems of values that impact health-based decision-making (Chaturvedi et al., 2015). Furthermore, ethical principles should guide the governance of sustainable development policies, which play a key role in building fair access to healthcare resources (US Partnership for the Decade of Education for Sustainable Development, 2006). In turn, embedding ethical considerations within health policy not only advances justice but ensures that global health governance sufficiently responds to the complexities of health inequities (Figure 15.14).

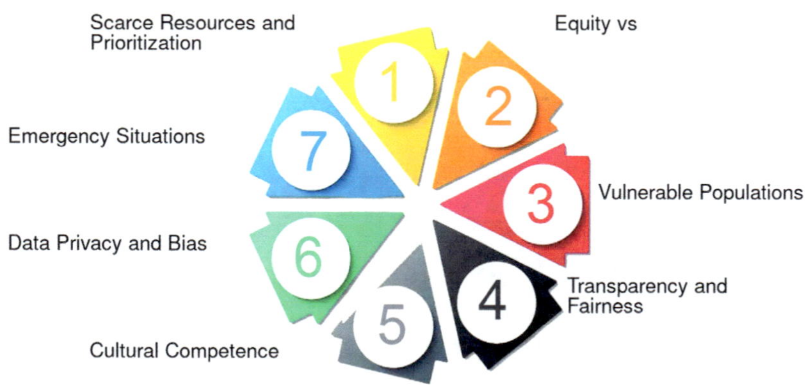
Scarce Resources and Prioritization
1
Equity vs
2
Vulnerable Populations
3
Transparency and Fairness
4
Cultural Competence
5
Data Privacy and Bias
6
Emergency Situations
7

Figure 15.14. Ethical considerations in health equity.

Source: FasterCapital. (n.d.). *Health Care Ethics: Navigating Ethical Dilemmas in Healthcare Startups—Ethical Considerations in Resource Allocation and Healthcare Equity.*

15.4. Emerging Global Health Issues

Rising global health challenges tend to be multifaceted, with common determinants often including globalization, climate change, and socioeconomic disparities. In response, these challenges require an international coordinated approach to strengthen public health governance and policy. For example, the interaction between health and sustainable environment is now evident, as manifested in the UNDAF strategic priority on health, sanitation, and nutrition, mirroring a devotion to comprehensive human capital development (Food and Agriculture Organization of the United Nations [FAO], 2014). In addition, the global health implications of globalization cannot be ignored, as they affect workers' rights and working conditions across the world, calling for the necessity of policy responses that are oriented toward equity and inclusiveness in health access (Dejardin et al., 2009). Effective response to these re-emerging challenges demands not just strong governance but also concerted action from multiple stakeholders so that health policy is kept responsive to the re-emerging challenges of the modern-day global scenario.

15.4.1. The Impact of Climate Change on Health

The deep impacts of climate change on health pose major challenges to global health governance, calling for policy action that responds to the complex risks of environmental changes. Rising temperatures and weather-related catastrophes heighten the occurrence of VBD, respiratory diseases, and food insecurity, thus taxing healthcare systems. Further, marginalized groups, especially in developing areas, are subject to greater risks due to compromised access to resources and adaptive potential, highlighting the importance of equitable health policy. As such health consequences become increasingly entangled with the socio-economic determinants of health, it is essential for policymakers to have a comprehensive approach that incorporates climate resilience into public health policy. All these demands concerted action among global institutions, governments, and communities to build adaptive capacities, strengthen surveillance systems, and institute sustainable practices that promote public health in a time of climate uncertainty (Figure 15.15).

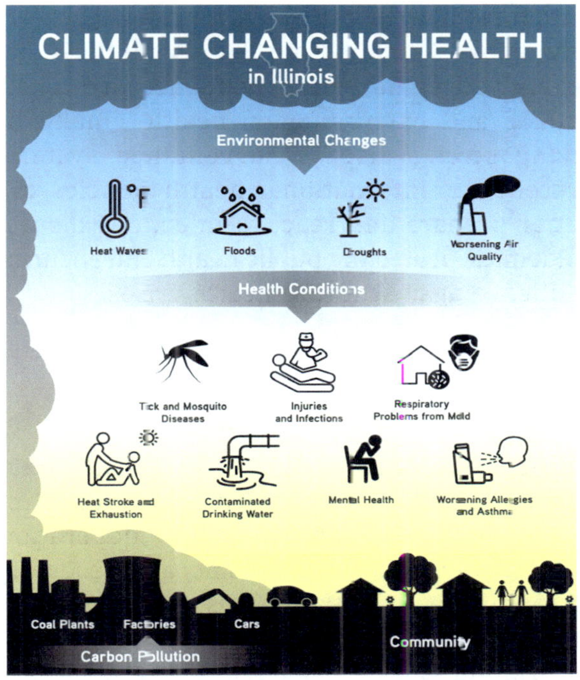

Figure 15.15. The profound effects of climate change on health present significant challenges for global health governance.

Source: BRACE-Illinois. (2020). *Climate Change Infographic*.

15.4.2. Infectious Disease Outbreaks and Responses

Infectious disease outbreaks pose considerable challenges to international health governance, requiring effective and timely response to their impact. The Rockefeller Foundations DSN Initiative is one such initiative aimed at improving disease monitoring and response capacity in poor countries, highlighting the importance of regional synergies and technical support (Ancheta et al., 2010). Through promoting partnerships and information sharing between transnational actors, the DSN seeks to enhance the capacities of local settings in disease surveillance, hence enabling a more appropriate response in public health (Ekirapa et al., 2011). All these efforts highlight the need for an integrated global health governance structure that incorporates multidisciplinary strategies—like the One Health model—that acknowledge the interdependence of human, animal, and environmental health. Finally, by giving strong disease surveillance systems precedence, international health policies can better prepare and react to infectious disease epidemics, protecting public health and ensuring resilience against future health crises.

15.4.3. Non-Communicable Diseases (NCDs) and Global Policy

Non-communicable diseases (NCDs) have become a key global health issue, requiring international and national policy cooperation. Good governance mechanisms are necessary to contain the effects of NCDs, as they tend to be the results of interrelated socio-economic determinants such as environmental factors and lifestyle.

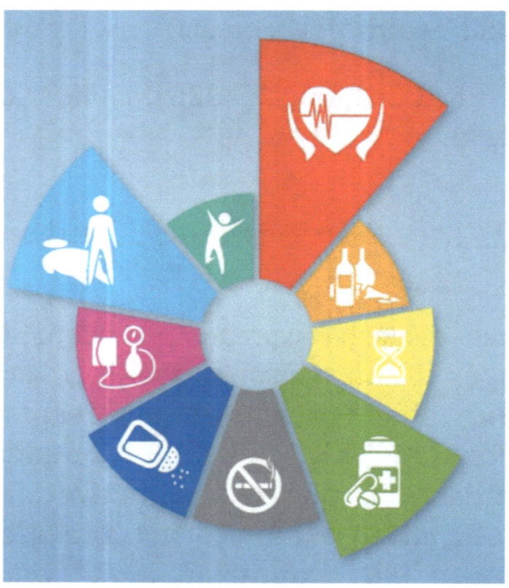

Figure 15.16. Non-communicable diseases (NCDs) and global policy.

Source: NCD Child. (2021). *Child Health and Noncommunicable Diseases Awareness Graphic.*

Some of the key obstacles in effective policy enforcement are the societal concept of individual responsibility in health behaviors and the possible conflicts from regulatory actions that might jeopardize the interests of industries like tobacco, alcohol, and processed foods (Gostin et al., 2011). To unravel these complexities, regional institutions such as the SADC have been seeking out inclusive social policies that improve access to healthcare and tackle social determinants of health through common action (Yeates et al., 2017). Therefore, a legally enlightened and holistic approach is essential for establishing policies that not only fight against NCDs but also promote social equity and sustainable development among affected communities (Figure 15.16).

15.4.4. Mental Health as a Global Health Priority

Mental illness has increasingly become a priority in international health governance, indicating a shift in policy priorities that recognizes its significant contribution to general well-being and development. The acknowledgment of mental health as a global health priority is not only for health at the individual level but also for economic stability and social cohesion. Global action, including the WHO's Comprehensive Mental Health Action Plan, seeks to strengthen mental health services where few resources are available, noting that mental disorders contribute significantly to the global burden of disease.

As the debate around the post-2015 Development Agenda unfolds, mental health inputs must be brought in to meet challenges that cut across countries for an environment to support equitable policies and sustainable interventions to thrive (Chaturvedi et al, 2015). Such a comprehensive approach is critical in fulfilling the potential for transformative change through effective mental healthcare to advance larger goals of health and development.

15.4.5. Antimicrobial Resistance (AMR) and Governance Challenges

The burgeoning crisis of antimicrobial resistance (AMR) highlights the urgency of having strong governance systems in international health policy. While the incidence of multidrug-resistant pathogens continues to rise, the failure to build new antibiotics and therapies combined with their abuse threatens formidable challenges (Bhagwandin et al., 2017). Successful responses call for concerted action in both public and private sectors, requiring governance systems that value innovation, awareness, and stewardship at every level (Busse et al., 2018). But mere policy-setting is not enough; the execution of these governance measures has to be accurate and subtle, harmonizing healthcare systems with the more general goals of prevention of AMR. This involves promoting collaborations among healthcare professionals (HCPs) and patients to increase accountability and democratized decision-making. Ultimately, a harmonious balance incorporating regulation with the power of persuasion will be critical in helping reduce AMR and assuring that health systems have the capacity to battle this growing threat.

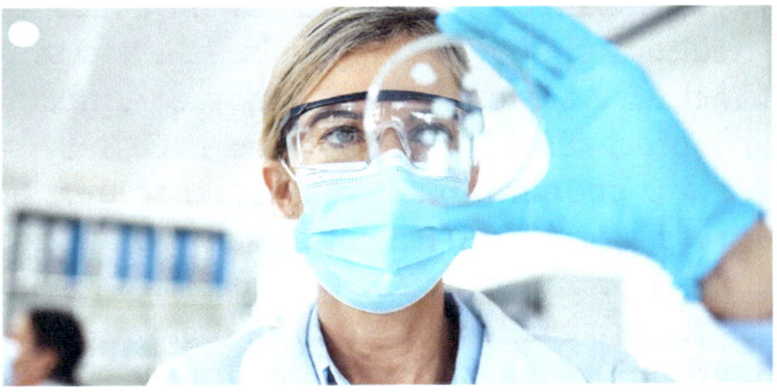

Source: IFPMA. (2022). *Areas of Work in Antimicrobial Resistance (AMR).*

15.4.6. Health Security and Preparedness

Security and readiness for health are essential aspects of international health governance, given the interdependence of states, which accentuates the threats of emerging infectious diseases and health disparities. The WHO is confronted with significant challenges, such as finance gaps and pressing the need to manage AMR and NCDs, which are accentuated by climate change and socio-economic inequalities (Friedman et al., 2017). Strong health security demands that countries prioritize fair access to care, strengthening their resilience in the face of crises by adopting solid health policies. By focusing on accountability and building intersectoral collaboration, WHO can become a strong institution that not only addresses current health emergencies but also advocates for long-term interventions toward UHC (Friedman et al., 2017). Strengthening these structures in public health will ensure preparedness, with vulnerable populations being safeguarded, thus decreasing the inequalities that usually hinder joint health developments.

15.4.7. The Role of Technology in Global Health

Technology's role in global health is ever more central, given its capacity to create new solutions for health policy and governance. New technologies in digital health, including telemedicine, mobile health tools, and electronic health records, make healthcare access and efficiency easier, especially in resource-scarce settings. These technologies allow for real-time data analysis and collection, which are critical in surveillance of disease trends and containment of health emergencies. In addition, they favor integration of epidemic surveillance systems to enable rapid public health interventions in the event of outbreaks. Yet, while technology has immense potential, there are challenges such as inequalities in access to digital capabilities and issues with data security and privacy. As noted in recent studies, failure to manage these challenges might erode the enormous health benefits gained in the past decades, making equitable application of technology in global health schemes a priority (Friedman et al., 2017) (Figure 15.17).

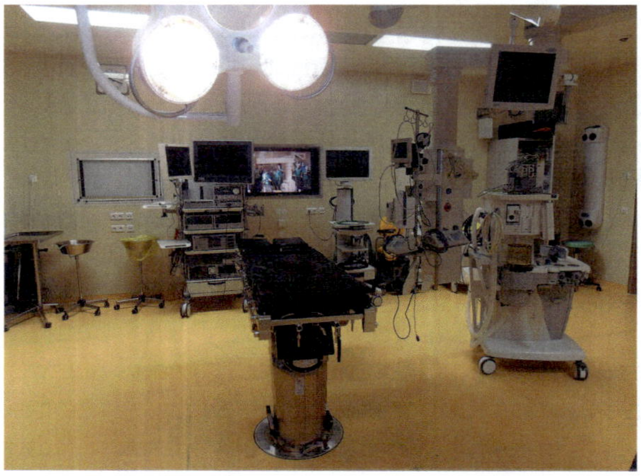

Figure 15.17. The role of technology in global health.

Source: By Дмитрий Кошелев - Own work, CC BY-SA 3.0, https://commons.wikimedia.org/w/index.php?curid=24408941

15.4.8. Global Health Financing and Resource Allocation

Effective global health financing and resource management are integral parts of effective health governance, as they have a direct influence on the ability to tackle urgent health issues globally. The advent of multi-bi aid has brought both opportunities and challenges within this landscape, providing earmarked resources for particular health programs while commonly displacing recipient country priorities and increasing aid fragmentation (Reinsberg et al., 2017). This was especially the case with the sudden HIV/AIDS funding ramp-up from 2002 to 2004, in which sudden flows of funds at times swamped public health budgets and strained local health systems (Maureen Lewis). To relieve such tensions, reform based on greater access to data, fee mechanisms to maximize impact, and more active involvement of recipient countries is necessary. Through alignment of financing institutions with overall health goals, international health governance can promote more sustainable health systems and ultimately healthier outcomes for populations in need.

15.4.9. Future Challenges in Global Health Governance

With continued transformation in global health governance, upcoming challenges are progressively compounded and call for interdisciplinary strategies. One of such urgent matters is HCPs migration, and it raises meaningful discrepancies between accessibility to healthcare among low-income sending countries and high-income recipient nations. Actions by multilateral institutions such as the WHO and the International Organization for Migration seek to redress these inequalities through policy interventions that accept the interlinked character of health, migration, and development (Pilpersist et al., 2013). Lastly, natural resource governance, more so the governance of soil and its influence on agricultural operations, emphasizes the necessity of inclusive structures that embrace differing viewpoints. Such structures are necessary to promote cooperation across stakeholders in addressing the intricacies of environmental health (Howard et al., 2014). Therefore, solving these future challenges entails increased global collaboration and communication tactics to facilitate effective governance for health and fair resource allocation in an interdependent globe.

CLOSER LOOK

Genomic Surveillance

Genomic surveillance refers to the sequencing and examination of the pathogen's genetic material, including viruses and bacteria, to track changes in their genome over time. This potent technique is important in understanding how diseases are transmitted, change, and react to interventions such as vaccines or drugs.

In the case of infectious diseases, genomic surveillance detects mutations, new variants, and drug resistance. For instance, during the COVID-19 pandemic, it played a crucial role in identifying and tracking variants such as Delta and Omicron and guiding public health policies and vaccine updates.

The process entails gathering samples from infected individuals, isolating genetic material (DNA or RNA), sequencing it, and comparing the outcome with reference genomes. The information assists scientists in tracing transmission routes, identifying outbreaks early, and determining whether prevailing diagnostics, vaccines, or treatments are still useful.

Genomic surveillance is also important in the monitoring of AMR, allowing health authorities to identify resistant bacteria strains and adjust antibiotic policies to respond. Such surveillance necessitates international cooperation, sharing of data, and robust laboratory infrastructure. WHO, CDC, and GISAID are among the organizations coordinating the making available and usability of genomic data. In conclusion, genomic surveillance improves our capacity to predict, prevent, and contain infectious disease threats in real time.

SUMMARY

The intricacies of global health governance and policy highlight the importance of synergy and multidimensional efforts to tackle urgent health issues. The interconnected nature of such concerns as youth unemployment and public health outbreaks illustrated by studies that reflect the influence of labor market forces on health (Betcherman et al., n.d.), emphasize the imperative for the synthesis of economic and health policy. In addition, the interconnection between health emergencies such as the HIV/AIDS epidemic and wider security issues highlights that public health cannot be separated from socioeconomic environments (Frerks et al., 2010). Through coordination across countries and sectors, stakeholders can build resilience and provide more effective responses to health crises. In the end, a holistic understanding of these interdependencies will inform future regulatory systems so that they can more effectively deal with the changing context of global health threats and promote sustainable policy-making.

Analysis of global health governance affords us critical understanding about the policy-discourse-stakeholder interface. The most seminal finding identifies the powerful role of the pharmaceutical industry in determining health policy as a reaction to public pressure for affordable HIV/AIDS drugs. This intricate dynamic is marked by politicized communication with a strategic focus on maintaining elite agreement surrounding prevailing intellectual property structures while, in the process, pursuing corporate social responsibility initiatives (Aronczyk et al., 2016). Furthermore, the importance of epistemic communities surfaces as pivotal in informing the reaction to outbreaks of infectious disease, for instance, SARS, where disputed discourses guided public health measures over time (Yoon et al., 2015). Collectively, these findings show that global health governance is not solely the result of technocratic decision-making; instead, it is characterized by ideological conflicts and power relations that define health priorities and shape policy action globally.

KEY TERMS FROM THIS CHAPTER

- Public health policy
- Health systems strengthening
- Health governance
- Regulation
- Public-private partnership (PPP)
- Pandemic preparedness
- Strategic planning
- Policy advocacy
- Sustainable development goals (SDGs)
- Climate-resilient health systems
- Universal health coverage (UHC)
- Policy implementation
- Evidence-based policy
- Health financing
- Global health diplomacy
- Health in All Policies (HiAP)
- Legislation
- Ethics in public health
- One Health approach
- Digital health

REFERENCES

1. Aguanno, R., Al Ariqi, L., Elkholy, A., Gardner, E., Grant, R., Pavade, G., Dobschuetz, S., et al. (2022). Global technical meeting on MERS-CoV and other emerging zoonotic coronaviruses. https://www.semanticscholar.org/paper/790b96b556e091d6b646ce9b569dfc5735fae8fc (accessed on 6 May 2025).
2. Aronczyk, M., Castells, M., Clark, A., Cottle, S., Davis, A., Drahos, P., Fraser, N., et al. (2016). Losing the media battle, waging the policy war: The pharmaceutical industry's response to the access to medicines crisis in the Global South. *SAGE Publications*. https://core.ac.uk/download/77027575.pdf (accessed on 6 May 2025).
3. Aziz, R., Roomi, J., Chan, K., John, E. A., Kapilashrami, A., et al. (2023). Bridging the gap: Using CHNRI to align migration health research priorities in India with local expertise and global perspectives. *International Society of Global Health, 13,* 04148. https://core.ac.uk/download/603246233.pdf (accessed on 6 May 2025).
4. Bento, A., Paolotti, D., Falkenbach, M., & Kuhlmann, E. (2024). 1.Q. Round table: Primary healthcare workforce crisis in Europe: Global policy discourse and national implementation. *34*. https://www.semanticscholar.org/paper/b330fc5523f1ec657c657f74919ac019b1d7e9a0 (accessed on 6 May 2025).
5. Betcherman,Gordon; Godfrey,Martin E.; Puerto, Susana; Rother,Friederike Uta; Manova Stavreska,Antoneta. A review of interventions to support young workers : findings of the youth employment inventory (English). Social Protection discussion paper ; no. SP 0715 Washington, DC: World Bank. http://documents.worldbank.org/curated/en/498381468779418249(accessed on 6 May 2025).
6. Chaturvedi, S., Ladikas, M., Stemerding, D., Zhao, Y., et al. (2015). Science and technology governance and ethics–A global perspective from Europe, India, and China. *Springer Science and Business Media LLC*. https://core.ac.uk/download/42136809.pdf (accessed on 6 May 2025).
7. Chen, Y., & Ely, A. (2011). Health biotechnology innovation for social sustainability: A perspective from China. *STEPS Centre*. This is one of a series of Working Papers from the STEPS Centre www.steps-centre.org. ISBN-978 1 78118 018 1 https://core.ac.uk/download/2731317.pdf.
8. Clapp, R., Dawit, S., Eagle, N., Fromkin, et al. (2010). Africa 2060: Good news from Africa, April 16, 2010. *Boston University Frederick S. Pardee Center for the Study of the Longer-Range Future*. https://open.bu.edu/bitstream/2144/22891/1/Conf_GoodNewsforAfrica.pdf (accessed on 6 May 2025).
9. Clifton, C., Hatada, Y., Koene, A., Richardson, et al. (2019). A governance framework for algorithmic accountability and transparency. *European Parliamentary Research Service*. https://core.ac.uk/download/288430163.pdf (accessed on 6 May 2025).
10. Cogill, B., Fanzo, J. C., & Johnston, J. L. (2015). Understanding sustainable diets: A descriptive analysis of the determinants and processes that influence diets and their impact on health, food security, and environmental sustainability. *American Society for Nutrition, 5,* 418–429. https://core.ac.uk/download/132676312.pdf (accessed on 6 May 2025).
11. Collin, J., da Silva Gomes, F., Hill, S., Ralston, et al. (2020). Towards preventing and managing conflict of interest in nutrition policy? An analysis of submissions to a consultation on a draft WHO tool. *International Journal of Health Policy and Management*. https://core.ac.uk/download/322484892.pdf (accessed on 6 May 2025).

12. Mathews, C., Goga, A., Loveday, M., Zembe, W., Daviaud, E., Siegfried, N., & Lewin, S. (2019). Moving towards universal health coverage: Strengthening the evidence ecosystem for the South African health system. *South African medical journal = Suid-Afrikaanse tydskrif vir geneeskunde, 109*(11b), 8–14. https://doi.org/10.7196/SAMJ.2019.v109i11b.14245

13. Dennis, S. (2009). Making aid effectiveness work for family planning and reproductive health. *Population Action International*. https://core.ac.uk/download/71342625.pdf (accessed on 6 May 2025).

14. Franek, A., Loucks, D. P., Koncagul, E., Unver, O., Connor, R., Grego, S., Abete, V., et al. (2012). Managing water under uncertainty and risk: The United Nations World Water Development Report 4. UN-Water. https://core.ac.uk/download/71360160.pdf (accessed on 6 May 2025).

15. Frerks, G., Huber, D., Klot, J., & M'Boup, et al. (2010). HIV/AIDS, security and conflict: New realities, new responses. *SSRC/Clingendael Institute for ASCI*. https://core.ac.uk/download/pdf/29237791.pdf (accessed on 6 May 2025).

16. Friedman, E. A., & Gostin, L. O. (2017). Reimagining WHO: Leadership and action for a new director-general. *Scholarship @ Georgetown Law*. https://core.ac.uk/download/74539395.pdf (accessed on 6 May 2025).

17. Grandvoinnet, H., Aslam, G., & Raha, S. (2015). Opening the black box: The contextual drivers of social accountability. https://doi.org/10.1596/978-1-4648-0481-6.

18. Gugushvili, D., Roche, J. M., Wise, L., & Hanna, L. (2015). The lottery of birth: Giving all children an equal chance to survive. *Save the Children*. https://core.ac.uk/download/75780374.pdf (accessed on 6 May 2025).

19. Kilibarda, B. (2024). Global challenges and opportunities in health promotion. https://www.semanticscholar.org/paper/bce0d1aea33eb6a60140ae55c6a164aab5840c49 (accessed on 6 May 2025).

20. Kotecha, P. (2011). Engaging universities in the regional integration project in Southern Africa. Volunteer and Service Enquiry Southern Africa (VOSESA). https://core.ac.uk/download/75779498.pdf (accessed on 6 May 2025).

21. Maureen Lewis, 2005. "Addressing the Challenge of HIV/AIDS: Macroeconomic, Fiscal and Institutional Issues," Working Papers 58, Center for Global Development.https://core.ac.uk/download/pdf/7089759.pdf (accessed on 6 May 2025).

22. Monachino, M. S., & Moreira, P. K. (2016). CSR: A catalyst for corporate contribution to global health governance? A case study from the pharmaceutical industry. Hygiea Internationalis: An Interdisciplinary Journal for the History of Public Health, 12(2), 73–91. https://doi.org/10.3384/hygiea.1403-8668.1612273.

23. Ralston, R. (2019). Politics of partnership in UK and Scotland: Understanding governance in obesity policy. *The University of Edinburgh*. https://core.ac.uk/download/429705865.pdf (accessed on 6 May 2025).

24. Reinsberg, B. (2017). Five steps to smarter multi-bi aid: A new way forward for earmarked finance. *Overseas Development Institute*. https://core.ac.uk/download/161770908.pdf (accessed on 6 May 2025).

25. Riggirozzi, P. (2015). Regional integration and poverty: How do southern regionalisms embed norms and practices of social development through health governance and diplomacy? *The*

Open University. https://core.ac.uk/download/613541245.pdf (accessed on 6 May 2025).

26. Schultz-Haudt, P. (2022). Translation of WHO-policy in Norway and Cuba: Directives from The World Health Organization in states with different governance systems and economies. *University of Agder*. https://core.ac.uk/download/542357454.pdf (accessed on 6 May 2025).

27. Singh, B., Kaur, J., & Chattu, V. K. (2022). Global vaccine inequities and multilateralism amid COVID-19: Reconnaissance of global health diplomacy as a panacea? *Health Promotion Perspectives, 12*(4), 315–324. https://core.ac.uk/download/555562306.pdf (accessed on 6 May 2025).

28. Stone, S., Myers, S. S., & Golden, C. D. (2018). Cross-cutting principles for planetary health education. *The Lancet Planetary Health, 2*, 192, 193. https://doi.org/10.1016/s2542-5196(18)30022-6.

29. Subtil, I., Estrada, J., Gomes, L., Morais, M., Correia, M., Correia, P., Durão, J., Quelhas, Q., Adrego, T., & Alho, A. M. (2024). Strengthening Global Health Security: The Role of the International Health Regulations in Monitoring and Controlling Vector-Borne Diseases. *The European Journal of Public Health, 34*(Suppl 3), ckae144.767. https://doi.org/10.1093/eurpub/ckae144.767 (accessed on 6 May 2025).

30. Upton, M. E. (2011). The Politics of Health: Community Engagement in South African HIV Vaccine Trial Sites. PhD thesis The Open University. DOI: https://doi.org/10.21954/ou.ro.000082d6 Walkenhorst, P., & Fries, T. (2011). Sharing global governance: The role of civil society organizations. *Bertelsmann Foundation*. https://core.ac.uk/download/71359915.pdf (accessed on 6 May 2025).

31. White, C., Allendes, D., Wyrwoll, P., & Grafton, R. Q. (2014). Global water: Issues and insights. *ANU Press*. https://core.ac.uk/download/pdf/30674516.pdf (accessed on 6 May 2025).

32. Witter, S. (2013). Implementing the agenda for global action on human resources for health: Analysis from an international tracking survey. *Journal of Hospital Administration, 2*(1), 77–87. https://core.ac.uk/download/11303985.pdf (accessed on 6 May 2025).

33. Yang, R. (2024). Pathways and significance of soil new pollutants management under the context of carbon neutrality. https://www.semanticscholar.org/paper/a6a36d659b4f10ca8c874f5a1ac33840a73029fc (accessed on 6 May 2025).

34. Yeates, N. (2015). A hundred key questions for the post-2015 development agenda. *United Nations Research Institute for Social Development-Sheffield Institute for International Development*. https://core.ac.uk/download/20667233.pdf (accessed on 6 May 2025).

35. Yoon, S; (2015) The Role of Epistemic Communities in the Global Response to Severe Acute Respiratory Syndrome: Implications for Global Health Governance. PhD thesis, London School of Hygiene & Tropical Medicine. DOI: https://doi.org/10.17037/PUBS.02163000(accessed on 6 May 2025).

INDEX